T0331124

Alzheimer's Disease Drug Development

Alzheimer's Disease Drug Development

Research and Development Ecosystem

Edited by

Jeffrey Cummings
University of Nevada, Las Vegas

Jefferson Kinney
University of Nevada, Las Vegas

Howard Fillit
Alzheimer's Drug Discovery Foundation

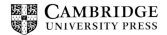

CAMBRIDGE
UNIVERSITY PRESS

University Printing House, Cambridge CB2 8BS, United Kingdom

One Liberty Plaza, 20th Floor, New York, NY 10006, USA

477 Williamstown Road, Port Melbourne, VIC 3207, Australia

314–321, 3rd Floor, Plot 3, Splendor Forum, Jasola District Centre, New Delhi – 110025, India

103 Penang Road, #05–06/07, Visioncrest Commercial, Singapore 238467

Cambridge University Press is part of the University of Cambridge.

It furthers the University's mission by disseminating knowledge in the pursuit of
education, learning, and research at the highest international levels of excellence.

www.cambridge.org
Information on this title: www.cambridge.org/9781108838665
DOI: 10.1017/9781108975759

First published 2022

A catalogue record for this publication is available from the British Library.

ISBN 978-1-108-83866-5 Hardback

The editors dedicate this book to all those doing the hard work of developing new therapies for Alzheimer's disease and to all those who will join the battle and contribute to the emergence of new therapies to improve the lives of those with Alzheimer's disease and those at risk for this mind-robbing disease.

Jeffrey Cummings dedicates this book to Kate Zhong, life partner, best friend, and incomparable traveling companion on life's journey.

Jefferson Kinney dedicates this book to his wife Debi Kinney and son Parker Kinney for all the inspiration they have provided.

Howard Fillit dedicates this book to his wife and best friend, Susan Kind, for her many years of support and love. He also thanks Leonard and Ronald Lauder and all his colleagues at the Alzheimer's Drug Discovery Foundation for their partnership and their efforts in conquering Alzheimer's disease.

Contents

Contributors

Paul S. Aisen, MD
University of Southern California Alzheimer's
Therapeutic Research Institute
San Diego, CA, USA

Arturo Aliaga
Translational Neuroimaging Laboratory
Research Centre for Studying in Aging
Douglas Mental Health Research Institute
McConnell Brain Imaging Centre
McGill University
Quebec, Canada

Cara Altimus, PhD
Center for Strategic Philanthropy
Milken Institute
Washington, DC, USA

Rhoda Au, PhD
Department of Anatomy and Neurobiology
Boston University School of Medicine
Boston, MA, USA

Clive Ballard, MD, MRC Psych
College of Medicine and Health
University of Exeter
Exeter, United Kingdom

Carlo Ballatore, PhD
Skaggs School of Pharmacy and Pharmaceutical
Sciences
University of California San Diego
La Jolla, CA, USA

Laurence Barker, PhD, MBA
Dementia Discovery Fund at SV Health
Investors
London, United Kingdom

Russell L. Barton, MS
PharmaSagacity Consulting, LLC
Carmel, IN, USA

Gil Bashe
Finn Partners
New York, NY, USA

Jonathan Behr, PhD
Dementia Discovery Fund at SV Health Investors
London, United Kingdom

Frank J. Belas, Jr., PhD
IUSM–Perdue TREAT-AD Center
Indiana University School of Medicine
Biotechnology Research and Training Center
Indianapolis, IN, USA

Charles Bernick, MD, MPH
Memory and Brain Wellness Center
University of Washington School of Medicine
Seattle, WA, USA

Kaj Blennow, MD, PhD
Clinical Neurochemistry Laboratory
Institute of Neuroscience and Physiology
The Sahlgrenska Academy at University of
Gothenbburg, Molndal Campus
Sahlgrenska University Hospital
Molndal, Sweden

Jason Bork, BS
Global Alzheimer's Platform
Washington, DC, USA

Adam Boxer, MD, PhD
Weill Institute for Neurosciences
Memory and Aging Center
University of California San Francisco
San Francisco, CA, USA

Kurt R. Brunden, PhD
Center for Neurodegenerative Disease Research
University of Pennsylvania, Perelman School of
Medicine
Philadelphia, PA, USA

Ramon Cacabelos, MD, PhD
EuroEspes Biomedical Research Center
International Center of Neuroscience and
Genomic Medicine
Bergondo, Corunna, Spain

Maria C. Carrillo, PhD
Alzheimer's Association
Chicago, IL, USA

Susan Catalano, PhD
Cognition Therapeutics
Pittsburgh, PA, USA

Feixiong Cheng, PhD
Genomic Medicine Institute, Lerner Research
Institute
Cleveland Clinic
Cleveland, OH, USA

Emily D. Clark, DO
Alzheimer's Disease Care, Research Education
Program (AD-CARE)
University of Rochester School of Medicine and
Dentistry
Rochester, NY, USA

Cyndy Cordell, MBA
Global Alzheimer's Platform
Washington, DC, USA

A. Claudio Cuello, MD
Department of Pharmacology and Therapeutics
McGill University
Quebec, Canada

Jayna Cummings, MBA
Laboratory for Financial Engineering
Sloan School of Management
Massachusetts Institute of Technology
Cambridge, MA, USA

Jeffrey Cummings, MD, ScD
Chambers–Grundy Center for Transformative
Neuroscience
Department of Brain Health
School of Integrated Health Sciences
University of Nevada Las Vegas
Las Vegas, NV, USA

Neal R. Cutler, MD
Worldwide Clinical Trials
Beverly Hills, CA/Wayne, PA, USA

Robert A. Dean, PhD, MD
Robert A. Dean Consulting, LLC
Whitestown, IN, USA

Samuel P. Dickson, PhD
Pentara Corporation
Millcreek, UT, USA

John Dwyer, JD
Global Alzheimer's Platform
Washington, DC, USA

Howard Fillit, MD
Alzheimer's Drug Discovery Foundation
New York, NY, USA

Lauren G. Friedman, PhD
Alzheimer's Drug Discovery Foundation
New York, NY, USA

Serge Gauthier, MD, FRCPC
Translational Neuroimaging Laboratory
Research Centre for Studying in Aging
Douglas Mental Health Research Institute
McGill University
Quebec, Canada

Armineh L. Ghazarian, MSF
National Institute on Aging
Bethesda, MD, USA

Gabe Goldfeder, MA
Global Alzheimer's Platform
Washington, DC, USA

Joshua Grill, PhD
Institute for Memory Impairments and
Neurological Disorders
Department of Psychiatry and Human Behavior;
Department of Neurobiology
Alzheimer's Disease Research Center
University of California Irvine
Irvine, CA, USA

Kevin V. Grimes, MD
Department of Chemical and Systems Biology
Stanford University School of Medicine
Stanford, CA, USA

George Grossberg, MD
Department of Psychiatry and Behavioral
Neuroscience
Saint Louis University School of Medicine
St. Louis, MO, USA

Willem de Haan, MD, PhD
Department of Neurology and Alzheimer Center;
Department of Clinical Neurophysiology
Amsterdam University Medical Center
Amsterdam, The Netherlands

Todd Haim, PhD
National Institute on Aging
Bethesda, MD, USA

John Harrison, PhD
Metis Cognition, Ltd
Wiltshire, UK

Suzanne Hendrix, PhD
Pentara Corporation
Millcreek, UT, USA

Sean P. Hennessey, MS
Pentara Corporation
Millcreek, UT, USA

Janice M. Hitchcock, PhD
Hitchcock Regulatory Consulting, Inc.
Fishers, IN, USA

Amanda Hu
Laboratory for Financial Engineering
Sloan School of Management
Massachusetts Institute of Technology (MIT)
Cambridge, MA, USA

Brenda Hug, BS
Veterans Administrative San Diego Healthcare
System
La Jolla, CA, USA

Samantha E. John, PhD
Department of Brain Health
School of Integrated Health Sciences
University of Nevada Las Vegas
Las Vegas, NV, USA

Christian Jung, PhD
Dementia Discovery Fund at SV Health
Investors
London, United Kingdom

Roos J. Jutten, PhD
Department of Neurology and Alzheimer Center
Amsterdam University Medical Center
Amsterdam, The Netherlands
and
Department of Neurology

Massachusetts General Hospital, Harvard Medical
School
Boston, MA, USA

Amir Kalali, MD
The Decentralized Trials and Research Alliance;
CNS Summit; The International Society for CNS
Drug Development; The International Society for
CNS Clinical Trials and Methodology
San Diego, CA, USA

Min Su Kang, PhD
Translational Neuroimaging Laboratory
Research Centre for Studying in Aging
Douglas Mental Health Research Institute
McConnell Brain Imaging Centre
McGill University
Quebec, Canada

Pragati Katiyar, PhD
National Institute on Aging
Bethesda, MD, USA

Diana Kerwin, MD
Kerwin Medical Center
Dallas, TX, USA

Jefferson Kinney, PhD
Department of Brain Health
School of Integrated Health Sciences
University of Nevada Las Vegas
Las Vegas, NV, USA

Dr Logan Kowallis, PhD
AltaSciences, Laval, QC, Canada

Newman T. Knowlton, MS
Pentara Corporation
Millcreek, UT, USA

Vijaya B. Kolachalama, PhD
Section of Computational Biomedicine
Department of Medicine
Boston University School of Medicine
Boston, MA, USA

Bruce Lamb, PhD
Stark Neuroscience Research Institute
Indiana University School of Medicine
Indianapolis, IN, USA

Jessica Langbaum, PhD
Banner Alzheimer's Institute
Phoenix, AZ, USA

Debra R. Lappin, JD
Faegre Drinker Consulting
Washington, DC, USA

Emily A. Largent, JD, PhD, RN
Department of Medical Ethics and Health Policy
University of Pennsylvania, Perelman School of Medicine
Philadelphia, PA, USA

Amanda M. Leisgang Osse
Department of Brain Health
School of Integrated Health Sciences
University of Nevada Las Vegas
Las Vegas, NV, USA

Honghuang Lin, PhD
Section of Computational Biomedicine, Department of Medicine
Boston University School of Medicine
Boston, MA, USA

Peter A. Ljubenkov, MD
Weill Institute for Neurosciences, Memory and Aging Center
University of California San Francisco
San Francisco, CA, USA

Andrew W. Lo, PhD
Laboratory for Financial Engineering, Sloan School of Management
Computer Science and Artificial Intelligence Laboratory
Massachusetts Institute of Technology
Cambridge, MA, USA

Zane Martin, PhD
National Institute on Aging
Bethesda, MD, USA

Gassan Massarweh, PhD
McConnell Brain Imaging Centre
McGill University
Quebec, Canada

Dawn C. Matthews, MS, MBA
ADM Diagnostics, Inc.
Northbrook, IL, USA

Soeren Mattke, MD, DSc
The USC Brain Health Observatory
University of Southern California
Los Angeles, CA, USA

J. Simon Mazza-Lunn, PhD
Harrington Discovery Institute
University Hospitals Health System
Cleveland, OH, USA

Emily A. S. Meyers, PhD
Alzheimer's Association
Chicago, IL, USA

Daria Mochly-Rosen, PhD
Department of Chemical and Systems Biology
Stanford University School of Medicine
Stanford, CA, USA

Richard Mohs, PhD
Global Alzheimer's Platform
Washington, DC, USA

Michael F. Murphy, MD, PhD
Worldwide Clinical Trials
Beverly Hills, CA/Wayne, PA, USA

Julie Neild, MTSC
Global Alzheimer's Platform
Washington, DC, USA

Scott C. Neu, PhD
Laboratory of Neuro Imaging
USC Stevens Neuroimaging and Informatics Institute
Keck School of Medicine
University of Southern California
Los Angeles, CA, USA

Jessie Nicodemus-Johnson, PhD
Pentara Corporation
Millcreek, UT, USA

Rachel Nosheny, PhD
Department of Psychiatry
University of California San Francisco/San Francisco Veteran's Administration Medical Center
San Francisco, CA, USA

Goodwell Nzou, PhD
Center for Neurodegenerative Disease Research
University of Pennsylvania, Perelman School of Medicine
Philadelphia, PA, USA

Adrian Oblack, PhD
Stark Neuroscience Research Institute

Indiana University School of Medicine
Indianapolis, IN, USA

Julie Ottoy, PhD
Translational Neuroimaging Laboratory
Research Centre for Studying in Aging
McGill University
Quebec, Canada

Meriel Owen, PhD
Alzheimer's Drug Discovery Foundation
New York, NY, USA

Alan D. Palkowitz, PhD
IUSM–Perdue TREAT-AD Center
Indiana University School of Medicine
Indiana Biosciences Research Institute
Indianapolis, IN, USA

Saif-Ur-Rahman Paracha, MD
Department of Psychiatry and Behavioral
Neuroscience
Saint Louis University School of Medicine
St. Louis, MO, USA

Suzana Petanceska, PhD
National Institute on Aging
Bethesda, MD, USA

Ronald C. Petersen, MD, PhD
Mayo Clinic
Rochester, MN, USA

Andrew A. Pieper, MD, PhD
Harrington Discovery Institute
University Hospitals Health System
Cleveland, OH, USA
and
Department of Psychiatry, Case Western Reserve
University
Louis Stokes VA Medical Center of Cleveland
Cleveland, OH, USA

Anton P. Porsteinsson, MD
Alzheimer's Disease Care, Research, and
Education Program (AD-CARE)
University of Rochester School of Medicine and
Dentistry
Rochester, NY, USA

Niels Prins, MD, PhD
Alzheimer Center

Amsterdam University Medical Center
Amsterdam, The Netherlands

Michael S. Rafii, MD, PhD
USC Alzheimer's Therapeutic Research Institute
San Diego, CA, USA

Rema Raman, PhD
USC Alzheimer's Therapeutic Research Institute
San Diego, CA, USA

William Maurice Redden, MD
Department of Psychiatry and Behavioral
Neuroscience
Saint Louis University School of Medicine
St. Louis, MO, USA

Lorenzo Refolo, PhD
National Institute on Aging
Bethesda, MD, USA

Henry Riordan, PhD
Worldwide Clinical Trials
Beverly Hills, CA/Wayne, PA, USA

Craig W. Ritchie, MD, PhD
Centre for Dementia Prevention
The University of Edinburgh
Edinburgh, United Kingdom

Pedro Rosa-Neto, MD, PhD
Translational Neuroimaging Laboratory
Research Centre for Studying in Aging
Douglas Mental Health Research Institute
McConnell Brain Imaging Centre
McGill University
Quebec, Canada

Laurie Ryan, PhD
National Institute on Aging
Bethesda, MD, USA

Marwan Sabbagh, MD
Alzheimer's and Memory Disorders Division
Barrow Neurological Institute
Phoenix, AZ, USA

Arnold Salazar, PhD
Department of Brain Health
School of Integrated Health Sciences
University of Nevada Las Vegas
Las Vegas, NV, USA

Cristina Sampaio, MD, PhD
CHDI Management/CHDI Foundation, Inc.
Princeton, NJ, USA
and
Laboratory of Clinical Pharmacology
Lisbon School of Medicine
University of Lisbon
Lisbon, Portugal

Swati Sathe, MD
CHDI Management/CHDI Foundation, Inc.
Princeton, NJ, USA
and
Rutgers University
Newark, NJ, USA

Philip Scheltens, MD, PhD
Alzheimer Center
Amsterdam University Medical Center; Life
Science Partners
Amsterdam, The Netherlands

Rona Schillinger, BS
Global Alzheimer's Platform
Washington, DC, USA

Mark E. Schmidt, MD
Neuroscience Therapeutic Area
Janssen Research and Development
Division of Janssen Pharmaceutica, NV
Beerse, Belgium

James E. Senetar, PharmD
JES Consulting, LLC
Zionsville, IN, USA

Jiong Shi, MD, PhD
Cleveland Clinic Lou Ruvo Center for Brain
Health
Las Vegas, NV, USA

Monica Shin, MS
Translational Neuroimaging Laboratory
Research Centre for Studying in Aging
McGill University
Quebec, Canada

Eric Siemers, MD
Siemers Integration, LLC
Zionsville, IN, USA

Jill Smith, MA
Global Alzheimer's Platform
Washington, DC, USA

Katy Smith, MA
Global Alzheimer's Platform
Washington, DC, USA

Heather M. Snyder, PhD
Alzheimer's Association
Chicago, IL, USA

Reisa A. Sperling, MD
Harvard Medical School
Boston, MA, USA

John J. Sramek, Pharm D
Worldwide Clinical Trials
Beverly Hills, CA/Wayne, PA, USA

Angela Su
Laboratory for Financial Engineering
Sloan School of Management
Massachusetts Institute of Technology
Cambridge, MA, USA

Janet Sultana, B Pharm, MSc, PhD
College of Medicine and Health, University of
Exeter
Exeter, United Kingdom

Rudolph E. Tanzi, PhD
Genetics and Aging Research Unit
Department of Neurology
Massachusetts General Hospital
Boston, MA, USA

Arthur W. Toga, PhD
Laboratory of Neuro Imaging
USC Stevens Neuroimaging and Informatics
Institute
Keck School of Medicine
University of Southern California
Los Angeles, CA, USA

Alessio Travaglia, PhD
Alzheimer's Drug Discovery Foundation
New York, NY, USA

Everhard Vijverberg, MD, PhD
Department of Neurology and Alzheimer Center

Amsterdam University Medical Center; Brain
Research Center
Amsterdam, The Netherlands

George Vradenburg, JD
Global Alzheimer's Platform
USAgainstAlzheimer's
Washington, DC, USA

Steven L. Wagner, PhD
Department of Neurosciences
School of Medicine
University of California San Diego
San Diego, CA, USA

Sarah Walter, MSc
Alzheimer's Therapeutic Research Institute
University of Southern California
San Diego, CA, USA

Huali Wang, MD, PhD
Dementia Care and Research Center
Clinical Research Division
Peking University Institute of Mental Health
Beijing, China

Tao Wang, MD, PhD
Department of Geriatric Psychiatry
Shanghai Mental Health Center
Shanghai Jiao Tong University School of Medicine
Shanghai, China

Diana R. Wetmore, PhD
Harrington Discovery Institute
University Hospitals Health System
Cleveland, OH, USA

Arno de Wilde, MD, PhD
Department of Neurology and Alzheimer Center
Amsterdam University Medical Center; Life
Science Partners
Amsterdam, The Netherlands

Manfred Windisch, PhD
NeuroScios GmbH
St. Radegund/Graz
Austria

Marcel Seungsu Woo, MD
Translational Neuroimaging Laboratory
Research Centre for Studying in Aging
McGill University
Quebec, Canada

Cally Xiao, PhD
Laboratory of Neuro Imaging
USC Stevens Neuroimaging and Informatics
Institute
Keck School of Medicine
University of Southern California
Los Angeles, CA, USA

Shifu Xiao, MD, PhD
Department of Geriatric Psychiatry
Shanghai Mental Health Center
Shanghai Jiao Tong University School
of Medicine
Shanghai, China

Xin Yu, MD
Beijing Municipal Key Laboratory of
Translational Research on Diagnosis and
Treatment of Dementia
Dementia Care and Research Center
Peking University Institute of Mental Health
Beijing, China

Eduardo R. Zimmer, PhD
Department of Pharmacology
Univerisdade Federal do Rio Grande do Sul
Porto Alegre, Rio Grande do Sul, Brazil

Leigh Zisko, MPH
Global Alzheimer's Platform
Washington, DC, USA

Foreword

Alzheimer's Disease Drug Development: A Research and Development Ecosystem captures the complexity of Alzheimer's disease (AD) drug development and provides a comprehensive set of perspectives from the many stakeholders involved in discovering and developing new therapies for AD.

There is no greater unmet therapeutic need for humanity than effective therapies for brain disorders. The suffering caused by these conditions and other neurodegenerative disorders is overwhelming and is burdened with substantial stigma. Therefore, I have devoted my professional life to changing the way brain disorders such as schizophrenia, depression, AD, among others are not only treated, but also viewed by society. From my time with the National Institutes of Health, Janssen and Johnson & Johnson, where I serve as the Global Head of Science for Minds, my colleagues and I recognize there is still much to uncover about brain disorders due to the rich complexity of the brain and the challenges in accessing it. But that is not a reason to stop – especially as we enter the golden age of neuroscience, driven largely by scientific breakthroughs and accelerated regulatory pathways.

Through our continued commitment in neuroscience, we have uncovered new tools which promise to help us succeed in brain disorder and AD drug development. Fluid biomarkers from blood and spinal fluid, as well as imaging biomarkers, are increasingly allowing us to identify proper populations for inclusion in clinical trials and to more comprehensively understand the effects of our drugs on the biology of complex brain disorders. These advances are described in detail in *Alzheimer's Disease Drug Development: A Research and Development Ecosystem*.

I believe that therapeutic efforts coupled with education will have a marked effect on the lives of those living with brain disorders and their caregivers, but also recognize the importance and value of collaborations and perspectives from key stakeholders in the industry. *Alzheimer's Disease Drug Development: A Research and Development Ecosystem* provides a roadmap for creating this collaborative foundation that will ultimately lead to success for our enterprise and the patient population.

Husseini Manji, MD, FRCPC
Global Head, Science for Minds, Johnson & Johnson

Acknowledgments

The editors gratefully acknowledge the tremendous effort, organizational expertise, and enthusiasm of Mary Kay Tarkanian brought to bear throughout the process of developing this volume.

Dr. Cummings and Dr. Kinney acknowledge the tremendous support of Joy Chambers-Grundy whose generosity has accelerated the study of drug development and expanded the ecosystem required to advance urgently needed new therapies for patients with brain disorders.

Alzheimer's Disease Drug Development: A Research and Development Ecosystem

Jeffrey Cummings, Jefferson Kinney, and Howard Fillit

1.1 Introduction

Alzheimer's disease (AD) is a progressive neurodegenerative disease with a long preclinical asymptomatic period followed by progressive decline in cognition manifested as mild cognitive impairment (MCI) and then by mild, moderate, and severe dementia [1, 2]. The key pathologies include amyloid (A), tau (T), and neurodegeneration (N) (A/T/N). A myriad of contributing factors have been identified including inflammation, oxidation, genetic and epigenetic factors, hormonal factors, metabolic and bioenergetic changes, autophagy dysfunction, proteostasis, apolipoprotein E (ApoE) effects and lipid abnormalities, and vascular factors.

AD can occur in individuals as young as their 30s but is more commonly of late onset, with AD dementia doubling in frequency every 5 years after age 60 from affecting approximately 1% of individuals at age 60 and increasing to affect approximately 40% of those 85 and older [3]. The current global population of 46.8 million AD dementia patients worldwide is projected to rise to 74.7 million by 2030 with a corresponding increase in cost of care from the current $1 trillion to $2 trillion [4].

Despite the urgent need for treatment for this burgeoning population, until 2021 there were only five drugs approved and on the market (donepezil; rivastigmine; galantamine, memantine, Namzaric™) with no new drugs approved in the United States or Europe since 2003 [5]. One additional agent was approved in China in 2019 (GV-971 [oligomannate]) [6]. In 2021, the ecosystem delivered a new treatment – aducanumab – approved for treatment by the US Food and Drug Administration (FDA) for treatment of MCI due to AD and mild AD dementia. Approval of aducanumab is a breakthrough in AD treatment and a milestone in development of disease-modifying therapies (DMTs) for neurodegenerative disorders

(NDDs). This is an important step forward, while still leaving many phases and aspects of AD untreated and introducing an agent that makes exceptional demands on healthcare systems [7]. Aducanumab is expected to have modest impact on the needs of the broader AD population and continuous involvement in new drug discovery for AD is required.

AD drug development takes a long period of time to progress from laboratory studies to possible human availability, is very expensive, and requires a complex ecosystem spanning the translational journey from non-clinical studies, to clinical trials, through regulatory review, to market. The process begins with an unmet medical need and ends with an agent that begins to address the problem; the solution is then subject to reiterative refinement and more unmet needs are identified and addressed (Figure 1.1). The ecosystem has scientific, patient and caregiver, healthcare delivery,

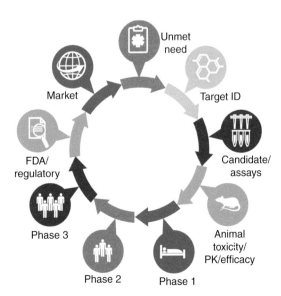

Figure 1.1 The drug-development process from identifying an unmet need to its resolution and reiterative refinement.

business/financial, advocacy, governmental, and policy dimensions that interact dynamically as the candidate agent progresses from molecule to market. Aducanumab is an example of the successful traversal of this complex process to success. Here we provide an overview of the steps in AD drug development and consider the complex multidimensional infrastructure that supports the process. We begin with a description of the phases of drug discovery and development, followed by the resources needed to advance the process including the funding. We end with a discussion of how the process might be improved.

1.2 Alzheimer's Disease Drug Discovery and Development

1.2.1 Overview of Drug Discovery and Development

Development of a new drug begins with identification of a target for treatment and progresses through development of assays for drugs that may modulate target-related processes, and assessment of the candidate(s) in relevant animal models for efficacy, toxicity, and pharmacokinetics (PK). Agents with desirable drug-like properties are then advanced to Phase 1 first-in-human (FIH) trials to assess PK, safety, and tolerability. Drugs with acceptable features in FIH trials are advanced to Phase 2 proof-of-concept (POC) and dose-ranging studies and then to Phase 3 if the Phase 2 studies suggest that the agent is efficacious and safe. If Phase 3 trials confirm efficacy, the drug is submitted for review to the FDA or other regulatory agencies [8]. A successful review results in marketing approval and the ability to make the agent available to patients and prescribing clinicians [8]. Figure 1.2 shows the elements of this process.

1.2.2 Target Identification and Drug Discovery

Common targets for DMTs in AD are processes that eventually lead to cell dysfunction and death

[9, 10]. Targets for cognitive-enhancing agents and treatment for behavioral syndromes of AD commonly include receptors, enzymes, and ion channels. Targets must be "druggable" with properties that can be modulated by small molecules (e.g., drugs) or antibodies, or other biologicals such as antisense oligonucleotides, and other forms of gene therapy [11].

After a target has been identified, an assay with a reporter for interactions suggesting that candidate agents are modulating the target is developed and used to screen candidate therapies. Libraries of compounds are screened for "hits" that have the desired effects in the assay. These libraries are constructed from agents with similar structures and multiple molecular forms, traditional medications (e.g., Chinese traditional medications), natural sources (e.g., bark, seaweed, etc.), repurposed agents that may have AD-related effects, and compounds designed computationally *in silico* [12]. Several hundred thousand compounds may be screened to identify a sufficient number of hits for further development. The hits are reviewed by medicinal chemists for "drug-likeness" including features that predict good absorption and membrane penetration [13, 14]. Compounds with promising characteristics are optimized for molecular features that enhance the likelihood of success as a human therapy – potency, half-life, blood–brain barrier (BBB) penetration, etc. Once a lead compound and several backups are identified testing in animals can begin [15].

An alternative to high-throughput screening with mechanistic assays is high content analysis, conducted in intact cells using automated microscopy and image analysis. High content analysis can be used to screen for effects on protein aggregation, synaptic integrity, and neuron and synapse number or survival as well as other cellular processes relevant to AD treatment [16].

1.2.3 Non-clinical Assessment

Assessment of the lead candidate in animals establishes the PK characteristics, toxicity, and preliminary efficacy of the molecule. These studies may

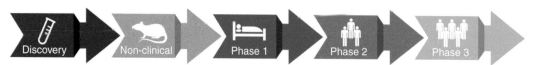

Figure 1.2 Phases in the discovery and development of therapeutic agents.

be done in parallel with or following evidence of proof of mechanism in an animal model (discussed below). Testing involves both short-term and long-term treatment in a wide range of doses to establish the absorption, distribution, metabolism, excretion (ADME), and toxicity of the potential treatment [17]. Testing is required in at least two species – usually mice and rats. Dogs are sensitive to cardiac effects of drugs and are used to assess possible cardiac toxicity [18]. Laboratory and necropsy studies are performed to thoroughly assess any off-target adverse effects in the animals; special attention is paid to liver, cardiac, bone-marrow, and reproductive organ toxicity. Panels of enzymes, ion channels, and other biological mechanisms are used to search for unanticipated off-target effects of the candidate therapy [19]. If no unusual toxicity is identified, the highest drug dose level at which no adverse events are seen is determined and becomes the basis for dose calculations for the recommended safe starting dose for FIH studies [20].

Development of monoclonal antibodies (mAbs) differs from developing small molecules. Monoclonal antibodies are manufactured to interact with a specific epitope of a target such as a portion of amyloid beta protein (Aβ) or tau protein [21, 22]. Monoclonal antibodies have fewer risks for off-target effects since they are exquisitely targeted to specific molecular sites.

Animal species are used to explore the proof of mechanism of candidate therapies. Although success in animal models has not yet predicted success of a DMT in humans, failure to see the desired effect on AD pathology in an animal model system would make one hesitant to advance the agent to human testing [23]. The most commonly used animal model systems are transgenic (Tg) mice that carry one or more human genes known to cause familial AD. Anti-Aβ approaches can be tested in this model. Tau transgenic model animals as well as many types of gene knock-in (KI) and knock-out (KO) models are available. The National Institute on Aging (NIA) and the National Institutes of Health (NIH) Library have created a publicly available data repository of non-clinical/preclinical studies (AlzPED) that includes the available animal models of AD. The model animals exhibit specific aspects of the AD pathology but not the complex multifactorial AD process observed in humans [24].

Human-derived induced pluripotent stem cells are increasingly used to move the early drug screening process toward a more humanized biological context with the hope of having greater predictability for human responses [25, 26]. The induced pluripotent stem cell models show both Aβ and tau protein accumulation, recapitulating the human disease and creating a more ecologically valid system for drug efficacy studies [25].

1.2.4 Phase 1 Clinical Trials

Phase 1 clinical trials involve the FIH exposure of the drug. In small molecule development programs, the persons participating in the Phase 1 trial are healthy volunteers [27]. If a vaccine is being developed, the FIH testing is usually done with patients with AD dementia. Vaccines can permanently alter the immune system and the unknown consequences of this cannot be risked in young healthy individuals.

At the end of Phase 1, the maximum tolerated dose (MTD), human PK, preliminary drug safety and tolerability, and BBB penetration should be known [28]. Single ascending dose (SAD) studies where cohorts of individuals are exposed to progressively higher doses of the agent are followed by multiple ascending dose (MAD) studies where cohorts are treated for 14–28 days with increasing doses of the agent [29]. A cohort is typically 8–12 individuals randomized in a 4:1 ratio of active agent to placebo. In some MAD approaches, at least one cohort of elderly individuals is included to assess PK, ADME, and toxicity differences in older adults. Phase 1b or 1/2 programs may include cohorts of individuals with AD to gather preliminary information on the effects in patients with the disease state.

Ideally, an MTD is determined at this stage of drug development. Maximum doses can be determined by tolerability and safety limits, volume of administration limits, receptor occupancy studies which show that increasing the dose no longer increases occupancy of a positron emission tomography (PET) ligand, or PK studies that demonstrate that increasing the dose no longer increases the maximum serum concentration or area under the curve. Failure to establish an MTD/maximal dose in Phase 1 can lead to future challenges in the development process; if later trials are negative, it may be difficult to know whether the agent is ineffective or was not given in a sufficient dose [30].

Assessing cerebrospinal fluid (CSF) drug levels in Phase 1 is critical to establishing the candidate compound's ability to penetrate the human BBB and exert central nervous system (CNS) effects. Treatments should not exit Phase 1 without evidence of BBB penetration and an understanding of plasma/CSF ratios.

1.2.5   Phase 2 Clinical Trials

Phase 2 generally encompasses Phase 2a POC trials and Phase 2b dose-determination studies. At the end of Phase 2, doses to be advanced to Phase 3, target engagement, preliminary information on biomarker or clinical responses, and insight into safety and tolerability in the population of interest should be available [28]. Phase 2 involves patients with AD dementia or prodromal AD/MCI due to AD [31]. The decision to advance an agent to Phase 3 may be based on a clinical outcome or on changes in a biomarker or repertoire of biomarkers considered likely to predict a clinical outcome (no biomarker is currently proven to predict clinical benefit). Alternatively, one can require clinical POC with benefit on a traditional clinical measure such as the AD Assessment Scale – cognitive subscale (ADAS-cog) [32] or Clinical Dementia Rating – sum of boxes (CDR-sb) [33]. Demonstration of clinical benefit typically requires a large long trial virtually equivalent to a Phase 3 trial [34]. Thus, some development programs move from Phase 1 directly to Phase 3, advancing an agent with limited information regarding safety, tolerability, biomarker effects, or dosing.

Biomarkers may be used as Phase 2 outcomes to support decision making for development programs [35]. Target engagement biomarkers are critical to demonstrating that the drug is having the desired pharmacological effect on a near-term target. Without evidence of target engagement, the potential disease-related biological impact of a putative DMT cannot be assessed [36, 37]. Examples of POC studies in AD drug development include demonstration of reduced Aβ production following administration of beta-site amyloid precursor protein cleaving enzyme (BACE) inhibitors or gamma-secretase inhibitors using stable isotope labeled kinetics (SILK) [38], reduced CSF Aβ with BACE inhibitors [39], and increased Aβ fragments in plasma and CSF with gamma-secretase inhibitors and modulators [40]. Candidate target engagement/proof-of-pharmacology (POP) biomarkers include peripheral indicators of inflammation and oxidation for use in trials of anti-inflammatory and antioxidant compounds. Demonstration of target

engagement does not guarantee efficacy in later stages of development but provides important de-risking of a candidate agent by showing biological effects that may translate into clinical efficacy.

Populations in AD trials are typically characterized by ApoE genotype to identify the *APOE-4* allele carriers and non-carriers. *APOE-4* carriers have earlier onset of AD and progress more rapidly in the early phases of the illness. Allele status may affect efficacy and side effects and often influences dosing in mAb trials [41–43]. Trials are not typically stratified by genotype, but the statistical analysis plans compare carriers and non-carriers for efficacy and toxicity. Approximately, 65% of biomarker-confirmed AD patients are *APOE-4* carriers; if proportions are markedly lower in trials where biomarkers were not used to verify the diagnosis, the number of non-AD patients inadvertently included in the trial may be high.

Growing information on blood biomarkers suggests that measurement of the $A\beta_{42}/A\beta_{40}$ ratio and plasma levels of hyperphosphorylated tau (p-tau$_{181}$, p-tau$_{217}$), total tau, and neurofilament light chain (NfL) may be useful in screening populations for more advanced testing (e.g., Aβ PET imaging) and may eventually be sufficiently accurate to allow their use in diagnosis and trial enrollment. Their possible role in monitoring Aβ-targeted or tau-target therapies is being assessed.

Cognition is mediated by integrated cerebral circuits, and interventions to preserve neurons and synapses – mediated by anti-Aβ, anti-tau, or other mechanisms – will succeed to the extent that they preserve circuit function. Circuit integrity can be assessed by functional MRI (fMRI), quantitative electroencephalography (QEEG), magnetoencephalography (MEG), or fluorodeoxyglucose (FDG) PET [44, 45]. Neurogranin, synaptotagmin, and synaptophysin are synaptic proteins that may represent CSF biomarkers of circuit involvement. These circuit measures can assess the impact of treatment on circuits and may better predict or correlate with the outcome of either cognitive-enhancing agents or DMTs [46].

Biomarkers are used to confirm the diagnosis of AD. The clinical diagnosis of AD dementia based solely on the phenotype of amnestic dementia is not confirmed by Aβ PET or CSF amyloid and tau measures in approximately 25% of patients [41], indicating that they do not have the pathobiology of AD. Approximately 50% of MCI patients have abnormal Aβ measures and constitute a prodromal AD population; 50% do not have early AD [47]. AD trials must be comprised of individuals with AD to draw accurate conclusions about efficacy of AD-directed therapies.

MRI is a measure of cerebral atrophy and neurodegeneration. It is used in DMT trials to assess effects on neuronal loss but the results have often been counter-intuitive with greater atrophy in patients for whom other evidence suggests a treatment benefit. MRI is used to monitor amyloid-related imaging abnormalities (ARIA) occurring as a side effect in patients treated with some anti-Aβ mAbs [42]. Other biomarkers commonly used to monitor adverse effects of medications include liver functions, hematological measures, and electrocardiography (ECG).

1.2.6 Phase 3 Clinical Trials

Phase 2 and Phase 3 are often conceived as "learn" (Phase 2) and "confirm" (Phase 3) trials [48]. The learnings of Phase 2 are tested in Phase 3 and, if

benefits are confirmed, the agent will be submitted to the FDA for review. Phase 3 trials for DMTs are 12–24 months in duration and typically involve 600–1,000 patients per arm of the study (doses and the placebo comprise 1 arm each). Prevention trials of individuals without cognitive symptoms may be up to 5 years in duration.

1.2.6.1 Phase 3 Trial Populations

Clinical trials in Phase 3 may include preclinical populations of participants with no cognitive symptoms but genetic or biomarker evidence (Aβ PET; CSF amyloid or p-tau changes) of high risk for developing symptomatic AD; prodromal AD populations comprised of participants with MCI and biomarker evidence of AD; or AD dementia with participants exhibiting mild, moderate, or severe AD [8, 49].

The FDA has provided guidance for trials involving early AD – those in the preclinical and prodromal phases [50] (Figure 1.3). FDA Stage 1 describes individuals with positive biomarkers of AD pathophysiology and no symptoms detectable

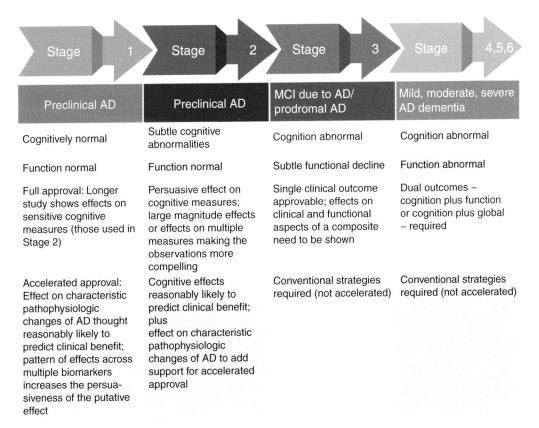

Stage 1	Stage 2	Stage 3	Stage 4,5,6
Preclinical AD	Preclinical AD	MCI due to AD/ prodromal AD	Mild, moderate, severe AD dementia
Cognitively normal	Subtle cognitive abnormalities	Cognition abnormal	Cognition abnormal
Function normal	Function normal	Subtle functional decline	Function abnormal
Full approval: Longer study shows effects on sensitive cognitive measures (those used in Stage 2)	Persuasive effect on cognitive measures; large magnitude effects or effects on multiple measures making the observations more compelling	Single clinical outcome approvable; effects on clinical and functional aspects of a composite need to be shown	Dual outcomes – cognition plus function or cognition plus global – required
Accelerated approval: Effect on characteristic pathophysiologic changes of AD thought reasonably likely to predict clinical benefit; pattern of effects across multiple biomarkers increases the persuasiveness of the putative effect	Cognitive effects reasonably likely to predict clinical benefit; plus effect on characteristic pathophysiologic changes of AD to add support for accelerated approval	Conventional strategies required (not accelerated)	Conventional strategies required (not accelerated)

Figure 1.3 FDA stages of Alzheimer's disease.

by even the most sensitive measures; Stage 2 individuals have positive biomarkers and cognitive symptoms that are detectable with very sensitive measures; Stage 3 is characterized by positive biomarkers, abnormal cognition and functional deficits detectable with only the most sensitive measures (this stage is traditionally known as MCI); Stages 4–6 are mild, moderate, and severe AD dementia. The FDA staging creates a framework for assessing treatments in very early AD with outcomes on sensitive measures (biomarkers or clinical assessments) or impact on progression to the next stage.

1.2.6.2 Biomarkers in Phase 3 Trials

Biomarkers are used in Phase 3 to diagnose participants, support disease-modifying activity, and to monitor ARIA in mAb studies. Biomarker evidence of less degeneration and more neuroprotection by the active agent suggests that the drug is a DMT [9, 51]. Biomarkers currently considered as indicative of disease modification in AD include volumetric MRI, FDG PET, CSF NfL chain and total tau, and blood NfL and total tau [52,53]. Changes on Aβ PET, tau PET, or CSF or blood measures of Aβ protein or p-tau may contribute to the weight of evidence informing the understanding of drug activity and building a narrative for how the agent is achieving

disease modification. Aβ and p-tau protein abnormalities are mediators of cell death and changes in these intermediate biomarkers are supportive but not definitive evidence of disease modification.

1.2.6.3 Clinical Outcomes in Phase 3 Trials

The standards for trials of patients with mild-to-moderate AD were created when tacrine – the first agent approved for the treatment of AD – trials were conducted, and these approaches have remained highly influential. The approval process is based on draft guidelines from the FDA of 1990 [54]. These guidelines require that anti-dementia agents show improvement on the core symptoms of AD – memory and cognition – and that the effect is clinically meaningful as shown by a significant drug–placebo difference on a global or a functional rating. Dual outcome requirements are the standard for both DMTs and cognitive enhancer trials for AD dementia trial populations.

New instruments have been added to the repertoire of tools available to assess different trial populations (Table 1.1). The CDR and CDR-sb are composites of cognitive and functional items that have become the standard global outcome for DMT trials [33]. In trials of prodromal AD, the CDR-sb may serve as a single outcome although regulatory authorities consider the contribution

Table 1.1 Clinical assessments commonly used in AD clinical trials

Population	Domain	Instruments
Preclinical (normal cognitive function)	Cognition	Preclinical Alzheimer's Cognitive Composite (PACC)
		API Preclinical Composite Cognitive (PCC) Test Battery
		DIAN-TU Cognitive Composite
	Function	Amsterdam Instrumental ADL scale
	Behavior	Neuropsychiatric Inventory (NPI)
		Mild Behavioral Impairment (MBI) Checklist
Prodromal	Global	Clinical Dementia Rating – sum of boxes (CDR-sb)
	Cognition	Neuropsychological Test Battery (NTB)
		Alzheimer's Disease Assessment Scale – cognitive subscale (ADAS-cog)
	Function	Amsterdam Instrumental ADL scale
		ADCS ADL scale (MCI version)
	Behavior	NPI
		MBI checklist

Table 1.1 (cont.)

Population	Domain	Instruments
Mild-to-moderate AD dementia	Global	CDR-sb
		Clinical Global Impression of Change (CGIC)
	Cognition	NTB
		ADAS-cog
	Function	Amsterdam Instrumental ADL Scale
		ADCS ADL scale
	Behavior	NPI
Severe AD dementia	Global	CDR-sb
		CGIC
	Cognition	Severe Impairment Battery (SIB)
	Function	ADCS ADL scale (severe)
	Behavior	NPI

ADCS – Alzheimer's Disease Cooperative Study; ADL – activities of daily living; API – Alzheimer's Prevention Initiative; DIAN-TU – Dominantly Inherited Alzheimer Network Treatment Unit; MCI – mild cognitive impairment.

of changes in cognition and changes in function to the total score change. The Neuropsychological Test Battery (NTB) has been shown to work well as an as an alternative to the ADAS-cog [55]. The Severe Impairment Battery (SIB) is most commonly used to assess cognition in patients with severe dementia [56]. The Neuropsychiatric Inventory (NPI) is the tool most commonly used to assess behavioral changes in trials of AD and other neurodegenerative disorders. Function is assessed with the Alzheimer's Disease Cooperative Study (ADCS) activities of daily living (ADL) scale [57] or the Amsterdam Instrumental ADL scale [58]. In some trials the Clinical Global Impression of Change (CGIC; or one of its variants) is used as a global measure instead of or in addition to the CDR. Measures of caregiver burden [59], quality of life [60], and resource utilization [61] are commonly included as outcome measures in Phase 3 trials in anticipation of payer discussions.

The emergence of prevention trials involving participants with normal cognitive function requires the use of tools that are very sensitive to small changes in cognition in older adults. Tools in this category include the Preclinical Alzheimer's Cognitive Composite (PACC) [62], Preclinical Composite Cognitive (PCC) Test Battery used in the Alzheimer's Prevention Initiative (API) [63], the Cognitive Composite of the Dominantly Inherited

Alzheimer Network Treatment Unit (DIAN-TU) [64], and the European Prevention of AD (EPAD) Neuropsychological Examination (EPE) [65].

1.2.7 Phase 4 Clinical Trials and Post-marketing Studies

Phase 4 studies occur after a drug has been approved by the FDA or other regulatory agency and is available on the market. Regulatory agencies may request a risk evaluation and mitigation strategy to assess safety after marketing approval. Phase 4 studies may be used to extend treatment to a new indication or can be used to extend an indication within the same disease [66, 67]. These strategies comprise life-cycle management of an asset once it is approved. Phase 4 studies may be required to confirm efficacy in agents marketed on the basis of accelerated approval and effects on a biomarker.

1.3 Organization and Funding of the Alzheimer's Disease Drug-Development Ecosystem

1.3.1 Drug Discovery

No agent progresses from discovery in the laboratory to approval for marketing under the stewardship of a single individual or team. The skills sets are too diverse and the financial infrastructure required too complex to be accommodated without a mosaic of stakeholders in an ecosystem of support [68].

Target identification begins with study of the neuropathology of AD where the key pathological aspects of AD are evaluated [69]. This type of research is typically conducted in university settings funded by the NIA of the NIH. Philanthropists and advocacy organizations with funding capacity such as the Alzheimer's Association play important roles in supporting basic research directed at the biology of AD. Within the pathology of AD, there are an array of possible drug targets. These are captured in the Common Alzheimer's Disease Research Ontology (CADRO) (https://iadrp.nia .nih.gov/about/cadro) (Table 1.2).

Once a target has been identified, assays are developed, and libraries screened for "hits" that begin the process of developing a candidate agent. This type of screening is done in academic laboratories, biotechnology companies, and pharmaceutical companies. Over the past 10–15 years there has been a shift in pharmaceutical company strategy away from being vertically organized, end-to-end discovery-to-marketing organizations to focusing more on late-stage compounds and Phase 3 opportunities. This shift has been accompanied by an increased emphasis on partnering with academic medical centers (AMCs) and biotechnology companies [70–72]. Products of value in collaborations between biopharmaceutical companies

and AMCs include information exchange and intellectual growth, drug candidates, new technology and laboratory processes, data, and biomarker development. Clinical trials are often conducted in AMCs and provide another conduit for collaboration. Academic trainees become familiar with the pharmaceutical industry, an experience that diversifies career choices for them [73]. Independent confirmation and validation of studies performed in academic laboratories are required before investments are made in a promising agent. The Academic Drug Discovery Consortium (ADDC) (www.addconsortium.org) facilitates information exchanges among AMCs with drug discovery programs [74].

Pharmaceutical companies have active landscape surveillance teams searching for promising emerging compounds that can be licensed, purchased (the compound or the company), partnered, or acquired through merger [75]. Some biotechnology companies specialize in performing assay and screening activities and may create libraries of compounds that can be purchased for further development. Some larger biotechnology companies can escort a compound from early-stage development to later-stage trials. Biopharmaceutical "deals" consist of upfront payment and have risk reduction strategies such as milestone payments that depend on satisfactory progress of the asset. Shared governance is common with assumption of some degree of oversight of the biotech by the pharmaceutical partner with participation in the board of the biotechnology company. Biotechnology companies may be able to take advantage of the partner's expertise in regulatory, legal, commercialization, operations, manufacturing, clinical and medical affairs, and drug safety and pharmacovigilance.

Biotechnology companies typically begin as "spin-offs" from academic programs. The "start-up" focuses on a single product and accesses federal funding through the Small Business Innovation Research (SBIR) program, angel investors, philanthropists, or friends and family investors. Success may attract venture capital that allows the development of the asset to the level where it may attract interest from another biotech, a pharmaceutical company, or larger scale venture capital investments. Venture capital may come from general funds, funds that specialize in biomedical and life science areas, or dementia-specific funds that specialize in dementia-related investments (e.g.,

Table 1.2 CADRO summary of possible therapeutic targets or treatment of AD

Amyloid beta	Tau	ApoE, lipids, and lipoprotein receptors
Neurotransmitter receptors	Neurogenesis	Inflammation
Oxidative stress	Cell death	Proteostasis/ proteinopathies
Metabolism and bioenergetics	Vasculature	Growth factors and hormones
Synaptic plasticity/ neuroprotection	Gut–brain axis	Circadian rhythm
Environmental factors	Epigenetic regulators	Multi-target
Unknown target	Other	

Source: https://iadrp.nia.nih.gov/about/cadro.

Dementia Discovery Fund, Dolby Ventures, LSP Dementia Fund).

Compounds may languish from lack of support in the early stages of development. Once a compound has been shown to be efficacious in animals, its promise can by explored and eventually realized only if it can be tested in humans. The cost of Phase 1 studies is substantial (~$1,000,000 to $2,500,000) per agent. The studies are typically conducted in healthy volunteers and focus on safety, tolerability, and PK. The information gained in Phase 1 is essential for advancing an agent further, but because it tends to be "recipe like" and does not provide information on treatment of a diseased population, it is often difficult to fund. This creates the "valley of death," where promising agents may not be advanced because of lack of funding, expertise, and infrastructure [76, 77]. Difficulty with fundraising may extend to early Phase 2 testing prior to the generation of disease-related information and beginning clarification of the commercial promise of the agent. Funding agencies have realized and responded to this challenge and support for very early-stage development is increasingly available through the NIA, National Center for Advancing Translational Science, and philanthropic organizations such as the Alzheimer's Drug Discovery Foundation (ADDF) [78, 79].

1.3.2 The Alzheimer's Disease Neuroimaging Initiative

The Alzheimer's Disease Neuroimaging Initiative (ADNI) began in 2004 as a public–private partnership between the NIA and more than 30 private (e.g., pharmaceutical) and not-for-profit enterprises. ADNI has a trial-like structure and was designed to collect brain imaging and biomarker data that could be used to understand the natural history of AD and to model trajectories relevant to planning clinical trials. ADNI has enrolled approximately 325 cognitively normal controls, 425 participants with MCI, and 215 participants with mild AD dementia. Biomarkers collected at 6-month intervals include MRI (structural, diffusion, perfusion, resting state), amyloid PET, tau PET, FDG PET, and genetic and autopsy data. CSF (for measures of Aβ, tau, p-tau, and other proteins) is collected annually. All participants have cognitive and clinical assessments with commonly used clinical trials instruments (Mini-Mental State Examination [MMSE], ADAS-cog, CDR, Everyday

Cognition [Ecog], NPI Questionnaire [NPI-Q], and others). Data are collected at 60 participating sites and added to a publicly available database in real time. Trial-like site monitoring and data management ensure data quality.

Among its most important contributions has been ADNI's provision of data to trials sponsors which can be used to model clinical trials and determine necessary sample sizes. Sample sizes for different populations using different clinical instruments have been calculated [80], and the utility of biomarkers, genetic assessments, and MRI atrophy measures in identifying patients with MCI likely to progress to AD dementia has been demonstrated [81–83].

ADNI has worldwide collaborators including ADNI-like organizations in Europe, Japan, Australia, Korea, and Argentina [84]. The similarity of the participants recruited in different global regions has been assessed and the feasibility of using data from different regions shown [85]. Most late-stage trials require globally distributed sites to achieve adequate recruitment, and the baseline features of participants in non-Western countries vary [86, 87] making global data valuable for trial planning.

1.3.3 The Dominantly Inherited Alzheimer's Network – Treatment Unit

The DIAN is an international multi-site study characterizing early clinical and biomarker changes occurring in persons inheriting autosomal-dominant AD (ADAD) mutations. All subjects in the DIAN are either affected by or known to be at 50% risk for inheriting pathogenic presenilin 1 (*PSEN1*), amyloid precursor protein (*APP*), or presenilin 2 (*PSEN2*) mutations. Washington University (St. Louis, Missouri, USA) is the lead site (John Morris, Principal Investigator) and there are 19 participating sites in eight countries recruiting and assessing ADAD participants.

DIAN-TU leverages the existing infrastructure of the ongoing DIAN longitudinal study and builds on important DIAN baseline and rate-of-change data. DIAN-TU has a platform trial design that can introduce new candidate treatments sequentially as each is shown to be effective and matriculates to other studies or is shown to be ineffective and is discontinued. DIAN-TU is led by Randall Bateman of Washington University. Governance is by a steering committee comprised of clinical trial experts, regulatory advisors, and ADAD family-member

9

representatives. Funding for the DIAN-TU is provided by the NIA, Alzheimer's Association, and the DIAN Pharma Consortium. The Pharma Consortium was created by the DIAN-TU and collaborating pharmaceutical companies to provide funds, expertise, and drug candidates for the platform [88].

The DIAN-TU platform was initiated as a randomized, blinded, placebo-controlled four-arm trial with a target of 160 asymptomatic to mildly symptomatic mutation carrier participants who are −15 to +10 years of their estimated age at onset of AD dementia [88]. A pooled placebo group derived from the placebo arm for each agent greatly increases efficiency and enhances the participant's likelihood of receiving the active drug compared with traditional designs; this makes participating in the trial more attractive to potential volunteers.

DIAN-TU has introduced innovations including construction of a disease progression model (DPM) to detect changes in cognition with fewer participants, self-administered cognitive testing, a predefined dose escalation algorithm to safely maximize target engagement, adaptive trial design strategies that include both early biomarker and later cognitive interim analyses to inform early efficacy or futility, and novel biomarkers [64].

1.3.4 Alzheimer's Prevention Initiative

The API, led by researchers from Banner Alzheimer's Institute (BAI; Drs. Reiman, Tariot, Langbaum) in partnership with leaders from academia, industry, and other public and private stakeholder organizations was initiated to accelerate the evaluation and approval of prevention therapies. The API ADAD Colombia trial is studying the use of an anti-amyloid treatment – crenezumab – in cognitively normal *PSEN1* mutation carriers and non-carriers from the world's largest ADAD kindred [89]. Mutation carriers are at virtually certain risk for developing AD at young ages. The study is conducted in conjunction with the University of Antioquia in Colombia and Genentech/Roche.

The API Generation Program aims to prevent or delay the onset of symptoms associated with AD in cognitively healthy people with two *APOE-4* alleles, making them at particularly high risk for developing the AD [90]. These studies are part of a collaboration between BAI, Novartis, Amgen, and the NIA. The API has pioneered new cognitive assessments for cognitively normal

individuals at risk for AD [91] and developed innovative approaches to genetic counseling [92].

1.3.5 European Prevention of Alzheimer's Disease

The EPAD project, funded by the Innovative Medicines Initiative (IMI), was established to overcome the major hurdles hampering drug development for secondary prevention of AD [65, 93, 94]. EPAD is led by Craig Ritchie at the University of Edinburgh and trial delivery centers throughout Europe participate in the consortium. EPAD incorporates several drug-development innovations: collaborative access to existing European cohorts and registries; development of the EPAD Registry of people at increased risk of developing AD dementia; establishment of the EPAD Longitudinal Cohort Study (LCS) to serve as a trial-ready cohort for POC studies; and establishment of an adaptive, POC trial platform. In addition to providing patients for trials, the LCS provides run-in data for the pre-randomization period in the EPAD POC study, gathers longitudinal data for AD modeling of probability of decline, and generates models that place individuals on the disease probability spectrum [93].

The EPAD POC study emphasizes biomarker effects of candidate agents, but success in the EPAD POC study requires the demonstration of clinical benefit. Drugs deemed successful in the POC study will, therefore, be more likely to achieve clinical and regulatory success in Phase 3. The POC study employs a Bayesian adaptive design that learns from data accrued as the trial progresses. Frequent interim analyses, done in accordance with predefined algorithms and blinded to all trial personnel, allow adaptive randomization of individuals to interventions that appear to show the greatest clinical efficacy, and, potentially, in subpopulations defined by clinical status, biomarkers, or genetics. These interim analyses are used to test for early signals of drug success or futility [93]. The trial design utilizes a shared placebo group to minimize the number of participants assigned to placebo without compromising trial integrity. EPAD has structured involvement of participants as collaborators recognizing the participants' key role [95]. Participant panels establish accountability and transparency between the study goals and the study population, provide an opportunity for researchers to respond to participants' concerns, and create a conduit for participants to provide input into the research processes, consent procedures, and dissemination of study results. The EPAD infrastructure may comprise the European component of the Global Alzheimer Platform (discussed below).

1.3.6 Coalition Against Major Disease

The Critical Path Institute (C-Path) is a nonprofit, public–private partnership with the FDA created under the auspices of the FDA's Critical Path Initiative program in 2005. The goal of C-Path is to accelerate the pace and reduce the costs of medical product development through the creation of new measurements, methods, and data standards that aid in the scientific evaluation of the efficacy and safety of new therapies. The Coalition Against Major Diseases (CAMD) was a founding consortium within C-Path and gave rise to the Critical Path for Alzheimer's Disease (CPAD) [96]. CPAD focuses on: (1) regulatory qualification of biomarkers (fluid, imaging, and digital/biosensor observational- and performance-based); (2) Clinical Data Interchange Standards Consortium (CDISC) data standards for AD endpoint assessments; (3) integrated databases for observational and clinical trials data; and (4) quantitative model-based tools for drug development. CPAD efforts led to the qualification by the European Medicines Agency (EMA) for the use of low baseline hippocampal volume for patient enrichment in pre-dementia trials; the creation of an AD drug–disease trial model and clinical trial simulation tool endorsed by the FDA and qualified by the EMA [97]; and the launch of an open database of aggregated CDISC-standardized clinical trial data for AD.

1.3.7 Clinical Trial Infrastructure

Phase 2 clinical trials typically include several hundred participants and Phase 3 trials may require several thousand. Recruitment of large numbers of participants can be achieved only if many sites are involved in the recruitment process; most sites randomize ~0.5 patients per trial per month, contributing six or fewer patients annually to trials [98]. Sites are typically comprised of a site principal investigator (PI), several research coordinators and research assistants, a research nurse, budget manager/financial officer, and a regulatory/institutional review board (IRB) specialist. Sites may be situated in AMCs associated with memory clinics or may be "commercial sites" whose purpose is to attract participants through advertisements and community events for the purpose of conducting trials. Most trials include both academic and commercial sites. Sites must have IRB (local or central) approval to conduct trials and be knowledgeable about informed consent requirements. Sites are monitored for quality during the conduct of the trial by site monitors from the sponsor, the sponsor's contract research organization (CRO), or both.

There are several clinical trial consortia that facilitate trials. The US Alzheimer Clinical Trial Consortium (ACTC) has 30 core academic sites and an extended group of academic and commercial collaborators that conduct NIA-sponsored and industry-sponsored trials. The ACTC is funded by the NIA and consists of a steering committee of the site PIs and cores addressing recruitment, statistics, bioinformatics, imaging, biomarkers, and clinical operations. Paul Aisen (University of Southern California), Reisa Sperling (Harvard University), and Ronald Petersen (Mayo Clinic) provide leadership to the ACTC. The ACTC collaborates with the NIA-funded Trial-Ready Cohort for Preclinical and Prodromal AD (TRC-PAD), a registry of individuals interested in trials who are prescreened through online testing, referred to sites for biomarker confirmation of AD, and comprise a trial-ready cohort for ongoing and emerging trials [99].

The Consortium of Canadian Centres for Clinical Cognitive Research (C5R) is a not-for-profit research network that facilitates collaboration and partnerships between pharmaceutical companies and Canadian dementia researchers. C5R research sites conduct clinical trials and develop treatments for patients with MCI, AD dementia, and other forms of dementia.

The Global Alzheimer Platform (GAP) is a network of over 80 clinical trial sites across North America whose goal is to conduct clinical trials of AD and to optimize clinical trial conduct [100]. GAP provides assistance with site activation, site optimization, recruitment, participant transportation, and participant engagement activities for GAP-enabled trials. GAP has a global vision for more international collaboration and trial conduct.

Neuronet is a European program that connects 18 research projects launched by the IMI, Europe's largest public–private partnership in the life sciences. To enhance the productivity and visibility of the IMI neurodegeneration portfolio, Neuronet created a platform for efficient collaboration, communication, and operational synergies among present and future IMI neurodegenerative disease projects. Neuronet is designing systems to map and analyze information regarding actions, initiatives, and partnerships to assess the impact of individual projects, identify remaining gaps, and determine the global value of the program for stakeholders. Neuronet supports the management of the program projects (timelines, dependencies, synergies and key results across projects). Neuronet provides support to the projects by organizing services, expert advice and guidelines/recommendations, opportunities, and transferable best practices. Neuronet promotes enhancement and coordination of communication across the IMI neurodegeneration projects, increasing program visibility, engaging key stakeholders, and establishing relationships with other initiatives in the field.

1.3.8 Contract Research Organizations

CROs play a major role in AD therapeutic and biomarker development and comprise important components of the AD drug-development ecosystem. The growth of CROs reflects the decision of pharmaceutical companies to reduce in-house work forces and rely more on outsourcing. Some pharmaceutical companies have internal trial conduct capability but a majority of them depend on CROs. Trial CROs conduct feasibility studies to assess site capabilities; engage the sites for trials; work with sites to achieve IRB approval; manage contract negotiations and contract review; monitor the sites once the trial is initiated; oversee data collection, capture, and transfer to the sponsor; identify members for data safety monitoring boards; and close sites when the trial is terminated [101]. Some CROs have biostatistical expertise and are contracted to do database management and data analysis. Most Phase 3 trials and some Phase 2 trials are conducted with multi-regional sites, and trial CROs must have multi-regional capability or affiliations with national or regional CROs [102].

Specialty CROs are available for a wide range of services including transgenic mouse testing, Phase 1 clinical trials, regulatory strategy formulation, biomarker measurement, brain imaging interpretation, rater training, and product manufacturing and supply chain management.

1.3.9 Advocacy Organizations

The Alzheimer's Association supports caregivers, funds research, and advocates on the behalf of AD patients and caregivers. It works on a national and local level (through chapters) to provide care and support for those affected by AD and related dementias. As the largest non-profit funder of AD research, the Alzheimer's Association supports research on methods of treatment, prevention, and, ultimately, a cure for AD. From the advocacy perspective, it fights for critical AD research and care initiatives at the state and federal level. In partnership with Bill Gates, the Alzheimer's Association funds the Part the Cloud program that promotes human studies to advance innovative ideas for early-phase human trials (Phase 1 or Phase 2). The association sponsors TrialMatch, a clinical study matching service that connects individuals living with AD, caregivers, and healthy volunteers with research studies. The Alzheimer's Association has partnered with a variety of organizations to support research on amyloid imaging and standardization of CSF biomarker measures, and it has sponsored work groups that advance diagnostic standards [52, 103]. It plays a key role in advocating for better care of AD patients and was a leader in the effort to gain FDA approval for aducanumab.

Alzheimer's Disease International (ADI) is a UK-based globally focused advocacy organization whose goal is to strengthen and support AD and dementia associations worldwide, raise awareness and lower stigma about dementia, make dementia a global health priority, support and empower people living with dementia and their care partners, and increase investment and innovation in dementia research. ADI sponsors the Alzheimer University, a series of workshops for volunteers to help them strengthen their local and national associations. ADI sponsors international and local meetings; publishes globally oriented reports and reviews, helps countries develop national plans for AD and other dementias, promotes "dementia friendly" community programs, and supports research with global impact such as the 10/66 research group [104–106].

Alzheimer Europe is a non-profit non-governmental organization aiming to provide a voice to people with dementia and their caregivers, make dementia a European priority, promote a rights-based approach to dementia, support dementia research, and strengthen the European dementia movement. Alzheimer Europe convenes European and local meetings, publishes reports, promotes and collaborates on research [107], and conducts surveys to influence policy and funding decisions [108].

UsAgainstAlzheimer's is a non-profit organization committed to stopping AD by creating urgency from government, industry, and the scientific community in the quest for an AD cure – accomplishing this through leadership, collaboration, advocacy, and strategic investments. Goals of UsAgainstAlzheimer's include improving brain health; increasing the speed, efficiency, and diversity of clinical trials (in collaboration with GAP); advancing national care goals and policies to support caregivers; and mobilizing advocates in many communities (e.g., Women Against AD, Latinos Against AD, etc.).

The Alzheimer's Foundation of America (AFA) provides support, services, and education to individuals, families, and caregivers affected by AD and related dementias nationwide. The AFA conducts support groups (face-to-face and online), webinars, and education programs for patients and caregivers. A signature program is the National Memory Screening Program, which provides, free, confidential memory screenings at sites across the country.

1.3.10　Philanthropy

Advocacy enterprises are one conduit for organized philanthropy. Philanthropists may also make direct contributions to scientists and their laboratories or make contributions as part of a philanthropy group that raises funds and identifies individual scientists or programs worthy of support. Philanthropy often provides seed funds for projects that require preliminary data before proposals for federal or other types of grant support can be developed. Similarly, philanthropy can help overcome "valley of death" challenges (described above) to advance candidate agents to an investment level of development. The Cure Alzheimer's Fund is a non-profit organization dedicated to funding research with the highest probability of preventing, slowing, or reversing AD. The Milken Institute Center for Strategic Philanthropy develops Giving Smarter Guides to help guide philanthropists to high-impact philanthropy. A Giving Smarter Guide for AD has been developed [109].

ADDF (Howard Fillit, Chief Scientific Officer) is a venture philanthropy enterprise that funds treatment-related research at the basic and clinical level. ADDF invests in development of new drugs, biomarkers, and digital technology relevant to drug development. The organization funds early laboratory studies of emerging therapeutics as well as early-stage clinical trials. ADDF emphasizes the importance of an experimental medicine approach to drug development, with early trials focusing on POC and biomarker effects with appropriate statistics for small trials with exploratory aims. ADDF is the largest non-federal funder of clinical trials in the United States and has a shaping influence on AD drug development through its investment strategy [78, 110]. Venture philanthropy invests in early-stage companies, is a company partner, benefits from profits generated, and re-invests any profits in the philanthropy [111].

1.3.11　Regulatory Agencies

Regulatory authorities include the FDA, EMA, Chinese National Medical Products Agency (NMPA), Japanese Pharmaceuticals and Medical Devices Agency (PMDA), and similar agencies in other countries. A key interaction with the FDA is submission of the investigational new drug (IND) when a new agent is to be studied, when an approved product is to be assessed for a new indication, or when a new patient population is to be included in trials. The IND application must include information on animal pharmacology and toxicology studies, product manufacturing, and clinical protocols and investigator information (www.fda.gov/drugs/types-applications/investigational-new-drug-ind-application). The new drug application (NDA) is the vehicle through which drug sponsors formally propose that the FDA approve a new pharmaceutical for sale and marketing in the USA.

The FDA corresponds and meets regularly with sponsors throughout the drug-development process. Planned meetings typically occur in the pre-IND period, with the initial IND submission, at end of Phase 2, prior to NDA submission, and with the drug marketing application (Figure 1.4). There is ongoing communication and updates throughout the trial and development process [112].

13

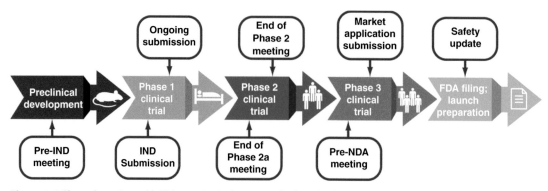

Figure 1.4 Planned meetings with FDA occurring in the course of a drug-development program.

The FDA issues "Guidances" to help sponsors understand FDA policies. Guidance documents usually discuss design, production, labeling, promotion, manufacturing, and testing of regulated products. Guidances provide information on the processing, content and evaluation or approval of submissions, as well as on inspection and enforcement policies. The FDA recently issued an influential Guidance on developing drugs for treatment of early AD [50] describing the stages of early AD to facilitate drug development for the preliminary stages of the illness (see Figure 1.3).

1.3.12 Media and Drug-Development Press

The public becomes aware of scientific advances through media coverage. Members of the lay public are concerned about AD and the consequences of cognitive decline; they do not read the scientific literature and depend on the press and media for scientific information. Social media channels have grown in importance as a source of information [113]. Direct-to-consumer advertising is a source of information for patients and families supported by pharmaceutical companies and providing information about their products. Media releases often have agendas beyond education: scientists want to draw attention to their work; biotechnology companies seek to influence investors; and pharmaceutical companies use media to attract patients in need of their products. Citizens often have no reliable way to assess the accuracy of health information found in the media (social or traditional), on the Internet, or in direct-to-consumer advertising [114]. News on

drug development can influence decisions to seek care, invest, join advocacy efforts, or donate funds. For this reason, it is particularly important for scientists to communicate clearly and for citizens to seek informed, objective advice when evaluating news and drawing conclusions based on media releases.

1.3.13 Scientific Publication of Drug-Development Information and Clinical Trials

Scientific publication in peer-reviewed journals is a key part of the life cycle of drug development. Publication of trial results is an ethical responsibility given that participants have taken risks with altruistic motivations to advance the public good. Most journals require that trials submitted for publication have been registered prior to conduct on approved registries such as ClinicalTrials.gov. Nearly all journals expect use of the Consolidated Standards of Reporting Trials (CONSORT) criteria with a checklist of essential elements (Table 1.3) and a figure showing the disposition of participants in the trial (enrollment, intervention, allocation, attrition, completion) [115]. The standardization of trial reporting allows the reader to evaluate the quality of the trial and to compare trials. The CONSORT criteria represent a useful planning document and checklist for trial protocol planning since publication of the trial results will require meeting this standard. Publication of trials in peer-reviewed journals is the principal means of getting treatment-related information into the public domain.

Table 1.3 CONSORT checklist

Section/topic	Checklist item
Title	Identification as a randomized trial in the title
Abstract	Structured summary of trial design, methods, results, and conclusions (for specific guidance, see CONSORT for abstracts)
Background and objectives	Scientific background and explanation of rationale; specific objectives or hypotheses
Trial design	Description of trial design (such as parallel, factorial) including allocation ratio; important changes to methods after trial commencement (such as eligibility criteria), with reasons
Participants	Eligibility criteria for participants; settings and locations where the data were collected
Interventions	The interventions for each group with sufficient details to allow replication, including how and when they were actually administered
Outcomes	Completely defined pre-specified primary and secondary outcome measures, including how and when they were assessed; any changes to trial outcomes after the trial commenced, with reasons
Sample size	How sample size was determined; when applicable, explanation of any interim analyses and stopping guidelines
Sequence generation	Method used to generate the random allocation sequence; type of randomization; details of any restriction (such as blocking and block size)
Allocation concealment mechanism	Mechanism used to implement the random allocation sequence (such as sequentially numbered containers), describing any steps taken to conceal the sequence until interventions were assigned
Implementation	Who generated the random allocation sequence, who enrolled the participants, and who assigned participants to interventions
Blinding	If done, who was blinded after assignment to interventions (for example, participants, care providers, those assessing outcomes) and how; if relevant, description of the similarity of interventions
Statistical methods	Statistical methods used to compare groups for primary and secondary outcomes; methods for additional analyses, such as subgroup analyses and adjusted analyses
Participant flow (with diagram)	For each group, the number of participants who were randomly assigned, received intended treatment, and were analyzed for the primary outcome; for each group, losses and exclusions after randomization, together with reasons
Recruitment	Dates defining the periods of recruitment and follow-up; why the trial ended or was stopped
Baseline data	A table showing baseline demographic and clinical characteristics for each group
Numbers analyzed	For each group, number of participants (denominator) included in each analysis and whether the analysis was by original assigned groups
Outcomes and estimation	For each primary and secondary outcome, results for each group, and the estimated effect size, and its precision (such as 95%); for binary outcomes, presentation of both absolute and relative effect sizes is recommended
Ancillary analyses	Results of any other analyses performed, including subgroup analyses and adjusted analyses, distinguishing pre-specified from exploratory
Harms	All important harms or unintended effects in each group
Limitations	Trial limitations, addressing sources of potential bias, impression, and, if relevant, multiplicity of analyses
Generalizability	Generalizability (external validity, applicability) of the trial findings
Interpretation	Interpretation consistent with results, balancing benefits and harms, and considering other relevant evidence
Registration	Registration number and name of trial registry
Protocol	Where the full trial protocol can be accessed, if available
Funding	Sources of funding and other support (such as supply of drugs), role of funders

Adapted from Ref. [115].

1.4 Aducanumab: The Ecosystem Delivers

Aducanumab (marketed as Aduhelm™) was approved by the FDA on June 4, 2021, as a means of lowering Aβ in the brain. The approval of aducanumab shows the successful interaction of the many stakeholders comprising the AD drug-development ecosystem. Aducanumab emerged from university-based foundational studies involving reverse translation of clinical observations and was further optimized by Neurimmune, a biotechnology company. The rights to advanced development were obtained by Biogen. Trials involving CROs and academic and commercial trial sites were conducted; new biomarkers including Aβ PET were incorporated in the trial design to better define the participant population and the outcome; the FDA conducted extensive reviews of the trials; and the Alzheimer's Association and USAgainstAlzheimer's played key roles in advocating for the approval of aducanumab. The development program of aducanumab had irregularities and some opposed approval. Many lessons emerged from the aducanumab trials that will be applied to other drug-development efforts and will further enhance the AD drug-development ecosystem. The approval of aducanumab is likely to increase confidence in the ability to change the course of AD with pharmacological intervention attracting greater interest from biotechnology and pharmaceutical companies, venture capital, philanthropy, and other sources of financial support.

1.5 Discussion

The drug-development ecosystem described here is not unique to AD; it is characteristic – with some variations – of nearly all drugs. It is successful in the sense that many drugs have traversed the pathway and become approved treatments with major impact on the public health.

Of 210 new molecular entities (NMEs) approved by the FDA between 2010 and 2016, federal funding contributed to development of all. NIH funding was focused primarily on the drug targets rather than on the NMEs themselves [116]. These figures demonstrate the critical role of NIH funding in providing the foundation on which much of the rest of the ecosystem is built. Considering the relatively small number of NMEs entering the AD drug-development pipeline, enhanced investment in AD target discovery is likely to lead to eventual benefit in new therapies [117].

The low rate of successful drug development for AD and other CNS disorders has resulted in a flight of pharmaceutical companies from pursuing treatments for these disorders. From 2009 to 2014 there was a 50% decrease in the number of major pharmaceutical companies working in CNS therapeutic areas [72]. Improvements in the ecosystem including more promising targets and optimized trial processes are required to attract industry sponsors back to AD drug development. Success by companies working on AD therapeutics will encourage other companies to launch programs for AD, and legislative and policy adjustments to incentivize AD drug development will encourage sponsors to include AD drug development in their portfolios. The approval of aducanumab is expected to serve as a stimulus for AD drug-development innovation.

The absence of a well-developed, stable, high-capacity, high-quality clinical trial network with excellent sites throughout the world hinders AD drug development. Organizations such as the ACTC (described above) are funded to test five to six new drugs in each 5-year grant cycle, far below the capacity needed to meet the needs of patients and sponsors. GAP (described above) can manage four to five trials at a time; far below the capacity needed to advance Phase 2 and Phase 3 drugs with a wide range of sponsors. University-based Clinical and Translational Science Award (CTSA) centers in the United States conduct trials in multiple disease states but lack capacity to conduct the trials needed to advance a major portion of the AD drug-development portfolio. The result of these shortfalls is that the sponsor or CRO must identify sites and rebuild the trial network for each trial. This has been likened to rebuilding a soccer stadium for each game. A global continuously functioning trial network that optimizes site function, ensures site quality, and encourages new sites and new principal investigators is needed.

An efficient means of testing drugs in Phase 2 is the use of an adaptive platform trial design [118, 119]. EPAD and DIAN-TU (described above) are examples of this approach. Advantages of platforms include the simultaneous testing of several agents, the use of biomarkers as readouts to determine which agents will continue to be assessed for clinical efficacy and which will be terminated, the use of Bayesian statistics to minimize the size and duration of trials for each agent, the pooling of data from placebo groups to minimize the number of patients assigned to placebo, and the ability to study new clinical and biomarker measures. Registries and trial-ready cohorts can be organized to facilitate enrollment in the platform, and assessment of pre-enrollment cognitive trajectories can assist in evaluating drug effects on the course of the disease. Time between trials is minimized as new drugs are continuously introduced as test agents in the platform are terminated or continue to the next phase of development. Trials sites are continuously operational, and the site network can be grown over time. Figure 1.5 illustrates an adaptive platform design for trials. Such a structure requires continuous external financial support at least until the costs can be covered in part by sponsors whose drugs are being assessed. The improvement in patient and caregiver quality of life, continued innovation, eventual generic status of drugs shown to be successful, training opportunities, and economic gains (salaries, etc.) more than justify the costs of supporting such a platform trial enterprise.

The globalization of drug-development research, clinical trials, and the availability of drugs shown to be safe and efficacious is a critical aspect of the AD drug-development ecosystem. Fourteen percent of Phase 2 trials and 42 percent of Phase 3 currently involve sites both in North America and non-North American locations [98]. The United States is the preferred site for trials by sponsors because it has a well-developed trial infrastructure, and its large market and robust reimbursement of drug costs are attractive. Sponsors conduct their trials in the United States to ensure that the data are acceptable to the FDA. Once approved in the United States, some countries require a full development program in their own populations, some require at least safety trials to allow marketing of the agent in their country, and others allow marketing of the agent based on FDA or other regulatory agency approval. This means that treatments will be used by patients in many countries not participating in trials, including those with different body sizes, genetics, diets, nutritional history, and medical care not represented in trials. Even within countries,

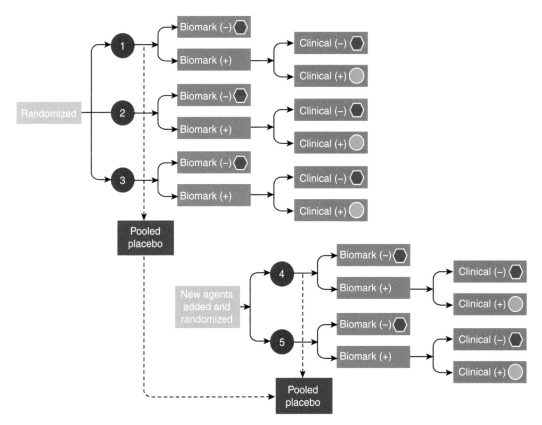

Figure 1.5 Adaptive clinical trial platform.

such as the United States, the participation in trials by minority members is low and extrapolation from majority-culture trial participants to minority-culture patients is hazardous [120]. Diversifying trial participants within countries and globally is an unmet need that must be resolved to advance health equity among the world's populations.

Training of translational neuroscientists with experience, knowledge, skills, and passion for drug development is another unmet need that must be addressed if future generations are to have ever better therapeutic options. Few training programs exist specifically for trialists, most residencies provide no exposure to trials, and although most academic dementia programs conduct trials, the involvement of trainees is variable. The need for new staff with trial skills far outstrips the current capacity to develop this workforce [121]. Many aspects of college curricula can be translated into contributions to drug development (Figure 1.6). Biology addresses drug targets; chemistry is key to candidate development; veterinary medicine is required for animal care; psychology contributes to outcomes; physicians trained in several

specialties are required for trials; and business, law, ethics, regulatory science, and governmental affairs all prepare students for potential roles in drug development. Few under-graduate or graduate programs acquaint students with career opportunities for drug development [122].

Clinical trials and drug development are key components of the larger concept of translational science or translational medicine that conceptualizes accelerating advances in science to improve public health [123]. There is a perceived gap between the increasing investment in science and the relative lack of new therapies in disorders such as AD; translational science aims to address this gap. In drug development, the translation from basic science to animal testing is T1; the translation of animal observation to humans in trials is T2; the translation from trials to care is T3; and the translation from care to public health and policy is T4 [124] (Figure 1.7). To achieve the laudable and important goal of improving public health, drug-development science must be complemented by advances in recruitment science, implementation science,

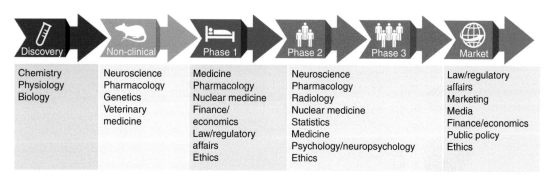

Figure 1.6 Alignment between skills needed for drug development and college curricula.

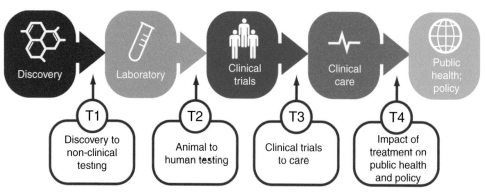

Figure 1.7 Steps in the translational research process.

regulatory science, science of behavior change, and other key approaches to ensure that new advances in treatment of AD and other related dementias reach all those in need of therapy [125–128].

1.6 Summary

Drug development for AD depends on a complex, dynamic, interactive ecosystem with many stakeholders (Figure 1.8). The system is successful in advancing drugs, biomarkers, and trials. The approval of aducanumab is an example of the successful working of the ecosystem to advance a new therapy for AD. Other promising agents are emerging from the pipeline and success will encourage more sponsors to enter the AD and related dementias therapeutic area. The ecosystem lacks optimal coordination among the many participants and accelerating drug development depends on building infrastructure and advancing training that will ensure the resources and expertise for future AD drug development.

Disclosures

Dr. Cummings has provided consultation to Acadia, Actinogen, Acumen, Alector, Alkahest, AriBio, Avanir, Axsome, Behren Therapeutics, Biogen, Biohaven, Cassava, Cerecin, Cerevel, Cortexyme, EIP Pharma, Eisai, Foresight, GemVax, Genentech, Green Valley, Grifols, Janssen, Karuna, LSP, Merck, Novo Nordisk, Ono, Otsuka, ReMYND, Resverlogix, Roche, Signant Health, Sunovion,

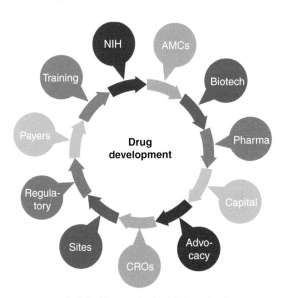

Figure 1.8 Stakeholders involved in AD drug development.

Suven, and Vaxxinity pharmaceutical, investment, and assessment companies. Dr. Cummings has stock options in ADAMAS, AnnovisBio, MedAvante, BiOasis. Dr. Cummings owns the copyright of the Neuropsychiatric Inventory. Dr. Cummings is supported by NIGMS grant P20GM109025; NINDS grant U01NS093334; NIA grant R01AG053798; NIA grant P20AG068053, and ADDF Goodes Prize.

Dr. Kinney has no disclosures.

Dr. Fillit has provided consultation to Axovant, vTv, Lundbeck, Otsuka, Lilly, Biogen, Roche, Genentech, Merck.

References

1. Scheltens P, Blennow K, Breteler MM, et al. Alzheimer's disease. *Lancet* 2016; **388**: 505–17.

2. Masters CL, Bateman R, Blennow K, et al. Alzheimer's disease. *Nat Rev Dis Primers* 2015; **1**: 15056.

3. Alzheimer's Association. Alzheimer's disease facts and figures. *Alzheimer Dement* 2019; **15**: 321–87.

4. Alzheimer's Disease International. *World Alzheimer Report 2015: The Global Impact of Dementia*. London: Alzheimer's Disease International; 2015.

5. Cummings JL, Morstorf T, Zhong K. Alzheimer's disease drug-development pipeline: few candidates, frequent failures. *Alzheimers Res Ther* 2014; **6**: 37.

6. Wang X, Sun G, Feng T, et al. Sodium oligomannate therapeutically remodels gut microbiota and suppresses gut bacterial amino acids-shaped neuroinflammation to inhibit Alzheimer's disease progression. *Cell Res* 2019; **29**: 787–803.

7. Servick K. Doubts persist for claimed Alzheimer's drug. *Science* 2019; **366**: 1298.

8. Cummings J, Ritter A, Zhong K. Clinical trials for disease-modifying therapies in Alzheimer's disease: a primer, lessons learned, and a blueprint for the future. *J Alzheimers Dis* 2018; **64**: S3–22.

9. Cummings J, Fox N. Defining disease modifying therapy for Alzheimer's disease. *J Prev Alzheimers Dis* 2017; **4**: 109–15.

10. Cummings J. Disease modification and neuroprotection in neurodegenerative disorders. *Transl Neurodegener* 2017; **6**: 25.

11. Fauman EB, Rai BK, Huang ES. Structure-based druggability assessment: identifying suitable targets for small molecule therapeutics. *Curr Opin Chem Biol* 2011; **15**: 463–8.

12. Ambure P, Roy K. Advances in quantitative structure–activity relationship models of anti-Alzheimer's agents. *Expert Opin Drug Discov* 2014; **9**: 697–723.

13. Gimenez BG, Santos MS, Ferrarini M, et al. Evaluation of blockbuster drugs under the rule-of-five. *Pharmazie* 2010; **65**: 148–52.

14. Leeson PD. Molecular inflation, attrition and the rule of five. *Adv Drug Deliv Rev* 2016; **101**: 22–33.

15. Hughes JP, Rees S, Kalindjian SB, et al. Principles of early drug discovery. *Br J Pharmacol* 2011; **162**: 1239–49.

16. Dragunow M. High-content analysis in neuroscience. *Nat Rev Neurosci* 2008; **9**: 779–88.

17. Alqahtani S, Mohamed LA, Kaddoumi A. Experimental models for predicting drug absorption and metabolism. *Expert Opin Drug Metab Toxicol* 2013; **9**: 1241–54.

18. Redfern WS, Carlsson L, Davis AS, et al. Relationships between preclinical cardiac electrophysiology, clinical QT interval prolongation and torsade de pointes for a broad range of drugs: evidence for a provisional safety margin in drug development. *Cardiovasc Res* 2003; **58**: 32–45.

19. Bass AS, Cartwright ME, Mahon C, et al. Exploratory drug safety: a discovery strategy to reduce attrition in development. *J Pharmacol Toxicol Methods* 2009; **60**: 69–78.

20. Freed LM. Dose selection for first-in-human (FIH) trials: regulatory perspective. In Krishna R, ed., *Dose Optimization in Drug Development*. New York, NY: Taylor & Francis Group, LLC; 2006: 45–60.

21. Presta LG. Selection, design, and engineering of therapeutic antibodies. *J Allergy Clin Immunol* 2005; **116**: 731–6.

22. Pul R, Dodel R, Stangel M. Antibody-based therapy in Alzheimer's disease. *Expert Opin Biol Ther* 2011; **11**: 343–57.

23. Sabbagh JJ, Kinney JW, Cummings JL. Alzheimer's disease biomarkers in animal models: closing the translational gap. *Am J Neurodegener Dis* 2013; **2**: 108–20.

24. Puzzo D, Gulisano W, Palmeri A, et al. Rodent models for Alzheimer's disease drug discovery. *Expert Opin Drug Discov* 2015; **10**: 703–11.

25. Choi SH, Kim YH, Hebisch M, et al. A three-dimensional human neural cell culture model of Alzheimer's disease. *Nature* 2014; **515**: 274–8.

26. Liu Q, Waltz S, Woodruff G, et al. Effect of potent gamma-secretase modulator in human neurons derived from multiple presenilin 1-induced pluripotent stem cell mutant carriers. *JAMA Neurol* 2014; **71**: 1481–9.

27. Umscheid CA, Margolis DJ, Grossman CE. Key concepts of clinical trials: a narrative review. *Postgrad Med* 2011; **123**: 194–204.

28. Cummings JL. Translational scoring of candidate treatments for Alzheimer's disease: a systematic approach. *Dement Geriatr Cogn Disord* 2020; **49**: 22–37.

29. Emilien G, van Meurs W, Maloteaux JM. The dose–response relationship in phase I clinical trials and beyond: use, meaning, and assessment. *Pharmacol Ther* 2000; **88**: 33–58.

30. Cummings J. Lessons learned from Alzheimer disease: clinical trials with negative outcomes. *Clin Transl Sci* 2018; **11**: 147–52.

31. Dubois B, Feldman HH, Jacova C, et al. Advancing research diagnostic criteria for Alzheimer's disease: the IWG-2 criteria. *Lancet Neurol* 2014; **13**: 614–29.

32. Rosen WG, Mohs RC, Davis KL. A new rating scale for Alzheimer's disease. *Am J Psychiatry* 1984; **141**: 1356–64.

33. Morris JC. The Clinical Dementia Rating (CDR): current version and scoring rules. *Neurology* 1993; **43**: 2412–14.

34. Cummings JL. Optimizing phase II of drug development for disease-modifying compounds. *Alzheimers Dement* 2008; **4**: S15–20.

35. Cummings J, Feldman HH, Scheltens P. The "rights" of precision drug development for Alzheimer's disease. *Alzheimers Res Ther* 2019; **11**: 76.

36. Greenberg BD, Carrillo MC, Ryan JM, et al. Improving Alzheimer's disease phase II clinical trials. *Alzheimers Dement* 2013; **9**: 39–49.

37. Gray JA, Fleet D, Winblad B. The need for thorough phase II studies in medicines development for Alzheimer's disease. *Alzheimers Res Ther* 2015; **7**: 67.

38. Bateman RJ, Munsell LY, Morris JC, et al. Human amyloid-beta synthesis and clearance rates as measured in cerebrospinal fluid in vivo. *Nat Med* 2006; **12**: 856–61.

39. Kennedy ME, Stamford AW, Chen X, et al. The BACE1 inhibitor verubecestat (MK-8931) reduces CNS beta-amyloid in animal models and in Alzheimer's disease patients. *Sci Transl Med* 2016; **8**: 363ra150.

40. Portelius E, Zetterberg H, Dean RA, et al. Amyloid-beta(1–15/16) as a marker for gamma-secretase inhibition in Alzheimer's disease. *J Alzheimers Dis* 2012; **31**: 335–41.

41. Sevigny J, Suhy J, Chiao P, et al. Amyloid PET screening for enrichment of early-stage Alzheimer disease clinical trials: experience in a Phase 1b clinical trial. *Alzheimer Dis Assoc Disord* 2016; **30**: 1–7.

42. Sperling RA, Jack CR, Jr., Black SE, et al. Amyloid-related imaging abnormalities in amyloid-modifying therapeutic trials: recommendations from the Alzheimer's Association Research Roundtable Workgroup. *Alzheimers Dement* 2011; **7**: 367–85.

43. Sperling R, Salloway S, Brooks DJ, et al. Amyloid-related imaging abnormalities in patients with Alzheimer's disease treated with bapineuzumab: a retrospective analysis. *Lancet Neurol* 2012; **11**: 241–9.

44. Babiloni C, Lizio R, Marzano N, et al. Brain neural synchronization and functional coupling in Alzheimer's disease as revealed by resting state EEG rhythms. *Int J Psychophysiol* 2016; **103**: 88–102.

45. Sperling RA, Dickerson BC, Pihlajamaki M, et al. Functional alterations in memory networks in early Alzheimer's disease. *Neuromolecular Med* 2010; **12**: 27–43.

46. Cummings J, Zhong K, Cordes D. Drug development in Alzheimer's disease: the role of default mode network assessment in phase II. *US Neurol* 2017; **13**: 67.

47. Sevigny J, Chiao P, Bussiere T, et al. The antibody aducanumab reduces Abeta plaques in Alzheimer's disease. *Nature* 2016; **537**: 50–6.

48. Sheiner LB. Learning versus confirming in clinical drug development. *Clin Pharmacol Ther* 1997; **61**: 275–91.

49. Crous-Bou M, Minguillon C, Gramunt N, et al. Alzheimer's disease prevention: from risk factors to early intervention. *Alzheimers Res Ther* 2017; **9**: 71.

50. Food and Drug Administration. *Early Alzheimer's Disease: Developing Drugs for Treatment. Guidance for Industry*. US Department of Health and Human Services Food and Drug Administration Center for Drug Evaluation and Research (CDER) Center for Biologics Evaluation and Research (CBER); 2018.

51. Cummings JL, Fox N. Defining disease modification for Alzheimer's disease clinical trials. *J Prev Alzheimers Dis* 2017; **4**: 109–15.

52. Jack CR, Jr., Bennett DA, Blennow K, et al. NIA-AA Research Framework: toward a biological definition of Alzheimer's disease. *Alzheimers Dement* 2018; **14**: 535–62.

53. Molinuevo JL, Ayton S, Batrla R, et al. Current state of Alzheimer's fluid biomarkers. *Acta Neuropathol* 2018; **136**: 821–53.

54. Leber P. *Guidelines for the Clinical Evaluation of Antidementia Drugs*. First draft. Technical Report. FDA Neuro-Pharm Group; 1990.

55. Karin A, Hannesdottir K, Jaeger J, et al. Psychometric evaluation of ADAS-cog and NTB for measuring drug response. *Acta Neurol Scand* 2014; **129**: 114–22.

56. Schmitt FA, Ashford W, Ernesto C, et al. The Severe Impairment Battery: concurrent validity and the assessment of longitudinal change in Alzheimer's disease. The Alzheimer's Disease Cooperative Study. *Alzheimer Dis Assoc Disord* 1997; **11**: S51–6.

57. Galasko D, Bennett D, Sano M, et al. An inventory to assess activities of daily living for clinical trials in Alzheimer's disease. The Alzheimer's Disease Cooperative Study. *Alzheimer Dis Assoc Disord* 1997; **11**: S33–9.

58. Sikkes SA, Pijnenburg YA, Knol DL, et al. Assessment of instrumental activities of daily living in dementia: diagnostic value of the Amsterdam Instrumental Activities of Daily Living Questionnaire. *J Geriatr Psychiatry Neurol* 2013; **26**: 244–50.

59. Zarit SH, Reever KE, Bach-Peterson J. Relatives of the impaired elderly: correlates of feelings of burden. *Gerontologist* 1980; **20**: 649–55.

60. Logsdon RG, Gibbons LE, McCurry SM, et al. Assessing quality of life in older adults with cognitive impairment. *Psychosom Med* 2002; **64**: 510–19.

61. Wimo A, Winblad B. Resource utilisation in dementia: RUD lite. *Brain Aging* 2003; **3**: 48–59.

62. Donohue MC, Sperling RA, Salmon DP, et al. The Preclinical Alzheimer Cognitive Composite: measuring amyloid-related decline. *JAMA Neurol* 2014; **71**: 961–70.

63. Langbaum JB, Ellison NN, Caputo A, et al. The Alzheimer's Prevention Initiative Composite Cognitive Test: a practical measure for tracking cognitive decline in preclinical Alzheimer's disease. *Alzheimers Res Ther* 2020; **12**: 66.

64. Bateman RJ, Benzinger TL, Berry S, et al. The DIAN-TU Next Generation Alzheimer's prevention trial: adaptive design and disease progression model. *Alzheimers Dement* 2017; **13**: 8–19.

65. Solomon A, Kivipelto M, Molinuevo JL, et al. European Prevention of Alzheimer's Dementia Longitudinal Cohort Study (EPAD LCS): study protocol. *BMJ Open* 2019; **8**: e021017.

66. Cummings JL, Froelich L, Black SE, et al. Randomized, double-blind, parallel-group, 48-week study for efficacy and safety of a higher-dose rivastigmine patch (15 vs. 10 cm(2)) in Alzheimer's disease. *Dement Geriatr Cogn Disord* 2012; **33**: 341–53.

67. Farlow M, Veloso F, Moline M, et al. Safety and tolerability of donepezil 23 mg in moderate to severe Alzheimer's disease. *BMC Neurol* 2011; **11**: 57–64.

68. Cummings J, Reiber C, Kumar P. The price of progress: funding and financing Alzheimer's disease drug development. *Alzheimers Dement (N Y)* 2018; **4**: 330–43.

69. DeTure MA, Dickson DW. The neuropathological diagnosis of Alzheimer's disease. *Mol Neurodegener* 2019; **14**: 32.

70. Gersdorf T, He VF, Schlesinger A, et al. Demystifying industry–academia collaboration. *Nat Rev Drug Discov* 2019; **18**: 743–4.

71. Silva PJ, Ramos KS. Academic medical centers as innovation ecosystems: evolution of industry partnership models beyond the Bayh–Dole Act. *Acad Med* 2018; **93**: 1135–41.

72. Yokley BH, Hartman M, Slusher BS. Role of academic drug discovery in the quest for new CNS therapeutics. *ACS Chem Neurosci* 2017; **8**: 429–31.

73. Ganem D. Physician–scientist careers in the biotechnology and pharmaceutical industries. *J Infect Dis* 2018; **218**: S20–4.

74. Slusher BS, Conn PJ, Frye S, et al. Bringing together the academic drug discovery community. *Nat Rev Drug Discov* 2013; **12**: 811–12.

75. Wiederrecht GJ, Hill RG, Beer MS. Partnership between small biotech and big pharma. *IDrugs* 2006; **9**: 560–4.

76. Finkbeiner S. Bridging the valley of death of therapeutics for neurodegeneration. *Nat Med* 2010; **16**: 1227–32.

77. Parrish MC, Tan YJ, Grimes KV, et al. Surviving in the valley of death: opportunities and challenges in translating academic drug discoveries. *Annu Rev Pharmacol Toxicol* 2019; **59**: 405–21.

78. Goldman DP, Fillit H, Neumann P. Accelerating Alzheimer's disease drug innovations from the research pipeline to patients. *Alzheimers Dement* 2018; **14**: 833–6.

79. Reis SE, Berglund L, Bernard GR, et al. Reengineering the national clinical and translational research enterprise: the strategic plan of the National Clinical and Translational Science Awards Consortium. *Acad Med* 2010; **85**: 463–9.

80. Grill JD, Di L, Lu PH, et al. Estimating sample sizes for predementia Alzheimer's trials based on the Alzheimer's Disease Neuroimaging Initiative. *Neurobiol Aging* 2013; **34**: 62–72.

81. Holland D, McEvoy LK, Desikan RS, et al. Enrichment and stratification for predementia Alzheimer disease clinical trials. *PLoS One* 2012; **7**: e47739.

82. Kohannim O, Hua X, Hibar DP, et al. Boosting power for clinical trials using classifiers based on multiple biomarkers. *Neurobiol Aging* 2010; **31**: 1429–42.

83. McEvoy LK, Edland SD, Holland D, et al. Neuroimaging enrichment strategy for secondary prevention trials in Alzheimer disease. *Alzheimer Dis Assoc Disord* 2010; **24**(3): 269–77.

84. Hendrix JA, Finger B, Weiner MW, et al. The Worldwide Alzheimer's Disease Neuroimaging Initiative: an update. *Alzheimers Dement* 2015; **11**: 850–9.

85. Iwatsubo T, Iwata A, Suzuki K, et al. Japanese and North American Alzheimer's Disease Neuroimaging Initiative studies: harmonization for international trials. *Alzheimers Dement* 2018; **14**: 1077–87.

86. Grill JD, Raman R, Ernstrom K, et al. Comparing recruitment, retention, and safety reporting among geographic regions in multinational Alzheimer's disease clinical trials. *Alzheimers Res Ther* 2015; **7**: 39.

87. Henley DB, Dowsett SA, Chen YF, et al. Alzheimer's disease progression by geographical region in a clinical trial setting. *Alzheimers Res Ther* 2015; **7**: 43.

88. Moulder KL, Snider BJ, Mills SL, et al. Dominantly Inherited Alzheimer Network: facilitating research and clinical trials. *Alzheimers Res Ther* 2013; **5**: 48.

89. Tariot PN, Lopera F, Langbaum JB, et al. The Alzheimer's Prevention Initiative Autosomal-Dominant Alzheimer's Disease Trial: a study of crenezumab versus placebo in preclinical PSEN1 E280A mutation carriers to evaluate efficacy and safety in the treatment of autosomal-dominant Alzheimer's disease, including a placebo-treated noncarrier cohort. *Alzheimers Dement (N Y)* 2018; **4**: 150–60.

90. Lopez Lopez C, Tariot PN, Caputo A, et al. The Alzheimer's Prevention Initiative Generation Program: study design of two randomized controlled trials for individuals at risk for clinical onset of Alzheimer's disease. *Alzheimers Dement (N Y)* 2019; **5**: 216–27.

91. Ayutyanont N, Langbaum JB, Hendrix SB, et al. The Alzheimer's Prevention Initiative Composite Cognitive Test score: sample size estimates for the evaluation of preclinical Alzheimer's disease treatments in presenilin 1 E280A mutation carriers. *J Clin Psychiatry* 2014; **75**: 652–60.

92. Langlois CM, Bradbury A, Wood EM, et al. Alzheimer's Prevention Initiative Generation Program: development of an ApoE genetic counseling and disclosure process in the context of clinical trials. *Alzheimers Dement (N Y)* 2019; **5**: 705–16.

93. Ritchie CW, Molinuevo JL, Truyen L, et al. Development of interventions for the secondary prevention of Alzheimer's dementia: the European Prevention of Alzheimer's Dementia (EPAD) project. *Lancet Psychiatry* 2016; **3**: 179–86.

94. Vermunt L, Veal CD, Ter Meulen L, et al. European Prevention of Alzheimer's Dementia

Registry: recruitment and prescreening approach for a longitudinal cohort and prevention trials. *Alzheimers Dement* 2018; **14**: 837–42.

95. Gregory S, Wells K, Forysth K, et al. Research participants as collaborators: background, experience and policies from the PREVENT Dementia and EPAD programmes. *Dementia (London)* 2018; **17**: 1045–54.

96. Romero K, de Mars M, Frank D, et al. The Coalition Against Major Diseases: developing tools for an integrated drug development process for Alzheimer's and Parkinson's diseases. *Clin Pharmacol Ther* 2009; **86**: 365–7.

97. Romero K, Ito K, Rogers JA, et al. The future is now: model-based clinical trial design for Alzheimer's disease. *Clin Pharmacol Ther* 2015; **97**: 210–14.

98. Cummings J, Lee G, Ritter A, Sabbagh M, Zhong K. Alzheimer's disease drug development pipeline: 2020. *Alzheimers Dement (N Y)* 2020; **6**: e12050.

99. Aisen P, Sperling R, Cummings J, et al. The Trial-Ready Cohort for Preclinical/Prodromal Alzheimer's Disease (TRC-PAD) project: an overview. *J Prev Alzheimers Dis* 2020; **7**: 208–12.

100. Cummings J, Aisen P, Barton R, et al. Re-engineering Alzheimer clinical trials: Global Alzheimer's Platform network. *J Prev Alzheimers Dis* 2016; **3**: 114–20.

101. Lamberti MJ, Wilkinson M, Harper B, et al. Assessing study start-up practices, performance, and perceptions among sponsors and contract research organizations. *Ther Innov Regul Sci* 2018; **52**: 572–8.

102. Drabu S, Gupta A, Bhadauria A. Emerging trends in contract research industry in India. *Contemp Clin Trials* 2010; **31**: 419–22.

103. Jack CR, Jr., Albert MS, Knopman DS, et al. Introduction to the recommendations from the National Institute on Aging–Alzheimer's Association workgroups on diagnostic guidelines for Alzheimer's disease. *Alzheimers Dement* 2011; **7**: 257–62.

104. Prina AM, Mayston R, Wu YT, et al. A review of the 10/66 dementia research group. *Soc Psychiatry Psychiatr Epidemiol* 2019; **54**: 1–10.

105. Abdin E, Vaingankar JA, Picco L, et al. Validation of the short version of the 10/66 dementia diagnosis in multiethnic Asian older adults in Singapore. *BMC Geriatr* 2017; **17**: 94.

106. Stewart R, Guerchet M, Prince M. Development of a brief assessment and algorithm for ascertaining dementia in low-income and middle-income countries: the 10/66 short dementia diagnostic schedule. *BMJ Open* 2016; **6**: e010712.

107. Winblad B, Amouyel P, Andrieu S, et al. Defeating Alzheimer's disease and other dementias: a priority for European science and society. *Lancet Neurol* 2016; **15**: 455–532.

108. Georges J, Jansen S, Jackson J, et al. Alzheimer's disease in real life: the dementia carer's survey. *Int J Geriatr Psychiatry* 2008; **23**: 546–51.

109. Keller K, Briggs L, Riley E. *Alzheimer's Disease: A Center for Strategic Philanthropy Giving Smarter Guide*, 2018; Available at: https://milkeninstitute.org/sites/default/files/reports-pdf/FINAL-Alz-GSG2.pdf.

110. Hara Y, McKeehan N, Fillit HM. Translating the biology of aging into novel therapeutics for Alzheimer disease. *Neurology* 2019; **92**: 84–93.

111. Lopez JC, Suojanen C. Harnessing venture philanthropy to accelerate medical progress. *Nat Rev Drug Discov* 2019; **18**: 809–10.

112. Food and Drug Administration. *Formal Meetings Between the FDA and Sponsors or Applicants of PDUFA Products: Guidance for Industry.* US Department of Health and Human Services Food and Drug Administration. Center for Drug Evaluation and Research (CDER) Center for Biologics Evaluation and Research (CBER); 2017.

113. Orr D, Baram-Tsabari A, Landsman K. Social media as a platform for health-related public debates and discussions: the polio vaccine on Facebook. *Isr J Health Policy Res* 2016; **5**: 34.

114. Kravitz RL, Bell RA. Media, messages, and medication: strategies to reconcile what patients hear, what they want, and what they need from medications. *BMC Med Inform Decis Mak* 2013; **13**: S5.

115. Schulz KF, Altman DG, Moher D, et al. CONSORT 2010 statement: updated guidelines for reporting parallel group randomized trials. *Ann Intern Med* 2010; **152**: 726–32.

116. Galkina Cleary E, Beierlein JM, Khanuja NS, et al. Contribution of NIH funding to new drug approvals 2010–2016. *Proc Natl Acad Sci USA* 2018; **115**: 2329–34.

117. Kosik KS, Sejnowski TJ, Raichle ME, et al. A path toward understanding neurodegeneration. *Science* 2016; **353**: 872–3.

118. Saville BR, Berry SM. Efficiencies of platform clinical trials: a vision of the future. *Clin Trials* 2016; **13**: 358–66.

119. Adaptive Platform Trials C. Adaptive platform trials: definition, design, conduct and reporting considerations. *Nat Rev Drug Discov* 2019; **18**: 797–807.

120. Kennedy RE, Cutter GR, Wang G, et al. Challenging assumptions about African American participation in Alzheimer disease trials. *Am J Geriatr Psychiatry* 2017; **25**: 1150–9.

121. Hall AK, Mills SL, Lund PK. Clinician-investigator training and the need to pilot new approaches to recruiting and retaining this workforce. *Acad Med* 2017; **92**: 1382–9.

122. Gehr S, Garner CC, Kleinhans KN. Translating academic careers into industry healthcare professions. *Nat Biotechnol* 2020; **38**: 758–63.

123. Thornicroft G, Lempp H, Tansella M. The place of implementation science in the translational medicine continuum. *Psychol Med* 2011; **41**: 2015–21.

124. Fort DG, Herr TM, Shaw PL, et al. Mapping the evolving definitions of translational research. *J Clin Transl Sci* 2017; **1**: 60–6.

125. Dilworth-Anderson P. Introduction to the science of recruitment and retention among ethnically diverse populations. *Gerontologist* 2011; **51**: S1–4.

126. Bauer MS, Kirchner J. Implementation science: what is it and why should I care? *Psychiatry Res* 2020; **283**: 112376.

127. Sheeran P, Klein WM, Rothman AJ. Health behavior change: moving from observation to intervention. *Annu Rev Psychol* 2017; **68**: 573–600.

128. Rouse R, Zineh I, Strauss DG. Regulatory science: an underappreciated component of translational research. *Trends Pharmacol Sci* 2018; **39**: 225–9.

Chapter 2

Drug Development for Alzheimer's Disease: An Historical Perspective

Howard Fillit and Jeffrey Cummings

2.1 Alois Alzheimer and the First Case

To understand how we have gotten to where we are today in Alzheimer's disease (AD), what relatively rapid progress we have made, what accounted for the lack of recognition of the illness for so long, and for the historical delay in research, particularly drug research, a historical overview is necessary.

In 1906, Alois Alzheimer, a German scientist, did an autopsy on a 55-year-old woman named Auguste D., who suffered and died from "pre-senile dementia," with memory loss, disorientation and other more severe forms of cognitive and functional loss. Her illness had dramatically shrunk the brain. Dr. Alzheimer investigated tissue from the brain under the microscope with synthetic dyes such as the Nissl stain, and congo red, a dye that came from the German fashion industry and was used to stain women's clothes. The dyes revealed abnormal deposits in and around brain nerve cells (the senile plaques and neurofibrillary tangles that characterize the pathology of the disease). Alzheimer also described "congophilic angiopathy" and glial cells surrounding the senile plaques. The combination of newly revealed pathology and the clinical symptoms of dementia was subsequently given the name Alzheimer's disease, then considered a rare cause of pre-senile dementia, but little research on the newly discovered disease was done over subsequent decades. There were some reports, primarily in Europe, of case studies [1, 2].

Until the late 1960s, senility, or loss of mind with aging, was still considered a normal part of aging.

2.2 Alzheimer's Disease, Senile Dementia, and Aging

Critical studies on "senile dementia of the Alzheimer's type" (or SDAT as the illness was called initially) were done in the late 1960s, when a group of pathologists – Blessed, Tomlinson, and Roth – working in Newcastle upon Tyne, UK, studied the brains of elderly people. They showed the quantitative relationship between Alzheimer's pathology and cognition, and demonstrated that aged individuals with "senility" actually had AD [3–5]. It could be said that in this period of history, senility finally went from being considered a "normal" part of aging to be recognized as a disease of old age, or AD.

In the mid 1960s and early 1970s, Robert Katzman and Robert Terry investigated correlations of clinical and pathological parameters of Alzheimer's [6, 7]. In 1976, Katzman reported in an influential editorial entitled "the prevalence and malignancy of Alzheimer's disease" that AD was the most common form of dementia [7]. He recognized that given the aging of the population and the increasing prevalence of dementia in the aged, a crisis was inevitable.

2.3 Alzheimer's Disease as a Rare Disorder

Despite this nascent work, in the early 1970s, AD was not generally taught in most medical school curricula, and the only mention of it in medical textbooks was as a rare pre-senile form of dementia. During the authors' clinical training in the mid 1970s, we took care of hundreds of older people, many of whom no doubt had AD or dementia, but we never made the diagnosis per se. The term "organic brain syndrome" (OBS) was commonly used to refer to older people with cognitive impairment. It might have conflated the presence of delirium and dementia. OBS was often used in a derogatory manner to describe older patients who were senile. "Senility" was described in textbooks and in clinical practice as a normal part of aging.

It was early days. Nothing was really known about the disease, there were no diagnostic tests, there were certainly no treatments, and nothing was known about prevention. There was no awareness of the illness among lay persons; and there was no research.

2.4 Origins and Influence of the National Institute on Aging

But times were changing in the 1970s. Robert N. Butler, MD, a geriatric psychiatrist, saw his first patient with AD at Saint Elizabeth's Hospital in Washington, DC in the early 1970s. Butler realized the importance of the recent description of what was then beginning to be called senile dementia of the Alzheimer's type (SDAT) [4]. He forecast the coming "epidemic" of AD in a book: *Why Survive? Being Old in America* (Harper & Row, 1975), which won a Pulitzer Prize in 1976, which was announced the very day that he assumed office as the founding director of the National Institute on Aging (NIA) at the National Institutes of Health (NIH). The primary purpose of the new NIA institute was to oversee research on AD and other illnesses related to aging, ultimately becoming the primary source of research funds for AD and related dementias in the United States today.

One of the first things Dr. Butler did when he arrived at the NIA was to do a survey of its research efforts. He found that, at a time when the United States was spending billions of dollars in the war on cancer and heart disease, we spent ~$625,000 on 12 grants for research on dementia, with grants primarily directed at caregivers (personal communication to H. Fillit from R. N. Butler)

To put this time in the history of research in perspective, the Imperial Cancer Fund, now called the Cancer Research Fund UK, was established in 1902, to begin research in cancer, more than 100 years ago. Albert Lasker, Jr., one of the wealthiest Americans in the 1920s, established a private foundation to begin funding cancer research in America in the 1920s, after his first wife died of cancer. His second wife, Mary Lasker, lobbied for a congressional act to establish the NIH in 1948, and one of the main priorities of the new NIH was cancer research (www.lasker foundation.org/new-noteworthy/articles/catalyst-national-cancer-act-mary-lasker/).

Thus, AD research has had a "late start" compared to other major illnesses for which there are treatments available today. Cancer research started more than 60 years before any real research was done in AD. This is also true for diabetes. Insulin was discovered and made available for patients with diabetes in the 1920s, and we have many treatments for diabetes today. The same is true for hypertension. Drugs for the treatment of high blood pressure became available in the 1950s (diuretics) and 1960s (beta-adrenergic receptor blocking agents). Cholesterol was discovered as a risk factor for heart disease only in the 1950s, with the first statins coming to market in the 1980s. Thus, cancer, heart disease, diabetes, and hypertension, leading causes of death, had many decades of a head start in research compared to AD.

2.5 Setting the Stage with the First Clinical Trials: Acetylcholine, the Cholinergic Hypothesis, and Tacrine

Despite this historical lag of many decades, great strides have been made in AD research and therapeutic development. In the mid 1970s, Peter Davies and David Bowen documented a relatively selective loss of acetylcholine [8, 9] in AD, and Peter Whitehouse and colleagues demonstrated that there was a corresponding atrophy of the cholinergic source nuclei in the nucleus basalis of Meynert [10]. These observations suggested that treatment of AD with cholinergic agents might improve cognitive function and the development of cholinergic agents was initiated. Cholinergic agonists, acetylcholine precursors, nicotinic cholinergic agents, and cholinesterase inhibitors were tested in this time. An early study by William Summers suggested that oral tetrahydroaminoacridine (tacrine) was effective in ameliorating the cognitive deficits of AD [11]. Although many aspects of this trial could not be reproduced, the study was instrumental in spurring research of this agent (eventually approved as the first treatment for AD as Cognex™) and other cholinesterase inhibitors in widespread use today [12].

Current clinical trials continue to use the "tacrine formula" created to guide the development of cognitive enhancers for AD. The US Food and Drug Administration (FDA) created new guidelines for approval of AD therapies in this era. These guidelines required that anti-dementia agents show improvement on the core symptoms of AD – memory and cognition – and that the effect be clinically meaningful as shown on a global or a functional rating [13]. The clinical instrumentation for AD trials was defined by trials of tacrine. Patients were selected using the Mini-Mental State Examination (MMSE) developed in 1975 [14], and outcomes included the Clinical Global Impression of Change (CGIC) [15] published in 1975 and the Alzheimer's Diseases Assessment Scale (ADAS) [16] developed in 1984. The tacrine trials were conducted in 1992 and led to approval of tacrine by the FDA in 1993 [17, 18]. This approach to AD clinical trials and approval remains highly influential. Trial participants are defined by MMSE score range; the ADAS – cognitive subscale (ADAS-cog) is a commonly used outcome instrument in clinical trials for patients with AD dementia; and the CGIC or modified versions of the instrument are used in most trials of cognitive-enhancing agents being developed for AD. Dual outcomes (related to cognition and function) as defined by the original FDA guidelines are required for all agents assessed in trials of patients with AD dementia. Newer guidelines allow that single outcomes may be sufficient for patients with mild cognitive impairment (MCI) due to AD or preclinical AD [19]. This FDA approach developed for cognitive-enhancing agents such as tacrine is applied to disease-modifying agents if the trial involves patients in the dementia stage of the illness.

2.6 Early Disease-Modifying Studies: Amyloid Beta and the "Amyloid Hypothesis"

In 1984, George Glenner discovered that amyloid-beta protein was a major component of the blood vessel changes observed in patients with Down syndrome and further discovered that the same protein comprised the senile plaques first described by Alzheimer in 1906 [20, 21]. In 1986, 80 years after Dr. Alzheimer's identification of the tangles, researchers such as Iqbal and colleagues identified tau protein as a key component in the tangles that represent the diseased and dying neurons in AD [22]. Discovery and characterization of these two molecules, amyloid-beta protein and tau protein, have revolutionized the field, becoming primary drug targets and serving as biomarkers in clinical trials, neuroimaging, and spinal fluid and blood diagnostic tests.

The characterization of the amyloid-beta protein in plaques, the uniform occurrence of amyloid-beta plaques in AD, and the demonstration that mutations affecting amyloid-beta processing lead to amyloid-beta accumulation and

early-onset AD led to elegant studies of the biology of amyloid beta in AD. These studies defined a pathway in which the "normal" production of monomers leads to misfolding and aggregation of amyloid beta in the form of oligomers, and then fibrillization in insoluble amyloid plaques. The "amyloid hypothesis" constructed by Dennis Selkoe and John Hardy in 2002 became a dominant conceptual framework for understanding AD and for developing new therapies for the disease [23].

2.6.1 Immunotherapy for Alzheimer's Disease

As the amyloid hypothesis was evolving, Dale Schenck conducted experiments showing that vaccination with amyloid produced remarkable clearing of amyloid in transgenic mice overexpressing the amyloid protein [24]. These observations ushered in the era of immunotherapy and led to the first vaccination trial with AN1792; the trial was interrupted when a small number of participants developed an allergic meningitis [25]. Autopsy studies showed the individuals receiving the vaccination had marked clearing of amyloid from the brain although they continued to exhibit cognitive decline [26]. The demonstration that amyloid was subject to immunotherapeutic manipulation gave rise to trials with passive immunotherapy using monoclonal antibodies directed at various epitopes on the amyloid molecule. The first such trial involved bapineuzumab which failed to show a drug–placebo difference in Phase 3 despite somewhat promising effects in Phase 2 [27, 28]. Learnings from current immunotherapy trials suggest that bapineuzumab may have been underdosed, and this may have contributed to the negative outcome of this development program. Solanezumab trials were based on the "peripheral sink" hypothesis postulating that engagement of the amyloid-beta monomer in the blood would lead to passive removal of the amyloid from the brain and slowing of disease progression. No drug–placebo differences were seen in Phase 3 trials [29]. After many years in development, anti-amyloid strategies are now beginning to show promise [30], with some monoclonal anti-amyloid antibodies demonstrating the ability to remove amyloid-beta plaques from the brain of AD patients, which may be associated with slowing of the progression of the disease. The monoclonal antibodies in current trials – aducanumab, lecanemab, gantenerumab – have all been shown to remove amyloid plaques and have preliminary evidence of amelioration of cognitive decline [31]. Of this group, aducanumab has been approved for marketing by the FDA and other anti-amyloid monoclonal antibodies are under review by regulatory authorities. Table 2.1 provides details of the monoclonal antibodies in recent or current trials [31].

2.6.2   Enzyme Inhibitors/Modulators for Alzheimer's Disease

Monoclonal antibodies depend on activating microglia to remove amyloid-beta protein species from the brain. Another approach to AD therapy based on the amyloid hypothesis is to inhibit or modulate the enzymes – gamma secretase and beta-site amyloid precursor protein cleaving enzyme 1 (BACE1) – responsible for the production of amyloid from the amyloid precursor protein. An early trial of tarenflurbil, a putative gamma secretase modulator, failed to show a drug–placebo difference but may have had insufficient brain penetration [32, 33]. Trials of enzyme-inhibiting agents showed that amyloid production was effectively reduced but cognitive decline was greater in the groups receiving active therapy than those on placebo [34, 35]. Further testing of this approach awaits improved understanding of the biology of the adverse treatment effects.

2.7   The Evolution of Alzheimer's Disease Drug Development

This was just the beginning. Today, after 40 years of basic research and many billions of dollars in AD research with tens of thousands of published papers and patents, we know as much about the biology of AD as we do about cancer and heart disease; we haven't YET translated that research into new drugs. Research on the biology of aging is just being translated into new drugs for AD, and many of these mechanisms are shared with cancer and other chronic diseases of old age [36] for which drug discovery and development preceded the AD efforts [37]. Figure 2.1 shows the timeline for the major clinical trials for AD.

Studies have shown that an average time from a basic science discovery to an FDA approval is approximately 35 years [38]. For example, blood cholesterol was discovered as a risk factor for heart disease in the mid 1950s, and played a key role as a biomarker for drug development, but the first statins did not become available for patients until the mid 1980s, almost 30 years later [39].

Due to the many decades of historical lag in the recognition of AD as the cause of "senility," there was a delayed start in AD-related research. However, today we are right on schedule to translate the basic science we have learned about AD during the last 40 years into developing new drugs. If AD research started in earnest in 1980, then one could expect the first drugs to market in 2015. The first drug approved by the FDA to treat AD,

Table 2.1 Monoclonal antibodies in clinical trials, the epitope they target, and the species of amyloid affected

Antibody	Development status	Class	IgG type	Epitope (AA sequence)	Amyloid conformation targeted
Bapineuzumab	Terminated	Humanized	IgG1	1–5	Monomer; oligomer; fibril
Solanezumab	Clinical trial for preclinical AD	Humanized	IgG1	16–26	Monomer
Crenezumab	Clinical trial of autosomal dominant AD in Colombia	Humanized	IgG1	13–24	Monomer; oligomer; fibril
Gantenerumab	Phase 3	Human	IgG1	3–12, 18–27	Oligomer; fibril
Lecanamab	Phase 3	Humanized	IgG1	Protofibrils	Protofibril; fibril
Aducanumab	Approved	Human	IgG1	3–6	Oligomer; fibril
Donanemab	Phase 3	Humanized	IgG1	N-terminal pyroglutamate	Plaque

Abbreviations: AA, amino acid; IgG, immunoglobulin G.

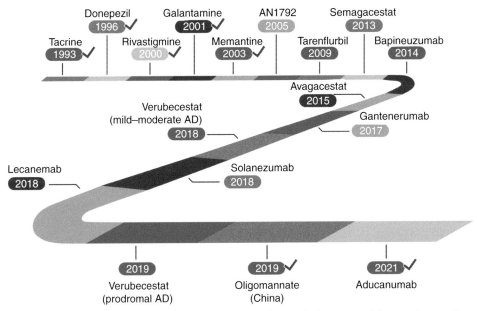

Figure 2.1 Timeline for the major clinical trials for Alzheimer's disease. Cholinesterase inhibitors and memantine were approved in the 1990s and early 2000s. Oligomannate was approved for use in China in 2019. Other trials were negative but highly informative regarding trial conduct, targets, populations, and biomarkers.

tacrine, was approved in 1993 (see above), about 25 years after the recognition of SDAT, and over the next decade tacrine was followed by four other drugs currently still on the market (donepezil, rivastigmine, galantamine, and memantine). These four drugs are cognitive enhancers, which are modestly effective in temporarily improving symptoms [40]. Between 1998 and 2017, almost 150 therapies failed in clinical trials. Much has been learned from these failed trials, and clinical trial methodology has improved greatly [41, 42]. Today, there are more than 120 drugs in clinical trials looking at new treatments for AD, many based on novel targets besides amyloid-beta targets such as tau, inflammation, metabolic disturbances, neuroprotection, epigenetics, and others [43].

Tau therapies include small molecules and monoclonal antibodies [44]. These agents are in Phase 1 and 2; large late-stage trials will depend on the outcomes observed in these early trials.

Inflammation is a compelling component of AD pathology and is posited to exacerbate the damage done by amyloid and tau [45]. Clinical trials of diclofenac/misoprostol, nimesulide, naproxen, rofecoxib, ibuprofen, indomethacin, and celecoxib have failed to show a drug–placebo

difference [46]. Understanding of the role of inflammation in AD is rapidly increasing and trial designs are improving, providing a foundation for more successful trials of anti-inflammatory agents for treatment of AD [47].

Oligomannate (GV-971), an agent with putative effects on neuroinflammation mediated through the microbiome, was approved for marketing in China in 2019 and is in a Phase 3 global trial [48]. GV-971 is an example of the diversified targets being addressed by agents in clinical trials for AD.

2.8 Biomarkers and Drug Development

Biomarkers are key to drug development; they convert "shots in the dark" to "shots on goal." Until relatively recently, the only way to confirm the diagnosis of AD was by an autopsy. From 2000 to 2004, the Alzheimer's Drug Discovery Foundation (ADDF) funded research at the University of Pennsylvania to develop a positron emission tomography (PET) amyloid-beta diagnostic test for AD (florbetapir/Amyvid™). The test was approved by the FDA in 2012 as the first diagnostic test for AD and detects the amyloid beta in senile plaques in living persons. No longer is an autopsy needed. Indeed, amyloid PET scans, and more recent tau PET imaging, have "revolutionized" AD research and care [49]. Other forms of neuroimaging, including MRI with volumetric quantitation and fluorodeoxyglucose (FDG) PET, have also contributed as quantitative biomarkers for more rigorous clinical trials in AD [50] .

The amyloid PET scan has remarkably improved the way we do clinical trials, making them more accurate and more efficient. Employing the PET scan in a clinical trial showed that up to 35% of people entered into clinical trials by dementia experts did not have positive scans, did not have AD, and did not even have amyloid beta in the brain, which was the focus of the therapy being tested [51]. Now, most studies use either the amyloid PET scan or a test for amyloid beta in the spinal fluid to ensure that all people entered into clinical trials have AD and have the target of anti-amyloid drugs under investigation.

Recent studies have used the amyloid PET scan to monitor whether anti-amyloid drugs remove amyloid beta from the brain, and the drug clearly worked. Over 80% of people treated with the amyloid monoclonal antibodies had all the PET signal removed from the brain [52], and this correlated with a slowing of the rate of cognitive and functional decline. These exciting studies of aducanumab were further studied in Phase 3 and are under consideration by the FDA for approval.

As we diversify targets, we will need even more biomarkers to enable us to study the effect of drugs in AD patients, such as neuroinflammation, epigenetic changes that lead to neurodegeneration, and other novel targets. This approach will enable precision medicine therapy for AD just as we have in cancer. Such biomarkers are currently in development.

Fluid biomarkers (plasma and cerebrospinal fluid), which are more affordable and non-invasive, are needed for diagnosis and clinical trials. Just as a simple cholesterol blood test revolutionized the treatment of heart disease, we need a simple, inexpensive blood test that will allow doctors to more easily screen patients for AD. These are in development. A blood test for amyloid beta was recently approved for clinical use by the US Centers for Disease Control and received the European Medicines Agency CE Mark (www.c2ndiagnostics .com/press/press) and other tests are anticipated to become clinically available in the next few years [53]. Blood tests for hyperphosphorylated tau protein (p-tau) that represents the tangles in the brain of patients are also in development [54]. These tests and others will further transform the field, greatly accelerating early diagnosis as well as screening, enrollment, and monitoring in clinical trials [55].

To facilitate AD biomarker development, the ADDF started a partnership, called the Diagnostics Accelerator (www.alzdiscovery.org/research-and-grants/diagnostics-accelerator), with Bill Gates, Jeff Bezos, and MacKenzie Scott, the Dolby Foundation, the Charles and Helen Schwab Foundation, and others. Our primary goal is to accelerate the development of novel biomarkers from blood to diagnose AD. Reliable, affordable, and novel biomarkers have the potential to further revolutionize how we approach AD by allowing us to better understand how the disease progresses, more easily identify people for clinical trials, and more accurately monitor their response to treatments. In addition to supporting blood biomarker development, ADDF's Diagnostic Accelerator is supporting the development of new digital biomarkers for the detection and monitoring of therapy in AD clinical trials.

2.9 Alzheimer's Prevention and Lifestyle Interventions

We have made tremendous progress toward preventing or delaying the onset of AD. Using the amyloid PET scan, we have discovered that AD begins in mid-life, up to 20 years before the first symptom of memory loss. Prevention research has shown that physical exercise, a healthy diet, not smoking or drinking excess alcohol, staying socially and occupationally involved, and managing obesity, hypertension, and diabetes are important in brain health and can delay the onset of cognitive decline [56]. Recent clinical trials employing these multifactorial interventions have shown that delaying or reducing the risk of AD are possible [57]. Clinical trials using biomarkers (genetic mutations or amyloid changes) in asymptomatic preclinical periods of the disease are now possible and prevention trials to delay the onset of AD or slow the progression are ongoing [58, 59]. Studies have shown that if we can delay the onset of AD by just 5 years, using both lifestyle prevention strategies and new drugs, we can reduce the population of people with dementia by 50% [60].

2.10 Looking Back, Looking Ahead

Dementia from AD affects an estimated 5.7 million Americans and is the fifth leading cause of death for those aged 65 or older. The Centers for Disease Control and Prevention (CDC) reported recently that the rates of death for AD are increasing, while heart disease and cancer death rates are on the decline. AD is already the most expensive disease in developed countries around the world. Today, people are well aware of the illness. We have certainly come a long way with AD since the 1970s. Improvements in understanding the biology of AD, identification of new drug targets and risk factors, development of candidate drugs for these new targets, biomarkers for early diagnosis and to show target engagement in clinical trials, better clinical trial design and conduct, and enhanced public awareness of the importance of the disease, all promise to deliver new, improved therapies to those with or at risk for AD. Though we got a late start, AD research is catching up with cancer, heart disease, and other chronic diseases of aging and old age, and new safe and effective drugs to prevent and treat AD are certainly on the way.

References

1. Newton RD. The identity of Alzheimer's disease and senile dementia and their relationship to senility. *J Ment Sci* 1948; **94**: 225–49.

2. Neumann MA, Cohn R. Incidence of Alzheimer's disease in large mental hospital; relation to senile psychosis and psychosis with cerebral arteriosclerosis. *AMA Arch Neurol Psychiatry* 1953; **69**: 615–36.

3. Roth M, Tomlinson BE, Blessed G. Correlation between scores for dementia and counts of 'senile plaques' in cerebral grey matter of elderly subjects. *Nature* 1966; **209**: 109–10.

4. Tomlinson BE, Blessed G, Roth M. Observations on the brains of demented old people. *J Neurol Sci* 1970; **11**: 205–42.

5. Tomlinson BE, Blessed G, Roth M. Observations on the brains of non-demented old people. *J Neurol Sci* 1968; **7**: 331–56.

6. Terry RD, Gonatas NK, Weiss M. The ultrastructure of the cerebral cortex in Alzheimer's disease. *Trans Am Neurol Assoc* 1964; **89**: 12.

7. Katzman R. Editorial: The prevalence and malignancy of Alzheimer disease. A major killer. *Arch Neurol* 1976; **33**: 217–18.

8. Davies P, Maloney AJ. Selective loss of central cholinergic neurons in Alzheimer's disease. *Lancet* 1976; **2**: 1403.

9. Bowen DM. Biochemistry of dementias. *Proc R Soc Med* 1977; **70**: 351–3.

10. Whitehouse PJ, Price DL, Clark AW, Coyle JT, DeLong MR. Alzheimer disease: evidence for selective loss of cholinergic neurons in the nucleus basalis. *Ann Neurol* 1981; **10**: 122–6.

11. Summers WK, Majovski LV, Marsh GM, Tachiki K, Kling A. Oral tetrahydroaminoacridine in long-term treatment of senile dementia, Alzheimer type. *N Engl J Med* 1986; **315**: 1241–5.

12. Atri A. Current and future treatments in Alzheimer's disease. *Semin Neurol* 2019; **39**: 227–40.

13. Leber P. *Guidelines for the Clinical Evaluation of Antidementia Drugs*. First draft. Technical Report. FDA Neuro-Pharm Group; 1990.

14. Folstein MF, Folstein SE, McHugh PR. "Mini-mental state". A practical method for grading the cognitive state of patients for the clinician. *J Psychiatr Res* 1975; **12**: 189–98.

15. Guy W. *Clinical Global Impressions. ECDEU Assessment Manual for Psychopharmacology – Revised*. Rockville, MD: US Department of Health, Education, and Welfare, Public Health Service, Alcohol, Drug Abuse, and Mental Health Administration, National Institute of Mental Health, Psychopharmacology Research Branch, Division of Extramural Research Programs; 1976: 218–22.

16. Rosen WG, Mohs RC, Davis KL. A new rating scale for Alzheimer's disease. *Am J Psychiatry* 1984; **141**: 1356–64.

17. Farlow M, Gracon SI, Hershey LA, et al. A controlled trial of tacrine in Alzheimer's disease. The Tacrine Study Group. *JAMA* 1992; **268**: 2523–9.

18. Davis KL, Thal LJ, Gamzu ER, et al. A double-blind, placebo-controlled multicenter study of tacrine for Alzheimer's disease. The Tacrine Collaborative Study Group. *N Engl J Med* 1992; **327**: 1253–9.

19. Food and Drug Administration. *Early Alzheimer's Disease: Developing Drugs for Treatment. Guidance for Industry*. US Department of Health and Human Services Food and Drug Administration Center for Drug Evaluation and Research (CDER) Center for Biologics Evaluation and Research (CBER); 2018.

20. Glenner GG, Wong CW. Alzheimer's disease: initial report of the purification and characterization of a novel cerebrovascular amyloid protein. *Biochem Biophys Res Commun* 1984; **120**: 885–90.

21. Glenner GG. Alzheimer's disease. The commonest form of amyloidosis. *Arch Pathol Lab Med* 1983; **107**: 281–2.

22. Grundke-Iqbal I, Iqbal K, Quinlan M, et al. Microtubule-associated protein tau. A component of Alzheimer paired helical filaments. *J Biol Chem* 1986; **261**: 6084–9.

23. Hardy J, Selkoe DJ. The amyloid hypothesis of Alzheimer's disease: progress and problems on the road to therapeutics. *Science* 2002; **297**: 353–6.

24. Schenk D, Barbour R, Dunn W, et al. Immunization with amyloid-beta attenuates Alzheimer-disease-like pathology in the PDAPP mouse. *Nature* 1999; **400**: 173–7.

25. Gilman S, Koller M, Black RS, et al. Clinical effects of Abeta immunization (AN1792) in patients with AD in an interrupted trial. *Neurology* 2005; **64**: 1553–62.

26. Holmes C, Boche D, Wilkinson D, et al. Long-term effects of Abeta42 immunisation in Alzheimer's disease: follow-up of a randomised, placebo-controlled phase I trial. *Lancet* 2008; **372**: 216–23.

27. Salloway S, Sperling R, Fox NC, et al. Two phase 3 trials of bapineuzumab in mild-to-moderate Alzheimer's disease. *N Engl J Med* 2014; **370**: 322–33.

28. Salloway S, Sperling R, Gilman S, et al. A phase 2 multiple ascending dose trial of bapineuzumab in mild to moderate Alzheimer disease. *Neurology* 2009; **73**: 2061–70.

29. Doody RS, Farlow M, Aisen PS, et al. Phase 3 trials of solanezumab for mild-to-moderate Alzheimer's disease. *N Engl J Med* 2014; **370**: 311–21.

30. Bullain S, Doody R. What works and what does not work in Alzheimer's disease? From interventions on risk factors to anti-amyloid trials. *J Neurochem* 2020; **155**: https://doi.org/10.1111/jnc.15023.

31. van Dyck CH. Anti-amyloid-β monoclonal antibodies for Alzheimer's disease: pitfalls and promise. *Psychiatry* 2018; **83**: 311–19.

32. Green RC, Schneider LS, Amato DA, et al. Effect of tarenflurbil on cognitive decline and activities of daily living in patients with mild Alzheimer disease: a randomized controlled trial. *JAMA* 2009; **302**: 2557–64.

33. Imbimbo BP. Why did tarenflurbil fail in Alzheimer's disease? *J Alzheimers Dis* 2009; **17**: 757–60.

34. Doody RS, Raman R, Farlow M, et al. A phase 3 trial of semagacestat for treatment of Alzheimer's disease. *N Engl J Med* 2013; **369**: 341–50.

35. Egan MF, Kost J, Voss T, et al. Randomized trial of verubecestat for prodromal Alzheimer's disease. *N Engl J Med* 2019; **380**: 1408–20.

36. Hara Y, McKeehan N, Fillit HM. Translating the biology of aging into novel therapeutics for Alzheimer disease. *Neurology* 2019; **92**: 84–93.

37. Clark CM, Pontecorvo MJ, Beach TG, et al. Cerebral PET with florbetapir compared with neuropathology at autopsy for detection of neuritic amyloid-beta plaques: a prospective cohort study. *Lancet Neurol* 2012; **11**: 669–78.

38. McNamee LM, Walsh MJ, Ledley FD. Timelines of translational science: from technology initiation to FDA approval. *PLoS One* 2017; **12**: e0177371.

39. Endo A. A historical perspective on the discovery of statins. *Proc Jpn Acad Ser B Phys Biol Sci* 2010; **86**: 484–93.

40. Qaseem A, Snow V, Cross TJ, Jr., et al. Current pharmacologic treatment of dementia: a clinical practice guideline from the American College of Physicians and the American Academy of Family Physicians. *Ann Intern Med* 2008; **148**: 370–8.

41. Cummings J, Ritter A, Zhong K. Clinical trials for disease-modifying therapies in Alzheimer's disease: a primer, lessons learned, and a blueprint for the future. *J Alzheimers Dis* 2018; **64**: S3–22.

42. Cummings J. Lessons learned from Alzheimer disease: clinical trials with negative outcomes. *Clin Transl Sci* 2018; **11**: 147–52.

43. Cummings J, Lee G, Ritter A, Sabbagh M, Zhong K. Alzheimer's disease drug development pipeline: 2020. *Alzheimers Dement (N Y)* 2020; **6**: e12050.

44. Cummings J, Blennow K, Johnson K, et al. Anti-tau trials for Alzheimer's disease: a report from the EU/US/CTAD Task Force. *J Prev Alzheimers Dis* 2019; **6**: 157–63.

45. Heneka MT, Carson MJ, El Khoury J, et al. Neuroinflammation in Alzheimer's disease. *Lancet Neurol* 2015; **14**: 388–405.

46. Miguel-Alvarez M, Santos-Lozano A, Sanchis-Gomar F, et al. Non-steroidal anti-inflammatory drugs as a treatment for Alzheimer's disease: a systematic review and meta-analysis of treatment effect. *Drugs Aging* 2015; **32**: 139–47.

47. Hampel H, Caraci F, Cuello AC, et al. A path toward precision medicine for neuroinflammatory mechanisms in Alzheimer's disease. *Front Immunol* 2020; **11**: 456.

48. Wang X, Sun G, Geng M. Sodium oligomannate therapeutically remodels gut microbiota and suppresses gut bacterial amino acids: shaped neuroinflammation to inhibit Alzheimer's disease progression. *Cell Res* 2019; **29**: 787–803.

49. Xia C, Dickerson BC. Multimodal PET imaging of amyloid and tau pathology in Alzheimer disease and non-Alzheimer disease dementias. *PET Clin* 2017; **12**: 351–9.

50. Risacher SL, Saykin AJ. Neuroimaging in aging and neurologic diseases. *Handb Clin Neurol* 2019; **167**: 191–227.

51. Sevigny J, Suhy J, Chiao P, et al. Amyloid PET screening for enrichment of early-stage Alzheimer disease clinical trials: experience in a phase 1b clinical trial. *Alzheimer Dis Assoc Disord* 2016; **30**: 1–7.

52. Sevigny J, Chiao P, Bussière T, et al. The antibody aducanumab reduces Abeta plaques in Alzheimer's disease. *Nature* 2016; **537**: 50–6.

53. Schindler SE, Bollinger JG, Ovod V, et al. High-precision plasma beta-amyloid 42/40 predicts current and future brain amyloidosis. *Neurology* 2019; **93**: e1647–59.

54. Barthelemy NR, Bateman RJ, Hirtz C, et al. Cerebrospinal fluid phospho-tau T217 outperforms T181 as a biomarker for the differential diagnosis of Alzheimer's disease and PET amyloid-positive patient identification. *Alzheimers Res Ther* 2020; **12**: 26.

55. Jack CR, Jr., Bennett DA, Blennow K, et al. NIA–AA Research Framework: toward a biological definition of Alzheimer's disease. *Alzheimers Dement* 2018; **14**: 535–62.

56. Dhana K, Evans DA, Rajan KB, Bennett DA, Morris MC. Healthy lifestyle and the risk of Alzheimer dementia: findings from 2 longitudinal studies. *Neurology* 2020; **95**: e374–83.

57. Kivipelto M, Ngandu T. Good for the heart and good for the brain? *Lancet Neurol* 2019; **18**: 327–8.

58. Andrieu S, Coley N, Lovestone S, Aisen PS, Bruno Vellas B. Prevention of sporadic Alzheimer's disease: lessons learned from clinical trials and future directions. *Lancet Neurol* 2015; **14**: 926–44.

59. Lopez Lopez C, Tariot PN, Caputo A, et al. The Alzheimer's Prevention Initiative Generation Program: study design of two randomized controlled trials for individuals at risk for clinical onset of Alzheimer's disease. *Alzheimers Dement (N Y)* 2019; **5**: 216–27.

60. Alzheimer's Association. *Changing the Trajectory of Alzheimer's Disease: How a treatment by 2025 Saves Lives and Dollars.* Chicago, IL: Alzheimer's Association; 2015.

Chapter 3

Alzheimer's Disease Drug Discovery in Academia: From High-Throughput Screening to In Vivo Testing

Kurt R. Brunden, Goodwell Nzou, and Carlo Ballatore

3.1 Introduction

Alzheimer's disease (AD) is the most prevalent neurodegenerative disease in the world, with an estimated 5.8 million cases in the USA and a projected increase to >13 million cases by 2050. Although a small percentage of early-onset AD (EOAD) cases result from inheritance of a genetic mutation [1], the vast majority of patients present with sporadic late-onset AD (LOAD) that manifests in the eighth and ninth decades of life. The cost of AD to society is enormous, affecting not only the patients but also caregivers who are often family members. Thus, there is a tremendous need for treatments that will slow AD onset and disease progression, although there are presently no disease-modifying therapeutics and only palliative treatments are available that temporarily modify symptoms [2].

The absence of drugs to treat the underlying disease course of AD does not reflect pharmaceutical efforts. There are presently >100 drug candidates in AD clinical trials [3], and these were preceded by many unsuccessful AD trials. To date, the majority of pharmaceutical efforts have been guided by the "amyloid cascade" hypothesis of AD [4], which postulates that the hallmark amyloid-beta (Aβ) senile plaque pathology within AD brain initiates events that ultimately promote neuronal tau neurofibrillary tangle (NFT) pathology and the onset of dementia. The amyloid cascade hypothesis is supported by the findings that inherited EOAD can result from mutations in the amyloid precursor protein (*APP*) gene, which encodes the APP from which Aβ peptides are derived [4], and from mutations in presenilin proteins that promote the cleavage of Aβ from APP [5].

An increased understanding of AD disease progression through biomarker and imaging studies suggests that the multiple failures of Aβ-directed candidates may, at least in part, be the result of Aβ plaque pathology developing 15–20 years before symptom onset [6, 7]. Thus, downstream events triggered by senile plaques may be ongoing for over a decade before clinical presentation, progressing to a stage where Aβ-directed drugs have limited effectiveness. Although disappointing, the failure of Aβ-directed drug programs has led to more recent interest in alternative AD targets and mechanisms, including programs directed to reducing the development of tau pathology [8] since there is a strong positive correlation between tau pathological burden and AD cognitive status [9, 10]. Moreover, there is increased interest in the role that glia may play in AD disease progression, as a number of microglial gene loci are associated with increased risk of LOAD [11].

Whereas there is incentive for industry to explore non-Aβ drug targets for AD, there has also been a decreased investment by industry in the earlier stages of drug discovery, including identification of new targets and associated assay systems. Moreover, the large number of AD clinical trial failures have led several pharmaceutical companies to eliminate or greatly reduce investment in AD. Finally, those with continuing AD programs have generally become more risk averse. In this climate, academic drug discovery can play an important role in complementing the efforts of the commercial sector, particularly in the earlier stages of the drug discovery process.

3.2 Academic AD Drug Discovery: Complementing but Not Competing with Industry Efforts

Reductions in discovery research within the pharmaceutical sector provide unique opportunities for academic laboratories, whether funded through traditional government grant sources or through collaborations with corporate partners. The growing need for academic participation in the drug discovery process has been recognized by federal funding agencies, which have developed a number of grant mechanisms to support target identification and drug discovery activities. This is particularly true in AD and related neurodegenerative diseases, and there are now many examples where academic research laboratories with expertise in AD biology have teamed with medicinal chemistry colleagues to pursue AD drug discovery.

Although increased grant support for academic AD drug discovery programs is critical and welcomed, it would be ill-advised for academic programs to compete directly with the medicinal chemistry and later development capabilities of pharmaceutical companies. Thus, it would seem advisable that academic drug discovery programs focus on higher-risk targets that are not under active pursuit in the commercial sector. In addition, academic groups can provide value through the creation of new disease-relevant assays that are suitable for compound screening, which in the context of AD drug discovery could include protein-, DNA/RNA-, or cell-based assays to new targets emerging from basic AD research, as well as cellular phenotypic screens that model one or more key aspects of AD neurodegeneration or pathology. Such assays, if appropriately optimized for compound screening, can lead to the identification of new chemical matter that may have potential for further optimization and development. Although certain academic teams may have the wherewithal to advance a lead compound to human clinical testing, this goal may not be achievable for many academic groups. Thus, the identification and optimization of probe molecules that provide proof of principle in animal disease models often represent a worthy accomplishment, particularly if this provides incentive for new pharmaceutical drug discovery efforts.

We review here the general process by which academic laboratories can identify molecules directed to new AD drug targets. This includes a brief discussion of assay types, as exemplified by tau-directed compound screens, followed by key principles of assay optimization and the types of compound libraries that might be used for screening. A discussion then follows on the steps taken after screening to identify compounds that are worthy of follow-up analyses in orthogonal and secondary assays, and the iterative process of medicinal chemistry optimization of confirmed hits. Finally, we briefly review the pharmacokinetic and preliminary safety testing that can be done to advance a lead candidate compound to a stage suitable for testing in mouse models of AD.

3.3 Academic AD Drug Discovery: Fundamentals of Lead Candidate Identification

3.3.1 Example Tau-Directed Assays Used for Compound Screening

We restrict the discussion here to examples of tau-directed assays used for compound screening, as they provide a general representation of assay types used in AD research. In particular, examples of protein-, cell-, and animal-based tau screens are provided that represent three tau-based therapeutic strategies: decreasing tau inclusions; reducing tau phosphorylation; or decreasing overall tau protein levels.

There have been a number of variations on compound screens that measure the inhibition of recombinant tau protein fibrillization, as tau fibrils can be created in vitro that bear similarity to those found within NFTs in AD brain. These include tau fibrillization assays where the recombinant tau was either full length [12, 13] or comprised of truncated tau species [14–16]. The net result of these screening efforts has been the identification of a number of small molecules that inhibit recombinant tau fibril formation, although many of these compounds have chemical liabilities that preclude development as drug candidates [8, 14, 17].

Small-molecule screens have also been conducted with cells that develop tau NFT-like inclusions. In most instances, these models have relied on the overexpression of full-length or truncated tau in cell lines [16, 18–20]. These cellular assays allow for the identification of molecules that inhibit tau inclusion formation as well as those that might enhance tau inclusion degradation. Our laboratory has recently compared HEK293 cell and primary rat neuron models of tau inclusion formation [20]. Whereas the HEK293 cell assay relies on overexpression of mutated tau, the neuron assay is unique in that there is no tau overexpression, with endogenous rat tau converted to inclusions upon seeding by insoluble tau isolated from AD brain [21]. Upon screening of the Prestwick library of mostly approved drugs, this neuronal assay yielded hits that were not identified in the HEK293 cell assay, including several dopamine D2 receptor antagonists [20]. Interestingly, D2 receptor antagonists were also identified in a small molecule screen utilizing *Caenorhabditis elegans* that develop tau inclusions [22], with the mechanisms by which such compounds reduce tau pathology still under investigation [23].

Another AD therapeutic strategy that has been actively pursued has been to identify inhibitors of tau phosphorylation. The hyperphosphorylation of tau leads to a reduction of normal microtubule binding, and can promote the formation of tau inclusions [24]. A number of kinases have been identified that can phosphorylate tau, leading to many enzyme-based screens directed to individual kinases, such as glycogen synthase kinase-3β (GSK-3β) and CDK5, which are summarized in other review articles [25, 26]. Recent screening efforts have consisted of virtual *in silico* screens, in which compound structures within databases have been computationally docked to known tau kinase crystal structures, leading to the identification of candidate inhibitors [27, 28]. This strategy led to the identification and subsequent testing of a relatively limited number of GSK-3β candidate compounds in HEK293 cells overexpressing tau [29]. Although substantial resources and efforts have gone into the identification of tau kinase inhibitors, the clinical results have thus far proven disappointing, as there are selectivity and safety challenges associated with this strategy [30].

Finally, an alternative strategy pursued to attenuate the negative consequences of tau in AD is to reduce total tau protein levels. One of the first screening assays developed to identify tau-lowering molecules utilized SH-SY5Y cells, with endogenous tau measured via AlphaLISA and homogeneous time-resolved fluorescence methodologies [31]. This led to the identification of four compounds from a Library of Pharmacologically Active Compounds (LOPAC) library screen that were active in both assay formats. An induced pluripotent stem cell (iPSC) neuronal assay was subsequently developed to identify compounds that lower tau levels. The neurons were pre-differentiated prior to plating in a 384-well format to reduce the total assay time to 21 days, leading to the identification of two active alpha-adrenergic agonists after screening the LOPAC library [32]. Very recently, iPSC-derived neuronal progenitor cells (NPCs) were screened with a selected library of putative autophagy modulators, with hits from this screen then further tested in iPSC-derived neurons from both control and inherited frontotemporal lobar degeneration (FTLD) patients [33]. Three inhibitors that inhibit the mechanistic target of rapamycin (mTOR) were identified, which lowered total and phosphorylated tau in differentiated patient neurons via enhanced autophagy, with evidence of lowered accumulation of insoluble tau.

3.3.2 Assay Optimization for Compound Screening

There are certain fundamental aspects of assay optimization that can be applied to most assay types when the goal is medium- to high-throughput compound screening, as discussed briefly below. For a more comprehensive discussion the reader is referred to the helpful *Assay Guidance Manual* [34].

Medium- to high-throughput screening assays are typically conducted in 96-, 384-, or 1,536-well plates. Regardless of plate format, screening assays should show uniform signal and sensitivity across plate wells so as to reduce intraplate variability. A common objective for all screening assays is a minimization of handling steps, as each manipulation can contribute to the overall assay variability. Another important aspect of a successful screening assay is proper validation of key reagents. This could include specifications for the purity of protein or RNA/DNA used in the assay, standardization of enzyme activity, and confirmation of proper cellular response in cell-based assays. Ideally, large batches of reagents should be pre-validated so that they can be used over multiple assay runs, although attention should be paid to reagent stability.

Once assay conditions have been optimized to yield the highest achievable signal that remains within the linear range of detection, with the lowest possible background signal (i.e., optimal signal-to-noise ratio), it is useful to determine the Z′-value [35] for the assay by running a large number of replicate wells of both high and low signal controls in the chosen plate format. The Z′-value is a statistical measure of assay robustness that incorporates the mean of the high and low signals along with the coefficient of variation for these measures. In general, a Z′-value of >0.5 is desirable for an assay in which compounds will be evaluated in single wells without replicates. The ability to reproducibly achieve appropriate Z′-values across independent assay plates over multiple days is critical. Similarly, the reproducibility of high- and low-control signals and half maximal inhibitory concentration (IC_{50}) or half maximal effective concentration (EC_{50}) values of positive control compounds is important. In this regard, another parameter that should be defined in assay validation tests is sensitivity to compound solvent. In most instances, this would be an assessment of assay sensitivity to dimethyl sulfoxide (DMSO) concentration since compound libraries are typically dissolved in 100% DMSO.

After validating that a chosen assay meets the fundamental requirements described above, it is often useful to determine the false-positive and false-negative hit rate for the assay. The former is readily determined by running an assay plate with a large number of high-control wells (i.e., compound vehicle only). This will yield a sense of the number of outlier wells that would meet the predetermined assay hit definition (e.g., >3SD [standard deviation] decrease in signal). The objective is to have an optimized assay with a low false-positive rate (e.g., ~0.1%). Assessment of false-negative rates can be done with a reference compound that is known to have appreciable activity within the assay, where again a large number of wells are examined and the percentage of wells that would be defined as inactive are defined by the assay hit criterion. In practice, false negatives are more problematic in compound screening than false positives, as the latter can be eliminated upon confirmation testing whereas the former will never be identified.

Finally, before embarking on a full-fledged high-throughput screening campaign, a smaller trial screen should be conducted with either an existing small library (e.g., Prestwick or LOPAC [20]), or with a subset of the full library to be screened. Multiple compound concentrations should be assessed in this trial screen to gain an understanding of compound hit rate, and potential toxicity rates in cell-based assays. Ideally, a compound concentration is identified in which a reasonable hit rate (e.g., 0.2–0.5%) is obtained without significant compound-induced toxicities.

3.3.3 Considerations in Designing and Accessing Compound Libraries

Library design and acquisition is a critical aspect of drug and probe discovery programs. In addition to practical cost considerations, several other important issues are generally examined [36]. Depending on the particular laboratory set-up, as well as the type of screening assay and its associated

throughput and anticipated hit rate, the desired library may vary greatly both in terms of size and composition. For example, if the target of interest belongs to a prominent target class, such as protein kinases or G-protein coupled receptors (GPCRs), libraries can be purchased that are enriched in chemotypes known to interact with these classes of biological targets. Alternatively, if structural information (e.g., X-ray data or homology models) exists for the target, a preliminary *in silico* screening [37] of large collections of commercially available compounds may be helpful to identify a more focused subset of compounds with high predicted target binding affinity. A number of suppliers now offer a variety of target-based libraries that have been generated based on predicted binding affinities for different targets.

Although the common scenarios mentioned above often result in the selection of relatively focused and perhaps structurally biased compound libraries, there are instances where structural diversity is an important requisite. For example, phenotypic assays are typically aimed at identifying potentially druggable targets that may be directly or indirectly associated with a particular disease phenotype. In these cases, libraries comprising structurally diverse compounds with known pharmacology/mechanism of actions may be most appropriate, as this could help the post-screening deconvolution of hits and ultimately facilitate the identification of target(s).

Finally, since blood–brain barrier (BBB) permeability is a major challenge shared by AD drug discovery programs [38], one additional critical aspect to be considered when designing libraries for AD and central nervous system (CNS) programs is the issue of brain penetration [39]. The property space of CNS-active drugs is generally a subset of the overall drug-like space defined by the Lipinski's rule of five [40], requiring compounds with relatively lower molecular weight (MW < 400 Da) and polar surface area (PSA < 100 Å^2).

3.3.4 Compound Triaging and Medicinal Chemistry Optimization

Initial hits from a screening campaign are usually not optimized for the assay target(s), and a chemical optimization process is almost always necessary to identify candidate leads. In addition to eliminating/de-prioritizing hit series that are known or suspected to be promiscuous assay-interfering compounds (e.g., pan-assay interference compounds [PAINS] [41]), including molecules featuring chemically reactive moieties, additional aspects are considered in determining the overall tractability of compounds and compound series. After elimination of problematic compounds by one or more medicinal chemists with prior drug discovery experience, assisted by existing molecular descriptors [41, 42], hit compounds should be confirmed through repeat analysis, typically in triplicate, in the primary screening assay. Confirmed hits should then undergo concentration–response analyses in the primary assay, and compounds that meet specified IC_{50}/EC_{50} values should then be assessed in an orthogonal assay in which activity is determined through a readout that differs from that of the primary screen. For example, if the primary screen relies on the measurement of a fluorescent signal, an orthogonal assay might measure compound activity via a colorimetric or biochemical readout to provide confidence that the identified compound is not a false positive due to an artifact related to the primary assay readout (e.g., fluorescence quencher).

The hit-to-lead optimization process is typically based on an iterative process, schematically outlined in Figure 3.1, which begins with the design and synthesis of analogs, and is followed by the evaluation of biological activity and physicochemical properties to reveal critical elements of structure–activity as well as structure–property relationships (SAR/SPRs). In addition to primary and orthogonal assays, for target-based drug discovery programs these evaluations will often also employ secondary assays, such as those that measure related-target interactions. Information on the SAR/SPR will then provide the basis for the design of new series of analogs. As each iteration often involves an incremental increase of molecular size and functionalization relative to the parent compound, monitoring of physicochemical properties, including solubility, will be required to ensure that analogs fall within ranges conducive to BBB permeability and CNS drug-like properties [43]. Thus, a judicious assessment of the quality/desirability of hits as starting points for optimization should always include an evaluation of size and physicochemical properties, and sole reliance on compound potency as the primary driver for hit selection should be avoided. In this context, several intuitive metrics, including ligand efficiency (LE) and lipophilic ligand efficiency (LLE) that normalize compound activity to its size (e.g., number of non-hydrogen atoms) and lipophilicity (logP), have been introduced to facilitate an appropriate prioritization of hits [44, 45].

3.3.5 Advancement of Molecules to In Vivo Testing

In many instances, the objective of an academic AD drug discovery program is the identification of a probe compound suitable for proof-of-principle

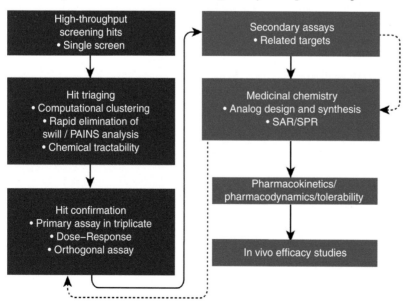

Figure 3.1 Schematic outline of the iterative process underlying the optimization of screening hits to lead candidate compounds.

testing in one or more animal models of AD pathology. In most cases this will be a mouse model, although other model systems such as *C. elegans* [46] or *Drosophila* [47] might be employed. We focus here on steps that can be taken to validate the suitability of a probe compound for in vivo efficacy testing in mice.

A compound suitable for efficacy testing in mouse models of AD must have certain key characteristics, including adequate brain exposure, reasonable metabolic stability, and an absence of significant dose-limiting side effects. Accordingly, certain in vivo studies are recommended that will validate that a probe compound meets these requirements (Figure 3.1). First among these is the determination of compound BBB permeability. Certain in vitro tests, such as PAMPA or MDCK cell assays [48], can be used to predict BBB permeability, but our laboratory typically conducts a small study in wild-type mice in which plasma and brain compound levels are determined 1 hour after compound dosing (intraveneous [IV] or intraperitoneal [IP]) [49]. These analyses require liquid chromatography–mass spectrometry (LC-MS) determinations of compound concentrations in these tissues, and many academic core facilities provide this service, as do several contract laboratories. It should be noted that an assessment of total compound in the brain and plasma provides only an approximation of BBB permeability, and determination of fractional free drug concentration (i.e., non-protein or -lipid bound) in plasma and brain homogenates by methods such as equilibrium dialysis [50] is required to accurately determine the BBB permeability of a compound [51].

Compounds with adequate brain exposure can be assessed for their pharmacokinetic (PK) properties by analyzing plasma and brain compound concentrations at multiple time points after administration (e.g., from 15 minutes to 16 hours) to allow for a determination of key PK parameters such as clearance and half-life [52]. A compound that is rapidly eliminated from plasma and brain will be difficult to utilize as a probe molecule in mouse efficacy studies since very frequent dosing would be required. Although longer half-lives are preferred, the need for frequent dosing can be mitigated by providing compound in drinking water or feed. As mice eat and drink many times throughout a 24-hour period, they will receive multiple small daily doses of compound. However, this requires that a compound has good oral bioavailability (e.g., >30% of administered dose absorbed into blood),

and thus PK studies will also need to be conducted in which the compound is administered orally, with the total compound exposure compared to that from IV dosing to determine the fraction of compound that is orally absorbed [52].

After the identification of a probe compound with suitable brain exposure and PK, key remaining questions are: (1) What is the projected efficacy dose?; and (2) Can the compound be tolerated by mice at efficacy dose? The projected efficacy dose is ideally determined through a biomarker of target engagement, such as substantial inhibition of a target enzyme activity or significant occupancy of a target receptor. If a direct measurement of target engagement is difficult, indirect measures can be employed, such as changes in target substrates or downstream signaling pathways. Once a minimal effective dose (MED) is established, it is helpful to determine the duration of the compound effect on the biomarker to inform dosing frequency, as it is possible that the biological effect exceeds the compound half-life. Finally, dose tolerability studies should be considered in which mice are dosed for 2–4 weeks at the MED and multiples of the MED to confirm that prolonged treatment, as is typically required for efficacy studies in AD mouse models, is tolerated without negative behavioral or physiological responses.

Efficacy study design will depend on the chosen AD model, but these studies are typically either of a preventative design in which compound dosing begins prior to the development of disease pathology, or an interventional design in which compound administration is started after the initial formation of pathology. A critical aspect of efficacy study design is ensuring that treatment group sizes are adequate to ensure that statistically significant data will be obtained, as determined through a power analysis [53]. In addition, many transgenic mouse models of AD show sex-dependent differences in the rate of disease pathology formation, which should be taken into consideration when conducting power analyses. The reader is referred to the useful review by Snyder et al. [54] that further discusses key aspects of efficacy study design.

3.4 Academic–Pharmaceutical Company AD Drug Discovery Collaborations

Although the drug discovery processes described above are well within the capabilities of many academic centers in which biology/pharmacology and medicinal chemistry colleagues work collaboratively, such activities can also be carried out jointly with a pharmaceutical company partner. There are many benefits to working with a pharmaceutical or biotechnology team, including financial support, drug discovery expertise, and access to company resources. However, there are also certain cautions that should be considered when entering such partnerships (Figure 3.2), as discussed further below.

3.4.1 Collaborative Small-Molecule Compound Screening and Hit Optimization Programs

We have undertaken several collaborative AD drug discovery programs with pharmaceutical partners based on the utilization of high-throughput screening assays developed in our laboratory. These have included recombinant tau fibrillization assays [15], as well as cell-line [55] and primary neuron [20] assays that modeled tau inclusion formation. In one instance, the assay was taught to the partner high-throughput screening group so that screening could be conducted within the pharmaceutical company facilities, with subsequent orthogonal and secondary assay testing of screening hits conducted within our laboratory. Conversely, in other programs the pharmaceutical partner has provided compound libraries for screening within cell-based assays in our laboratory. Subsequent orthogonal and secondary assays have typically been conducted jointly by both teams, leading to a collaborative scientific exchange. In all of these programs, medicinal chemistry optimization activities resided solely with the pharmaceutical partner, an acknowledgment to the generally greater chemistry staffing available within the pharmaceutical sector.

Potential Benefits	Potential Cautions
• Access to drug discovery expertise	• Strict timelines and milestones
• Healthcare impact	• Frequent reporting
• Financial support	• Publication restrictions
• Access to company resources	• Narrow research focus
• Sense of teamwork	• Misaligned research interests
• Patent filings	• Short-term funding
• Publications	
• Licensing revenue	

Figure 3.2 Considerations before embarking on a collaborative drug discovery program with a pharmaceutical/biotechnology company.

However, academic laboratories can remain engaged in the chemical optimization phase of the program through participation in the iterative cycle of compound testing in primary and secondary assays.

There are multiple issues for an academic laboratory to consider when contemplating a collaborative drug discovery program that starts with compound screening. Many of these relate to the tension between the academic mission and the commercialization objectives of the pharmaceutical company. A primary goal of academic research is to publish results in a timely manner, whereas there is often considerable benefit and at times a necessity for pharmaceutical drug discovery results to remain confidential, certainly until patent applications are filed. Thus, there can be restrictions within the governing sponsored research agreement (SRA) on publications or presentations that rely on the disclosure of chemical structures. A potential solution that allows the academic team to publish study results is to allow disclosure of non-lead molecules that provide sufficient proof of principle for quality publications.

Other issues that should be discussed during SRA negotiations between academic laboratories and potential commercial partners are those related to timelines, milestones, and reporting. Most academic laboratory heads are familiar with federal or other non-profit grant reporting requirements, which are typically once per year and relatively straightforward. In contrast, pharmaceutical company projects are timeline and milestone driven, and typically require monthly meetings, regular data uploads, and 6-month progress reports. Thus, the administrative time required of the academic principal investigator in an industry collaboration is usually much greater than for grant-funded programs.

Finally, a key issue in contract negotiations for early-stage drug discovery collaborations is recognition of program success through licensing of intellectual property and downstream financial rewards linked to clinical development. Thus, there should be specific language in the SRA describing the handling of joint inventions. This typically entails providing the commercial entity certain licensing options, such as an exclusive first right to negotiate for a commercial license to joint intellectual property. Such a license agreement typically contains milestone-dependent financial rewards linked to advancement to clinical stages and to regulatory approval. The negotiation of these financial terms is usually outside the expertise of academic investigators and is the bailiwick of the university technology transfer office.

3.4.2 Collaborative Programs Characterizing Identified Pharmaceutical Assets

A second type of drug discovery program in which academic laboratories can assist pharmaceutical company programs is in the further characterization and validation of already identified drug candidates. In these programs, the pharmaceutical partner typically seeks additional scientific expertise and/or unique assays that are presently lacking in their internal program. For example, we have examined previously identified drug candidates in neuronal assays of AD pathology and in mouse models that develop AD-like pathology [56–58].

Contractual agreement on issues such as publication rights become especially important in programs of this type, as there may not be licensing opportunities since patent filings likely occurred prior to the initiation of the collaboration. It is important that the academic group ask whether the proposed studies are aligned with their overall research interests and objectives, as in our experience there is less satisfaction in programs in which the academic laboratory is not involved in inventive work.

Finally, another type of collaboration that can form around already identified molecular assets is that in which the academic group has discovered lead molecules that are of interest to a pharmaceutical partner. In these instances, the nature of the collaboration can vary depending on the stage of advancement of the academic program. Well-characterized drug candidates are often licensed by the pharmaceutical partner, who will then undertake further preclinical and clinical advancement. In earlier-stage programs, the pharmaceutical partner may work collaboratively with the academic team to further optimize, characterize, and advance early lead molecules, with possible medicinal chemistry contributions. Such alliances will again require licensing agreements and possibly SRAs.

3.4.3 Lessons from Industry Drug Discovery Collaborations

Perhaps the foremost benefit of working with a commercial drug discovery partner is the sense of making a true difference in healthcare and patient outcomes. Many scientists find gratification in working on projects that might directly impact human disease. However, such programs often require a relatively narrow focus on key objectives with defined timelines, and not all academic scientists thrive in a work environment where interesting tangential observations are often left untouched so as to keep on a linear path to maximize the odds of drug discovery/development success.

In our experience, the most satisfying partnerships have been those where both the academic and pharmaceutical researchers work closely together, with regular exchanges that focus on data sharing, troubleshooting, and new ideas that might enhance the drug discovery program. The sense of teamwork that arises from a strong collaborative program is something that many academic researchers have not previously experienced. One key to developing and maintaining comradery and productivity between industry and academic groups is an alignment of vision and shared respect. This can also lead to greater appreciation of the success metrics of both groups; i.e., the need of academic scientists to publish and the company desire for timely program advancement.

Drug discovery and development is characterized by a high attrition rate and most programs will not result in the identification of a true drug candidate. Accordingly, we have found that industry is hesitant to commit to more than 2 years of funding, and in many instances prefers year-to-year agreements. This can be problematic for academic laboratories, as graduate students and post-doctoral fellows typically require longer time commitments. Finally, academic laboratories should also be aware that their perceived value will likely diminish over time, even in successful collaborative programs. If a drug candidate has been identified, subsequent testing to meet regulatory requirements and future clinical studies will be conducted by the pharmaceutical company, and the academic group usually adds less value from this stage forward. Nonetheless, the identification of a clinical drug candidate is a significant accomplishment that few academic researchers can claim, pointing to another of the several potential advantages to collaborative programs with pharmaceutical partners.

References

1. Cacace R, Sleegers K, Van Broeckhoven C. Molecular genetics of early-onset Alzheimer's disease revisited. *Alzheimers Dement* 2016; **12**: 733–48.

2. Joe E, Ringman JM. Cognitive symptoms of Alzheimer's disease: clinical management and prevention. *BMJ* 2019; **367**: l6217.

3. Cummings J, Lee G, Ritter A, Sabbagh M, Zhong K. Alzheimer's disease drug development pipeline: 2019. *Alzheimers Dement (N Y)* 2019; **5**: 272–93.

4. Hardy J. The discovery of Alzheimer-causing mutations in the *APP* gene and the formulation of the "amyloid cascade hypothesis". *FEBS J* 2017; **284**: 1040–4.

5. George-Hyslop PH, Petit A. Molecular biology and genetics of Alzheimer's disease. *CR Biol* 2005; **328**: 119–30.

6. Jack CR, Jr., Knopman DS, Jagust WJ, et al. Tracking pathophysiological processes in Alzheimer's disease: an updated hypothetical model of dynamic biomarkers. *Lancet Neurol* 2013; **12**: 207–16.

7. McDade E, Wang G, Gordon BA, et al. Longitudinal cognitive and biomarker changes in dominantly inherited Alzheimer disease. *Neurology* 2018; **91**: e1295–306.

8. Khanna MR, Kovalevich J, Lee VM, Trojanowski JQ, Brunden KR. Therapeutic strategies for the treatment of tauopathies: hopes and challenges. *Alzheimers Dement* 2016; **12**: 1051–65.

9. Arriagada PV, Growdon JH, Hedleywhytc ET, Hyman BT. Neurofibrillary tangles but not senile plaques parallel duration and severity of Alzheimers disease. *Neurology* 1992; **42**: 631–9.

10. Teng E, Ward M, Manser PT, et al. Cross-sectional associations between [(18)F]GTP1 tau PET and cognition in Alzheimer's disease. *Neurobiol Aging* 2019; **81**: 138–45.

11. Malik M, Parikh I, Vasquez JB, et al. Genetics ignite focus on microglial inflammation in Alzheimer's disease. *Mol Neurodegener* 2015; **10**: 52.

12. Taniguchi S, Suzuki N, Masuda M, et al. Inhibition of heparin-induced tau filament formation by phenothiazines, polyphenols, and porphyrins. *J Biol Chem* 2005; **280**: 7614–23.

13. Honson NS, Johnson RL, Huang WW, et al. Differentiating Alzheimer disease-associated aggregates with small molecules. *Neurobiol Dis* 2007; **28**: 251–60.

14. Crowe A, Ballatore C, Hyde E, Trojanowski JQ, Lee VMY. High throughput screening for small molecule inhibitors of heparin-induced tau fibril formation. *Biochem Biophys Res Commun* 2007; **358**: 1–6.

15. Crowe A, Huang W, Ballatore C, et al. The identification of aminothienopyridazine inhibitors of tau assembly by quantitative high-throughput screening. *Biochemistry* 2009; **48**: 7732–45.

16. Pickhardt M, Gazova Z, von Bergen M, et al. Anthraquinones inhibit tau aggregation and dissolve Alzheimer's paired helical filaments in vitro and in cells. *J Biol Chem* 2005; **280**: 3628–35.

17. Crowe A, James MJ, Lee VM, et al. Aminothienopyridazines and methylene blue affect tau fibrillization via cysteine oxidation. *J Biol Chem* 2013; **288**: 11024–37.

18. Pickhardt M, Tassoni M, Denner P, et al. Screening of a neuronal cell model of tau pathology for therapeutic compounds. *Neurobiol Aging* 2019; **76**: 24–34.

19. Khlistunova I, Biernat J, Wang YP, et al. Inducible expression of tau repeat domain in cell models of tauopathy: aggregation is toxic to cells but can be reversed by inhibitor drugs. *J Biol Chem* 2006; **281**: 1205–14.

20. Crowe A, Henderson MJ, Anderson J, et al. Compound screening in cell-based models of tau inclusion formation: comparison of primary neuron and HEK293 cell assays. *J Biol Chem* 2020; **295**: 4001–13.

21. Guo JL, Narasimhan S, Changolkar L, et al. Unique pathological tau conformers from Alzheimer's brains transmit tau pathology in nontransgenic mice. *J Exp Med* 2016; **213**: 2635–54.

22. McCormick AV, Wheeler JM, Guthrie CR, Liachko NF, Kraemer BC. Dopamine D2 receptor antagonism suppresses tau aggregation and neurotoxicity. *Biol Psychiatry* 2013; **73**: 464–71.

23. Kow RL, Sikkema C, Wheeler JM, et al. DOPA decarboxylase modulates tau toxicity. *Biol Psychiatry* 2018; **83**: 438–46.

24. Ballatore C, Lee VMY, Trojanowski JQ. Tau-mediated neurodegeneration in Alzheimer's disease and related disorders. *Nat Rev Neurosci* 2007; **8**: 663–72.

25. Tell V, Hilgeroth A. Recent developments of protein kinase inhibitors as potential AD therapeutics. *Front Cell Neurosci* 2013; **7**:189.

26. Martin L, Latypova X, Wilson CM, et al. Tau protein kinases: involvement in Alzheimer's disease. *Ageing Res Rev* 2013; **12**: 289–309.

27. Zeb A, Son M, Yoon S, et al. Computational simulations identified two candidate inhibitors of CDK5/p25 to abrogate tau-associated neurological disorders. *Comput Struct Biotechnol J* 2019; **17**: 579–90.

28. Shukla R, Munjal NS, Singh TR. Identification of novel small molecules against GSK3beta for Alzheimer's disease using chemoinformatics approach. *J Mol Graph Model* 2019; **91**: 91–104.

29. Lin CH, Hsieh YS, Wu YR, et al. Identifying GSK-3beta kinase inhibitors of Alzheimer's disease: virtual screening, enzyme, and cell assays. *Eur J Pharm Sci* 2016; **89**: 11–19.

30. Bhat RV, Andersson U, Andersson S, et al. The conundrum of GSK3 inhibitors: is it the dawn of a new beginning? *J Alzheimers Dis* 2018; **64**: S547–54.

31. Dehdashti SJ, Zheng W, Gever JR, et al. A high-throughput screening assay for determining cellular levels of total tau protein. *Curr Alzheimer Res* 2013; **10**: 679–87.

32. Wang C, Ward ME, Chen R, et al. Scalable production of iPSC-derived human neurons to identify tau-lowering compounds by high-content screening. *Stem Cell Reports* 2017; **9**: 1221–33.

33. Silva MC, Nandi GA, Tentarelli S, et al. Prolonged tau clearance and stress vulnerability rescue by pharmacological activation of autophagy in tauopathy neurons. *Nat Commun* 2020; **11**: 3258.

34. Coussens NP, Sittampalam GS, Guha R, et al. Assay Guidance Manual: quantitative biology and pharmacology in preclinical drug discovery. *Clin Transl Sci* 2018; **11**: 461–70.

35. Zhang JH, Chung TDY, Oldenburg KR. A simple statistical parameter for use in evaluation and validation of high throughput screening assays. *J Biomol Screen* 1999; **4**: 67–73.

36. Dandapani S, Rosse G, Southall N, Salvino JM, Thomas CJ. Selecting, acquiring, and using small molecule libraries for high-throughput screening. *Curr Protocol Chem Biol* 2012; **4**: 177–91.

37. Caldwell GW. *In silico* tools used for compound selection during target-based drug discovery and development. *Expert Opin Drug Discov* 2015; **10**: 901–23.

38. Pardridge WM. The blood–brain barrier: bottleneck in brain drug development. *NeuroRx* 2005; **2**: 3–14.

39. Hitchcock SA. Blood–brain barrier permeability considerations for CNS-targeted compound library design. *Curr Opin Chem Biol* 2008; **12**: 318–23.

40. Lipinski CA, Lombardo F, Dominy BW, Feeney PJ. Experimental and computational approaches to estimate solubility and permeability in drug discovery and development settings. *Adv Drug Deliver Rev* 1997; **23**: 3–25.

41. Dahlin JL, Nissink JW, Strasser JM, et al. PAINS in the assay: chemical mechanisms of assay interference and promiscuous enzymatic

42. Bruns RF, Watson IA. Rules for identifying potentially reactive or promiscuous compounds. *J Med Chem* 2012; **55**: 9763–72.

43. Wager TT, Hou X, Verhoest PR, Villalobos A. Central nervous system multiparameter optimization desirability: application in drug discovery. *ACS Chem Neurosci* 2016; **7**: 767–75.

44. Hopkins AL, Keseru GM, Leeson PD, Rees DC, Reynolds CH. The role of ligand efficiency metrics in drug discovery. *Nat Rev Drug Discov* 2014; **13**: 105–21.

45. Meanwell NA. Improving drug design: an update on recent applications of efficiency metrics, strategies for replacing problematic elements, and compounds in nontraditional drug space. *Chem Res Toxicol* 2016; **29**: 564–616.

46. Dimitriadi M, Hart AC. Neurodegenerative disorders: insights from the nematode *Caenorhabditis elegans*. *Neurobiol Dis* 2010; **40**: 4–11.

47. McGurk L, Berson A, Bonini NM. *Drosophila* as an in vivo model for human neurodegenerative disease. *Genetics* 2015; **201**: 377–402.

48. Bicker J, Alves G, Fortuna A, Falcao A. Blood–brain barrier models and their relevance for a successful development of CNS drug delivery systems: a review. *Eur J Pharm Biopharm* 2014; **87**: 409–32.

49. Kovalevich J, Cornec AS, Yao Y, et al. Characterization of brain-penetrant pyrimidine-containing molecules with differential microtubule-stabilizing activities developed as potential therapeutic agents for Alzheimer's disease and related tauopathies. *J Pharmacol Exp Ther* 2016; **357**: 432–50.

50. Di L, Umland JP, Chang G, et al. Species independence in brain tissue binding using brain homogenates. *Drug Metab Dispos* 2011; **39**: 1270–7.

51. Di L, Rong H, Feng B. Demystifying brain penetration in central nervous system drug discovery. Miniperspective. *J Med Chem* 2013; **56**: 2–12.

52. Benet LZ, Zia-Amirhosseini P. Basic principles of pharmacokinetics. *Toxicol Pathol* 1995; **23**: 115–23.

53. Gaskill BN, Garner JP. Power to the people: power, negative results and sample size. *J Am Assoc Lab Anim Sci* 2020; **59**: 9–16.

54. Snyder HM, Shineman DW, Friedman LG, et al. Guidelines to improve animal study design and reproducibility for Alzheimer's disease and related

43

dementias: for funders and researchers. *Alzheimers Dement* 2016; **12**: 1177–85.

55. Guo JL, Buist A, Soares A, et al. The dynamics and turnover of tau aggregates in cultured cells: insights into therapies for tauopathies. *J Biol Chem* 2016; **291**: 13175–93.

56. Sankaranarayanan S, Barten DM, Vana L, et al. Passive immunization with phospho-tau antibodies reduces tau pathology and functional deficits in two distinct mouse tauopathy models. *PLoS One* 2015; **10**: e0125614.

57. He Z, Guo JL, McBride JD, et al. Amyloid-beta plaques enhance Alzheimer's brain tau-seeded pathologies by facilitating neuritic plaque tau aggregation. *Nat Med* 2018; **24**: 29–38.

58. Sopko R, Golonzhka O, Arndt J, et al. Characterization of tau binding by gosuranemab. *Neurobiol Dis* 2020; **146**: 105120.

The Harrington Discovery Institute and Alzheimer's Disease Drug Development

Andrew A. Pieper, J. Simon Mazza-Lunn, and Diana R. Wetmore

4.1 Scope of the Problem

Society is currently suffering from a dearth of effective medicines for patients with Alzheimer's disease (AD) or AD-related dementias (ADRD). This problem is becoming increasingly important as people are living longer, and senior citizens are the fastest growing segment of our population. At present, some form of dementia afflicts approximately 11% of those in the United States over age 65, with the incidence roughly doubling every 5 years, peaking around 40–60% when people reach their 90s. About two-thirds of these patients suffer from AD and ADRD [1], and the number of people living beyond 90 is projected to increase from 2 million up to 10 million by 2050 [2]. Since age is the greatest risk factor for developing AD, this portends an imminent health crisis related to the debilitating effects of AD on patients, caregivers, and society. Indeed, it is projected that by 2050 there will be 13.8 million cases of AD in the United States alone, reaching a financial cost of more than $1 trillion per year. Despite the magnitude of the problem, however, only five medicines have been approved for AD since its discovery almost 120 years ago [3, 4], and the last time a Phase 3 trial for a wholly novel treatment succeeded (not just a combination of two already approved drugs) was about 16 years ago. To date, more than 99% of AD clinical trials have failed [5], and existing therapies are limited primarily to acetylcholine or N-methyl-D-aspartate (NMDA) glutamatergic mechanisms. Unfortunately, these medicines provide only mild symptomatic benefit and do not halt, or even slow, disease progression [6]. Simply put, society will soon be facing a devastating humanitarian crisis unless new and effective treatments for AD are developed. The Harrington Discovery Institute is addressing this crisis by diversifying and accelerating the development path of new medicines for the treatment and prevention of AD, from laboratory discovery into the clinic for patients.

4.2 AD Drug Discovery

The classic pathological findings of AD, stereotyped progressive neurodegeneration with accumulation of hyperphosphorylated tau (p-tau) and amyloid-beta (Aβ)-containing plaques, have traditionally driven the bulk of drug-development efforts in the field. The p-tau protein accumulates in intracellular neurofibrillary tangles (NFTs), which originate within the nucleus basalis of Meynert–entorhinal cortex circuitry and then spread to the hippocampus, remainder of the limbic system, neocortex, and primary motor and sensory cortices [7]. Aβ, by contrast, forms extracellular plaques in cortical and deep brain areas [8]. Despite our understanding of the pathology, however, there is still no consensus as to whether these pathological findings actually correlate with AD severity or progression. Indeed, the same pathologies are widespread in the aging brain even in the absence of clinical dementia [1, 9]. Thus, it is not surprising that enormous efforts over past decades from both academia and industry to target these pathological phenomena have failed to produce disease-modifying therapies.

The historical focus on these pathologies in drug discovery has arisen largely because they are seen in rare and early-onset forms of AD associated with single gene mutations. Pathways related to such genes have lent themselves readily to laboratory study through genetic manipulation of animal and cell model systems. As a consequence, the bulk of AD research has focused on very rare forms of the disease. However, the vast majority of AD cases are sporadic and late-onset, with minimal familial clustering, and likely result from a complex interaction of many genes, the environment, and the normal physiological processes of aging [10]. This suggests utility for new discovery approaches involving diverse targets that complement and move beyond the traditional hypotheses. For example, broadly targeting neurodegeneration or synaptic function may prove beneficial. Likewise, preserving vascular function for optimal

45

brain health, particularly at the level of the neurovascular unit that coordinates the blood–brain barrier and neurovascular coupling, may help protect the brain from AD. It is entirely likely that concurrent inhibition of multiple aspects of AD will be necessary for sustained long-lasting neuroprotection throughout the course of this chronic disease. Offering hope, it has recently been shown that directly blocking nerve cell death in a preclinical model of AD is able to prevent both cognitive decline and depression-like behavior, two of the most salient and debilitating features of AD, without altering amyloid or tau pathology [11].

4.3   The AD Challenge

Supported by billions of dollars of government funding, many medical research institutions in the United States have a primary mission of advancing medicine by producing breakthrough scientific discoveries. One of the critical gaps in translating these scientific discoveries to the clinic, however, is finding the right commercial partners to advance through the costly process of clinical trials. A broadly accepted analysis has estimated the out-of-pocket cost per new drug approval to be approximately $1.4 billion [12]. Academic institutes are particularly challenged to meet the expectations required to attract attention from for-profit entities capable of supporting the substantial investment required to bring a new medicine to market. In the past, breakthrough discoveries from academic labs could be readily licensed to venture capital firms or pharmaceutical companies for financing and development into medicines. Today, however, many of these commercial entities have diminished interest in therapeutic products that have not yet demonstrated human clinical proof of concept. This has become particularly evident in the field of neuroprotection and AD. The specific challenges surrounding programs for AD further increases the rigor required to de-risk any program to the level where typical investors will enter into partnerships. As a result, a large money and knowledge gap separates the two sides of the medicine development process, particularly in the field of AD where the numerous clinical failures have prompted the pharmaceutical industry to drastically reduce its internal neurotherapeutic discovery research. The Harrington Discovery Institute is uniquely positioned to guide academic researchers along the path to commercial partnership by maximizing value creation from both a fast-to-clinic and a de-risked-for-partnership approach.

4.4   The Harrington Discovery Institute

The Neurotherapeutics Center of the Harrington Discovery Institute, housed at the University Hospitals Health System of Cleveland, is pursuing diversified therapeutic targets for AD, based on cutting-edge discoveries originating from academic laboratories across the United States, Canada, and United Kingdom. Generating the medicines of tomorrow requires an appetite for risk, bona fide access to novel targets, and collaboration between academic and industry-oriented professional teams. The Harrington Discovery Institute, through working with partners such as the Alzheimer's Drug Discovery Foundation (ADDF), has pioneered this approach to pursue potentially paradigm-shifting therapies for patients. The objective of the Harrington Discovery Institute is to shorten the time between the discovery of potential drug targets and the development of new medicines for patients by facilitating the translation of discoveries from laboratory bench to patient bedside. By leveraging philanthropic funds and providing critical drug-development know-how, the Harrington Discovery Institute de-risks programs centered on novel targets to foster their progression to critical inflection points. Such de-risking is key to advancing novel discoveries to where they are attractive for further investment from biotechnology and pharmaceutical companies.

Founded in 2012, and powered by an initial $50 million gift to University Hospitals Cleveland Medical Center from local philanthropists Ron and Nancy Harrington and their family, the Harrington Discovery Institute was created to implement the Harringtons' vision of bridging the ever-widening gap between academic scientific discovery at the laboratory bench and development of commercially viable medicines for patients in the clinic. Today, the Harrington Discovery Institute and its mission-aligned for-profit partners that together comprise the Harrington Project is a United States, Canada, and United Kingdom-wide disease- and institutional-agnostic initiative that is accelerating the development of scientific breakthroughs into medicines for multiple areas of unmet need, including AD and other neurological and psychiatric disorders. The Harrington Discovery Institute

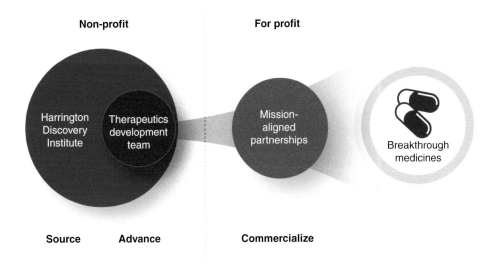

Figure 4.1 The Harrington Project Model.

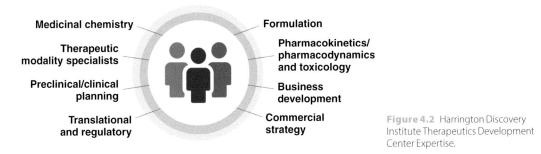

Figure 4.2 Harrington Discovery Institute Therapeutics Development Center Expertise.

utilizes a multi-vector approach that promotes cutting-edge science, critical-path planning for proof of concept between preclinical models and clinical endpoints, and commercial partnering strategies to cross the so-called "valley of death" that separates discoveries in the laboratory from clinical testing in human trials. This unique model aligns, through mission and structure, non-profit and for-profit resources to address the major challenges in medicine creating the current development gap that has contributed to a long-term decline in new medicine approvals for areas of unmet need, including AD (Figure 4.1).

4.5 The Harrington Discovery Institute Approach

A deeper look into the Harrington Discovery Institute model begins with project selection. Scientists with an exceptionally innovative and early therapeutic discovery are identified through a call for applications. The rigorous selection process is advised by a panel of academic and industry scientists, each of whom are themselves innovators in the fields of medicine and therapeutics development. Once accepted into a Harrington Discovery Institute scholar program, the Harrington Discovery Institute immediately begins to bridge the knowledge gap by forming a supporting project team around each scholar with the know-how to evaluate, plan, and advance the program (Figure 4.2). Through direct interaction with eminent drug developers who were formerly heads of departments and executive leaders in the pharmaceutical industry, the scholars' laboratory team is able to access key drug-development knowledge areas that would typically be available only at a large pharmaceutical company. The de-risking strategies followed by pharmaceutical industry teams are often based on broad institutional knowledge informed by both successes and failures in clinical development, but most of this knowledge is not published and is thus difficult or impossible for academic researchers to access. The advisors in each project support team have deep and intimate knowledge of drug discovery and development from target validation through US Food and Drug Administration (FDA) approval and marketing, which they have acquired from their own experiences in developing new medicines, and which they use to guide the scholars. In addition, each team has a project manager, who works with the scholars' team to delineate a path for commercial and clinical success, ensuring that the critical knowledge gap is addressed as needed.

Collectively, the Harrington Discovery Institute advisory experts and project managers are known as the Therapeutic Development Center (TDC). The TDC directs academic investigators through drug-development-stage gated processes that mirror the rigor of a major pharmaceutical company. TDC guidance adds significant value to the academic discovery technology, thereby positioning it more strongly for ultimate advancement into a medicine for patients. The commercial path to FDA approval is typically through either licensing of the technology to a pharmaceutical company, or by securing investor funding for a new biotechnology company based around the discovery, including investment by the Harrington Project. Thus, the Harrington Discovery Institute provides academic scientists who have made breakthrough basic science discoveries related to disease with both financial capital for advancement and human capital in the form of expert industry guidance to manage the translation and development of their projects. All of this is done without the Harrington Discovery Institute taking rights to the technology.

In the 8 years since its formation, the Harrington Project has already demonstrated the success of its innovative model by sourcing and developing breakthrough technologies and establishing strategic partnerships with disease foundations and pharmaceutical companies. To date, this has progressed the individual scientific discoveries of Harrington Discovery Institute scholars into 8 medicines in clinical trials, 29 new companies launched with institutional investment funding, and 9 medicines licensed to major pharmaceutical companies.

4.6 Harrington Discovery Institute Programmatic Structure: Supporting the Physician-Scientist

The Harrington Discovery Institute is a stand-alone institute at University Hospitals Cleveland Medical Center that instantiates its discovery mission and provides services in the realm of unmet need. It is also an international organization that manages a large set of transatlantic programs (~40 at any given time). Launched at the inception of the Harrington Discovery Institute, the flagship Harrington Scholar-Innovator program recognizes the unique and often underfunded role of physician-scientists in drug discovery. This disease- and institution-agnostic program has supported approximately 80 physician-scientists thus far. The annual call for applications attracts ~150 (range 100–550) unique high-caliber submissions from leading institutions across the United States and Canada, demonstrating the high demand for this unique program. The more recently developed Harrington Investigator Program identifies and recruits to Cleveland exceptionally innovative and translationally minded physician-scientists to anchor the Harrington Discovery Institute's areas of focus within the institute itself. Harrington investigators benefit from institutional support for their laboratories and are committed to fundamental scientific discovery, scholarship, community, and patient care. Through these physician-scientists, who are currently working in neuroprotection, mental health, rare disease, oncology, and vascular biology, the Harrington Discovery Institute is a growing center of excellence in translational medicine that is leveraging internal research leadership to support its growing network of external programs. The Harrington Discovery Institute's commitment to supporting excellence in translation of academic drug discovery is further emphasized by its partnership with the American Society for Clinical Investigation (ASCI). The ASCI is dedicated to advancing research that extends understanding and improves treatment of human diseases, and its members are committed to mentoring future generations of physician-scientists. Together, ASCI and the Harrington Discovery Institute annually award The Harrington Prize for Innovation in Medicine to an exceptionally inventive physician-scientist who has advanced the field through novel research with clear potential for clinical impact.

More recent programs launched include: the Harrington Medical Scientist Training Program (MSTP) Award, which supports novel discoveries by MSTP students at Case Western Reserve University (CWRU), and the Harrington Fellows program, which recognizes and supports other physician-scientists within the Cleveland academic community.

4.7 Partnerships for Impacting Neurodegenerative Diseases

Since its inception, the Harrington Discovery Institute has recognized the critical need for new and novel technologies for treating neurodegenerative disease. Starting with two of the first cohort of Harrington Scholar-Innovators, the Harrington Discovery Institute has now supported over 30 projects aiming to improve brain health (Figure 4.3). The institute expanded its commitment to this critical area of unmet need by first partnering with the ADDF and later by launching the Harrington Discovery Institute Neurotherapeutics Center, which focuses on discovering new ways to protect the brain from mental illness and neurodegenerative disease, including AD. In 2014, the Harrington Discovery Institute and ADDF created the Harrington–ADDF Scholar program in order to leverage the Harrington Discovery Institute model to provide a meaningful paradigm-shifting impact in therapeutic development of disease-modifying therapies in AD. The goal was to support research on novel targets for AD and to advance the development of therapeutic interventions against those targets toward candidates for clinical studies. Of the 12 Harrington Discovery Institute-supported scientists to date with a specific focus on AD, 9 have received support through this joint program (Table 4.1). The most advanced example of the success of this program is represented by ADDF–Harrington Scholar Dr. Jerri Rook, PhD of Vanderbilt University. Together with collaborator Dr. Paul Newhouse of Vanderbilt University Medical Center, Dr. Rook has progressed the discovery of a novel small-molecule highly selective positive allosteric modulator of the muscarinic M1 receptor drug candidate, VU319, into clinical trials. Specifically, her 2015 ADDF–Harrington award supported critical early safety pharmacology and toxicology studies, which enabled a first-in-human Phase 1 clinical safety study in 2017 [13]. TDC advisor expertise was critical for the formulation and interpretation of safety pharmacology and toxicology data, and in 2020 ACADIA Pharmaceuticals acquired exclusive worldwide rights to VU319.

In addition, Harrington Discovery Institute programs and partnerships in neurotherapeutics development with a primary focus on rare diseases are anticipated to yield medical interventions that work through mechanisms that may also have therapeutic benefit for patients with AD. For example, in 2017, the Harrington Discovery Institute announced a call for applications in partnership with Takeda Pharmaceutical Company, with a particular emphasis on novel approaches to neurological, oncological, and gastrointestinal diseases. Eight academic investigators were selected in 2018 as Harrington Rare Disease Scholars, including several whose technology was potentially applicable broadly in neuroprotection and AD (Table 4.1).

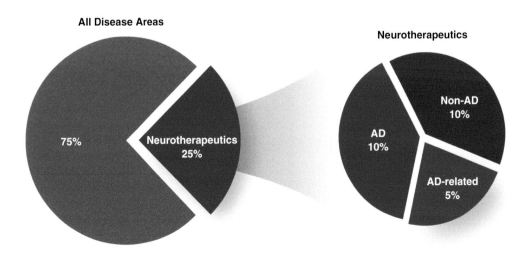

All Disease Areas

75%

Neurotherapeutics
25%

Neurotherapeutics

Non-AD
10%

AD
10%

AD-related
5%

Figure 4.3 Harrington Discovery Institute emphasizes Neurotherapeutics.

Table 4.1 Selected Harrington Discovery Institute scholars in AD and AD-related (ADR) projects

Name	Institution	Harrington Discovery Institute program	Year	Project title	AD vs. ADR	Harrington Discovery Institute advisor expertise accessed
Colton, Carol	Duke University	ADDF–Harrington	2015	Slowing arginine utilization by inhibiting arginase	AD	Target validation and preclinical proof of concept
Diamond, Marc	University of Texas, Southwestern	Scholar-Innovator	2013	Development of new treatments for Alzheimer's Disease	AD	Medicinal chemistry
Dunckley, Travis	Arizona State University	ADDF–Harrington	2016	Testing of selective DYRK1A inhibitors as a novel treatment for AD	AD	Medicinal chemistry
Ganesh, Thota	Emory University	ADDF–Harrington	2014	EP2 antagonists for the suppression of inflammation and neuropathology in Alzheimer's model	AD	Pharmacokinetics/ pharmacodynamics, toxicology
Hodgetts, Kevin	The Brigham & Women's Hospital	ADDF–Harrington	2018	Novel benzoxazines for the treatment of AD	AD	Medicinal chemistry
Lin, Chien-liang	Ohio State University	ADDF–Harrington	2014	Development of small-molecule activators of glutamate transporter EAAT2	AD	Target validation, medicinal chemistry
Perez, Dianne	Cleveland Clinic Foundation	ADDF–Harrington	2017	Optimization of novel positive allosteric modulators of the alpha 1A-adrenergic receptor to treat AD	AD	Medicinal chemistry, proof-of-concept study design
Rook, Jerri	Vanderbilt University	ADDF–Harrington	2015	Development of novel M1 PAMs	AD	Formulation, IND-enabling studies
Strittmatter, Stephen	Yale University	Scholar-Innovator	2020	Prion protein antagonist for AD and Creutzfeldt–Jakob disease	AD	Medicinal chemistry
Trushina, Eugenia	Mayo Clinic	ADDF–Harrington	2019	Development of small-molecule modulators of mitochondrial function	AD	Medicinal chemistry
Weaver, Donald	University Health Network	Scholar-Innovator	2020	Targeting immunopathy to treat AD	AD	Medicinal chemistry
Yoon, Sung Ok	Ohio State University	ADDF–Harrington	2016	Discovery and preclinical development of isoform selective JNK inhibitors for AD	AD	Medicinal chemistry, proof-of-concept study design
Letterio, John	Case Western Reserve University	Scholar-Innovator	2017	Design and development of the first highly specific bisubstrate inhibitors of CDK5	ADR	Compound design, manufacturing
Dorn, Gerald	Washington University	Scholar-Innovator	2019	Small-molecule mitofusin agonists to treat Charcot Marie Tooth and other neurodegenerative diseases	ADR	Medicinal chemistry, preclinical planning, IND-enabling studies
Gould, Todd	University of Maryland	Scholar-Innovator	2017	(2R, 6R)-Hydroxynorketamine for the treatment of major depressive disorder	ADR	Preclinical planning, IND-enabling studies

Table 4.1 (cont.)

Name	Institution	Harrington Discovery Institute program	Year	Project title	AD vs. ADR	Harrington Discovery Institute advisor expertise accessed
Ichida, Justin	University of Southern California	Harrington Rare Disease	2018	Validation of PIKFYVE inhibition as a therapeutic target for amyotrophic lateral sclerosis	ADR	In vivo model study design, ASO design
Marshall, John	Brown University	Harrington Rare Disease	2018	Early-phase clinical development of a lead cyclic-PDZ-enhancer drug for Angelman syndrome	ADR	Compound design, manufacturing
Qi, Xin	Case Western Reserve University	Harrington Rare Disease	2018	Identification of mitochondrial functional enhancers as candidate therapeutics for Huntington's disease	ADR	Medicinal chemistry, target validation
Shayman, James	University of Michigan	Harrington Rare Disease	2018	Brain penetrant glucosylceramide synthase inhibitors for the treatment of central nervous system-based glycosphingolipidoses	ADR	Medicinal chemistry, candidate selection

Finally, in 2018, the University of Oxford, UK, and University Hospitals Cleveland Medical Center announced an affiliation to form the Oxford–Harrington Rare Disease Centre (OHC), which leverages combined resources from the two institutions to advance drug discovery projects for cures and therapies in rare disease. The OHC focuses on three themes: neurotherapeutics, oncology, and developmental diseases, and it takes a strategic approach to selecting drug-development projects with potential for a broad impact beyond their initial rare indications. In this regard, new technologies in neuroprotection are of particular interest. To date, the Harrington Scholar-Innovator, ADDF–Harrington, and Neurotherapeutics Center programs have supported 12 scientists in the field of AD drug development (Table 4.1).

4.8 The Harrington Discovery Institute Process

There are two unique but intimately related considerations in meeting the challenge of translating academic discovery science to the clinic. First: What makes a good drug? Academic scientists are well trained to test a hypothesis on mechanistic insight into unique biological processes and paradigms. However, these are not the only questions that need to be addressed when making a medicine. Second: What is required to obtain capital investment in a project aiming to develop a new therapeutic? This latter question becomes increasingly important the closer a discovery gets to the clinic, as the costs increase exponentially. The Harrington Discovery Institute aims to align scholars on both of these considerations, from the earliest steps in the drug-development process, through supporting both science and commercial translation.

4.9 Scientific Support through the Harrington Discovery Institute

Each scientist's experience with the Harrington Discovery Institute is uniquely shaped by their own personal experiences, their home-institutional support, and the near-term goal for their discovery. The first step for any project supported by the Harrington Discovery Institute's TDC is to deploy standard project management tools to enable a comprehensive evaluation of the status of the discovery technology and identify areas where TDC advisors can help. TDC leadership assigns project managers and specific advisors to the scientists (usually a team of three to four per program), matching their background and scientific training to the type and stage of the technology. These individuals effectively become the scientist's own team, and together they undertake a deep evaluation of the existing science in order to construct a translation roadmap for reaching the clinical steps of testing a new medicine. The key question that drives this process is: "What is needed to get to the clinic?" Thus, Harrington Discovery Institute-supported scientists benefit from key know-how and operational experience in real time.

Importantly, the Harrington Discovery Institute implements a diverse portfolio-based platform with strategically defined milestones that either advance or terminate the program. Harrington Discovery Institute-supported scientists typically meet with their Harrington Discovery Institute project management team by teleconference or videoconference on a monthly basis for guidance and updates. The meeting agendas cover such topics as: structure–activity relationship studies to optimize therapeutic potency and efficacy while minimizing potential side effects, dosing formulation for optimal human exposure, generation and protection of new intellectual property, preclinical toxicity analysis, pharmacokinetics and pharmacodynamics, and the composition of an application package to present to the United States Food and Drug Administration for Investigational New Drug (IND) status. Importantly, 100% of any contribution to intellectual property provided through this process remains with the academic inventor's institution

4.10   Commercial Translation

A typical challenge for most scientists is understanding the key value inflection points in their program and how they will be viewed by potential investors. In addition to scientific drug-development support, the Harrington Discovery Institute and its TDC also help the scientist and their home institution's technology transfer office attract business partners and capital investment. Scientists in Harrington Discovery Institute scholar programs benefit from commercial analysis and strategy for the anticipated new drug, business development support, and professional coaching on how to pitch the project idea to investors and plan for diligence activities for licensing negotiation. Furthermore, Harrington Discovery Institute scholars are connected with mission-aligned for-profit partners within the Harrington Project. Together, the access to investment and pharmaceutical industry know-how

and the application of a rigorous value-incurring approach to drug development and business strategy strategically address the major challenges encountered in the academic environment. Importantly, the Harrington Discovery Institute proactively collaborates with the scientist's home-institution technology transfer office to work toward successful commercialization of an asset, again with all intellectual property remaining with the scientist and their home institution. Through its innovative approach, the Harrington Discovery Institute is thus bridging the translational gap to bring new medicines to patients, with keen and growing focus on AD.

4.11   Portfolio Approach

As outlined above, the dearth of new drug approvals for AD and related dementias does not reflect a lack of dedication in the field to conducting clinical trials [5]. Rather, the more than 200 clinical trials in AD to date have been too narrowly focused on presumed disease mechanisms. In order to increase the likelihood of breakthrough discoveries succeeding in the future, it is important for mission-driven organizations such as the Harrington Discovery Institute and ADDF to develop a broad set of supported discovery projects that are diversified and non-correlated. Thus, the ADDF–Harrington Discovery Institute partnership has invested in multiple new projects each year and has assembled a mechanistically diverse portfolio. Further, the ADDF–Harrington Discovery Institute program and the Harrington Discovery Institute Neurotherapeutics Center provide strategic oversight on a project-by-project basis, from selection informed by the latest scientific insights to co-investments in projects that meet critical developmental milestones.

4.12   Conclusions

Within universities, foundations, and philanthropic ventures, new and exciting potential cures to neurodegenerative diseases like AD are within reach, but not yet attained. Breakthrough technologies discovered by today's academic researcher could be advanced through a multitude of development partner options available. For example, traditional big pharmaceutical partnerships, venture capital investment, and local and national accelerator/development groups can all help advance a program once a licensing agreement is secured. However, it can be hard to know when and where to start the partnership quest. The field of AD is emblematic of this challenge and opportunity. The Harrington Discovery Institute is bridging the "valley of death" through its unique not-for-profit and for-profit partnership model for potential new drugs. Pharma-experienced advisors help the scientist by providing industry know-how to build value through de-risking their cutting-edge scientific discoveries. Business-oriented experts provide guidance on when, where, and how to approach partnering activities, and for-profit opportunity necessary to commercialize technology is identified. By applying the model to projects in partnership with non-profit partners such as ADDF, and building the Neurotherapeutics Center, the Harrington Discovery Institute is developing a diversified portfolio of new drug candidates for patients suffering from AD.

References

1. Gardner RC, Valcour V, Yaffe K. Dementia in the oldest old: a multi-factorial and growing public health issue. *Alzheimers Res Ther* 2013; **5**: 27.

2. Corrada MM, Berlau DJ, Kawas CH. A population-based clinicopathological study in the oldest-old: the 90+ study. *Curr Alzheimer Res* 2012; **9**: 709–17.

3. Alzheimer A. Über eine eigenartige Erkrankung der Hirnrinde. *Allg Z Psychiat* 1907; **64**: 146–8.

4. Fischer O. Miliare Nekrosen mit drusigen Wucherungen der Neurofibrillen, eine regelmässige Veränderung der Hirnrinde bei seniler Demenz. *Monatsschr Psychiatr Neurol* 1907; **22**: 361–72.

5. Cummings JL, Morstorf T, Zhong K. Alzheimer's disease drug-development pipeline: few candidates, frequent failures. *Alzheimers Res Ther* 2014; **6**: 37.

6. Allgaier M, Allgaier C. An update on drug treatment options of Alzheimer's disease. *Front Biosci* 2014; **19**: 1345–54.

7. Braak H, Braak E. Neuropathological stageing of Alzheimer-related changes. *Acta Neuropathol* 1991; **82**: 239–59.

8. Mirra SS, Heyman A, McKeel D, et al. The Consortium to Establish a Registry for Alzheimer's Disease (CERAD). Part II. Standardization of the neuropathologic assessment of Alzheimer's disease. *Neurology* 1991; **41**: 479–86.

9. Haroutunian V, Schnaider-Beeri M, Schmeidler J, et al. Role of the neuropathology of Alzheimer disease in dementia in the oldest-old. *Arch Neurol* 2008; **65**: 1211–17.

10. Boyle PA, Yu L, Wilson RS, et al. Person-specific contribution of neuropathologies to cognitive loss in old age. *Ann Neurol* 2018; **83**: 74–83.

11. Voorhees JR, Remy MT, McDaniel LM, et al. P7C3 compounds protect a rat model of Alzheimer's disease from cognitive decline, depressive-like behavior, and neuronal cell death without affecting neuroinflammation or amyloid–tau pathology. *Biol Psychiatry* 2018; **84**: 488–98.

12. DiMasi JA, Grabowski HG, Hansen RW. Innovation in the pharmaceutical industry: new estimates of R&D costs. *J Health Econ* 2016; **47**: 20–33.

13. Conley A, Key A, Blackford J, et al. Functional activity of the muscarinic positive allosteric modulator VU319 during a Phase 1 single ascending dose study. *Am J Geriatr Psychiatry* 2020; **28**: S114–15.

Repurposed Agents in Alzheimer's Disease Drug Development

Clive Ballard and Janet Sultana

5.1 Introduction

Drug repositioning concerns the development of a drug for an indication other than that in the marketing authorization, and drug repurposing is the use of known drugs for new indications. Both repositioning and repurposing are opportunities to complement traditional drug development and may shorten the time for a drug to reach the patient. Drug repurposing was key for the novel use of several drugs in various diseases, including cancer (e.g., thalidomide) and Parkinson's disease (e.g., amandatine). An important benefit of repurposing is that there is already a body of pre-marketing, and often, post-marketing, safety information available. There would also likely be no need for toxicology studies. Taken together, this available evidence, along with the results achieved regarding formulation and manufacturing, significantly reduces the costs and time of bringing successful treatments to the clinic.

5.2 Promising Pharmacological Agents

Expert Delphi consensuses were completed in 2012 and 2020, identifying the most promising candidates for repurposing as treatments for Alzheimer's disease (AD) or mild cognitive impairment (MCI). These drugs include fasudil, phenserine, antiviral drugs, and glucagon-like peptide 1 (GLP-1) analogs [1, 2]. The key factors used to identify drug candidates included biological plausibility, blood–brain-barrier (BBB) penetration and safety profile, including whether dosages used in preclinical studies would be safe in humans. In terms of efficacy, preclinical, clinical, and epidemiological evidence was considered.

5.2.1 Fasudil

Fasudil is a selective rho-kinase (ROCK) 1 and 2 inhibitor and has significant central nervous system (CNS) vasodilator properties. It is predicted to cross the BBB. Fasudil is licensed for cerebral vasospasm after subarachnoid hemorrhage in Japan and in China. There are several pharmacological mechanisms of interest in an AD context, including fasudil's ability to promote the dephosphorylation (inactivation) of LIM domain kinase 2 (LIMK2) and downstream dephosphorylation (activation) of cofilin/actin-depolymerizing factors, which have been associated with the maintenance of synapse structure and function [3]. Fasudil has also been found to protect neurons against the neurotoxic effects of amyloid beta (Aβ) [4], to reduce the deposition of Aβ, and to reduce levels of beta-secretase [5]. Overall, fasudil can be said to have multifaceted pharmacological properties that lend themselves well to a disease with a complex and multifaceted pathophysiology such as AD.

5.2.1.1 Preclinical Studies

In vivo, fasudil decreased tau phosphorylation in a cell model of tauopathy [6] and prevented synaptic loss due to Aβ [4]. Fasudil also modulates microglial activation, which is known to play a role in AD neuropathology [7] and reduces oxidative stress [8]. In vivo, fasudil has been found to reduce Aβ levels in triple transgenic AD mice [9] and to improve memory in amyloid precursor protein (APP)/presenilin 1(PS1) transgenic mice [10] as well as other mouse models of AD.

One of the main strengths of this body of preclinical evidence is that fasudil consistently improves learning and memory in a range of AD mouse models. These mouse models were also useful in demonstrating that fasudil crosses the BBB in AD and that the observed beneficial effects on cognition are supported by plausible mechanisms.

5.2.1.2 Clinical Studies

Fourteen randomized placebo-controlled trials have been reported using fasudil, with a total number of more than 500 patients with treatment indications ranging from coronary heart disease to pulmonary hypertension. Good tolerability has been reported with doses between 60 mg and 120 mg per day [11, 12]. One clinical trial of an extended release formulation of fasudil in seriously ill patients with pulmonary arterial hypertension [13] reported two serious adverse events in 12 patients receiving active treatment, one with renal impairment and one with heart failure leading to death. There is only one trial focusing on cognition [14], conducted in 106 people with MCI treated with nimodipine, who were randomly allocated to 30 mg fasudil intravenously (IV) or placebo for 3 months. Fasudil had a good tolerability profile and significant benefits were reported on the Mini-Mental State Examination (MMSE). The results are encouraging but need to be interpreted cautiously given the modest sample size and short duration.

5.2.1.3 Observational Studies

Fasudil has been used extensively in Japan and China, with safety reports suggesting good tolerability. There are currently no observational studies investigating the impact of fasudil on cognition or dementia in real-world populations.

5.2.2 Phenserine

Phenserine is a highly selective, reversible acetylcholinesterase (AChE) inhibitor with additional pharmacological properties compared to currently available AChEs such as donepezil and galantamine. Indeed, phenserine also has anti-amyloid activity, which is thought to confer disease-modifying effects in AD. Phenserine acts at the post-transcriptional phase at the level of the 5′-untranslated region of the APP messenger RNA to decrease APP translational efficiency and, as a result, decreases Aβ levels in mouse models of AD [15]. It is predicted to cross the BBB. It is currently not available commercially in any country. As a result, there are some lacunae considering the large-scale safety of this drug as well as pharmaceutical aspects such as ideal formulation, dosing regimen, and manufacturing processes. Generally speaking, the available preclinical and clinical information concerning phenserine can be considered to be much more limited compared to fasudil.

5.2.2.1 Preclinical Studies

Phenserine was found to decrease Aβ levels [16] and to inhibit AChE [17] in vitro. Phenserine increased neuron proliferation, reduced $A\beta_{1-42}$ levels in triple-transgenic AD mice, and increased

dendritic arborization in younger mice with mild neurodegeneration and decreased inflammatory markers in older mice with a higher plaque burden [18]. In this same mouse model, another study showed that phenserine promotes neurogenesis in the presence of brain-derived neurotrophic factor (BDNF) [19]. Phenserine also reduced APP levels in vivo, increasing neurogenesis and suppressing gliosis in APP transgenic mice [20].

While the available preclinical evidence consistently points toward the benefit of phenserine in AD, there is only one study which specifically investigates cognition as an outcome, which is a limitation. Another limitation is the lack of diversity in the murine AD models used. On the other hand, the published studies are very useful in providing several overlapping but distinct biological mechanisms to support the use of phenserine in AD. They also suggest that phenserine is well tolerated.

5.2.2.2 Clinical Studies

Phenserine was initially developed and evaluated as a AChE inhibitor, which is reflected in the clinical trial designs. Two Phase 2 trials have been conducted comparing phenserine to placebo in people with mild-to-moderate AD. A Phase 2, 12-week randomized controlled trial (RCT) in 164 patients reported a good tolerability profile and indicated that phenserine conferred significant benefits on cognitive function. There was no significant benefit in global outcome, although there was a numerical advantage for phenserine and this needs to be interpreted in the context of the limited power of Phase 2 trials to examine global and functional outcomes in dementia studies [15, 21], There were no direct measures of biomarker outcomes, and the duration of the study was too short to examine the potential impact of any disease-modifying properties of phenserine. Over 12 weeks, the Cohen's d effect sizes of 0.3–0.4 are similar to the symptomatic benefits reported for other AChE inhibitors. A second smaller RCT compared 20 patients randomized equally to phenserine or placebo for 3 months. The placebo group then received donepezil after 12 weeks in an open design. Participants receiving phenserine had significantly greater improvements in cognition and cerebral glucose metabolism compared to those receiving placebo. The duration of the trial is again too short to evaluate any disease-modifying effects, and cautious interpretation is needed given the small sample size. A subsequent Phase 3 trial was discontinued early for commercial reasons, having only recruited 284 participants and using doses of 10–15 mg, which are probably suboptimal. These results have not been reported in full but there was no significant benefit on the primary outcome measure [22].

Overall, there is some encouragement to suggest some symptomatic benefits upon 3 months of treatment with phenserine, but the short duration of trials and the absence of biomarker data makes it difficult to make any inferences about potential disease-modifying effects.

5.2.2.3 Observational Studies

Phenserine is not a licensed drug, and there are hence no observational studies concerning phenserine in an AD/MCI context.

5.2.3 Antiviral Drugs

Some antiviral drugs used in herpes simplex virus (HSV), specifically aciclovir, famciclovir, and valaciclovir, have been highlighted as being of potential interest in AD. All three drugs are commercially available. It is not known if aciclovir crosses the BBB, but it has been suggested that this is unlikely as aciclovir is lipophobic, a physicochemical property that does not favor BBB penetration. Famciclovir and valaciclovir are predicted to cross the BBB. HSV type 1 (HSV-1) is found in an active form in the brains of a large number of elderly people. It has also been suggested that HSV-1 may induce the deposition of amyloid plaques and neurofibrillary tangles in the brain; these are hallmarks of AD.

5.2.3.1 Preclinical Studies

There is limited information on the benefits or safety of antiviral drugs in a preclinical setting when used for AD. In primary adult mouse hippocampal neurons infected with HSV-1, aciclovir reduced but did not prevent the accumulation of Aβ [23]. Aciclovir, penciclovir, and foscarnet reduced Aβ and hyperphosphorylated-tau (p-tau) build-up, as well as HSV-1 load in a human osteosarcoma cell line, while foscarnet was less effective [24]. There are no studies in murine models of AD. The available preclinical evidence suggests that there are plausible biological mechanisms by which antiviral drugs may act in AD and both the available studies are in favor of antiviral drugs.

However, it is a limitation that there is no information on how these drugs affect cognition in murine models of AD.

5.2.3.2 Clinical Studies

There are no fully reported clinical trials focusing on people with AD or related conditions. A small open-label study of 33 patients with AD has recently been completed in Sweden, focusing on cerebrospinal fluid (CSF) and positron emission tomography (PET) biomarkers, but no results have yet been reported (ClinicalTrials.gov, ID: NCT02997982). There is also an ongoing Phase 2 study of valaciclovir underway, led by Columbia University in New York. The study aims to recruit 130 participants with mild AD, focusing on cognitive and biomarker outcomes (NCT03282916).

5.2.3.3 Observational Studies

There are three observational studies that investigate the protective effect of antiviral drugs against dementia, all of which use large claims databases. A retrospective cohort study identified over 8,000 persons with HSV from the Taiwan National Health Insurance Research Database and matched them on age and sex to controls without HSV [25]. HSV infection was associated with a significantly higher 2.5-fold risk of dementia. However, the use of anti-herpetic medications reduced this risk. Another retrospective cohort study used the same database to identify patients with new herpes zoster, identifying almost 40,000 persons with herpes zoster [26]. This study confirmed the association between HSV and dementia and the reduced risk of dementia after treatment with antiviral agents. The third study is also a retrospective cohort study using the South Korean National Health Insurance Service–National Sample Cohort [27]. This study identified over 34,000 persons with HSV, finding that these patients had a higher risk of dementia compared to persons without HSV. In line with the previous two studies, treatment with antiviral drugs had a protective effect against dementia.

It is of interest that all three studies with similar methodologies and data sources all point to the same protective effect of antiviral drugs against dementia. Such studies have very large population sizes and reflect clinical practice, making them very useful. On the other hand, although some methods such as the propensity score matching method attempt to mimic randomization, confounding remains an issue in observational studies.

5.2.4 Glucagon-Like Peptide 1 Receptor Agonists

The GLP-1 receptor agonists exenatide and liraglutide were identified as having potential for repurposing in AD as far back as 2012 [2]. Both drugs are available commercially. Liraglutide and exenatide cross the BBB and act on the APP and other pathways of relevance to AD, such as inflammation and tau phosphorylation.

5.2.4.1 Preclinical Studies

In diabetic mice, exenatide reduced tau hyperphosphorylation in the hippocampus [28]. It also reduced APP levels in cultured neurons and ex vivo in diabetic mouse brains [29]. In wild-type (tau(+/+)) and tau knockout (tau(−/−)) mice, exenatide restored BDNF levels and rescued axonal transport [30]. In male C57BL/6 mice, exenatide administered intranasally improved cognition [31]. Exenatide also improved cognition in mice treated with streptozotocin [32]. It also improved cognition in APP/PS1 [33] but not in triple-transgenic AD mice [33]. Liraglutide reduced astrogliosis in this same mouse model [34] and improved cognition in mice injected intracerebroventricularly with $A\beta_{1-42}$ [35] as well as in other mice models, including senescence-accelerated mouse prone 8 (SAMP8) mice, in mice injected intracerebroventricularly with streptozotocin, and in APP/PS1 mice.

Overall, the preclinical studies concerning liraglutide and exenatide all suggest a beneficial effect on cognition in AD, spanning several different mouse models. Since both drugs are available commercially, the lack of information on safety outcomes in a preclinical setting is not a significant limitation as there is a body of clinical/observational pre- and post-marketing studies.

5.2.4.2 Clinical Studies

Several preliminary studies have examined the impact of GLP-1 receptor agonists in people with AD, indicating potential benefit. A small 6-month placebo-controlled RCT in 38 patients with AD suggested that liraglutide (1.8 mg/day, subcutaneous injection) conferred benefits compared to placebo in reducing the decline in glucose metabolism on fluorodeoxyglucose PET [36]. A larger Phase 2 RCT of 200 patients has been presented at a conference but not yet fully reported, but the results are promising and indicate a significant benefit on cognition compared to placebo [37]. A further 18-month double-blind RCT of exenatide in 21 participants did not identify any benefits on clinical, cognitive, neuroimaging, or CSF measures, but is very difficult to interpret given the very small sample size. In a further analysis of exploratory biomarkers, a reduction of $A\beta_{42}$ in extracellular neuronal vesicles extracted from plasma was reported in patients receiving exenatide compared to placebo-treated patients [38].

A further cluster of trials provide additional supportive evidence from the evaluation of secondary outcomes focused on cognition in RCTs examining cardiovascular outcomes in patients with diabetes. For example, an exploratory analysis of the Researching cardiovascular Events with a Weekly Incretin in Diabetes (REWIND) 5-year trial of 8,828 people over 50 with type 2 diabetes and cardiovascular risk suggested that dulaglutide conferred cognitive benefits compared to placebo, with MCI occurring at a rate of 4·05 per 100 patient-years in participants treated with dulaglutide and 4·35 per 100 patient-years in people receiving placebo, with a 14% reduction in the hazard of substantive cognitive impairment in those assigned dulaglutide (hazard ratio [HR] 0·86, 95% confidence interval [CI]: 0·79–0·95; $p = 0.0018$) [39]. A similar study reported as a conference abstract compared incident dementia between patients taking liraglutide or semaglutide compared to placebo from three double-blind RCTs examining cardiovascular outcomes in more than 15,000 people with type 2 diabetes (LEADER, SUSTAIN 6, PIONEER 6) followed up for a median of 3.6 years, with an estimated HR of 0.47 (95% CI: 0.25–0.86) in favor of the GLP-1 treatment [40]. The findings are encouraging but need to be interpreted cautiously, and the full publication is awaited with interest.

Overall, there is promising emerging evidence both from small Phase 2 studies of GLP-1 agonists in people with AD, supported by exploratory analyses of large Phase 2 trials in people with type 2 diabetes examining cognition or dementia as a secondary outcome. Whilst there are important caveats for the interpretation of each individual study, it is a convincing body of evidence and appears to clearly merit a Phase 3 RCT.

5.2.4.3 Observational Studies

A recent conference abstract presented data indicating a reduction in the incidence of dementia in people with type 2 diabetes treated with GLP-1 analogs compared to people receiving treatments at a comparable stage of the treatment pathway [40]. The full publication of the results is awaited.

5.3 Future Developments

5.3.1 Transcriptional Approaches to Drug Repositioning in AD

To identify novel compounds for repurposing or repositioning, additional strategies are needed. One such approach is transcriptional profiling. A disease or injury will alter gene expression in a characteristic manner in a cell or tissue, which will produce a "transcriptional signature." A transcriptional hypothesis proposes that a drug altering the transcriptome in an opposing manner to the disease may have a therapeutic benefit by counteracting potential pathological pathways. The Connectivity Map (CMAP) collaboration produced transcriptional signatures or 1,300 drugs or natural compound profiled on three cancer cell lines [41]. CMAP has been complemented by the Library of Integrated Network-based Cellular Signatures (LINCS) program, which examined changes in 1,000 "landmark" transcripts for an additional 20,000 compounds, using algorithms to impute changes in expression of transcripts that were not quantified directly [42].

Transcriptional profiles are widely published and available through meta-analysis platforms such as SPIED for early, mid, and late stages of AD and other dementias, and for preclinical mouse models [43]. Using this approach in CMAP, 153 drugs were identified with signatures that significantly inversely correlate with the AD transcription signature, the majority of which retained this profile in further studies using human induced pluripotent stem cell-derived cortical neurons [44]. Based on these studies, the top 78 candidate drugs were taken forward to an in vitro screening program with six independent assays evaluating the impact on different aspects of AD pathology. Nineteen (24%) of the agents were hits in at least two assays, with 15 being novel or emerging candidates known or likely to be brain penetrant (some examples are shown in Table 5.1). Importantly, in addition to identifying novel candidates for

further evaluation, this supports the hypothesis that transcriptional profiling may be a useful way of identifying or triaging compounds for in vitro screening. Other hits included drugs already highlighted as potential repositioning candidates in AD, including metformin, nabumetone, and several flavonoids.

The global transcriptional signatures identified above were generated without considering the functions of the individual transcripts or the established mechanism of drug action. In other words, this is a "black-box" approach that operates independently of any mechanism-based hypothesis. Almost 30 risk genes have now been identified for AD [45], and the identification of drugs that alter the expression of some of these, or another endogenous gene with known therapeutic potential, provides for a hypothesis-driven approach to drug repositioning. There are no well-developed cases for this in AD yet, but there are promising emerging candidates for other neurodegenerative diseases using this approach [46, 47].

5.3.2 Targeting Risk Genes and Growth Factors

Rather than increasing the expression of a protective gene, other studies have sought to identify candidate drugs that reduce the expression of a risk gene. Although this approach has not yet been widely used for AD, there is an interesting recent example of this strategy for Parkinson's disease (PD) where reducing beta-synuclein transcription may have therapeutic benefits [48]. A screen of the Food and Drug Administration (FDA) library demonstrated that alpha-2-adrenergic agonists such as salbutamol suppress this transcription, and subsequent work has also suggested that salbutamol offers some protection in a preclinical model of PD [49]. Future clinical trials will be needed to verify this approach, but nonetheless similar approaches targeting risk genes in AD may offer a use strategy of identifying further candidate therapies.

5.4 Conclusion

Repurposing has proven useful in identifying novel drugs or novel indications for existing drugs in several diseases. The potential of repurposing in the context of AD is highlighted by the number of drugs being studied, including the documented targeted pharmacology and preclinical and clinical

Table 5.1 Examples of novel compounds emerging from a CMAP transcript analysis which were positive hits on at least two in vitro assays

Compound	Current use	BBB penetration	Novel	Safety	Drug–drug interactions	Proposed drug target
Imatinib	Tyrosine-kinase inhibitor	Yes	Yes	Side effects at dose used for chemotherapy	Risk with CYP3A4 inhibitors/inducers e.g. rifampicin	Kinase-independent inhibitor of the interaction between gamma-secretase and the gamma-secretase activating protein
Mitoxantrone	Anthracenedione antineoplastic agent	Unknown	Yes	Side effects at dose used for chemotherapy	Risk with anti-neoplastic agents, cardiotoxic drugs, and immunosupressants	Reduces/blocks $A\beta_{42}$ oligomerization, antifibrillogenic
Thiostrepton	Oligopeptide antibiotic	Unknown	Yes	Unknown	Unknown	Proteosome inhibition
Famotidine	Histamine H_2 receptor antagonist	Unknown	Yes	Good	None established	Histamine H_2 receptor inhibitor
Doxazosin mesylate	Adrenergic alpha-1 receptor antagonist	Yes	Yes	Possible hypotension	Avoid PDE-5 inhibitors	Potential antihypertensive effect in AD
Hexestrol	Non-steroidal estrogen	Unknown	No	Unknown	Unknown	Unknown, DNA/RNA interaction
Pyrantel	Antinematodal thiophene	Unknown	Yes	Unknown	Avoid AChE inhibitors, levamisole, piperazine	Nicotinic receptor agonist
Nabumetone	NSAID	Yes	No	Some GI/CV effects with long-term use	Possible interactions with anticoagulants etc., as for all NSAIDs	COX2 inhibitor

Abbreviations: AChE, acetylcholinesterase; AD, Alzheimer's disease; BBB, blood–brain barrier; COX2, cyclooxygenase 2; CV, cardio/cerebrovascular; CYP3A4, cytochrome P450 3A4; GI, gastrointestinal; NSAID, non-steroidal anti-inflammatory drug; PDE-5: phosphodiesterase-5.

benefits. The importance of repurposing in AD is highlighted by the high level of drug attrition seen in clinical trials, resulting in a lack of novel therapeutic options and reluctance by pharmaceutical companies in investing in drug development. The next 5–10 years will be critical in discovering whether the drugs currently being considered for repurposing in AD will be used in clinical practice. It is, however, certain that the clinical and commercial value of repurposing in AD is increasingly clear.

References

1. Ballard C, Aarsland D, Cummings J, et al. Drug repositioning and repurposing for Alzheimer disease. *Nat Rev Neurol* 2020; **16**: 661–73.

2. Corbett A, Pickett J, Burns A, et al. Drug repositioning for Alzheimer's disease. *Nat Rev Drug Discov* 2012; **11**: 833–46.

3. Hou Y, Zhou L, Yang QD, et al. Changes in hippocampal synapses and learning-memory abilities in a streptozotocin treated rat model and intervention by using fasudil hydrochloride. *Neuroscience* 2012; **200**: 120–9.

4. Rush T, Martinez-Hernandez J, Dollmeyer M, et al. Synaptotoxicity in Alzheimer's disease involved a dysregulation of actin cytoskeleton dynamics through cofilin 1 phosphorylation. *J Neurosci* 2018; **38**: 10349–61.

5. Yu JZ, Li YH, Liu CY, et al. Multitarget therapeutic effect of fasudil in APP/PS1transgenic mice. *CNS Neurol Disord Drug Targets* 2017; **16**: 199–209.

6. Hamano T, Shirafuji N, Yen SH, et al. Rho-kinase ROCK inhibitors reduce oligomeric tau protein. *Neurobiol Aging* 2020; **89**: 41–54.

7. Zhang X, Ye P, Wang D, et al. Involvement of RhoA/ROCK signaling in Aβ-induced chemotaxis, cytotoxicity and inflammatory response of

microglial BV2 cells. *Cell Mol Neurobiol* 2019; **39**: 637–50.

8. Chen J, Sun Z, Jin M, et al. Inhibition of AGEs/RAGE/Rho/ROCK pathway suppresses non-specific neuroinflammation by regulating BV2 microglial M1/M2 polarization through the NF-κB pathway. *J Neuroimmunol* 2017; **305**: 108–14.

9. Elliott C, Rojo AI, Ribe E, et al. A role for APP in Wnt signalling links synapse loss with β-amyloid production. *Transl Psychiatry* 2018; **8**: 179.

10. Guo MF, Zhang HY, Li YH, et al. Fasudil inhibits the activation of microglia and astrocytes of transgenic Alzheimer's disease mice via the downregulation of TLR4/Myd88/NF-κB pathway. *J Neuroimmunol* 2020; **346**: 577284.

11. Vicari RM, Chaitman B, Keefe D, et al.; Fasudil study group. Efficacy and safety of fasudil in patients with stable angina: a double-blind, placebo-controlled, phase 2 trial. *J Am Coll Cardiol* 2005; **46**: 1803–11.

12. Kamei S, Oishi M, Takasu T. Evaluation of fasudil hydrochloride treatment for wandering symptoms in cerebrovascular dementia with ^{31}P-magnetic resonance spectroscopy and Xe-computed tomography. *Clin Neuropharmacol* 1996; **19**: 428–38.

13. Fukumoto Y, Yamada N, Matsubara H, et al. Double-blind, placebo-controlled clinical trial with a rho-kinase inhibitor in pulmonary arterial hypertension. *Circ J* 2013; **77**: 2619–25.

14. Yan B, Sun F, Duan L, et al. Curative effect of fasudil injection combined with nimodipine on Alzheimer disease of elderly patients. *J Clin Med Pract* 2011; **14**: 36.

15. Winblad B. Giacobini E. Frölich L. et al. Phenserine efficacy in Alzheimer's disease. *J Alzheimers Dis* 2010; **22**: 1201–8.

16. Lahiri DK, Alley GM, Tweedie D, et al. Differential effects of two hexahydropyrroloindole carbamate-based anticholinesterase drugs on the amyloid beta protein pathway involved in Alzheimer's disease. *Neuromol Med* 2007; **9**: 157–68.

17. Tabrez S, Damanhouri GA. Computational and kinetic studies of acetylcholine esterase inhibition by phenserine. *Curr Pharm Des* 2019; **25**: 2108–12.

18. Lilja AM, Röjdner J, Mustafiz T, et al. Age-dependent neuroplasticity mechanisms in Alzheimer Tg2576 mice following modulation of brain amyloid-β levels. *PLoS One* 2013; **8**: e58752.

19. Lilja AM, Luo Y, Yu QS, et al. Neurotrophic and neuroprotective actions of (−)- and (+)-phenserine, candidate drugs for Alzheimer's disease. *PLoS One* 2013; **8**: e54887.

20. Sugaya K, Kwak YD, Ohmitsu O, et al. Practical issues in stem cell therapy for Alzheimer's disease. *Curr Alzheimer Res* 2007; **4**: 370–7.

21. Greig NH, Sambamurti K, Yu QS, et al. An overview of phenserine tartrate, a novel acetylcholinesterase inhibitor for the treatment of Alzheimer's disease. *Curr Alzheimer Res* 2005; **2**: 281–90.

22. Schneider LS, Lahiri, DK. The perils of Alzheimer's drug development. *Curr Alzheimer Res* 2009; **6**: 77–8.

23. Powell-Doherty RD, Abbott ARN, Nelson LA, Bertke AS. Amyloid-β and p-tau anti-threat response to herpes simplex virus 1 infection in primary adult murine hippocampal neurons. *J Virol* 2020; **94**: e01874–19.

24. Wozniak MA, Frost AL, Preston CM, Itzhaki RF. Antivirals reduce the formation of key Alzheimer's disease molecules in cell cultures acutely infected with herpes simplex virus type 1. *PLoS One* 2011; **6**: e25152.

25. Tzeng NS, Chung CH, Lin FH, et al. Anti-herpetic medications and reduced risk of dementia in patients with herpes simplex virus infections: a nationwide, population based cohort study in Taiwan. *Neurotherapeutics* 2008; **15**: 417–29.

26. Chen VC, Wu SI, Huang KY, et al. Herpes zoster and dementia: a nationwide population-based cohort study. *J Clin Psychiatry* 2018; **79**: 16m11312;DOI: http://doi.org/10.4088/JCP.16m11312.

27. Bae S, Yun SC, Kim MC, et al. Association of herpes zoster with dementia and effect of antiviral therapy on dementia: a population-based cohort study. *Eur Arch Psychiatry Clin Neurosci* 2020;DOI: http://doi.org/10.1007/s00406-020-01157-4.

28. Xu W, Yang Y, Yuan G, et al. Exendin-4, a glucagon-like peptide-1 receptor agonist, reduces Alzheimer disease-associated tau hyperphosphorylation in the hippocampus of rats with type 2 diabetes. *J Investig Med* 2015; **63**: 267–72.

29. Perry T, Lahiri DK, Sambamurti K, et al. Glucagon-like peptide-1 decreases endogenous amyloid-beta peptide (Abeta) levels and protects hippocampal neurons from death induced by Abeta and iron. *J Neurosci Res* 2003; **72**: 603–12.

30. Takach O, Gill TB, Silverman MA. Modulation of insulin signaling rescues BDNF transport defects independent of tau in amyloid-β oligomer-treated hippocampal neurons. *Neurobiol Aging* 2015; **36**: 1378–82.

31. Wang X, Wang L, Xu Y, et al. Intranasal administration of exendin-4 antagonizes Aβ31-35-induced disruption of circadian rhythm and impairment of learning and memory. *Aging Clin Exp Res* 2016; **28**: 1259–66.

32. Solmaz V, Çınar BP, Yiğittürk G, et al. Exenatide reduces TNF-α expression and improves hippocampal neuron numbers and memory in streptozotocin treated rats. *Eur J Pharmacol* 2015; **765**: 482–7.

33. Bomba M, Ciavardelli D, Silvestri E, et al. Exenatide promotes cognitive enhancement and positive brain metabolic changes in PS1-KI mice but has no effects in 3×Tg-AD animals. *Cell Death Dis* 2013; **4**: e612.

34. Long-Smith CM, Manning S, McClean PL, et al. The diabetes drug liraglutide ameliorates aberrant insulin receptor localisation and signalling in parallel with decreasing both amyloid-β plaque and glial pathology in a mouse model of Alzheimer's disease. *Neuromol Med* 2013; **15**: 102–14.

35. Qi L, Ke L, Liu X, et al. Subcutaneous administration of liraglutide ameliorates learning and memory impairment by modulating tau hyperphosphorylation via the glycogen synthase kinase-3β pathway in an amyloid β protein induced Alzheimer disease mouse model. *Eur J Pharmacol* 2016; **15**: 23–32.

36. Gejl M, Brock B, Egefjord L, et al. Blood–brain glucose transfer in Alzheimer's disease: effect of GLP-1 analog treatment. *Sci Rep* 2017; **7**: 17490.

37. Edison P, Femminella G, Holmes C, et al. Evaluation of liraglutide in treatment for Alzheimer's disease. Clinical Trials in Alzheimer's Disease (CTAD) Congress, November 4–7, 2020.

38. Mullins RJ, Mustapic M, Chia CW, et al. A pilot study of exenatide actions in Alzheimer's disease. *Curr Alzheimer Res* 2019; **16**: 741–52.

39. Gerstein HC, Colhoun HM, Dagenais GR, et al Dulaglutide and cardiovascular outcomes in type 2 diabetes (REWIND): a double-blind, randomised placebo-controlled trial. *Lancet* 2019; **394**: 121–30.

40. Ballard C, Nørgaard CH, Friedrich S, et al. Liraglutide and semaglutide: pooled post-hoc analysis to evaluate risk of dementia in patients with type 2 diabetes. Alzheimer's Association International Conference, 2020.

41. Lamb J, Crawford ED, Peck D, et al. The Connectivity Map: using gene-expression signatures to connect small molecules, genes, and disease. *Science* 2006; **313**: 1929–35.

42. Subramanian A, Narayan R, Corsello SM, et al. A next generation connectivity map: L1000 platform and the first 1,000,000 profiles. *Cell* 2017; **171**: 1437–52.

43. Williams, G. SPIEDw: a searchable platform-independent expression database web tool. *BMC Genomics* 2013; **14**: 765.

44. Williams G, Gatt A, Clarke E, et al. Drug repurposing for Alzheimer's disease based on transcriptional profiling of human iPSC-derived cortical neurons. *Transl Psychiatry* 2019; **9**: 220.

45. Bertram, L, Tanzi RE. Alzheimer disease risk genes: 29 and counting. *Nat Rev Neurol* 2019; **15**: 191–2.

46. Rothstein JD, Patel S, Regan MR, et al. Beta-lactam antibiotics offer neuroprotection by increasing glutamate transporter expression. *Nature* 2005; **433**: 73–7.

47. Cudkowicz ME, Titus S, Kearney M, et al. Safety and efficacy of ceftriaxone for amyotrophic lateral sclerosis: a multi-stage, randomised, double-blind, placebo-controlled trial. *Lancet Neurol* 2014; **13**: 1083–91.

48. Singleton AB, Farrer M, Johnson J, et al. Alpha-synuclein locus triplication causes Parkinson's disease. *Science* 2003; **302**: 841.

49. Mittal S, Bjørnevik K, Im DS, et al. β$_2$-Adrenoreceptor is a regulator of the α-synuclein gene driving risk of Parkinson's disease. Science 2017; **357**: 891–8.

Chapter 6

Artificial Intelligence in Alzheimer's Drug Discovery

Feixiong Cheng and Jeffrey Cummings

6.1 Introduction

Alzheimer's disease (AD), first described in 1906 by Alois Alzheimer, is a highly prevalent and progressive neurodegenerative disorder with gradual cognitive decline and memory loss [1]. AD and AD-related dementias (AD/ADRD) are a major global health challenge, with 43.8 million affected people worldwide in 2016 [2, 3]. An estimated 6.2 million Americans age 65 and older are living with AD/ADRD today and the population of those with AD dementia in the United States is expected to be 13.6 million by 2060 [4]. New treatments for AD are needed but development programs have an attrition rate of 99.6% [5]. A recent study estimated that pharmaceutical companies spent $2.6 billion in 2015, up from $802 million in 2003, for the development of a US Food and Drug Administration (FDA)-approved new chemical entity [6]. The cost of development of drugs for AD is higher than this industry average. The increasing cost of drug development is due to the high failure rate of randomized control trials, especially for AD where pathobiological processes and biological risk factors are under-determined.

The rapid growth in computing power and memory storage, an unprecedented wealth of big data, and the development of advanced algorithms have led to significant breakthroughs in artificial intelligence (AI) [7]. AI-enabled solutions are emerging as crucial tools for transforming the process of improving small-molecule compound design and optimization; identifying drug mechanisms of action; revolutionizing the understanding of the disease variants/genes, pathways, and networks; developing actionable biomarkers for disease prognosis and progression; improving drug efficacy; and enhancing clinical trials design [8–10]. AI applications in drug discovery and development have already delivered new candidate therapeutics, in some cases in months rather than decades or years required for other approaches [8, 10]. If broadly applied to the drug discovery pipeline, AI strategies have the possibility of kick-starting the productivity of the entire research and development (R&D) process, which will help reduce attrition rates and costs for AD drug development. For example, AI has the potential to:

- **Reduce timelines for drug discovery and improve the efficiency of the research process.** The successful application of innovative AI technologies could accelerate the discovery and non-clinical stages significantly.

- **Enhance the accuracy of predictions of pharmacokinetics and pharmacodynamics (PK/PD) and the clinical efficacy of drugs.** Only 10% of drugs from Phase 1 are approved in Phase 3. Most failures are due to lack of efficacy and poor PK/PD properties. Accurate prediction of PK/PD and the efficacy of drugs before clinical trials using innovative AI technologies and big data approaches could save billions of dollars spent on drug development.

- **Improve the opportunities to diversify drug pipelines.** Big data and AI-driven modeling tools could increase the speed and precision of discovery and non-clinical testing of candidate therapeutic agents, opening up new research avenues and enabling more competitive R&D strategies.

In this chapter, we focus on AI technologies for specific domains in drug discovery, where they offer rapid and cost-effective solutions for therapeutic development in AD. We provide an overview of current AI tools and techniques (the toolbox) used in various stages of drug discovery and development (Figure 6.1), including machine learning (ML) and deep learning (DL), and we describe several examples of the application of AI for key AD pharmaceutical applications.

6.2 Big Data in AD Drug Discovery

Over the past few years, there has been a drastic increase in "omic" data generation, including genomics, transcriptomics, proteomics, lipidomics, and metabolomics, and data digitalization in

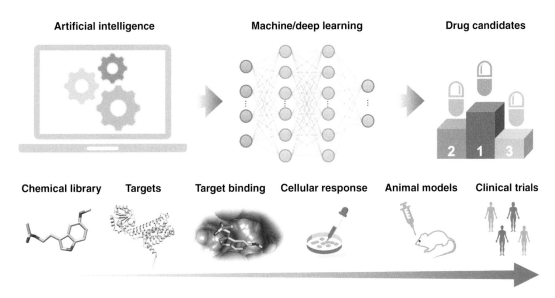

Figure 6.1 Overview of AI-assisted drug discovery for AD. AI can accelerate drug discovery through traditional ML and DL approaches. These approaches can guide the drug discovery pipeline utilizing biological knowledge and real-world evidence (e.g., animal models and electronic health records).

patient care and the pharmaceutical sectors. Yet, the availability of big data has prompted the emergence of multiple challenges for personalized diagnosis and treatment in the clinical settings for AD based on the FAIR (Findable, Accessible, Interoperable, and Reusable digital objects) principle. These challenges have motivated the use of multiple advanced AI and informatics tools to mimic human intelligence. Databases that collect and store high-throughput experimental data play crucial roles in development of AI-based solutions to identify novel drug targets, offer evidence for target–disease associations, and improve understanding of disease biology and drug mechanism of action for the treatment of AD. For instance, high-throughput DNA/RNA sequencing technologies have rapidly led to a robust body of genomic data in multiple national genome projects in AD, including the Alzheimer's Disease Sequencing Project (ADSP) [11] and the Alzheimer's Disease Neuroimaging Initiative (ADNI) [12]. The Genetics of Alzheimer's Disease Data Storage Site (NIAGADS, www.niagads.org), funded by the National Institute on Aging (NIA), is a national genetic and genomic data repository for AD. By June 2021, NIAGADS had collected 75 data sets, 90,644 samples, and 33,900,227,055 genotypes. The ADSP, launched in 2012, has sequenced and analyzed genomes to identify a wide range of AD risk or protective gene variants, including whole-exome sequencing

(WES) data from brain tissues (i.e., hippocampus and prefrontal cortex) from nearly 11,000 individuals and whole-genome sequencing (WGS) data of brain tissues from nearly 600 individuals [11]. The Accelerating Medicines Partnership® Program for Alzheimer's Disease (AMP® AD) concentrates on identifying novel, clinically relevant therapeutic targets and discovering biomarkers to validate existing therapeutic targets. The AMP® AD data and analysis results are stored in the AMP® AD Knowledge Portal (https://agora.ampadportal.org/genes), including various genomic, metabolomic, and proteomic data for over 15,000 individuals.

There are several commonly used drug-target databases, such as DrugBank [13] and DrugCentral [14]. DrugBank is a comprehensive database with detailed drug and target information. The current version of DrugBank (v5.1.2) includes 11,934 drug entries containing 3,736 approved drugs (2,542 small molecules), 130 nutraceuticals, and over 5,767 experimental drugs [13]. DrugCentral, an open-access online drug compendium, integrates structure, target, and indication information for 4,531 approved drugs (2,094 FDA-approved drugs and 2,437 ones approved by other regulatory agencies; 2018 release) [14]. Our group recently developed AlzGPS (Genome-wide Positioning Systems platform for Alzheimer's Therapeutic Discovery, https://alzgps.lerner.ccf.org), a comprehensive systems biology tool to enable searching, visualizing, and analyzing multi-omics, various types of biological networks, and clinical databases for target identification and effective prevention and treatment of AD [15]. AlzGPS provides a systemic evaluation of 3,000 FDA-approved or investigational drugs with mechanisms compared against over 100 multi-omics data sets [15].

6.3 AI Algorithms, Recent Advancements, and the Toolbox

6.3.1 Representation Learning

Multiple efforts have been made to integrate learning methods into the design of feature representations of the input data that make it easier to extract the useful information. For molecules, a critical one-dimensional (1D) representation is SMILES [16], a text notation for the topological information based on chemical bonding rules. There are multiple types of features that can be used to code molecules, including physical descriptors and molecular fingerprints (Figure 6.2). Physicochemical descriptors are features representing physicochemical properties of compounds. For example, the RDKit (www.rdkit.org) molecular descriptors contain a set of 200 either experimental properties or theoretical descriptors, such as molar refractivity, octanol–water partition coefficient (logP), heavy-atom counts, bond counts, molecular weight, and topological polar surface area. Lipinski's rule of five [17], formulated by Christopher Lipinski, has been widely used in various processes of early drug discovery for evaluation of an orally active drug: (i) No more than five hydrogen bond donors; (ii) No more than

10 hydrogen bond acceptors; (iii) A molecular weight less than 500 daltons; and (iv) A logP does not exceed 5. These features of drug-likeness are among those embedded in the RDKit molecular descriptors.

Fingerprint-based features contain circular, path-based, and substructure keys, such as the extended-connectivity fingerprints (ECFPs) [18]. An ECFP consists of the element, number of heavy atoms, isotope, number of hydrogen atoms, and ring information. Inspired by the pre-trained language model in natural language processing (NLP), Mol2vec [19] was proposed and is recognized as the most representative method to consider molecular substructures as "words" and compounds as "sentences," and to generate the atom identifiers. These diverse representation learning methods offer powerful tools to encode a series of digital codes for molecules (compounds) as inputs for AI and ML algorithms (Figure 6.2).

6.3.2 Machine-Learning Toolbox

There are two main types of ML technologies that are widely used, including supervised and unsupervised learning methods. Unsupervised methods are used for clustering the data in an unbiased way that helps users to better understand the chemical or biological footprints of data. The unsupervised learning techniques (i.e., principal component analysis) can identify hidden patterns or intrinsic structures in the input data, which will illustrate the meaningful features.

Supervised methods are used to develop training models to predict future endpoints of data categories (i.e., classification) or continuous variables

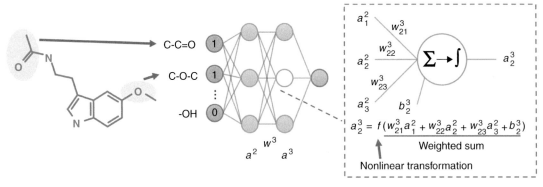

Figure 6.2 Fingerprint representation of molecules for the advanced AI algorithms. Molecules can be encoded using a series of binary digits that indicate the occurrence of certain substructures. Such representation can be used as input for various AI algorithms, such as fully connected deep neural networks. The example deep neural network has two hidden layers (green). Each neuron in the hidden layer performs a weighted sum of its input and transforms the result using nonlinear transformations. A weighted sum is calculated for each neuron in the hidden layer and the result is found using nonlinear transformations.

(i.e., regression). Specifically, supervised learning trains a model using well-established labels (such as inhibitors vs. non-inhibitors on a specific target) to predict new meaning labels (i.e., biological activities) for new inputs. There are multiple well-established ML techniques, including k-nearest neighbors (k-NN), support vector machine (SVM), and random-forest (RF) decision tree, and naïve Bayes algorithms (Figure 6.3). The scikit-learn package (https://scikit-learn.org/stable/) includes 22 distinct ML algorithms.

6.3.3 Deep-Learning Architecture

DL is a subfield of ML that refers to the paradigm of exploring the data with layers of linear and nonlinear transformations organized hierarchically [20].

DL has promise as an emerging big-data-driven pharmaceutical research and drug discovery approach. A popular DL model is artificial neural networks (ANNs), wherein the basic building block is an artificial neuron that nonlinearly transforms the weighted sum of input feature variables. A more straightforward architecture is the fully connected feedforward neural networks (FNNs): the artificial neurons are connected layer by layer from input features to output endpoints [8]. In addition, a weight is associated with each connection and can be optimized by minimizing the predicted loss of the output endpoints by employing backpropagation on training samples [21]. More recently, graph neural networks (GNNs) have been developed as the state-of-the-art method for

(a) *K*-nearest neighbors (*K*-NN)

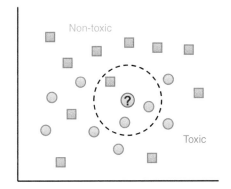

(b) Support vector machine (SVM)

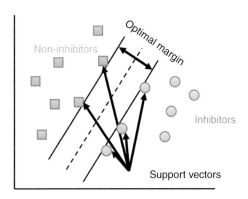

(c) Random forest (RF)

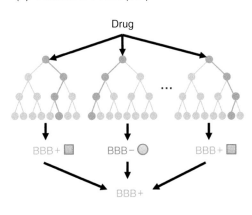

(d) Deep neural networks (DNN)

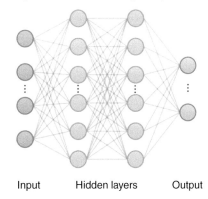

Figure 6.3 Example machine-learning and deep-learning algorithms. (a) The k-NN algorithm classifies samples using plurality voting of k closest neighbor samples. (b) The SVM algorithm separates different classes by finding an optimal hyperplane (dashed line) with maximum distances to the nearest samples. (c) The RF algorithm classifies samples through an ensemble of decision trees. (d) DNNs are composed of artificial neurons connected layer by layer from input features to output targets. BBB, Blood–brain barrier.

various graph-related tasks, such as node-level and graph-level classification. A recent study evaluated the ability to predict cardiotoxicity of small molecules using a multitask deep neural network (DNN) algorithm (Figure 6.3d), a single-task DNN, a naïve Bayes, a support vector machine, a random forest, and a graph convolutional neural network (GCNN) [22]. They showed that multitask DNNs outperformed other DL algorithms or traditional ML methods. DeepChem [23] is a popular framework for using ML and DL in drug discovery; it has implemented various DL algorithms, including DNNs and GNNs.

6.4 Applications of AI in Alzheimer's Drug Discovery

6.4.1 Pharmacokinetic/ Pharmacodynamic Evaluation

Over the past few decades, characterizing properties related to absorption, distribution, metabolism, excretion, and toxicity (ADMET) has been recognized as one of the crucial steps in drug discovery and development. The high attrition rate for AD clinical trials increased the pressure on the pharmaceutical industry to improve ADMET properties of candidate compounds, such as brain penetration [24]. Since in vivo and in vitro evaluations are costly and laborious, AI-based models have been widely used to estimate these properties [25]. For example, a classification model based on substructure pattern recognition was proposed to evaluate blood–brain barrier (BBB) penetration of molecules [26]. In this classification model, a substructure pattern fingerprint from a predefined substructure dictionary was used to code each molecule as an input to build SVM models. The overall predictive accuracies of the best BBB model on the test set were 98.4% [26], suggesting possible application of the BBB model in the early stage of drug discovery.

A light gradient boosting machine (LightGBM) model to predict BBB penetration has also been developed. The authors trained a LightGBM model using 5,453 BBB-permeable and 1,709 BBB-non-permeable molecules [27]. An overall accuracy of 89% during 10-fold cross validation and 90% accuracy on an external validation set of 74 central nerve system (CNS) compounds were achieved. Several new BBB models using the advanced AI algorithms have been proposed [28, 29].

More details about evaluation of ADMET properties using AI and ML methods can be found in recent reviews [25, 29].

6.4.2 Target Identification

Without complete drug-target information, development of promising and affordable approaches for effective treatment is challenging, owing to unintended therapeutic effects or multiple drug–target interactions including off-target adverse effects and suboptimal effectiveness [30]. A team utilized the IBM Watson knowledge base, to identify novel RNA-binding proteins (RBPs) in amyotrophic lateral sclerosis (ALS) [31]. IBM Watson is an AI-based computer system capable of addressing various questions, from drug discovery to healthcare, using the advanced NLP algorithms. Via IBM Watson, the authors searched published abstracts of previously known RBPs involved in ALS and then incorporated text-based knowledge of all possible RBPs in the human genome to prioritize candidate RBPs using a semantic similarity measure [31]. Among the top 10 predicted candidates, 5 novel RBPs were experimentally identified in ALS at the protein and RNA levels in tissues from ALS and non-neurological disease controls, as well as in patient-derived induced pluripotent stem cell neuron models [31].

Published by *Nature Neuroscience*, a team presented a novel network-based Bayesian approach that is capable of integrating multi-omics data along with gene networks to accurately infer risk genes and drug targets impacted by variants identified from genome-wide association studies (GWAS) [32]. They further applied this approach to the latest GWAS data in AD patients and identified 103 likely causal genes for AD by incorporating existing GWAS loci and large-scale multi-omics data [33]. Drug–target network analysis showed that the 103 predicted risk genes are likely to be drug targets for drug development in AD [33]. Our team established AlzGPS [15], a systems biology platform to enable searching, visualizing, and analyzing over 100 multi-omics (i.e., single-cell) data sets in prioritizing novel drug targets for AD.

Funded by the NIA, a multidisciplinary team is leveraging AI to find patterns in genetic, imaging, and clinical data from over 60,000 AD patients, with the goal of identifying new targets and biomarkers for AD/ADRD, called the Ultrascale Machine Learning to Empower Discovery in Alzheimer's Disease Biobanks (AI4AD) project.

6.4.3 Drug Repurposing

Drug repurposing, an effective drug discovery strategy based on discovering new applications for existing drugs, could significantly shorten the time and reduce the cost for random clinical trials and *de novo* drug discovery. Identification of molecular targets for known drugs is essential to drug repurposing to improve efficacy while minimizing side effects in clinical trials [34–36]. However, experimental determination of drug–target interactions is costly and time-consuming [37]. The capable and intelligent computer science-based ML and DL models offer novel testable hypotheses for unbiased identification of molecular targets of known drugs.

Our group recently developed a network-based DL methodology, denoted deepDTnet [38], for systematic identification of molecular targets for known drugs. Specifically, deepDTnet embeds 15 types of chemical, genomic, phenotypic, and cellular networks (Figure 6.4) to generate digital features via learning low-dimensional but informative vector representations for both drugs and targets. Compared to traditional "black box" ML methods, the prediction process of deepDTnet is chemical-biology intuitive, involving a medicinal chemist relating a drug to the drug-target database of similar drugs they have seen. deepDTnet computationally identifies thousands of novel drug–target interactions with high accuracy, outperforming previous state-of-the-art methodologies [38]. Importantly, via deepDTnet and experimental validation, topotecan, an approved topoisomerase inhibitor, was identified as a new, direct inhibitor (half maximal inhibitory concentration [IC_{50}] = 0.43 μM) of human retinoic-acid-receptor-related orphan receptor-gamma t (ROR-γt). Furthermore, by specifically targeting ROR-γt, topotecan reveals a potential therapeutic effect in a mouse model of multiple sclerosis [38]. Subsequently, the same team further adopted a multi-modal deep autoencoder algorithm to learn high-dimensional features of drugs and used a variational autoencoder to predict drug–disease pairs [39]. Using this new approach, termed deepDR, the authors identified several drug candidates, including risperidone and aripiprazole, for possible treatment of AD [39]. The detailed description of drug repurposing for AD can be found in a recent review [40].

6.4.4 Patient Stratification

The marked heterogeneity of patient populations, including clinical manifestations, disease progression, and genetic predisposition, make identifying effective treatments for individuals more challenging. Heterogeneity in patient population is also a challenge for clinical trial design. Accumulating clinical, biomarker expression, genetic, omic, and neuroimaging profiles can be fed into ML and DL algorithms for prediction of drug responses. For example, ML or DL models can identify patients who have different responses on a specific agent. As a proof of concept, a team proposed an AD precision medicine framework using unsupervised formal concept analysis to predict the response to blarcamesine, a selective sigma-1 receptor (SIGMAR1) agonist, using genomic biomarkers [41]. Similarly, Simpraga et al. applied ML models based on EEG recording data to predict clinical outcomes of scopolamine, a muscarinic acetylcholine receptor antagonist (mAChR) [42]. They showed that scopolamine is a valid model of AD pathophysiology based on an ML-based index from 14 EEG biomarkers between healthy elders and AD patients [42].

The application of ML and DL to longitudinal patient data collection and electronic health records have the potential to inform patient stratification. Park et al. built data-driven ML models with reasonable accuracy for risk assessment of AD using large-scale administrative health data [43]. Accumulating evidence demonstrates that clinicians often lack the best information to provide the optimal care for patients. AI-driven clinical care solutions have been especially successful in radiological and histopathological image analysis. For large-volume imaging data, AI has frequently been shown to outperform physicians both in diagnostic performance and efficiency. Importantly, AI-driven approaches can help identify high-risk patient groups, alerting physicians to pay greater attention to those who require urgent action. Rather than replacing physicians, such AI solutions currently assist healthcare professionals by providing analytical, diagnostic, and decision support for patient management and clinical trials.

6.5 Discussion, Perspective, and Future Directions

Despite the enthusiasm for AI-enabled discovery of AD treatments, questions and challenges abound. For decades, translational science has been facing a conundrum: how to translate research findings into new effective medicines and technologies

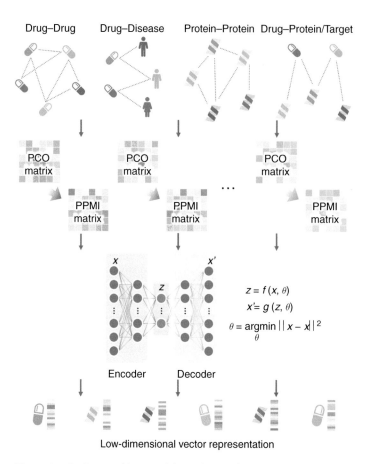

Drug–Drug   Drug–Disease   Protein–Protein   Drug–Protein/Target

$$z = f(x, \theta)$$
$$x' = g(z, \theta)$$
$$\theta = \operatorname*{argmin}_{\theta} || x - x' ||^2$$

Encoder   Decoder

Low-dimensional vector representation

Figure 6.4 An AI-assisted framework for prediction of drug–target interactions. Random surfing models can capture the information of various biological networks and generate probabilistic co-occurrence (PCO) matrices, which are further transformed to positive pointwise mutual information (PPMI) matrices. Autoencoder can generate a compressed, low-dimensional vector representation for the drug or target. The low-dimensional vectors encode the relational properties, association information, and topological context of drugs or targets, and are used as input for downstream computation, such as drug–target interaction prediction.

that rapidly deliver them. Responding to this problem has required collaboration of basic and translational sciences. Most AI models in drug discovery require large-volume data for training and validation, especially for DL models. A lack of adequate quality data and robust sharing practices is a key barrier to positively impact drug discovery. Inadequate data quality can lead to AD models that have poor generalizability and limited predictiveness. Data harmonization that improves data quality and utilization via the use of domain knowledge and ML techniques will play crucial roles in development and application of AI-based drug discovery. Given the sensitive nature of drug discovery data, privacy and security are vital to public trust.

Today's drug discovery platforms are quickly turning into big data factories. A robust enterprise architecture and infrastructure, including strong computing capacity, hardware, and connectivity, are a priority in national/international drug discovery data strategies among industry, academia, and governments. Strong data stewardship practices enable the realization of interoperability and standards. Three axes of big data stewardship are recommended: (i) data ownership rights (laying the groundwork for data-sharing models) must be operationalized and taken into consideration for data acquisition, use, and distribution practices; (ii) representative data (including diverse chemical and target coverage) are critical to allow AI models to cover a universal application domain; (iii) big data's volume, variety, velocity, and veracity (4Vs) require automated and rigorous data harmonization and validation. Data harmonization and extrenal validation can ensure data quality (completeness, consistency, integrity, fairness, and transparency) and accuracy. Data used for training AI models must therefore be annotated by a sufficient number of qualified medicinal chemists and pharmacologists to avoid "garbage-in, garbage-out." For AI models in drug discovery, three best practices are particularly important as they will ensure the integrity of training, validation, and test data sets.

Another limitation of AI models is that they are often "black boxes," that is, they cannot be used to understand the underlying problem by chemists and pharmacologists. Drug discovery is a complicated process involving multilevel interactions between the chemical compounds and biological systems. Therefore, a potential way of building an effective and explainable AI-based drug discovery model is to enrich the biologically inspired visible neural network model [44] with drug-related entities connecting drugs, targets, and disease status. In an explainable AI model, algorithms rationalize their prediction processes in a way that can be understood by humans. Resolving the challenges involved will require multidisciplinary collaborations among chemists, pharmacologists, biologists, computer scientists, and physicists [45].

For example, selection of the right chemical and biology data sets will need domain knowledge from well-trained chemists and pharmacologists. Selection of the most promising drug candidates for experimental or clinical validation will need input from disease biologists and physicians.

The predisposition to AD involves a complex, polygenic, and pleiotropic genetic architecture [46]. Traditional reductionist paradigms overlook the inherent complexity of AD biology and have often led to treatments that are inadequate or fraught with adverse effects. Existing data resources, including genomics, transcriptomics, proteomics, radiomics (imaging data), and interactomics (protein–protein interactions) [47], have not yet been fully utilized and integrated to explore their potential contributions to AD drug discovery. We propose an AI-based infrastructure for precision medicine drug discovery in AD by unique integration of genetic and multi-omic findings from human genomics, functional genomics, transcriptomics, and the human protein–protein interactome (Figure 6.5). Several recent studies have shown promising findings for precision medicine drug discovery for AD using this type of approach [48–50].

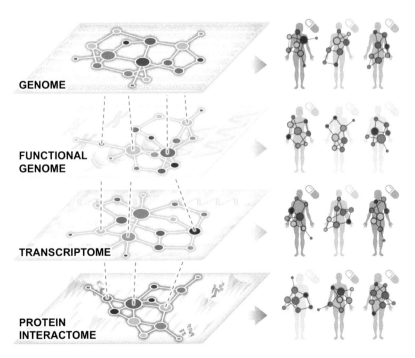

GENOME

FUNCTIONAL GENOME

TRANSCRIPTOME

PROTEIN INTERACTOME

Figure 6.5 A proposed AI framework for precision medicine drug discovery in AD. Traditional reductionist paradigm overlooks the inherent complexity of AD and has often led to treatments that are inadequate. Using AI methodologies, integration of the genome, transcriptome, proteome, and the human interactome are essential for novel target identification and precision medicine drug discovery for AD.

In summary, the application of AI solutions to AD drug discovery and development, as well as clinical trial design, is possible via cross-disciplinary collaborations to address existing gaps and challenges. If broadly applied, AI solutions can facilitate decision making for best-in-class AD drug discovery among academics, the pharmaceutical industry, and healthcare systems [45]. Important terms and concepts discussed in this chapters are summarized in Box 6.1.

Box 6.1   Terms and concepts

Artificial intelligence (AI): the study of building machines or programs that exhibit human intelligence in performing specific or general tasks.

Data harmonization: a process to improve data quality and utilization via the use of domain knowledge and ML techniques.

Deep neural networks (**DNNs**): general terms referring to multi-layer neural networks.

Graph convolutional neural networks (GCNNs): neural network architectures specifically designed for analyzing image data, which generally include multiple layers of convolutional layers and pooling layers.

Drug–target network: a bipartite graph composed of approved drugs and proteins linked by drug–target binary associations.

Machine learning (ML) algorithms: a subset of AI algorithms that can learn from data, therefore removing the need for explicit instructions on how to perform certain tasks.

Natural language processing (**NLP**): a subfield of AI that reads, deciphers, understands, processes, and analyzes large amounts of natural language data.

Visible neural network: a new generation of "visible" approaches that aim to guide the integration of ML models with increasing domain knowledge of a biological mechanism.

Training data: the data used to fit an AI model to solve a specific problem.

Validation data: the data used to offer an unbiased performance evaluation of an AI model while fine tuning the model's (hyper)parameters to enhance performance and robustness.

Test data: the data used to provide an unbiased final performance evaluation of an AI model.

Acknowledgments

We thank Yadi Zhou for assistance to prepare Figures. This work was supported by the National Institute on Aging (NIA) of the National Institutes of Health (NIH) under award number R01AG066707, U01AG073323, 1R56AG074001-01, 3R01AG066707-01S1 and 3R01AG066707-02S1 and the National Heart, Lung, and Blood Institute of the NIH under award number R00HL138272 to F.C. This work was supported, in part, by the VeloSano Pilot Program (Cleveland Clinic Taussig Cancer Institute) to F.C. Dr. Cummings is supported by NIGMS grant P20GM109025; NINDS grant U01NS093334; NIA grant R01AG053798; and NIA grant P20AG068053.

References

1. Hippius H, Neundorfer G. The discovery of Alzheimer's disease. *Dialogues Clin Neurosci* 2003; **5**: 101–8.

2. Corriveau RA, Koroshetz WJ, Gladman JT, et al. Alzheimer's Disease-Related Dementias Summit 2016: national research priorities. *Neurology* 2017; **89**: 2381–91.

3. Alzheimer's Association. 2016 Alzheimer's disease facts and figures. *Alzheimers Dement* 2016; **12**: 459–509.

4. Alzheimer's Association. 2020 Alzheimer's disease facts and figures. *Alzheimers Dement* 2020; **17**: 327–406.

5. Cummings JL, Morstorf T, Zhong K. Alzheimer's disease drug-development pipeline: few candidates, frequent failures. *Alzheimers Res Ther* 2014; **6**: 37.

6. Avorn J. The $2.6 billion pill: methodologic and policy considerations. *N Engl J Med* 2015; **372**: 1877–9.

7. Fleming N. How artificial intelligence is changing drug discovery. *Nature* 2018; **557**: S55–7.

8. Zhou Y, Wang F, Tang J, et al. Artificial intelligence in COVID-19 drug repurposing. *Lancet Digit Health* 2020; **2**: E667–76.

9. Vamathevan J, Clark D, Czodrowski P, et al. Applications of machine learning in drug discovery

and development. *Nat Rev Drug Discov* 2019; **18**: 463–77.

10. Schneider P, Walters WP, Plowright AT, et al. Rethinking drug design in the artificial intelligence era. *Nat Rev Drug Discov* 2020; **19**: 353–64.

11. Beecham GW, Bis JC, Martin ER, et al. The Alzheimer's Disease Sequencing Project: study design and sample selection. *Neurol Genet* 2017; **3**: e194.

12. Petersen RC, Aisen PS, Beckett LA, et al. Alzheimer's Disease Neuroimaging Initiative (ADNI): clinical characterization. *Neurology* 2010; **74**: 201–9.

13. Wishart DS, Feunang YD, Guo AC, et al. DrugBank 5.0: a major update to the DrugBank database for 2018. *Nucleic Acids Res* 2018; **46**: D1074–82.

14. Ursu O, Holmes J, Knockel J, et al. DrugCentral: online drug compendium. *Nucleic Acids Res* 2017; **45**: D932–9.

15. Zhou Y, Fang J, Bekris L, et al. AlzGPS: a genome-wide positioning systems platform to catalyze multi-omics for Alzheimer's therapeutic discovery. *Alzheimers Res Ther* 2021; **13**: 24.

16. O'Boyle NM. Towards a universal SMILES representation: a standard method to generate canonical SMILES based on the InChI. *J Cheminform* 2012; **4**: 22.

17. Lipinski CA. Lead- and drug-like compounds: the rule-of-five revolution. *Drug Discov Today Technol* 2004; **1**: 337–41.

18. Rogers D, Hahn M. Extended-connectivity fingerprints. *J Chem Inf Model* 2010; **50**: 742–54.

19. Jaeger S, Fulle S, Turk S. Mol2vec: unsupervised machine learning approach with chemical intuition. *J Chem Inf Model* 2018; **58**: 27–35.

20. LeCun Y, Bengio Y, Hinton G. Deep learning. *Nature* 2015; **521**: 436–44.

21. Rumelhart DE, Hinton GE, Williams RJ. Learning representations by back-propagating errors. *Nature* 1986; **323**: 533–6.

22. Cai C, Guo P, Zhou Y, *et al*. Deep learning-based prediction of drug-induced cardiotoxicity. *J Chem Inf Model* 2019; **59**: 1073–84.

23. Wu Z, Ramsundar B, Feinberg EN, et al. MoleculeNet: a benchmark for molecular machine learning. *Chem Sci* 2018; **9**: 513–30.

24. Pardridge WM. Alzheimer's disease drug development and the problem of the blood–brain barrier. *Alzheimers Dement* 2009; **5**: 427–32.

25. Cheng F, Li W, Liu G, et al. *In silico* ADMET prediction: recent advances, current challenges and future trends. *Curr Top Med Chem* 2013; **13**: 1273–89.

26. Shen J, Cheng F, Xu Y, et al. Estimation of ADME properties with substructure pattern recognition. *J Chem Inf Model* 2010; **50**: 1034–41.

27. Shaker B, Yu MS, Song JS, et al. LightBBB: computational prediction model of blood–brain-barrier penetration based on LightGBM. *Bioinformatics* 2021; **37**:1135–9.

28. Miao R, Xia LY, Chen HH, et al. Improved classification of blood–brain-barrier drugs using deep learning. *Sci Rep* 2019; **9**: 8802.

29. Saxena D, Sharma A, Siddiqui MH, et al. Blood brain barrier permeability prediction using machine learning techniques: an update. *Curr Pharm Biotechnol* 2019; **20**: 1163–71.

30. Cheng F, Kovacs IA, Barabasi AL. Network-based prediction of drug combinations. *Nat Commun* 2019; **10**: 1197.

31. Bakkar N, Kovalik T, Lorenzini I, et al. Artificial intelligence in neurodegenerative disease research: use of IBM Watson to identify additional RNA-binding proteins altered in amyotrophic lateral sclerosis. *Acta Neuropathol* 2018; **135**: 227–47.

32. Wang Q, Chen R, Cheng F, et al. A Bayesian framework that integrates multi-omics data and gene networks predicts risk genes from schizophrenia GWAS data. *Nat Neurosci* 2019; **22**: 691–9.

33. Fang J, Zhang P, Wang Q, et al. Network-based translation of GWAS findings to pathobiology and drug repurposing for Alzheimer's disease. *bioRxiv* 2020;DOI: http://doi.org/10.1101/2020.01.15.2001 7160.

34. Cheng F, Desai RJ, Handy DE, et al. Network-based approach to prediction and population-based validation of *in silico* drug repurposing. *Nat Commun* 2018; **9**: 2691.

35. Greene JA, Loscalzo J. Putting the patient back together: social medicine, network medicine, and the limits of reductionism. *N Engl J Med* 2017; **377**: 2493–9.

36. Zeng X, Song X, Ma T, et al. Repurpose open data to discover therapeutics for COVID-19 using deep learning. *J Proteome Res* 2020; **19**: 4624–36.

37. Santos R, Ursu O, Gaulton A, et al. A comprehensive map of molecular drug targets. *Nat Rev Drug Discov* 2017; **16**: 19–34.

38. Zeng X, Zhu S, Lu W, et al. Target identification among known drugs by deep learning from heterogeneous networks. *Chem Sci* 2020; **11**: 1775–97.

39. Zeng X, Zhu S, Liu X, et al. deepDR: a network-based deep learning approach to *in silico* drug repositioning. *Bioinformatics* 2019; **35**: 5191–8.

40. Fang J, Pieper AA, Nussinov R, et al. Harnessing endophenotypes and network medicine for

Alzheimer's drug repurposing. *Med Res Rev* 2020; **40**: 2386–426.

41. Hampel H, Williams C, Etcheto A, et al. A precision medicine framework using artificial intelligence for the identification and confirmation of genomic biomarkers of response to an Alzheimer's disease therapy: analysis of the blarcamesine (ANAVEX2-73) Phase 2a clinical study. *Alzheimers Dement (N Y)* 2020; **6**: e12013.

42. Simpraga S, Alvarez-Jimenez R, Mansvelder HD, et al. EEG machine learning for accurate detection of cholinergic intervention and Alzheimer's disease. *Sci Rep* 2017; **7**: 5775.

43. Park JH, Cho HE, Kim JH, et al. Machine learning prediction of incidence of Alzheimer's disease using large-scale administrative health data. *NPJ Digit Med* 2020; **3**: 46.

44. Ma J, Yu MK, Fong S, et al. Using deep learning to model the hierarchical structure and function of a cell. *Nat Methods* 2018; **15**: 290–8.

45. Cheng F, Ma Y, Uzzi B, et al. Importance of scientific collaboration in contemporary drug discovery and development: a detailed network analysis. *BMC Biol* 2020; **18**: 138.

46. Tasaki S, Gaiteri C, Mostafavi S, et al. The molecular and neuropathological consequences of genetic risk for Alzheimer's dementia. *Front Neurosci* 2018; **12**: 699.

47. Cheng F, Zhao J, Wang Y, et al. Comprehensive characterization of protein–protein interactions perturbed by disease mutations. *Nat Genet* 2021; **53**: 342–53.

48. Swarup V, Hinz FI, Rexach JE, et al. Identification of evolutionarily conserved gene networks mediating neurodegenerative dementia. *Nat Med* 2019; **25**: 152–64.

49. Wang M, Li A, Sekiya M, et al. Transformative network modeling of multi-omics data reveals detailed circuits, key regulators, and potential therapeutics for Alzheimer's disease. *Neuron* 2021; **109**: 257–72.

50. Xu J, Zhang P, Huang Y, et al. Multimodal single-cell/nucleus RNA-sequencing data analysis uncovers molecular networks between disease-associated microglia and astrocytes with implications for drug repurposing in Alzheimer's disease. *Genome Res* 2021;DOI: http://doi.org/10.1101/gr.272484.120.

Role of Animal Models in Alzheimer's Disease Drug Development

Jefferson Kinney, Amanda M. Leisgang Osse, Bruce Lamb, Adrian Oblack, Alan D. Palkowitz, and Frank J. Belas, Jr.

7.1 Introduction

It is critical to identify treatments capable of slowing or halting Alzheimer's disease (AD) progression. Prior to being able to test novel therapeutics in clinical populations, let alone to be used as a treatment, all candidate therapeutics require testing in animal model systems prior to any first-in-human (FIH) clinical trials. While animal models have not predicted success in humans, they constitute critically important means of establishing the biological effects of candidate agents, and no agent would be progressed to clinical trials without having shown benefit in animal models. Clinical trials for experimental drugs are composed of multiple phases, from Phase 0 to Phase 4, varying in sample size and allowing for evaluation of safety and efficacy. Earlier phases collect initial data on the human population regarding drug regimen, side effects, and outcome of the treatment. With positive results in each phase, the drug will continue through the phases to receive approval for use by the US Food and Drug Administration (FDA). However, even before the initiation of a novel therapeutic into clinical trials in humans, animal models are required and crucial for the evaluation of the mechanism of action and target engagement, and for the evaluation of numerous necessary measures ranging from drug absorption and distribution to the determination of side effects and toxicity. The examinations of candidate therapies in animal models serves as a vital decision step about whether to invest the time and resources in moving a therapeutic into the clinical trial workflow. In addition to the data required to make a decision about the feasibility of a novel therapeutic, these experiments have provided great advancements in the understanding of AD in areas that include genetics, cellular and molecular mechanisms, and clinical symptoms. This chapter highlights the process of preclinical evaluation of a therapeutic candidate in terms of the primary animal models used, the behavioral and biochemical assessments/endpoints measured, the considerations in selecting specific animal models, and the necessity and future directions of animal models in the AD drug-development ecosystem.

7.2 Background of Animal Use in AD Drug Development

The majority of AD drug-development research utilizes mouse models due to their similarity to human anatomy, physiology, and genetics. There also exist a wealth of well-established behavioral and cognitive testing approaches relevant to tests performed in clinical populations. In addition, the required housing and care of rodent models removes outside variability in data, and the shorter lifespan and well-characterized genetics provides the opportunity for generating models of aging and age-related diseases. There are numerous mouse models to select from (see below) that provide tremendous opportunity for evaluating potential therapeutics.

The use of animal models in drug discovery spans a considerable history with some variation in specific design, based on the clinical disorder being approached. However, a common thread relies on the availability of data indicating that a candidate therapy is well tolerated and is capable of disease-modifying effects in a model system. When a candidate ligand is discovered, a critical role of animal models in the drug-development pipeline is the evaluation of pharmacokinetics (PK) and pharmacodynamics (PD) prior to clinical trials. Commonly using wild-type animals (standard mice with no genetic alterations), the PK of the drug is tested by analyzing the time course and path of the compound (ligand) throughout the body and how it is processed, including absorption, distribution, metabolism, excretion, and bioavailability (ADME-PK). In addition, PD is studied to evaluate the effects the drug has on the body, such as dose toxicity and adverse side effects. PK and PD are critical for the determination of tolerability,

73

toxicity, and dose finding in a novel therapeutic, though administration considerations must also be taken, including route/method, location, timing, frequency, duration, and the metabolism of the animal [1]. PK and PD evaluation on animals has been shown to be translational to the human population and is essential before FIH trials, demonstrating its importance in the drug-development pipeline [2]. As an example, tacrine, an acetylcholinesterase inhibitor, was the first AD candidate ligand used in clinical trials in the 1980s, based on a promising role in the improvement of cognition. The preclinical characterization of tacrine was almost entirely based on drug toxicity and side effects, dose response, and additional assessments of behavior in wild-type rodents [3]. At the time, there did not exist the robust number of genetic and non-genetic animal model systems for AD, resulting in a more general safety and tolerability evaluation with minimal evaluation of disease specific modifications.

Separate from the tolerability and toxicity data required for any candidate ligand to move into human clinical trials, there has been a substantial effort to advance only candidates that have demonstrated some efficacy on AD-related features/pathology. In AD, there exist several central clinical presentations, with memory disturbances being a central feature. There are also a number of pathological features of AD, including plaques comprised of amyloid-beta (Aβ) protein, neurofibrillary tangles (NFTs) composed of hyperphosphorylated tau (p-tau), and, more recently, indications of alterations in inflammatory signaling. Each of these features must be modeled (alone or in combination) to allow for evaluation of candidate therapeutics that may demonstrate benefit in alleviating AD pathology. The demonstration that a candidate ligand is capable of impacting one or more of the above core features of AD provides the necessary rationale to move to FIH testing. However, for a number of reasons (see below) there is no one model that incorporates the entire AD pathobiology. As a result, in preclinical evaluations one or two preclinical models are selected as the testbed for a therapeutic, typically models that render an aspect of AD that the candidate ligand will alter.

Recently, there has been excitement surrounding the candidate ligand BIIB037 (aducanumab), which was recently approved by FDA. Aducanumab is a human monoclonal antibody that targets aggregated Aβ, particularly parenchymal amyloid, rather than vascular. With interest in this novel treatment, the drug has undergone multiple evaluations in animal models prior to FIH clinical trials, including evaluation of dose, toxicity, and effects on AD pathology. As amyloid is the primary target of aducanumab, an amyloid transgenic mouse model was selected to evaluate the impact of this novel ligand. It was reported that aged amyloid-bearing mice treated with aducanumab over the course of 13 weeks, with chronic dosing, showed reduction in parenchymal plaques and no microhemorrhages at doses up to 70 mg/kg. It was also important to note that plaque clearance began even at a low dose of 3 mg/kg. These animal model data demonstrate promise and further our understanding of the drug; aducanumab was then moved into Phase 1 clinical trials. The drug has continued to be evaluated through Phase 3, and is now approved. Over the last 40 years, there have been numerous similar examples in which compelling preclinical data indicated a candidate therapy should be moved to clinical trials. There have been far more candidate therapeutics that failed to show any impact on AD pathology or AD-related cognitive impairments in animal models, which were never advanced to clinical trials.

There has been tremendous growth in the number of animal models for study of AD, as well as discussions of which models are the most appropriate. These models range from the most commonly used genetic mouse models that are being derived from familial AD (FAD) genetic mutations, to models developed based on risk-factor genes, as well as alternative models that recapitulate other aspects of AD absent of genetic changes. Selection of the most appropriate model that best fits the candidate therapeutic profile is a vital step in this process, as it can influence whether the candidate is given the best opportunity to demonstrate efficacy and advance to FIH trials. Equally important is the selection of the appropriate behavioral and biochemical measures to demonstrate that a candidate therapeutic exhibits sufficient benefit to advance to human clinical trials [4]. Detailed below are some of the most frequently utilized models employed in the evaluation of candidate therapeutics, as well as the behavioral and biochemical measures utilized.

Figure 7.1 demonstrates the process of AD drug development and the evaluation of novel therapeutic candidates in animal models.

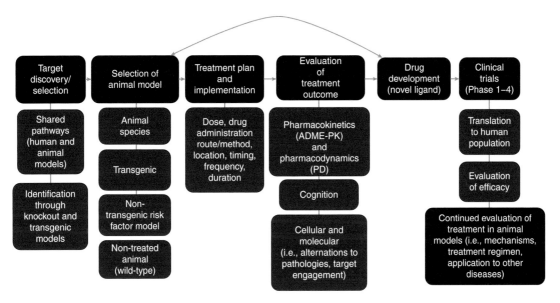

Figure 7.1 The process of activities for drug development and evaluation in animal models.

7.3   Familial AD Models

Due to differences within their genome, rodents do not naturally develop AD pathology. However, the identification of genetic mutations associated with FAD provided researchers the opportunity to induce these mutations in rodent models to mimic the hallmarks of AD, allowing investigations of AD pathobiology, as well as the opportunity to evaluate novel treatments in the AD models. The first genetic mutations recognized in patients as being involved in AD have shown direct links to early-onset AD (EOAD), accounting for 3–5% of all cases. The more prevalent form of AD, sporadic or late-onset AD (LOAD) (about 95–97% of all cases), cannot be solely attributed to genetic mutations, however, both types are characterized by the presence of Aβ, NFTs, and chronic neuroinflammation [5, 6], allowing EOAD rodent models to be used in research targeting the pathological features of the disease. Given the several pathological features of AD, the selection of the most appropriate model system is made based on the mechanism of drug action and/or pathological feature impacted. Discussed below are the major categories of genetic mouse models based on AD specific pathology.

Aβ has been the most prevalently investigated AD pathology, and data indicating it is present in the brain up to a decade or more prior to cognitive decline made it the most investigated target in drug development. Insertion of amyloid FAD mutations, including mutations in the amyloid precursor protein (*APP*), presenilin 1 (*PSEN1*), and presenilin 2 (*PSEN2*) genes in rodents, led to the development of Aβ pathology, allowing initial models to be used for investigations into amyloidosis and the impact of Aβ on disease progression. The first successful amyloid AD mouse model was the PDAPP mouse, developed using the *APP* mutation, V717F. In this model, there is a presence of Aβ at age 6 months, with aggregation to plaques by age 9 months. The PDAPP mouse was used in the first immunization studies, injecting mice with Aβ$_{42}$ at two time points, before the deposition of Aβ and after. The therapy was successful in the PDAPP model, demonstrating that immunization in young animals prevented the formation of Aβ plaques, neurotic dystrophy, and astrogliosis [7]. With the positive outcome from this study, immunization with a synthetic Aβ$_{42}$, AN1792, along with QS-21 adjuvant, was used in clinical trials. Unfortunately, the Phase 2 trial was halted due to development of subacute aseptic meningoencephalitis in patients following the treatment [8]. However, even with the disappointing result, there were a number of similarities documented between the PDAPP and patient studies. As observed in the mouse model, patients treated with the Aβ immunotherapy had decreased plaque density in the cerebral cortex. In addition, these areas were absent of plaque-related dystrophic neurites, as well as reactive astrocytes [9]. There are disadvantages to using this model, with Aβ$_{42}$ levels and vascular amyloid deposition varying between the PDAPP model and human

LOAD. A number of other amyloid models using *APP* mutations are available, including the Tg2576 and APP23 models, utilizing mutations in presenilin, a component of the gamma-secretase complex, involved in the digestion of APP. One of the most well-established amyloid models, designed with both APP and presenilin 1 (PS1), the APP/PS1 model, has Aβ deposition reported earlier than age 3 months, considerable neuron loss, and cognitive impairments by age 6 months, allowing studies to be performed at a relatively young age. Additional amyloid mouse models have been generated that better reflect/differentially reflect amyloid pathology (see the 5×FAD model that includes several familial AD mutations) in an effort to better understand the underlying biology but also to provide a more appropriate testbed for LOAD treatment approaches. Several candidate therapies have been evaluated using this model, including cholinesterase inhibitors commonly prescribed for AD and a number of drugs currently in clinical trials.

Within tissue samples, the effectiveness of disease-modifying therapies (DMTs) on deposition of Aβ can be evaluated by many ways in these models, including quantification of plaques, plaque density, and the sizes of the Aβ peptides. While these animals provide an ideal testbed for these measures, it remains to be determined if reduction in amyloid plaques is necessarily a positive response given evidence that some amyloid aggregation may be a defense mechanism in the brain. These animal models also assist with analyses of the pathways involved in the accumulation of Aβ in the brain and evaluation of a novel ligand being able to target Aβ accumulation. In addition, the $A\beta_{42}$ peptide has demonstrated increased toxicity and the ratio between the $A\beta_{40}$ and $A\beta_{42}$ peptides has been shown to be an indicator of the disease [10, 11]. Aβ animal models vary in the degree that each of the peptides are expelled/removed and these differences can provide insight into interventions that may alter specific Aβ clearance [12]. The absence of NFT pathology in this model limits them to Aβ-specific targeted treatments; however, NFTs are vital for evaluation of amyloid models in understanding the initiation and progression of Aβ deposition and aggregation, as well as interventions to impact them in AD.

The presence of p-tau is a central pathological feature of AD and levels of specific epitopes' phosphorylation states are associated with AD. This provides a measure to be used to assess the impact of a drug on AD tau pathology. While far fewer novel drug candidates have been designed to directly decrease p-tau, several candidate therapies have been examined in p-tau models to determine if, in addition to the drug's primary mechanism of action, there may be some benefit on p-tau levels. Further, the phosphorylation of specific tau epitopes indicates increased risk for the disease and appear to be associated with onset and progression of AD. For example, recent data have demonstrated a link between levels of p-tau, particularly at the 181 and 217 epitopes, and patients with AD [13, 14]. These findings inform a promising target for the disease, in which animal models can assist with the search for novel ligands that could impact these specific mechanisms. During the development of models of tauopathy, research revealed that tau mutations accounted for the development of frontotemporal dementia and parkinsonism, specifically linked to human chromosome 17. These mutations were applied to the development of novel tau-specific mouse models, including P301S and JNPL3, which have made a considerable impact on drug development. Preclinical research on lithium, used to inhibit the glycogen synthase kinase-3β (GSK-3β) pathway known to serve a role in the hyperphosphorylation of tau, demonstrated promising results. In 2010, using the Tg30tau model, which is a double tau mutant through cross of the P301S and another tau model, G272 V, treatment with lithium showed decreases in tau phosphorylation, tau aggregation, and NFTs [15]. Researchers have reported mixed results regarding the use of lithium in the human population; however, it remains a promising candidate, with studies showing the drug may delay the onset of dementia and remains a treatment in clinical trials [16]. One of the more common approaches in screening novel compounds, which may impact one of the core pathological features of AD (Aβ and tau), has been to include models that combine both pathological features. This provides the opportunity to both evaluate the therapeutic potential of a ligand directed at one of these discrete targets, as well as measure of target effects related to other pathological features.

The incorporation of both Aβ and tau mutations in animal models assists with the consideration of pathology interactions during drug development. By the early 2000s, the first model combining both Aβ and tau mutations emerged. The 3×Tg, which included mutations in the *APP*, *PSEN1*, and microtubule associated protein tau (*MAPT*) genes, develops Aβ plaques at age 6 months, NFTs by 12 months, and demonstrates impairment in cognition [17]. This model continues to be one of the most frequently utilized lines in AD research in the evaluation of novel therapeutics. For example, memantine was approved by the FDA in 2003, and was the first approved treatment for patients with moderate-to-severe AD [15]. However, even by 2010, the mechanisms behind memantine's ability to enhance cognition and the effects on AD pathology remained unclear [18]. An investigation into the mechanism of memantine was performed on the 3×Tg mouse model, demonstrating improvement in learning and memory, as well as alterations in Aβ and NFTs, depending on age of treatment [15, 18]. In the last two decades, there have been numerous animal model systems developed to follow the 3×Tg model, which typically involve the combination of additional FAD mutations. This has resulted in models such as the 5×Tg, 7×Tg, and other variations. Each of these models have been developed in an effort to better understand the pathophysiology of AD but have also served as the testbed for novel therapeutics. While there has been substantial progress in our understanding of AD biology in preclinical animal models systems, the limited progress of drugs that demonstrate safety, tolerability, and therapeutic benefit in the animal models surviving to FDA approval has created a push for the development of non-FAD animal models to more closely represent LOAD, allowing further translation to the human population and advancing drug development. These non-FAD models often are derived from risk genes in LOAD and/or from mutations that alter the underlying biology to mimic other features of AD. Below are some of the more common non-FAD models currently being utilized.

7.4 Inflammation Models

As the role of neuroinflammation has become more of a focus in AD research, animal models are important in the identification of key targets of inflammatory pathways and evaluating novel compounds to intervene in AD. With substantial data demonstrating a sustained immune response in the brain (neuroinflammation) as a core part of AD pathology [6], as well as data showing that neuroinflammation promotes both Aβ and NFT pathologies, animal models of inflammation have emerged. These models have been extensively used to understand AD mechanisms but are now also testbeds for a group of completely novel candidate therapies targeting inflammation.

One avenue of inducing neuroinflammation for evaluation of a candidate ligand is through a systemic immune challenge. Lipopolysaccharide (LPS), an endotoxin, is composed of the membrane of gram-negative bacteria. When injected into the body, LPS activates toll-like receptor (TLR) 4, causing microglial activation and the production of pro-inflammatory cytokines. TLR4 has been reported to be increased in Aβ mouse models, as well as in the brains of human AD patients [19]. A deficiency in this receptor in rodent models leads to an increase in Aβ, as well as a reduction in microglial activation and cognitive function [19]. Mice treated with LPS have a deficit in spatial learning and memory, neuronal loss in the hippocampus, and accumulation of $A\beta_{42}$ [20]. Varied results of TLR4 being beneficial versus detrimental in AD require further investigation into this pathway; these studies may help resolve the controversy surrounding the role of microglia in the disease. Currently, a clinical trial using an LPS challenge is underway to investigate the ability of positron emission tomography (PET) to identify microglial activation in patients with AD, as significant differences between AD patients and normal controls could reveal mechanisms altered in the disease and potential targets for treatment (ClinicalTrials.gov, ID: NCT04057807).

Another peripheral immune challenge drug that evokes neuroinflammation is polyriboinosinic-polyribocytidilic acid, a double-stranded RNA with similarity to a viral infection, which induces inflammation through the activation of TLR3 and promoting release of pro-inflammatory cytokines, including interleukin 1 beta (IL-1β), IL-6, and tumor necrosis factor alpha (TNF-α). This model results in increased $A\beta_{42}$ and cognitive impairments in a fear conditioning task [21]. In human AD patients' brains, an increase in TLR3 was observed on phagocytic microglia. This study demonstrated a significant positive correlation between TLR3 transcript levels and plaque load as well [22]. The neuroinflammatory response in these models and the impact of a candidate ligand is often measured through the quantification of pro- and anti-inflammatory cytokines, as well as markers and morphological changes in the activation of glial cells. Analysis of the pathways involved, including assessment of gene transcription and protein expression, is also crucial to the evaluation of the immune response. In the clinical population, through imaging techniques of the brain, such as PET, identification of Aβ, NFTs, and neuroinflammation can be performed. However, the direct and immediate effects of novel ligands cannot be fully evaluated in AD patients, with animal models providing that ability. Research into the specificity of inflammatory pathways and inflammation-related therapeutic targets in animal models assist in evaluating the connection between inflammation and neurodegeneration. There has been some concern raised in the use of the inflammation models above that the TLR3 and TLR4 receptor activation via these approaches is more robust than what is observed in LOAD populations, and this has resulted in other inflammatory approaches in more recent mouse genetic models (see below).

7.5 Environmental and Non-genetic Risk Factor Models

There are several risk factors associated with AD, which may be beneficial targets in the advancement of novel therapeutics to slow or halt disease progression, or even as preventative measures. Animals assist in therapeutic testing by providing a model for many of the risk factors, including aging, diabetes mellitus (DM) and obesity, and cardiovascular disease.

The greatest risk factor for developing AD is age; 10% of individuals over the age of 65 have AD, and the risk doubles every additional 5 years [23]. Through the process of aging, there are several alterations in the body that can impact the risk of developing AD, such as alterations in neuro- and systematic inflammation, reduction in neuronal spine density and neuronal connections, and metabolic alterations [24]. In addition, behavior changes, including deficits in spatial learning, motor function, and cerebellar function can be observed. Studies have established similarities in rodent and human aging, allowing aged mice and rats to be a model for investigating this process [24]. In addition, genetically modified models of accelerated aging, such as the senescence-accelerated mouse-prone (SAMP) models, assist with the study of aging by accelerating the process, reducing cost and time for investigation. The SAMP8 mouse specifically displays changes in cognition and behavior, alterations in circadian rhythms, immune responses, and

changes in multiple neurotransmitter systems, as well as increased Aβ and p-tau [25], making it a beneficial model for AD drug development targeting age-related changes.

Females have an increased risk for developing AD, making up two-thirds of the AD human patient population [23]. Studies have shown a relationship between the transition to menopause and AD, possibly being attributed to the alteration of hormones later in life. To assist in research surrounding this link, one of the most common animal models to mimic human menopause is ovariectomized rodents, used to evaluate the loss of ovarian hormones on the initiation and progression of the disease. The ovariectomized model has been beneficial in the investigation of hormone therapy, including treatment with progesterone, estrogen, and leuprolide acetate (for reduction of luteinizing hormone) [26, 27], and is currently a promising target being tested in clinical trials (NCT043312399, NCT00066157). With the disproportion of gender in AD, development of candidate ligands specifically targeting the female population is a necessity, and animal models will be vital in this process.

DM, characterized as having hyperglycemia due to dysregulation in insulin signaling [28], has also been shown to be a risk factor for cognitive decline and AD; individuals with DM have a 1.5–4-fold increase in risk for developing dementia [29]. Autopsies of individuals with DM reveal increases in Aβ plaques and NFTs in the hippocampus [29], linking abnormal insulin signaling with AD pathologies. In addition, impairment in insulin signaling and glucose metabolism has been described in AD, making DM an appealing target in novel therapeutics [30, 31]. While there are several details to be delineated in understanding the association between DM and AD, the development of animal models provides the opportunity to examine novel therapeutic approaches. Streptozotocin (STZ) is a chemical that is specifically toxic to insulin-producing beta cells when given at a high dose, mimicking type 1 DM; however, with a staggered dose, STZ results in a sustained hyperglycemia and mild impairment of insulin secretion, more comparable to type 2 DM. Murtishaw et al. demonstrated that the use of this drug in rodents led to cognitive impairments in novel object recognition tasks and increases in both p-tau and neuroinflammation [29]. The STZ model is not limited to rodents; there have been studies with non-human primates that utilize STZ as a diabetic model [32, 33]. The presence of neurodegeneration in these animals makes the STZ model an excellent platform for investigations into the link between DM and AD. The STZ model is vital to the AD drug-development pipeline with six antidiabetic drugs currently in clinical trials as repurposed drugs for AD [34].

Related and sometimes overlapping approaches have emerged for other risk factors for AD, including obesity and cardiovascular impairments. Often, obesity and cardiovascular disorders can be attributed to high fat diets, and research indicates that diets high in saturated fats increase the risk for developing AD, with an even higher risk for patients carrying an apolipoprotein E ε4 (APOE-4) allele [35]. Obese individuals show alterations in neuroanatomy and cognition relevant to AD [36, 37]. Animal models are vital to drug development targeting the impact of obesity on the brain and links to AD. Using rodent models fed a high-fat diet, studies have demonstrated increased synaptic pruning by activated microglia and alterations in the gut microbiome, resulting in changes in inflammation and short-term memory [36]. In addition, AD animal models fed a high-fat diet have demonstrated increased Aβ deposition and neuroinflammation, with some (not all) studies demonstrating changes in p-tau levels [35, 38–40].

7.6 Alternatives to Rodent Models

Drosophila (e.g., fruit fly) is a well-characterized animal model, with its whole genome sequenced and annotated. With rapid generation time and short lifespans, *Drosophila* allow the ability to perform quick studies, especially in AD, where aging is an important component of the disease. *Drosophila* are also inexpensive and easy to maintain. Comparable to AD patients, *Drosophila* with overexpression of $Aβ_{42}$ and tau show neuronal decline, leading to shortened lifespan, reduction in locomotion and flight, and alterations in vision and eye phenotype [41]. In addition, simple behavioral tests can be used to evaluate the learning and memory in flies, a key component in AD. Pathologies of the disease have been represented by expression of AD genes, such as in the 3×Tg model, including humanized *APP* and beta-site APP cleaving enzyme (*BACE*) genes, as well as *Drosophila* presenilin. This model exhibits $Aβ_{40}$ and $Aβ_{42}$ plaques with neurodegeneration [42]. Having an impact

on drug development, both beta-secretase and gamma-secretase inhibitors have been tested in the 3×Tg model, showing amelioration of Aβ toxicity [42]. *Drosophila* are also beneficial in studies of tau pathology. A relationship was observed between abnormal tau and neurodegeneration in flies overexpressing the humanized tau gene, and earlier mortality rate [41]. Investigations into the roles of specific tau phosphorylation sites would provide details into possible therapeutic ligands in AD and utilizing the *Drosophila* model could assist with understanding these mechanisms. Research into novel treatments can benefit from the fly model; however, studies on *Drosophila* alone are insufficient to move into FIH trials, and typically serve as a very early stage of ligand engagement. Since the flies' body systems differ greatly from humans, the processing of drugs cannot be reliably tested in *Drosophila*. In addition, complex behaviors cannot be evaluated as clearly in the fly model as in mammals.

On the other end of the spectrum, non-human primates have higher translational relevance to humans, with about 99% genetic similarity overall. In addition, non-human primates have 100% sequence homology with human Aβ and 99–100% sequence homology with human tau [43]. Though there are fewer studies on non-human primates, due to a number of factors, these models have played a role in the drug-development ecosystem. For instance, testing of the FDA-approved AD drug donepezil was performed in non-human primates demonstrating a rescue in cognitive impairment [44, 45]. Most non-human primate studies have used rhesus monkeys, which naturally develop Aβ accumulation in the cortex and hippocampus, similar to that observed in human AD. These changes are typically reported only in rhesus monkeys at least 25 years old, making these models a large investment in time and cost. Even with the accumulation of Aβ plaques in aged rhesus monkeys, there are no reports of extensive neuronal loss, even in areas with substantial plaque load [43]. One major difficulty in the rhesus monkey model is the lack of tauopathy, even with the genetic consistency in non-human primates and humans, demonstrating that no animal model thus far is a perfect representation of LOAD. In addition to these pathological limitations, the cost of housing and the care for non-human primates are high due to their size, lifespan, and need for mentally stimulating housing.

79

Additional species have been used in AD therapeutic research including fish, worms, rabbits, rats, guinea pigs, dogs, and pigs, varying in ease of use and translation to the human population [15, 43, 46–48]; nevertheless, mice remain the most commonly used animal model due to the balance of low cost, short lifespan, and translation to human physiology and behavior. There is debate about the most appropriate model(s) in the evaluation of a therapeutics potential to advance to human clinical trials. Over the last decade there has been a stronger emphasis on testing any new therapeutic in more than one model, typically one that is related to the mechanism of the candidate therapy, and one more broad model. Equally important in the drug discovery process is the selection of appropriate endpoints in the preclinical evaluation of a candidate therapy. The endpoints have evolved in the last 30 years from initially being primarily behavioral measures relevant to AD (cognitive/learning and memory measures) to more sophisticated combinations of behavioral improvement and evidence of benefit on AD-specific pathologies (Aβ, tau, inflammation, and others). In this chapter, we will further discuss the measures most frequently utilized, necessary in the evaluation of a candidate therapeutic's potential to impact one or more features of AD.

7.7 Cognitive Evaluation in Rodent Models

Progressive cognitive decline is the primary criterion for the diagnosis of neurodegenerative dementia and the evaluation of disease progression. AD patients present with many impairments, including in learning and memory, making cognitive testing an important evaluation of novel therapeutics. Cognitive assessments can similarly be used in the evaluation of animal models and assist in the investigation of relationships between biological and clinical hallmarks of AD. Similarities in behavior between rodents and humans make testing relatable between the species. The concordance between mouse and human is particularly useful for hippocampal-mediated learning and memory and – given that the hippocampus is one of the earliest areas impacted in AD – for the examination of therapeutics in mice.

One of the most common hippocampally dependent spatial learning and memory tasks in rodents for the evaluation of candidate ligands is the Morris water maze (MWM). During this task,

the animal is placed into a circular pool of water and allowed to openly swim to a hidden platform. Rodents are capable swimmers; however, they will actively search to escape the water, which serves as motivation to complete the task. Spatial cues are placed around the swim tank for the rodent to learn the spatial location of the platform in reference to the cues over the course of several training days. If learning and memory is unimpaired, the latency for the animal to find the platform will decrease over the test days. For evaluation of memory, the platform is removed, and the time spent in the platform's previous location is recorded (probe trial). Rodents with intact memory will spend more time swimming in that area, whereas animals that have not learned the spatial location (cognitively impaired) will search around the entire arena. A number of AD mouse models, including PDAPP, APP/PS1, P301S, and STZ models, demonstrate impairments in learning and memory using the MWM task [49–52]. Recently, a virtual MWM approach has been utilized in human AD patients, to evaluate the validity of this task. A study by Possin et al. compared amyloid mouse models to AD patients with mild cognitive impairments in a virtual MWM setting [53]. They reported that both the mouse model and AD human patients showed similar impairments in locating the target, demonstrating cross-species validity.

Another example of a simple, but effective task used for the evaluation of recognition memory in rodents is novel-object recognition (NOR). During this task, rodents are given two identical objects to explore. After a retention period, the rodents are again given one of the familiar objects and one novel object. Using the rodents' innate preference for novelty, the rodents that have intact cognition will spend more time with the novel object, since it will recognize the familiar object. Numerous studies have demonstrated NOR deficits in most of the animal models of AD discussed [29, 54, 55]. Differences in recognition memory have also been performed in human participants, with AD patients demonstrating similar deficits as those observed in the preclinical models [56, 57]. Both MWM and NOR studies have been shown to be effective in the evaluation of drugs in AD rodent models, including in drugs such as the FDA-approved AD drugs donepezil [58] and galantamine [59, 60] demonstrating cognitive improvement. Numerous other hippocampal-dependent tests have been employed in the process of therapeutic benefit evaluation [61], as well as other behavioral tasks that tap into alternative learning and memory systems altered in AD. This includes Pavlovian conditioning, working memory, and operant learning approaches [61]. Learning and memory assessment in animal models, and application to the human population, are essential to the drug-development pipeline.

7.8 Cellular and Molecular Techniques for Evaluation of Drug Effectiveness

Numerous cellular and molecular techniques are used during the evaluation of drug effectiveness in AD animal models. The detection and quantification of proteins in a biological sample is critical in studies of drug development. This approach is vitally important as these same measures are impossible to assess with the same accuracy and precision in clinical samples until relevant biomarkers are more capable of detection and quantification. In addition, the evaluation of specific tissues provides both opportunities to evaluate the extent that a potential therapeutic engaged the target of interest and/or altered AD pathobiology; it also serves to greatly enhance our understanding of AD. Techniques including enzyme-linked immunosorbent assay (ELISA) and western blot are common in the analysis of proteins in drug discovery. Both techniques use antibody detection methods. ELISA is a sensitive method in the detection of novel proteins and investigation into protein interaction, having a higher throughput of samples. Though requiring more complex laboratory skills, western blots have higher specificity in the analysis of protein levels. In a study investigating the effects of resveratrol, a grape seed polyphenolic extract that may have neuroprotective properties, researchers evaluated the treatment through both ELISA and western blot techniques [62]. Using the 5×FAD mouse model, resveratrol was administered orally for 60 days and the mice were assessed through a series of cognitive tests, including MWM. Subsequently, the brain tissue was evaluated for the levels of $A\beta_{40}$ and $A\beta_{42}$ through ELISA, demonstrating a decrease in both peptides with treatment, compared to a control group. In addition, western blotting was used to measure enzymes related to the $A\beta$ formation, to better understand the mechanisms involved in $A\beta$ processing and their treatment-related features. Not only does this approach provide data on the ability of a therapeutic to alter AD specific pathology, but it also allows for the determination of whether the therapeutic alters discrete protein levels in associated pathways, affecting the severity or progression of the disease. For example, upregulation of a specific protein such as GSK-3β (involved in tau phosphorylation) could demonstrate potential negative effects in tau phosphorylation pathways indicating exacerbation of the disease. In addition, downregulation of specific proteins, such as $A\beta$, could indicate a possible novel target for therapeutic development. As the capacity and sensitivity of techniques has advanced in the last 20 years, the number of targets, as well as the sensitivity of the assay, has improved significantly.

The next generation of this approach has moved toward multiplex assays for the quantification of multiple analytes in one sample. These more robust techniques not only provide information on whether the treatment impacts the mechanism of interest, but provide insight on numerous other related proteins. With the use of small animal models, biological samples are limited, and this technique provides large data sets from minimal amounts of sample. Smaller proteins, such as inflammatory cytokines, can be easily measured in a multiplex assay making it an ideal technique in the investigation of processes such as neuroinflammation. More and more preclinical investigations have been able to tap into the evaluation of off-target impacts of potential therapeutics utilizing the expanded approach of the multiplex assays.

Another frequently used procedure for the evaluation of treatment efficacy is immunohistochemistry. As the pathological hallmarks of AD are exhibited as structural changes in brain tissue (plaques and tangles), it is common for immunohistochemistry to be performed on the brain tissue of animal models. The sample is sectioned, stained or probed with antibodies, and imaged through microscopy. Immunohistochemistry allows a visual analysis of the tissue, including the evaluation of tissue integrity, detection and comparison of pathological expression, as well as investigation into the cell morphology. It also allows the exploration into the interactions and relationships between cells or cells with AD pathologies. These approaches have become more sensitive at the identification of changes in discrete proteins in both the brain and in other tissues where they may provide biomarkers to be monitored in human clinical trials.

Additional biochemical approaches are emerging that provide far greater sensitivity and insight into AD pathobiology; these assessments are beginning to be included in the evaluation of novel therapies. For example, a very specialized and sensitive technique that is increasingly popular is flow cytometry. In this method, live cells are utilized for the quantification of specific proteins. This approach allows for very specific changes to be detected. Flow cytometry facilitates the analysis of specific cell populations; in neuroinflammation research, for example, the analysis of targets involved in specific cells, such as glia, can be achieved. The ability to design novel therapeutics for discrete cell types and to effectively measure disease-relevant changes represents the next leap forward in several fields, including AD. A specialized flow cytometry technique known as fluorescence-activated cell sorting allows the population of cells of interest to be isolated and used in additional studies. With complex, precise, and specialized techniques, such as flow cytometry, come an investment of resources and training. Although many of these techniques are used to analyze human AD samples including cerebrospinal fluid (CSF), blood, plasma, and tissue biopsies, animal models provide the opportunity to directly and immediately test brain tissue, enabling further understanding of AD and the efficacy of a novel therapeutic.

7.9 Emerging Approaches

The above highlighted approaches have yielded a robust program for the examination of potential therapeutics in AD. However, given that numerous candidates that have met the criteria (go versus no-go) required in preclinical systems to move to humans have ultimately failed in clinical trials, there is a need to improve the process. Several factors have been highlighted as potential limiting factors in the available approaches, which include the use of FAD models, the lack of an integrated multi-technique approach in phenotyping models, and refined approaches to evaluate candidate ligands. Highlighted below are examples of the coordinated efforts underway to advance the process of preclinical testing in AD.

7.10 Model Organism Development and Evaluation for Late-Onset AD (MODEL-AD)

As indicated above, AD is generally classified as early-onset (EOAD) or late-onset (LOAD), based on factors including age of onset and genetic markers. The majority of cases of EOAD are caused by mutations in the *APP*, *PSEN1*, and *PSEN2* genes, but EOAD accounts for a small fraction of AD cases. The use of animal models of EOAD has been raised as a concern in the evaluation of candidate therapeutics given that it differs from the more common LOAD. To this end, there has been considerable effort dedicated to emerging approaches to LOAD. Genetic susceptibility to LOAD is more complex, with variations in many genes significantly associated with increased risk. The greatest and most common genetic risk factor is the ε4 allele, *APOE-4*, which accounts for ~30% of risk. Next generation sequencing has more recently determined that the R47 H variant in triggering receptor expressed on myeloid cells 2 (*TREM2*) – $TREM2^{R47H}$ – conferred increased risk for AD [63]. Animal models for these LOAD risk genes have been generated and are now making their way into the novel ligand testing domain, in particular for agents that target downstream changes of the mutations (for example, inflammation).

Based on EOAD studies, as highlighted above, many approaches toward therapies aimed at reducing the Aβ burden in the brains of AD patients have been developed and tested in clinical trials, including active and passive Aβ immunization [64], gamma- and beta-secretase inhibitors, gamma-secretase modulator [65], and Aβ aggregation inhibitors. Unfortunately, these strategies have failed in AD clinical trials [66]. There are numerous potential explanations as to why these clinical trials have failed, including the stage of disease targeted, mechanism of delivery, effective engagement of target and off-target effects, face and construct validity of the animal models, and others [67, 68]. However, the exact reasons for failures of the clinical trials remain to be established.

In 2015, a recommendation of the National Institute on Aging (NIA) Alzheimer's Research Summit was to develop and characterize novel animal models of AD that would facilitate the development of novel AD therapies, from genetics and systems biology to animal model development to preclinical drug testing. This approach has yielded numerous promising animal models to better understand AD pathology, but also a wealth of new model systems for drug evaluation. One of the forerunners in the approach is the MODEL-AD Center.

7.10.1 The Aims of MODEL-AD

In 2016, the first Model Organism Development and Evaluation for Late-Onset AD (MODEL-AD) center was established; a second center was funded in 2017. The MODEL-AD center is a consortium consisting of two centers: one is a collaboration between Indiana University, the Jackson Laboratory, the University of Pittsburgh, and Sage Bionetworks; the second is at the University of California, Irvine. The major aims of MODEL-AD are to develop, create, characterize, and distribute models for LOAD, and establish robust preclinical pipelines for testing new therapies. Their strategy will be to create new rodent models, initially in the mouse. Mice will be engineered using clustered regularly interspaced short palindromic repeats (CRISPR) and other traditional methods to carry combinations of human variants identified using computational analyses of human data sets made available from Accelerating Medicines Partnership® Program for Alzheimer's Disease (AMP® AD) Molecular Mechanisms of the Vascular Etiology – AD (M²OVE-AD), AD Sequencing Project (ADSP), AD Neuroimaging Initiative (ADNI), and other sources. New models will be "staged" and must pass through a "go/no-go" gate, which enables the center to determine the relevance to human AD using a transcriptomic approach. Human-relevant outcome measures, particularly transcriptional profiling, blood biomarkers, in vivo imaging, as well as traditional phenotyping methods including neuropathology, biochemistry, and behavioral assays, will be evaluated in a subset of models that pass through the initial staging phase. To maximize uptake of all resources created by MODEL-AD (mice, data, protocols, etc.) all data are made available via the AD Knowledge Portal (https://adknowledgeportal.synapse.org/). All mice are made available from the Jackson Laboratory AD Mouse Model Resource (www.jax.org/alzheimers).

7.10.2 Creating, Validating, and Disseminating New Models of LOAD

A primary goal of MODEL-AD is to create novel models for LOAD, and extensively characterize them using human-relevant and translatable outcome measures (Figure 7.2). New models will be assessed side by side with prominent existing EOAD models. The first model created (sensitized background strain) carries the two greatest genetic risk factors of LOAD – *APOE-4* and *Trem2^{R47H}* – on the C57BL/6 J (B6) mouse genetic background. AD-relevant genetic variants will be incorporated into this sensitizer "model." The consortium has now humanized the *APP* allele corresponding to the Aβ$_{42}$ region and are incorporating a humanized *MAPT* gene as well. To date, over 50 new models have been created and made available.

The Bioinformatics and Data Management Core (BDMC) leverages large data resources (e.g., ADNI, AMP® AD, M²OVE-AD, ADSP, and the International Genomics of Alzheimer's Project [IGAP]) to identify and prioritize candidate variants modeling LOAD. The consortium's initial strategy was to use sequencing studies to aid in prioritizing variants in existing genome-wide association studies (GWAS) loci. Once existing loci have been addressed, novel candidate genes and variants from the rapidly expanding efforts will be incorporated to understand the genetics of AD. MODEL-AD has expanded the modeling strategy to include modeling non-coding variants and integrating data from expression quantitative trait locus (eQTL) studies. The expanding availability of quantitative traits related to AD pathology from ADNI, eQTL, and other functional studies will enable greater statistical power and phenotypic resolution. Importantly, such studies facilitate the use of advanced computational strategies to infer epistatic and pleiotropic networks of genes that can aid in prioritizing polygenic animal models.

All new strains will initially be characterized at 4 and 12 months utilizing a transcriptomic approach to assess the relevance to human AD [69]. These data serve as a go/no-go gate for determining which models move into a "deep phenotyping" pipeline that includes more comprehensive phenotyping at multiple ages (up to 24 months) in male and female mice and, in addition to more traditional phenotyping assays (e.g., behavior, biochemistry, and neuropathology), will include in vivo imaging with autoradiography validation of tracer compounds, blood, and CSF biomarkers, and molecular profiling by RNA sequencing. Assays are designed to complement existing and forthcoming data from human studies, and the BDMC will systematically align the phenotypes of each mouse model with corresponding human data. For example, early gene expression signatures that appear in mouse models may be present in human brain samples, providing evidence for a particular pathway dysfunction in LOAD. The identification of such signatures in human subpopulations may further discriminate among heterogeneous etiologies within the human population [70]. These analyses will link precise genetic variation in the mouse

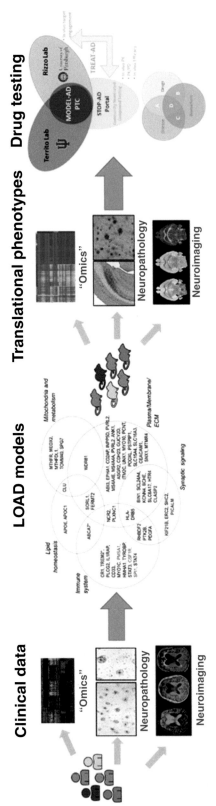

Figure 7.2 Pipeline of animal models being created by the MODEL-AD center. The goals of MODEL-AD are to create and characterize novel models of LOAD by prioritizing variants from human data sets. Once a variant is identified, CRISPR and other techniques are used to create the model and the model moves into a primary screening mechanism. The mouse models are aligned with human phenotypes. The preclinical testing core tests novel therapies in the new models of LOAD. All data and protocols are shared through the AD Knowledge Portal.

model with pathological outcomes that contribute to LOAD, which can be further assessed in human carriers of the homologous variants. These human/mouse comparisons will provide critical data to determine the most appropriate models to use in preclinical studies and also novel targets to test as therapies for LOAD.

7.10.3 The Preclinical Testing Core

MODEL-AD is comprehensively addressing many identified concerns related to preclinical screening of test compounds. The Preclinical Testing Core (PCT) will establish a streamlined preclinical strategy with go/no-go decision points allowing critical and unbiased assessments of potential therapeutic agents (Figure 7.3). The primary screen is the determination of appreciable PK and target tissue activity in the disease model and at the pathologically and disease-relevant age. Quantification of PK parameters for the parent compound will use standard moment theory (non-compartmental)

methods and parameters [71]. The compounds nominated for the pipeline will need to meet a strict set of criteria. In the absence of meeting the criteria, compounds will not move forward. Provided the compound meets the "go" criteria, the PK data will be used to model the dosing paradigm for the secondary screen where appropriate disease models at the pathological ages achieve target brain exposure levels to evaluate disease-modifying effects.

The secondary screen evaluates target engagement and disease-modifying activity of the test compound utilizing non-invasive PET/MRI as a pharmacodynamic readout of cerebral changes in metabolism, blood flow, and Aβ or tau deposition. Blood samples will be collected and processed for plasma to confirm the PK from the primary screen at the conclusions of the study. To permit secondary confirmation for PET and autoradiography studies, tissue sections will be immunostained with Aβ, tau, or neuroinflammation antibodies. Tertiary screening will evaluate both the dose–response

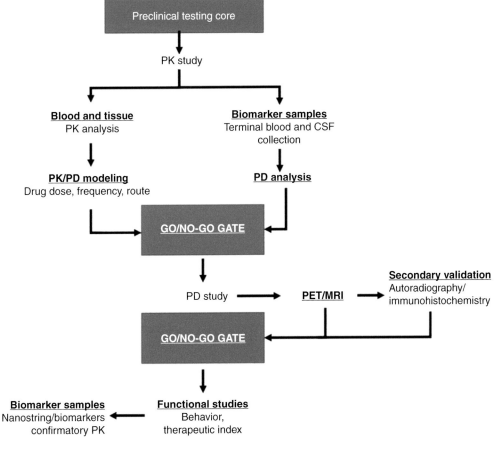

Figure 7.3 Preclinical screening of test compounds by the PCT of the MODEL-AD center.

curve and dose-range regimens to determined disease-modifying effects of the test compound in order to normalize a disease-related phenotype. Tertiary screening will include assessments of cognition (e.g., working memory, short-term memory) and activity measures (e.g., locomotor activity, motor coordination) to identify whether the dose range perceived to improve a functional (i.e., memory) deficit is without side effects that confound the interpretation of the data.

This approach is innovative, first by establishing this standardized, streamlined preclinical screening strategy, and by providing access to these resources to the AD research community.

7.10.4   Summary and Outlook

MODEL-AD is configured to fully exploit contemporary resources to create the next generation of LOAD models and, moving forward, will be augmented with novel information and technologies. The expanded efforts to quantify proteins and metabolites in addition to transcriptomes by AMP® AD can be readily reproduced in mouse models. This will allow multiscale molecular comparisons between novel models and human LOAD cohorts, possibly identifying subpopulations of AD patients with distinct neuropathology and/or genetic etiology. Alignment of multiscale phenotypes (molecular, histological, and behavioral) of these models to human data will likely identify key pathways and processes that drive neuropathology and LOAD.

7.11   TaRget Enablement to Accelerate Therapy Development for Alzheimer's Disease (TREAT-AD)

As part of long-range strategic planning, the NIA recently funded two drug discovery centers that comprise the TaRget Enablement to Accelerate Therapy Development for Alzheimer's Disease (TREAT-AD) consortium. The two centers, one led by Emory University, Sage Bionetworks, and the Structural Genomics Consortium; and the other led by the Indiana University School of Medicine (IUSM) and Purdue University, add to the growing number of NIA-sponsored initiatives that are collectively working to create breakthroughs for the diagnosis, management, and treatment of AD. The overarching purpose of the TREAT-AD program is to improve, diversify, and reinvigorate the AD drug-development pipeline by accelerating the

characterization and experimental validation of next-generation therapeutic targets and integrating the targets into drug discovery campaigns. In addition, this program aims to de-risk potential therapeutics to the point that industry will invest in them, accelerating the delivery of new drugs to AD patients. To this end, the funded centers will: (1) design, develop, and disseminate tools that support target-enabling packages for the experimental validation of novel, next-generation therapeutic targets, including those emanating from the NIA-funded, target discovery programs such AMP® AD; and (2) initiate early-stage drug discovery campaigns against the enabled targets. Central to this initiative is the open-access, rapid dissemination of data, methods, and computational and experimental tools generated by the centers to all qualified researchers for their use in advancing AD drug discovery and AD disease biology.

A more thorough description of the IUSM–Purdue TREAT-AD center provides insight into how this program will contribute to the overarching goals of the TREAT-AD consortium, as well as draw synergy with not only other NIA programs, but also the global scientific community working to find solutions to AD. In concert with the vision of the TREAT-AD consortium, the goal of the IUSM–Purdue TREAT-AD center is to advance the field of AD translational research by diversifying drug discovery efforts to explore novel emerging disease hypotheses and contribute to a pipeline of possible new treatments. Central to this approach is leveraging the foundational work of multiple NIA programs directed at AD research (Figure 7.4). Over the past several years, the NIA has made substantial investments in large, multi-site and multi-institutional consortia focused on developing key translational research infrastructure for accelerating the identification and characterization of novel therapeutic targets for LOAD and the development of testing of therapies based upon these targets. This has included the AMP® AD, M²OVE-AD, MODEL-AD, and Resilience-AD consortia, Alzheimer's Clinical Trial Consortium (ACTC), and the Religious Orders Study and Rush Memory and Aging Project (ROS/MAP), among others. Specifically, the IUSM–Purdue TREAT-AD center will work closely with the AMP® AD initiative to evaluate nominated disease targets through a strategy that will initially focus on neuroinflammatory signaling. This is driven by an emerging scientific understanding of the role of activated microglia in AD etiology and

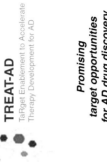

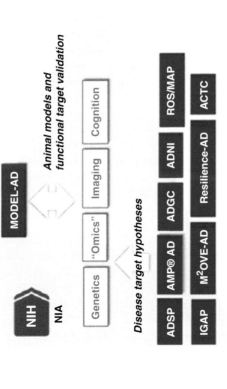

Figure 7.4 NIA programs directed at AD research.

an opportunity to establish a strong thematic drug discovery program through synergy with global researchers. Additionally, neuroinflammation pathways that contribute to AD phenotypes are represented by significant genetic diversity; this creates a framework to pursue the work in the context of precision medicine translational strategies. Thus, these efforts will contribute to important groundwork for the design of clinical studies for new classes of therapeutics in genetically defined patients. To this end, the IUSM–Purdue TREAT-AD center has also tightly integrated the MODEL-AD initiative into its strategy and operational plans. This provides direct access to cutting-edge animal models, reflective of variants observed in immune genes, for the purpose of target validation and prioritization of targets for drug discovery. Additionally, these same models can be used to evaluate potential therapeutics for efficacy, hopefully with improved translational prediction.

By design, the TREAT-AD centers bring together sophisticated scientific talent and capability to evaluate and prosecute prioritized drug discovery targets. For example, the IUSM–Purdue center's work is organized around an Administrative and Data Management Core and four technical cores that include Bioinformatics and Computational Biology, Structural Biology and Biophysics, Assay Development and High Throughput Screening, and Medicinal Chemistry and Chemical Biology (Figure 7.5). The technical cores work together as a highly integrated and collaborative scientific team to provide both ongoing evaluation of potential drug targets, and drug discovery enablement of select opportunities that align with the center's strategy.

As previously mentioned, an important function of the TREAT-AD initiative is to create a dynamic portfolio of prioritized targets for drug discovery enablement. While the focus on AMP® AD nominated targets representing a neuroinflammatory signature provides one level of filter, the IUSM–Purdue TREAT-AD center portfolio will be further refined to represent a risk balance of both nascent and more mature target hypotheses that map to the center's expertise and capacities. To differentiate between opportunities, drug targets will be continually assessed through the lens of target validation and druggability. This approach provides an evidentiary and dynamic framework to consider the status and innovation potential of each target, reflecting an understanding of connection to disease pathology (validation), and the likelihood of

identifying small-molecule modulators based on contemporary precedent and available technologies (druggability). In addition to data assembled by the AMP® AD and MODEL-AD scientific teams, multiple data sources are used to evaluate targets against these dimensions, including available "omics" databases, informatics, and computational biology analyses, as well as the general scientific and patent literature. When viewed two-dimensionally (Figure 7.6), this analysis permits the relative comparison of target validation and druggability for multiple targets and is thus a powerful strategic tool to create a risk-balanced portfolio. Taken collectively, the guiding principles for target prioritization for the IUSM–Purdue TREAT-AD center is to focus on AMP® AD nominated targets with high innovation potential (as informed by target validation and druggability) and well-defined biological hypotheses that will contribute to a systematic study of neuroimmune pathology in AD. Clinical studies will ultimately validate novel targets in patients; and therefore the targets we select also require a feasible experimental path to design molecules that engage the target sufficiently (in relevant models), in order to inform the discovery and development of a clinical candidate that is safe and effective enough to test in humans.

As evidence of this strategy, the first two neuroinflammation targets prioritized by the IUSM–Purdue TREAT-AD center are inositol polyphosphate-5-phosphatase D (INPP5D, also known as SHIP1) and 1-phosphatidylinositol-4,5-bisphosphate phosphodiesterase gamma-2 (PLCG2) (Figure 7.7). INPP5D is an AMP® AD nominated target and AD risk gene (identified by GWAS), preferentially expressed in lymphoid cells, including microglia. INPP5D is a negative modulator of TREM2 function; and researchers at the center are working with MODEL-AD to evaluate and develop animal models for PK/PD evaluation and to lead to optimization of promising inhibitor chemical series. The target class (phosphatase) represented by INPP5D poses significant druggability challenges; however, novel molecular and protein structural approaches will be explored that may provide innovative solutions for modulating phosphatase activity with high-quality selective inhibitors. Similarly, PLCG2 is an AMP® AD prioritized target and is also the focus of MODEL-AD animal model characterization studies. PLCG2 is a transmembrane signaling enzyme implicated in beta-cell activation and

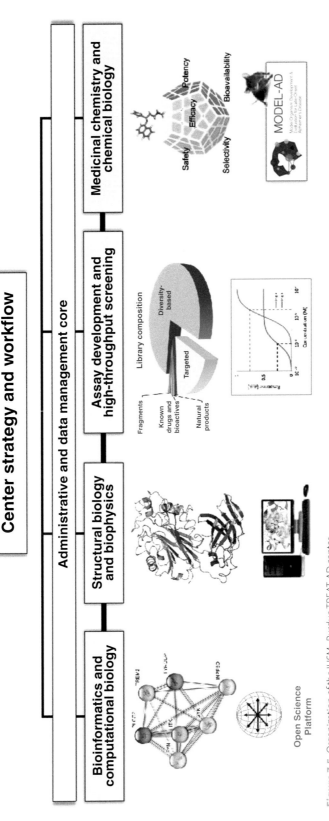

Figure 7.5 Organization of the IUSM–Purdue TREAT-AD center.

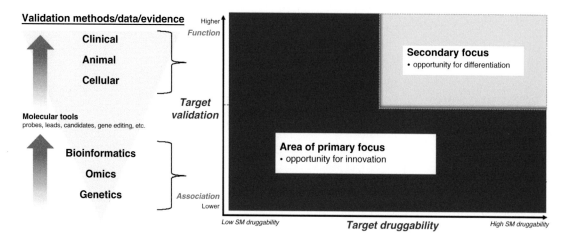

Figure 7.6 TREAT-AD center framework for considering the status and innovation potential of each target, reflecting a connection to disease pathology and the likelihood of identifying small-molecule (SM) modulators based on contemporary precedent and available technologies (druggability).

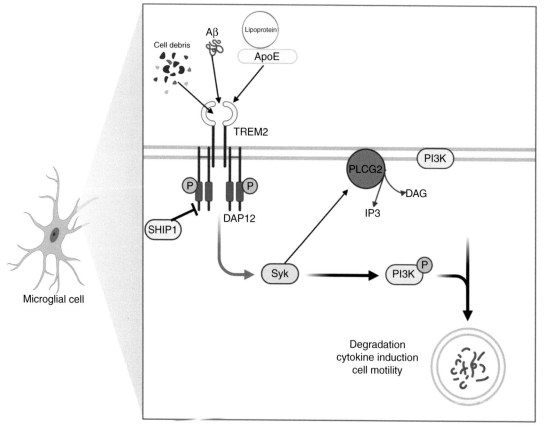

Figure 7.7 INPP5D (also known as SHIP1) and PLCG2: anti-inflammatory targets prioritized by the IUSM–Purdue TREAT-AD center as risk genes in microglia signaling [72]. DAG, diacylglycerol; DAP12, DNA activating protein 12; IP3, inositol trisphosphate; PI3K, phosphoinositide 3 kinase.

proliferation, with PLCG2 mRNA upregulated in the cortical tissue of LOAD patients. Interestingly, there is an activating mutation of the *PLCG2* gene (P522 R) that is protective against AD; and thus agonism of the enzyme in microglia is postulated to be a promising target for further exploration. There are no selective small-molecule activators known for PLCG2; however, recent structural data and insights into enzymatic activation through interactions with protein binding partners may provide a productive path to novel small-molecule modulators.

A key deliverable of the IUSM–Purdue TREAT-AD center is to contribute toward an increased translational understanding of AD while concomitantly providing a path to new innovative therapies. Therefore, an important measure of our performance will be the creation of high-quality lead molecules for prioritized targets with a trajectory for optimization into clinical candidates. The molecular optimization process will be issue-driven and will focus on multiparameter structure–activity relationship (SAR) studies with a view to human translation. The goal is not simply to produce lead molecules but to create molecules with a strong trajectory to a clinical candidate by anticipating and de-risking codependent performance variables that cover disease pharmacology and general pharmaceutical properties for centrally acting drugs. As a general rule, lead candidates from the IUSM–Purdue TREAT-AD center will meet the late stage entry criteria listed in the Alzheimer's Disease Drug Development Program funding opportunity (https://grants.nih.gov/grants/guide/pa-files/par-18-820.html). These rigorous criteria require a clear and convincing demonstration of preclinical efficacy in an established AD animal model along with in vivo target engagement at the clinically intended site of action. By design, the experimental testing paradigm to guide the discovery and optimization of promising chemical series, which includes PK/PD assays and the pairing of specific disease models and associated fluid and imaging biomarker endpoints, is an integral part of the IUSM–Purdue TREAT-AD approach to deliver on these outcomes.

Finally, as with all NIA AD initiatives, the timely sharing of experimental data generated by the IUSM–Purdue TREAT-AD center through an open-access portal is an essential part of creating synergy and collaboration with global scientific researchers searching for cures. These data and research tools (as part of target enablement packages) will enable external investigators to both reproduce and expand on the IUSM–Purdue TREAT-AD center's findings, as well as accelerate new and diverse research efforts to advance the field.

7.12 Considerations in Research Animal Use

The use of animal models is essential to the expansion of knowledge into AD and advancement of drug development. The testing of candidate ligands in animal models assists with the assessment of efficacy of novel treatments. However, drugs prescribed to AD patients currently target cognitive aspects of the disease without slowing or halting the progression of the disease pathologies. Many AD clinical trials have failed, partly due to the lack of translation between animal models and humans. As described throughout the chapter, no model completely encompasses all complexities of the disease; each represents a facet that can contribute to the overall understanding of AD. With the recent expansion of AD risk-factor models, and programs such as MODEL-AD and TREAT-AD, animal models will continue to represent keys aspects of the disease. Though researchers are responsible for choosing an appropriate animal model in a study, there should be consideration into the validation of the model and the questions asked. Three categories of validity should be evaluated before choosing a model: face validity, construct validity, and predictive validity. Face validity describes the extent to which a model represents the pathology, symptom, or mechanism being evaluated; construct validity evaluates how well the model reflects the disease in humans; predictive validity is defined by the degree to which the animal model predicts the outcome in humans. A good model should have validity in each of these three areas, though a model typically will not be able to encompass all three completely. Choosing the correct model to effectively evaluate a treatment is critical to the AD drug-development ecosystem. It is also important to ethically consider whether animal models are necessary to answer pressing questions, ways to limit the use by maintaining a minimal sample size required for statistical significance, and replacement of the use of animals with other methods when possible.

7.13 Contribution of Animal Models to the AD Drug-Development Ecosystem

Non-clinical assessment in animal models establishes preliminary safety and efficacy against targets of interest prior to advancing the agent to FIH trials with possible development of a viable therapy. Animal models have not predicted efficacy in humans but have validated efficacy against intended targets and have played a critically important role in AD drug development. The advances described in this chapter promise to provide better targets and more promising candidate therapies to advance to human trials.

References

1. Zhao M, Lepak AJ, Andes DR. Animal models in the pharmacokinetic/pharmacodynamic evaluation of antimicrobial agents. *Bioorg Med Chem* 2016; **24**: 6390–400.

2. Ambrose PG, Bhavnani SM, Rubino CM, et al. Pharmacokinetics–pharmacodynamics of antimicrobial therapy: it's not just for mice anymore. *Clin Infect Dis* 2007; **44**: 79–86.

3. Fitten LJ, Flood JF, Baxter CF, Tachiki KH, Perryman K. Long-term oral administration of memory-enhancing doses of tacrine in mice: a study of potential toxicity and side effects. *J. Gerontol* 1987; **42**: 681–5.

4. Scearce-Levie K, Sanchez PE, Lewcock JW. Leveraging preclinical models for the development of Alzheimer disease therapeutics. *Nat Rev Drug Discov* 2020; **19**: 447–62.

5. Fan L, Mao C, Hu X, et al. New insights into the pathogenesis of Alzheimer's disease. *Front Neurol* 2020; **10**:1312.

6. Kinney JW, Bemiller SM, Murtishaw AS, et al. Inflammation as a central mechanism in Alzheimer's disease. *Alzheimers Dement (N Y)* 2018; **4**: 575–90.

7. Schenk D, Barbour N, Dunn W, et al. Immunization with amyloid-β attenuates Alzheimer-disease-like pathology in the PDAPP mouse. *Nature* 1999; **400**: 173.

8. Orgogozo J-M, Gilman S, Dartigues J-F, et al. Subacute meningoencephalitis in a subset of patients with AD after Abeta42 immunization. *Neurology* 2003; **61**: 46–54.

9. Nicoll JAR, Wilkinson D, Holmes C, et al. Neuropathology of human Alzheimer disease after immunization with amyloid-β peptide: a case report. *Nat Med* 2003; **9**: 448–52.

10. Fandos N, Pérez-Grijalba V, Pesini P, et al. Plasma amyloid $\beta_{42/40}$ ratios as biomarkers for amyloid β cerebral deposition in cognitively normal individuals. *Alzheimers Dement (Amst)* 2017; **8**: 179–87.

11. Moore BD, Martin J, de Mena L, et al. Short Aβ peptides attenuate $A\beta_{42}$ toxicity in vivo. *J Exp Med* 2018; **215**: 283–301.

12. Salazar A, Leisgang A, Ortiz A, Kinney J. Dementia insights: what do animal models of Alzheimer's disease tell us? *Pract Neurol* 2019;July/August:23–34.

13. Janelidze S, Stomrud E, Smith R, et al. Cerebrospinal fluid p-tau217 performs better than p-tau181 as a biomarker of Alzheimer's disease. *Nat Commun* 2020; **11**: 1683.

14. Thijssen EH, La Joie R, Wolf A, et al. Diagnostic value of plasma phosphorylated tau_{181} in Alzheimer's disease and frontotemporal lobar degeneration. *Nat Med* 2020; **26**: 387–97.

15. Van Dam D, De Deyn PP. Animal models in the drug discovery pipeline for Alzheimer's disease. *Br J Pharmacol* 2011; **164**: 1285–300.

16. Cummings J, Lee G, Ritter A, Sabbagh M, Zhong K. Alzheimer's disease drug development pipeline: 2020. *Alzheimers Dement (N Y)* 2020; **6**: e12050.

17. Sterniczuk R, Antle MC, LaFerla FM, Dyck RH. Characterization of the 3×Tg-AD mouse model of Alzheimer's disease: part 2. Behavioral and cognitive changes. *Brain Res* 2010; **1348**: 149–55.

18. Martinez-Coria H, Green KN, Billings LM, et al. Memantine improves cognition and reduces Alzheimer's-like neuropathology in transgenic mice. *Am J Pathol* 2010; **176**: 870–80.

19. Fiebich BL, Batista CRA, Saliba SW, Yousif NM, de Oliveira ACP. Role of microglia TLRs in neurodegeneration. *Front Cell Neurosci* 2018; **12**: 329.

20. Zhao J, Bi W, Xiao S, et al. Neuroinflammation induced by lipopolysaccharide causes cognitive impairment in mice. *Sci Rep* 2019; **9**: 5790.

21. Weintraub MK, Kranjac D, Eimerbrink, MJ, et al. Peripheral administration of poly I:C leads to increased hippocampal amyloid-beta and cognitive deficits in a non-transgenic mouse. *Behav Brain Res* 2014; **266**: 183–7.

22. Walker DG, Tang TM, Lue L-F. Increased expression of toll-like receptor 3, an anti-viral signaling molecule, and related genes in Alzheimer's disease brains. *Exp Neurol* 2018; **309**: 91–106.

23. Alzheimer's Association. 2020 Alzheimer's disease facts and figures. *Alzheimers Dement* 2020; **16**: 391–460.

24. Yeoman M, Scutt G, Faragher R. Insights into CNS ageing from animal models of senescence. *Nat Rev Neurosci* 2012; **13**: 435–45.

25. Morley JE, Farr SA, Kuma VB, Armbrecht HJ. The SAMP8 mouse: a model to develop therapeutic interventions for Alzheimer's disease. *Curr Pharm Des* 2012; **18**: 1123–30.

26. Carroll JC, Roasrio ER, Chang L, et al. Progesterone and estrogen regulate Alzheimer-like neuropathology in female 3×Tg-AD mice. *J Neurosci* 2007; **27**: 13357–65.

27. Palm R, Chang J, Blair J, et al. Down-regulation of serum gonadotropins but not estrogen replacement improves cognition in aged-ovariectomized 3×Tg AD female mice. *J Neurochem* 2014; **130**: 115–25.

28. Rolo AP, Palmeira CM. Diabetes and mitochondrial function: role of hyperglycemia and oxidative stress. *Toxicol Appl Pharmacol* 2006; **212**: 167–78.

29. Murtishaw AS, Hearney CF, Bolton MM, et al. Intermittent streptozotocin administration induces behavioral and pathological features relevant to Alzheimer's disease and vascular dementia. *Neuropharmacology* 2018; **137**: 164–77.

30. Candeias E, Duarte AI, Carvalho C, et al. The impairment of insulin signaling in Alzheimer's disease. *IUBMB Life* 2012; **64**: 951–7.

31. Dineley KT, Jahrling JB, Denner L. Insulin resistance in Alzheimer's disease. *Neurobiol Dis* 2014; **72**: 92–103.

32. Lee Y, Kim Y-H, Park SJ, et al. Insulin/IGF signaling-related gene expression in the brain of a sporadic Alzheimer's disease monkey model induced by intracerebroventricular injection of streptozotocin. *J Alzheimers Dis* 2014; **38**: 251–67.

33. Yeo H-G, Lee Y, Jeon CY, et al. Characterization of cerebral damage in a monkey model of Alzheimer's disease induced by intracerebroventricular injection of streptozotocin. *J Alzheimers Dis* 2015; **46**: 989–1005.

34. Bauzon J, Lee G, Cummings J. Repurposed agents in the Alzheimer's disease drug development pipeline. *Alzheimers Res Ther* 2020; **12**: 98.

35. Knight EM, Martins VA, Gümüsgöz S, Allan SM, Lawrence CB. High-fat diet-induced memory impairment in triple-transgenic Alzheimer's disease (3×TgAD) mice is independent of changes in amyloid and tau pathology. *Neurobiol Aging* 2014; **35**: 1821–32.

36. Bracko O, Vinarcsik LK, Cruz Hernández JC, et al. High fat diet worsens Alzheimer's disease-related behavioral abnormalities and neuropathology in APP/PS1 mice, but not by synergistically decreasing cerebral blood flow. *Sci Rep* 2020; **10**: 9884.

37. Rollins CPE, Gallion D, Kong V, et al. Contributions of a high-fat diet to Alzheimer's disease-related decline: A longitudinal behavioural and structural neuroimaging study in mouse models. *Neuroimage Clin* 2019; **21**: 101606.

38. Bhat NR, Thirumangalakudi L. Increased tau phosphorylation and impaired brain insulin/IGF signaling in mice fed a high fat/high cholesterol diet. *J Alzheimers Dis* 2013; **36**: 781–9.

39. Busquets O, Ettcheto M, Pallàs M, et al. Long-term exposition to a high fat diet favors the appearance of β-amyloid depositions in the brain of C57BL/6 J mice. A potential model of sporadic Alzheimer's disease. *Mech Ageing Dev* 2017; **162**: 38–45.

40. Pugazhenthi S, Qin L, Reddy PH. Common neurodegenerative pathways in obesity, diabetes, and Alzheimer's disease. *Biochim Biophys Acta* 2017; **1863**: 1037–45.

41. Prüßing K, Voig, A, Schulz JB. *Drosophila melanogaster* as a model organism for Alzheimer's disease. *Mol Neurodegener* 2013; **8**: 35.

42. Tan FHP, Azzam G. *Drosophila melanogaster*: Deciphering Alzheimer's disease. *Malays J Med Sci* 2017; **24**: 6–20.

43. Drummond E, Wisniewski T. Alzheimer's disease: experimental models and reality. *Acta Neuropathol* 2017; **133**: 155–75.

44. Callahan PM, Hutchings EJ, Kille NJ, Chapman JM, Terry AV. Positive allosteric modulator of α7 nicotinic-acetylcholine receptors, PNU-120596 augments the effects of donepezil on learning and memory in aged rodents and non-human primates. *Neuropharmacology* 2013; **67**: 201–12.

45. Vardigan JD, Cannon CE, Puri V, et al. Improved cognition without adverse effects: novel M1 muscarinic potentiator compares favorably to donepezil and xanomeline in rhesus monkey. *Psychopharmacology (Berl)* 2015; **232**: 1859–66.

46. Link CD. Invertebrate models of Alzheimer's disease. *Genes Brain Behav* 2005; **4**: 147–56.

47. Tse FL, Laplanche R. Absorption, metabolism, and disposition of [14 C]SDZ ENA 713, an acetylcholinesterase inhibitor, in minipigs following oral, intravenous, and dermal administration. *Pharm Res* 1998; **15**: 1614–20.

48. Wang D. Tumor necrosis factor-alpha alters electrophysiological properties of rabbit hippocampal neurons. *J Alzheimers Dis* 2019; **68**: 1257–71.

49. Brody DL, Holtzman DM. Morris water maze search strategy analysis in PDAPP mice before and after experimental traumatic brain injury. *Exp Neurol* 2006; **197**: 330–40.

50. Li D, Huang Y, Cheng B, et al. Streptozotocin induces mild cognitive impairment at appropriate doses in mice as determined by long-term potentiation and the Morris water maze. *J Alzheimers Dis* 2016; **54**: 89–98.

51. Sadowski M, Pankiewicz J, Scholtzova H, et al. Amyloid-β deposition is associated with decreased hippocampal glucose metabolism and spatial memory impairment in *APP/PS1* mice. *J Neuropathol Exp Neurol* 2004; **63**: 418–28.

52. Xu H, Rösler TW, Carlsson T, et al. Memory deficits correlate with tau and spine pathology in P301S *MAPT* transgenic mice. *Neuropathol Appl Neurobiol* 2014; **40**: 833–43.

53. Possin KL, Kramer JH, Finkbeine S, et al. Cross-species translation of the Morris maze for Alzheimer's disease. *J Clin Invest* 2016; **126**: 779–83.

54. Dodart J-C, Bales KR, Gannon KS, et al. Immunization reverses memory deficits without reducing brain Aβ burden in Alzheimer's disease model. *Nat Neurosci* 2002; **5**: 452–7.

55. Shen L, Hang B, Geng Y, et al. Amelioration of cognitive impairments in APPswe/PS1dE9 mice is associated with metabolites alteration induced by total salvianolic acid. *PLoS One* 2017; **12**: e0174763.

56. Barbeau E, Didic M, Tramoni E, et al. Evaluation of visual recognition memory in MCI patients. *Neurology* 2004; **62**: 1317–22.

57. Didic M, Felician O, Barbeau E, et al. Impaired visual recognition memory predicts Alzheimer's disease in amnestic mild cognitive impairment. *Dement Geriatr Cogn Disord* 2013; **35**: 291–9.

58. Zhang R, Xue G, Wang S, et al. Novel object recognition as a facile behavior test for evaluating drug effects in AβPP/PS1 Alzheimer's disease mouse model. *J Alzheimers Dis* 2012; **31**: 801–12.

59. Koola MM. Galantamine–memantine combination in the treatment of Alzheimer's disease and beyond. *Psychiatry Res* 2020; **293**: 113409.

60. Wu Z, Zhao L, Chen X, Cheng X, Zhang Y. Galantamine attenuates amyloid-β deposition and astrocyte activation in APP/PS1 transgenic mice. *Exp Gerontol* 2015; **72**: 244–50.

61. Puzzo D, Lee L, Palmeri A, Calabrese G, Arancio O. Behavioral assays with mouse models of Alzheimer's disease: practical considerations and guidelines. *Biochem Pharmacol* 2014; **88**: 450–67.

62. Chen Y, Shi G-W, Liang Z-M, et al. Resveratrol improves cognition and decreases amyloid plaque formation in Tg6799 mice. *Mol Med Rep* 2019; **19**: 3783–90.

63. Guerreiro R, Wojtas A, Bras J, et al. *TREM2* variants in Alzheimer's disease. *N Engl J Med* 2013; **368**: 117–27.

64. Lannfelt L, Relkin NR, Siemers ER. Amyloid-ß-directed immunotherapy for Alzheimer's disease. *J Intern Med* 2014; **275**: 284–95.

65. De Strooper B, Vassar R, Golde T. The secretases: enzymes with therapeutic potential in Alzheimer disease. *Nat Rev Neurol* 2010; **6**: 99–107.

66. Cummings JL, Morstorf T, Zhong K. Alzheimer's disease drug-development pipeline: few candidates, frequent failures. *Alzheimers Res Ther* 2014; **6**: 37.

67. Bales KR. The value and limitations of transgenic mouse models used in drug discovery for Alzheimer's disease: an update. *Expert Opin Drug Discov* 2012; **7**: 281–97.

68. Shineman DW, Basi GS, Bizon JL, et al. Accelerating drug discovery for Alzheimer's disease: best practices for preclinical animal studies. *Alzheimers Res Ther* 2011; **3**: 28.

69. Preuss C, Pandey R, Piazza E, et al. A novel systems biology approach to evaluate mouse models of late-onset Alzheimer's disease. *Mol Neurodegener* 2020; **15**: 67.

70. Wan Y-W, Al-Ouran R, Mangleburg CG, et al. Meta-analysis of the Alzheimer's disease human brain transcriptome and functional dissection in mouse models. *Cell Reports* 2020; **32**: 107908.

71. Hayden KM, Jones RN, Zimmer C, et al. Factor structure of the National Alzheimer's Coordinating Centers uniform dataset neuropsychological battery: an evaluation of invariance between and within groups over time. *Alzheimer Dis Assoc Disord* 2011; **25**: 128–37.

72. Hansen DV, Hanson JE, Sheng M. Microglia in Alzheimer's disease. *J Cell Biol* 2018; **217**: 459–72.

Use of Induced Pluripotent Stem Cell-Derived Neuronal Disease Models from Patients with Familial Early-Onset Alzheimer's Disease in Drug Discovery

Brenda Hug, Rudolph E. Tanzi, and Steven L. Wagner

8.1 Introduction

Neuropathologically, Alzheimer's disease (AD) is characterized by an abundance of neuritic plaques and neurofibrillary tangles (NFTs) in specific regions of the brain critical for cognition [1]. AD is currently a huge health problem that imposes a severe social and economic burden; in the absence of an effective disease-modifying treatment, AD is projected to become a dominant source of health-care expenditures over the next several decades. Unfortunately, existing palliative treatments provide only temporary symptomatic benefit. Potential disease-modifying therapeutic approaches for AD have been and are currently being tested in the clinic; however, thus far, none have been shown to retard the rate of disease progression. Most treatments under active investigation are informed by the large body of data pointing to the amyloid precursor protein (APP) and its proteolytic processing to amyloid-beta (Aβ) peptides in the pathogenesis of AD. In particular, the Aβ peptide products of APP, especially $A\beta_{42}/A\beta_{43}$, the most fibril prone, are being targeted. Enzyme inhibition strategies (e.g., gamma-secretase inhibitors [GSIs] such as semagacestat and avagacestat) have focused on reducing the levels of all Aβ peptide species and, so far, have demonstrated significant side effects including a worsening of cognitive abilities relative to placebo [2, 3].

In contrast, immunization approaches which aim at clearing deposited Aβ peptides have recently shown potential as an AD therapy [4, 5]. Biogen Idec initially reported preliminary Phase 1b clinical trial results of an anti-Aβ human monoclonal antibody (mAb), aducanumab, which showed dose-dependent reduction of amyloid plaques as measured by amyloid PET imaging and significantly reduced cognitive decline as measured by Mini-Mental State Examination (MMSE) and Clinical Dementia Rating – Sum of Boxes scores, in prodromal or mildly affected AD patients, relative to patients treated with placebo [6].

More recent disclosures include a secondary-prevention clinical trial from the DIAN-TU (Dominantly Inherited Alzheimer's Network Trials Unit), involving escalated doses of another anti-Aβ mAb, gantenerumab. The magnitude of amyloid reduction in gantenerumab-treated subjects was a >200% reversal toward normal in presymptomatic and symptomatic ADAD (autosomal-dominant AD)-linked gene carriers, also known as familial early-onset AD (EOAD). The cerebrospinal fluid (CSF) $A\beta_{42}/A\beta_{40}$ ratio, which reflects active cerebral amyloid deposition, returned toward normal for those on gantenerumab and worsened for those on placebo. CSF total tau and CSF hyperphosphorylated tau ($p\text{-tau}_{181}$), biomarkers known to increase in AD, were down by nearly a third in familial-EOAD gene carriers receiving gantenerumab compared to those on placebo. In addition, CSF neurofilament light chain (NFL), considered a generic indicator of active neurodegeneration, rose significantly more in familial-EOAD gene carriers on placebo than on gantenerumab but stayed largely stable in non-carriers.

Even more recently, Eli Lilly disclosed that donanemab, a mAb that recognizes a pyroglutamated form of Aβ, slowed cognitive decline by a third relative to placebo, in people with early AD. In addition to stemming cognitive decline, the mAb also wiped out Aβ plaques, lowering them into the range seen in healthy volunteers.

Collectively, these encouraging passive immunization studies lend strong support to therapeutic strategies targeting the reduction/elimination of Aβ peptides, especially those comprising neuritic plaques (i.e., $A\beta_{42}/A\beta_{43}$) for the treatment of AD. Not only are neuritic plaques composed predominantly of $A\beta_{42}/A\beta_{43}$ [7], it is also known that the most common biochemical phenotype of the more than 200 different familial-EOAD or EOAD-linked genetic mutations is an increased ratio of $A\beta_{42}$ to $A\beta_{40}$ [8]. Moreover, a large body of data points to $A\beta_{42}$ as the most potently pathogenic of this family of peptides [1]. Thus, preferential attenuation of $A\beta_{42}$ relative to the shorter $A\beta$ peptides (i.e., $A\beta_{38}$ and $A\beta_{37}$) may prove most efficacious. An important additional therapeutic goal is the ability to prevent AD. This objective will be viewed as increasingly important if current passive immunization clinical trials reinforce evidence that intervening after the development of abundant neuritic plaque pathology severely limits efficacy. In which case, treatment of only relatively few individuals – i.e., those with familial EOAD or with Down syndrome (DS) and possibly apolipoprotein E ε4 (*APOE-4*) homozygotes – will be justified by use of agents that are costly and whose mode of administration is necessarily invasive. Far more practical would be a treatment that is much less expensive and can be administered orally and for years prior to the onset of AD in both genetically defined AD patients, as well as those deemed to be at risk in the general population.

A critical problem in AD small-molecule drug development is the high failure rate in clinical trials. Possible causes include: on- and off-target side effects, the lack of translatable animal models, and the fact that target engagement/engagement of mechanism in humans is not evaluated until Phase 1b/Phase 2 clinical trials. Improvement in the small-molecule drug-development process through the use of more appropriate cellular models for assessing efficacy and toxicity is the key to more successful drug development for AD and is a top priority of the National Alzheimer's Project Act (NAPA) [9].

The emergence of human-induced pluripotent stem cell (hiPSC) disease models, including three-dimensional organoids, is a result of the enormous progress in iPSC technology over the past decade [10]. Commensurate progress in reprogramming, transdifferentiation, and genome editing has enabled the ability to utilize iPSC technology in performing unbiased genetic and small-molecule screening, using patient-derived cells [11]. These hiPSC-derived neuronal cell models also have the potential to significantly advance

the drug-development process by enabling clinical candidates to be tested against human neurons from selected patient populations during the preclinical development phase, to avoid waiting until Phase 1 and 2 clinical trials to confirm engagement of mechanism with the human target.

iPSCs reprogrammed from familial-EOAD-patient fibroblasts and differentiated into neurons have been shown to model the alterations in $A\beta$ peptide variant levels known to occur in familial-EOAD patients. For example, iPSC-derived neurons from patients harboring missense mutations in the presenilin 1 (*PSEN1*) gene or the presenilin 2 (*PSEN2*) gene have been shown to secrete elevated levels of $A\beta_{42}$, recapitulating a critical biochemical element in the molecular pathogenesis of the over 200 familial-EOAD-linked *PSEN1* and *PSEN2* genetic mutations [12].

In one of the initial studies aimed at evaluating the utility of iPSC-derived neurons isolated from familial-EOAD patients in drug efficacy testing [13], Liu et al. showed, in iPSC-derived neuronal cultures from three different familial-EOAD-linked *PSEN1* mutation carriers (*PSEN1*^{A246E}, *PSEN1*^{H163R}, and *PSEN1*^{M146L}), elevated $A\beta_{42}/A\beta_{40}$ ratios compared to iPSC-derived neurons from non-demented control (NDC) subjects. In addition, when the various iPSC-derived neuronal cultures were treated with the GSI semagacestat in concentration response curve (CRC) experiments, to generate half maximal inhibitory concentration (IC$_{50}$) values for the ability to lower the various $A\beta$ peptides ($A\beta_{42}$, $A\beta_{40}$, $A\beta_{38}$, and total $A\beta$ levels), semagacestat was almost two times less effective against the familial-EOAD-linked *PSEN1*-mutant neurons compared to the NDC neurons. This study also showed, in identical CRC studies, using a previously published gamma-secretase modulator (GSM)[14], that unlike the GSI semagacestat, the GSM (compound 4) had no effect on secreted total $A\beta$ levels and inhibited secretion of $A\beta_{42}$ and $A\beta_{40}$ with equal or greater potency in *PSEN1*-mutant neurons compared to NDC neurons.

Importantly, hiPSC-derived disease models have been used in both the earliest phase of drug discovery and in later phases of preclinical drug development, in order to identify and characterize potential therapeutic molecules for AD and related neurodegenerative disorders. For example, phenotypic screens using iPSC-derived neurons from reprogrammed familial-EOAD- and sporadic-AD-patient fibroblasts have been carried out. Recently, van der Kant et al. performed a drug screen of a collection of US Food and Drug Administration (FDA)-approved compounds in iPSC-derived human familial-EOAD neurons [15], in order to identify compounds capable of preventing hyperphosphorylated tau$_{231}$ (p-tau) accumulation, which has been shown to occur in *APP* duplication (*APP^{dp}*) familial-EOAD neurons [16]. This so-called "repurposing screen" identified a number of hits, including a series of statins, which led to the deconvolution of the druggable cholesterol ester cholesterol 24S-hydroxylase (CYP46A1)–tau axis, whereby allosteric activation of CYP46A1, using the HIV drug efavirenz, lowered cholesterol ester levels and p-tau levels in familial-EOAD iPSC-derived neurons.

In addition, Kondo and colleagues conducted a screen of a pharmaceutical small-molecule library in induced neurons converted from iPSCs derived from familial EOAD and sporadic AD patients in order to identify Aβ-lowering compounds [17]. A small number of hits were prioritized based on structural diversity-biased clustering, and combinations of these were tested for synergistic lowering of Aβ levels in highly purified AD-patient-derived induced-neuron cultures. It was found that the combination of bromocriptine, cromalyn, and topiramate was an effective Aβ-lowering cocktail, demonstrating dose-dependent lowering of Aβ$_{42}$, Aβ$_{40}$, and Aβ$_{42}$/Aβ$_{40}$ ratios with half maximal effective concentration (EC$_{50}$) values in the low micromolar range and a maximum of 70% reduction compared to vehicle control values.

Finally, in pioneering work, Shi and colleagues isolated cortical neurons from iPSCs derived from DS patients and showed that, within a few months of being cultured, the iPSC-derived neurons developed both of the neuropathological hallmarks of AD: Aβ aggregates and NFTs containing p-tau filaments [18]. Since it is known that more than 75% of individuals affected with DS (caused by trisomy of chromosome 21; they also carry an extra copy of *APP*) develop full-blown AD by the time they reach the age of 65, these DS-patient iPSC-derived cortical neurons were proposed as a useful tool for AD drug discovery. This notion soon became realized when Brownjohn et al. [19] used iPSC-derived cortical neurons from a DS patient, in a screen of the Prestwick library of FDA- and European Medicines Agency (EMA)-approved drugs, and identified a family of macrocyclic lactone anthelminthic compounds known as avermectins, which

were shown to favorably affect APP proteolytic processing, yielding decreased levels of the longer, aggregation-prone Aβ$_{42}$ and Aβ$_{40}$ peptides, while increasing the shorter non-fibrillogenic Aβ$_{38}$ and Aβ$_{37}$ peptides. This rather appealing effect on the preferential attenuation of the most fibrillogenic Aβ peptide variants, in the absence of accumulating gamma-secretase substrates, is almost identical to the profile elicited by GSMs. However, unlike GSMs, the avermectins appeared not to bind the carboxy terminus of the APP substrate within the Aβ motif, like the initially described non-steroidal anti-inflammatory drug (NSAID)-like GSMs [20, 21], nor did they appear to allosterically modulate the gamma-secretase enzyme complex, like the methylimidazole class of GSMs [22]. Avermectins are known to have affinity for the mammalian ligand-gated chloride channels gamma-aminobutyric acid A and glycine, acting as positive allosteric modulators and direct partial agonists at nanomolar concentrations; however, a number of studies employing specific agonists and antagonists of these receptors definitively excluded binding to these receptors as a mechanism for the ability of avermectins to affect Aβ peptide production. These mechanistic conclusions, or rather a lack thereof, were also based on the inability of avermectins to show efficacy in a cell-free gamma-secretase assay system [19]. Although the avermectins phenocopy GSMs in iPSC-derived neurons from patients affected with DS, familial EOAD (*APP^{dp}*, *APP^{V717I}*, *PSEN1^{M146L}*), as well as in iPSC-derived neurons from NDC subjects, their poor physicochemical properties and poor oral bioavailability, combined with an unknown mechanism of action, make these much less attractive as candidates for further preclinical development. However, the discovery of the avermectins represents a proof of principle regarding the utility of DS and potentially familial-EOAD patient-based iPSC-derived neuronal models in phenotypic screening assays, and the ability to identify potentially disease-modifying small molecules acting through novel pathways and mechanisms.

Alternatively, GSMs remain as one of the most promising small-molecule-based, disease-modifying therapeutic approaches for AD. Our team has discovered and developed a series of highly potent GSMs. One of the more advanced of these, BPN-15606, has an in vitro IC$_{50}$ = 7 nM for lowering Aβ$_{42}$ levels in cell-based assays and an in vivo potency of ~5–10 mg/kg for lowering Aβ$_{42}$ levels in brains of rats and mice following oral adminis-tration. BPN-15606 has undergone in vivo efficacy studies in two different rodent models, as well as 7-day dose-range-finding toxicology studies in rats and non-human primates, which showed a no observed adverse effect level (NOAEL) of >30 mg/kg in both species and a therapeutic index (safety margin) of >20 [23]. As mentioned previously, we reported that treatment with a first-generation GSM (GSM-4) led to a reduction in $A\beta_{42}$ and $A\beta_{40}$ levels, as well as a reduction in the $A\beta_{42}/A\beta_{40}$ ratio in neurons derived from hiPSCs from two NDC subjects and from four patients harboring three different *PSEN1* genetic mutations which cause familial EOAD [13]. Below we will describe the preclinical development of a more recent GSM clinical candidate and how iPSC-derived neurons from familial-EOAD patients, as well as additional stem-cell-based human cellular disease models, can be utilized to improve this process.

8.2 Pharmacological Characterization of Clinical Candidate GSM Compounds

Over the past several years, our team has synthe-sized and characterized over 600 novel GSMs encompassing four closely related scaffolds [23–26]; approximately 200 of these have in vitro poten-cies for lowering $A\beta_{42}$ levels in cell-based assays with IC_{50} values < 100 nM. We have shown excellent in vivo pharmacokinetic (PK) and pharmacodynamic (PD) properties with one of our best-characterized GSMs, referred to as BPN-15606, and have dem-onstrated highly significant dose-dependent bio-chemical efficacy (lowering of CSF and brain $A\beta_{42}$ levels by ~40% at doses as low as 5–10 mg/kg in rats and mice, respectively; and dose proportional exposures of 5–50 mg/kg). At higher doses (25 mg/kg), this compound can almost totally eliminate $A\beta_{42}$ levels in brain and in CSF of mice and rats, respectively. These in vivo results are remarkably promising since the CSF $A\beta_{42}$ biomarker is cur-rently being used in clinical trials in order to assess target engagement and has been shown to inversely correlate with neuritic plaque load in the brain. Based on human studies and transgenic animal studies, CSF $A\beta_{42}$ levels begin to rise prior to plaque development and then begin to decrease once sig-nificant plaque load has been established due to the incorporation of soluble $A\beta_{42}$ into diffuse amyloid deposits and neuritic plaques in the brain [27].

Since the discovery of this novel pyridazine scaffold, as exemplified by BPN-15606, further optimization efforts have been undertaken with the goal of ultimately identifying a number of backup compounds with improved pharmaco-logical properties. A number of analogs of com-pound BPN-15606 have been synthesized to date, with several analogs displaying IC_{50} values below 10 nM and which demonstrate potencies equal or superior to BPN-15606. As we pursue a disease-modifying therapy for a challenging disorder such as AD, establishing a series of credible backup lead molecules is critical. The ultimate goal is to develop a series of GSMs, with at least one capable of ful-filling the properties depicted in the target product profile (Table 8.1).

This GSM-based, disease-modifying thera-peutic approach is targeted at the amyloid cas-cade hypothesis [28], which is supported by over 25 years of biomedical research and over 200 familial-EOAD-linked genetic mutations involv-ing three different genes, all of which are directly tied to $A\beta$ peptide production [1]. Previous small-molecule therapeutic approaches based on the amyloid cascade hypothesis have arguably been either toxic or have been administered too late in the disease process for therapeutic benefit. Both active and passive immunological approaches involving anti-$A\beta$ vaccines and antibodies, as well as non-selective inhibitors of gamma-secretase, have been previously developed with the aim of curbing brain levels of all $A\beta$ peptide species (e.g., $A\beta_{42}$, $A\beta_{40}$, $A\beta_{39}$, $A\beta_{38}$, $A\beta_{37}$, etc.) [2–5, 29]. Based on the fact that the vast majority of the more than 200 familial-EOAD-linked genetic mutations appear to cause a two-fold increase in the ratio of the longer more oligomeric-prone $A\beta_{42}$ peptide to the shorter $A\beta_{40}$ peptide, and a large body of data pointing specifically to $A\beta_{42}$ in pathogenesis, a therapeutic rationale that modulates gamma-secretase activity to reduce only the level of $A\beta_{42}$ without affecting overall gamma-secretase activ-ity may prove most efficacious [30]. These data provide evidence that an orally bioavailable small molecule with this activity does exist and can be optimized for use in vivo. We view the GSM approach as superior to the use of vaccines and immunization, which require invasive proced-ures and immune regulation. In addition, because GSMs preferentially attenuate the levels of $A\beta_{42}$, while potentiating the levels of $A\beta_{37}$ and $A\beta_{38}$, they may prove to be easier to test, evaluate, and monitor

Table 8.1 Target product profile of a disease-modifying GSM

Drug properties	Minimum acceptable result	Ideal result
Primary drug indication	Prevention or a statistically significant reduction in the accumulation in biomarkers of AD pathology and rate of cognitive decline per year in presymptomatic familial-EOAD carriers, *APOE-4* carriers, and AD-biomarker-positive (A+T−N−) subjects with AD pathological change	Prevention or statistically significant reduction in the accumulation in biomarkers of AD pathology and rate of cognitive decline per year in presymptomatic familial-EOAD carriers, *APOE-4* carriers, and AD-biomarker-positive (A+T±N±) AD patients
Patient population	AD biomarker negative (A−T−N−) familial EOAD, *APOE-4* carriers (primary prevention) Presymptomatic AD-biomarker-positive (A+T−N−) subjects with AD pathological change (secondary prevention)	Presymptomatic familial EOAD, *APOE-4* carriers, (primary prevention) Presymptomatic AD-biomarker-positive (A+T+N−) AD patients (secondary prevention)
Delivery mode	Oral	Oral
Treatment duration	Chronic	Chronic
Regimen	Twice a day	Once a day
Efficacy	Prevention or a ≥ 25% reduction in the accumulation in biomarkers of AD pathology and rate of cognitive decline per year	Prevention or a ≥ 50% reduction in the accumulation in biomarkers of AD pathology and the rate of cognitive decline per year

Abbreviations: A, aggregated Aβ or associated pathological state; T, aggregated tau (NFTs) or associated pathological state; N, neurodegeneration or neuronal injury.

clinically than ligands which inhibit the activities of either beta-secretase or gamma-secretase.

We have previously shown that the attenuation of $A\beta_{42}$ levels via the modulation of gamma-secretase over an extended period of time (7 months) dramatically reduces the number of neuritic plaques in Tg2576 transgenic mice [14]. These data were generated following chronic treatment with 50 mg/kg per day of a first-generation aminothiazole-bridged aromatic GSM (AGSM), similar in structure and function to the GSMs that we have been optimizing and characterizing over the past several years. The first-generation GSMs act through a mechanism similar to BPN-15606, by inhibiting production of $A\beta_{42}$ and $A\beta_{40}$ while potentiating production of $A\beta_{38}$ and $A\beta_{37}$, yet cause no signs of toxicity even after exposures of 50 mg/kg per day for seven consecutive months. We have demonstrated that our new and improved GSMs (bridged heterocycles) have dramatically superior physicochemical properties compared to the original bridged aromatics, and thus will substantially facilitate both the preclinical and clinical development of GSMs. We have also recently shown that the potent novel pyridazine-containing GSM, BPN-15606, is capable of statistically significant lowering of $A\beta_{42}$ levels in plasma and brain/CSF of mice and rats at doses 5–10-fold lower than doses previously required for the first-generation GSMs

or AGSMs, and is also able to significantly attenuate cerebral amyloidosis in a transgenic mouse model following chronic (6 months) administration [23].

The GSM mechanism of action is ideally suited for familial-EOAD prevention. Clinical studies [31] have demonstrated that familial-EOAD patients do indeed have increased fractional synthetic rates of $A\beta_{42}$ in their CSF when compared to non-carrier siblings, thus validating the clinical relevance of CSF $A\beta_{42}$ as a disease biomarker. Both the earlier reported AGSMs and our more recently discovered GSMs have been shown to bind directly to the highly purified gamma-secretase enzyme complex [14, 24], as well as reduce the $A\beta_{42}$ biomarker in CSF in acute in vivo rodent studies [23].

Table 8.1 depicts the target product profile that encompasses the desired key features of an acceptable or ideal disease-modifying GSM. Through rational chemical design, collaborative teams from University of California San Diego and Massachusetts General Hospital have identified a new family of small molecules which exhibit the proper modulating effects on a critical biochemical phenotype of the vast majority of familial-EOAD mutations (an increased $A\beta_{42}/A\beta_{40}$ ratio) and which also potently inhibit production of the most aggregation-prone Aβ species, $A\beta_{42}$. Previous clinical studies suggest that earlier intervention preventative strategies are far more likely to arrest disease progression than those targeting mildly or moderately affected patients. Thus, these types of molecules would be ideal for primary (familial-EOAD gene carriers) and secondary (presymptomatic $A\beta$-PET-positive individuals) prevention trials. While we envision the ultimate goal of the GSMs is to prevent AD, it is important also to eventually test an effective and safe GSM in those with mild-to-moderate AD as well. This compound has undergone extensive preclinical study, including five species metabolite profiling, which confirms the absence of unique human metabolites and without any major human metabolite (accounting for >10% of the parent compound). Additionally, BPN-15606 demonstrated a >20-fold safety margin over the lowest efficacious dose in a 7-day dose-range-finding and toxicokinetic study in male Sprague-Dawley rats. Similarly, BPN-15606 also demonstrated a >20-fold safety margin in a 7-day dose-range-finding and toxicokinetic study in male and female cynomolgus macaques. Furthermore, this latter toxicokinetic study also determined the NOAEL for BPN-15606 to be $\geq$30 mg/kg and the maximum tolerated dose to be $\geq$ 100 mg/kg in non-human primates.

Based on the balance of data summarized above, BPN-15606 progressed into advanced preclinical development including good laboratory practice, investigational new drug (IND)-enabling 28-day safety and toxicological analysis in both rats and non-human primates, along with a close structural analog, GSM-776890.

8.3 An In Vitro Clinical Trial Utilizing iPSC-Derived Neurons from Familial-EOAD Patients

A desirable plan going forward, provided successful IND filing with the FDA and positive safety and toxicity Phase 1 single ascending dose and multiple ascending dose clinical trials, would be to conduct a proof-of-concept Phase 2 primary prevention clinical trial in familial-EOAD carriers. Because the age of onset is relatively constant within each EOAD family and with each mutation, this study would enroll carriers who are asymptomatic and are within a specific window of time of expected age of onset for their family and/or mutation. Due to the fact that certain familial-EOAD-linked mutations have been shown to be resistant to some NSAID-based GSMs [32, 33], it is necessary to demonstrate target engagement/

engagement of mechanism using induced neurons from these EOAD patients prior to enrollment into a Phase 2 clinical trial. This will ensure that no familial-EOAD gene carriers harboring a GSM-resistant missense mutation are enrolled in the primary prevention trial. A number of iPSC lines derived from patient fibroblasts obtained from the Dominantly Inherited Alzheimer's Network (DIAN), which have been generated and characterized with *PSEN1* (A431E, H163R, and A79V), *PSEN2* (N141I), and *APP* (V717I) familial-EOAD-linked mutations, are listed in Table 8.2. We have also generated five stable, NDC iPSC lines from normal healthy human subjects followed in the longitudinal study at the Shiley–Marcos Alzheimer's Disease Research Center at the University of California, San Diego. Figure 8.1 schematically depicts the process deployed in generating these hiPSC lines. Fibroblasts were transduced with non-integrating Sendai virus encoding Oct3/4, Krüppel-like factor 4 (Klf4), Sox2, c-Myc, and iPSC lines were selected based on normal karyotype, harboring the characteristics of pluripotency by expression of biomarkers for pluripotency, both with immunofluorescent staining with pluripotency markers and by a quantitative polymerase chain reaction (PCR). Furthermore, the hiPSC lines were characterized for their ability to differentiate into cells of the three germ layers by embryoid body formation. Morphologically, the appearance of the hiPSC resembles human embryonic stem cells (hESCs), with a scanty cytoplasm and prominent nuclei. The iPSC lines can be differentiated to neural progenitors and sorted using several differentiation protocols. Yuan and colleagues developed an efficient differentiation protocol and purification method based on cell surface markers [34]. Using the CD24/CD184/CD44 cell surface signature, neural stem cells (NSCs), neurons, and glia can be enriched. Most of the sorted neurons (>90% mature) exhibit neuronal electrophysiological properties, including the presence of sodium and potassium channels, and the ability to fire action potentials [16]. Purified induced human neurons from *PSEN1* mutation carriers, when compared to the NDC-induced human neurons, consistently exhibit an elevated $A\beta_{42}/A\beta_{40}$ ratio [13]. As mentioned previously, the first-generation GSM-4 reduced the $A\beta_{42}/A\beta_{40}$ ratio, as well as $A\beta_{42}$ and $A\beta_{40}$ levels in fibroblasts, iPSCs, NSCs, and iPSC-derived neurons from *PSEN1*-mutation-harboring patients,

Table 8.2 iPSC cell lines from familial EOAD patient donors

Familial-EOAD-linked mutation	iPSC lines generated and analyzed	Karyotype	Pluripotency formation of three germ layers	Pluripotency markers
APP^{V717I}	2	Normal	Yes	Yes
$PSEN2^{N141I}$	2	Normal	Yes	Yes
$PSEN1^{A431E}$	2	Normal	Yes	Yes
$PSEN1^{H163R}$	2	Normal	Yes	Yes
$PSEN1^{A79V}$	2	Normal	Yes	Yes

while total Aβ levels were unchanged. GSM-4 was effective against all three *PSEN1* mutations (A246E, H163R, and M146L) tested. A distinct Aβ biomarker profile upon GSM-4 treatment (lowering of $A\beta_{42}$ and $A\beta_{40}$ levels and little if any effect on $A\beta_{38}$ levels or total Aβ levels) was observed in fibroblasts, NSCs, and neurons. This Aβ biomarker profile following GSM-4 treatment is slightly different from the one previously reported in Tg2576 transgenic mouse mixed brain cultures overexpressing mutant human "Swedish" APPswe (significant lowering of $A\beta_{42}$ and $A\beta_{40}$ levels, with highly significant potentiation of $A\beta_{38}$ levels and with no effect on total Aβ levels) [14]. This discrepancy, with respect to the effects of GSM-4 on $A\beta_{38}$ levels, is likely due to the artificially high APP expression level in these mixed brain cultures from Tg2576 transgenic mice, since all of the imidazole-containing GSMs we have studied

dramatically potentiate $A\beta_{38}$ levels in SHSY5Y human neuroblastoma cells stably overexpressing APP751, and in Chinese hamster ovary cells stably overexpressing either APP695 or APPswe. When testing BPN-15606 and another IND-stage GSM, GSM-776890 [35], in the iPSC-derived neurons listed in Table 8.2, we found very similar results to those reported previously for GSM-4. Importantly, none of the iPSC-derived neuronal cell lines from familial-EOAD patients carrying mutations in *APP*, *PSEN1*, or *PSEN2* were resistant to the effects of either BPN-15606 or GSM-776890 on lowering of $A\beta_{42}$ levels. These data demonstrate that patient neurons derived from hiPSCs can reproduce the properties typical of human neurons, and that this in vitro model system can be used effectively to test the in vitro efficacy of different drug candidates safely in the human background.

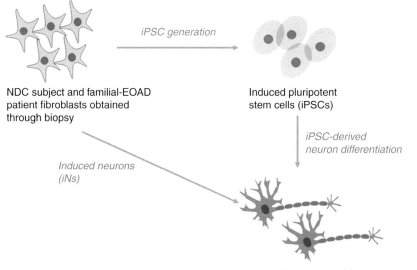

NDC subject and familial-EOAD patient fibroblasts obtained through biopsy

iPSC generation

Induced pluripotent stem cells (iPSCs)

iPSC-derived neuron differentiation

Induced neurons (iNs)

Purified human iPSC-derived neurons

Figure 8.1 Schematic diagram depicting the process of establishing iPSC-derived neuronal cell familial-EOAD disease models.

8.4 Using Familial-EOAD Patient iPSC-Derived Neurons in Systems Biology Approaches to Drug and Target Discovery

Going well beyond the utilization of these familial-EOAD-patient iPSC-derived neuronal models in the evaluation of the efficacy of small-molecule therapeutics against clinically relevant biomarkers such as $A\beta_{42}$, Caldwell and colleagues [36] recently used this familial-EOAD patient-specific iPSC-derived neuron model system and an integrative multi-omics approach to characterize the mechanistic changes occurring at the transcription factor (TF) and chromatin dynamics levels, leading to transcriptional dysregulation in familial-EOAD iPSC-derived neurons due to EOAD-linked *PSEN1* genetic mutations. When compared to iPSC-derived neurons from NDC subjects, expanded gene set enrichment analyses of *PSEN1* mutant neuron transcriptomics using RNA sequencing (RNA-seq), combined with chromatin dynamics analyses, assay for transposase-accessible chromatin sequencing (ATAC-seq), and histone methylation chromatin immunoprecipitation sequencing (ChIP-seq), revealed six modulated gene programs integral to the overall disease mechanism from a systems biological perspective: (1) pluripotency, (2) dedifferentiation, (3) cell cycle reentry, (4) inflammation, (5) lineage miRNA, and (6) neuronal specification encompassing lineage definition and synaptic function. Strikingly, all four *PSEN1* missense mutations (*PSEN1^{M146L}*, *PSEN1^{H163R}*, *PSEN1^{A246E}*, and *PSEN1^{A431E}*) demonstrated consistent dysregulation of these six endotypes by both RNA-seq and ATAC-seq analyses, reinforcing the consistency of these mechanisms to remodel the chromatin and gene expression landscape in mutant *PSEN1*-induced familial EOAD. The integration of differential RNA-seq and ATAC-seq or histone methylation ChIP-seq genes offers a mechanistic insight into the type of regulatory control of these gene programs; for example, while the "cell cycle reentry endotype" is significantly enriched in iPSC-derived neurons of all four EOAD-linked *PSEN1* mutants and particularly the *PSEN1^{A431E}* mutation, there is less observed directional overlap between the genes belonging to cell cycle reentry processes at the interface of RNA-seq and ATAC-seq. This may indicate more transient gene regulatory mechanisms of cell cycle

reentry genes alternative to chromatin modification and explains why there is less observed overlap between RNA-seq and ATAC-seq in the *PSEN1^{A431E}* iPSC-derived neurons, as this mutation has the most severe dysregulation of the cell cycle reentry endotype among the four *PSEN1* genetic mutations analyzed. The authors' analyses also revealed that *PSEN1^{M146L}* mutants had the most severe repression of neuronal lineage and synaptic function, whereas *PSEN1^{H163R}* and *PSEN1^{A246E}* mutations displayed the most significant upregulation of dedifferentiation and non-ectoderm lineage. The results of these transcriptomic analyses using the familial-EOAD-patient iPSC-derived neuronal model system were supported by the re-analysis of a previous transcriptomic study (GSE39420) of posterior cingulate cortex post-mortem brain tissue from NDC and *PSEN1*-mutation-harboring familial-EOAD donors [37]. The comparative expression analyses revealed a substantial number of differentially expressed genes (DEGs) in *PSEN1*-mutant post-mortem brains, even though these involved different *PSEN* mutations (*PSEN1^{M139T}*, *PSEN1^{V89L}*, and *PSEN1^{E120G}*), which overlapped with DEGs observed in the *PSEN1*-mutant iPSC-derived neurons. Interestingly, the National Institutes of Health Accelerating Medicines Partnership® Program for Alzheimer's Disease (AMP® AD) program's Agora list of sporadic AD susceptibility genes, identified by multiple omics approaches using post-mortem brain tissues from a large number of brain bank sources, shows an overlap with those observed in the familial-EOAD iPSC-derived neuronal model, at both the gene and gene program level, with key drivers and markers of neuronal dedifferentiation, including RE1-silencing transcription factor (REST), histone deacetylase 1 (HDAC1), ELAV-like RNA binding protein 4 (ELAVL4), gamma-aminobutyric acid type A receptor subunit alpha 4 (GABRA4), sodium voltage-gated alpha subunit 2 (SCN2A), and VGF (VGF nerve growth factor inducible), similarly identified. This commonality of cellular programs altered in both the familial EOAD and the more prevalent late-onset, sporadic forms of AD may offer a critical insight into the underlying mechanistic basis for neurodegeneration in AD, and provide a basis for innovative therapeutic intervention strategies, possibly targeting earlier stages of disease progression.

Finally, Figure 8.2 displays a schematic diagram depicting the blending of this RNA-seq transcriptome evaluation, using NDC versus

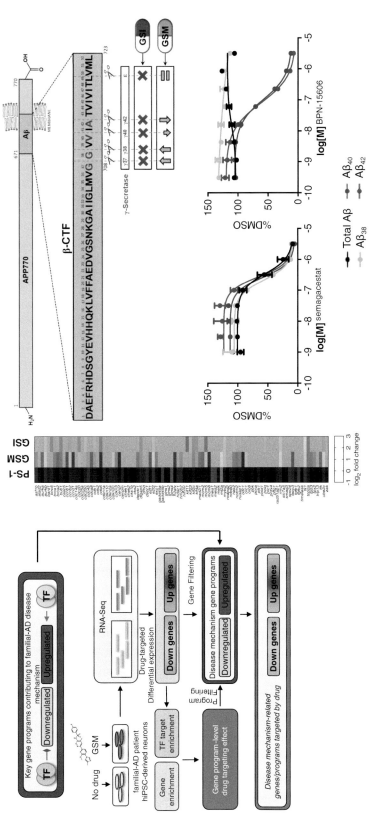

Figure 8.2 Schematic diagram depicting: the processes involved in combining of the RNA-seq transcriptome analyses of NDC versus familial-EOAD-patient-specific (*PSEN1^{A246E}*) iPSC-derived neurons, with the testing of the Aβ-peptide-lowering mechanisms and efficacies of the GSM, BPN-15606, and the GSI, semagacestat, enabling the simultaneous evaluation of the ability to attenuate Aβ-peptide-variant production and to modify the familial-EOAD-associated transcriptional state. β-CTF, beta-carboxyl-terminal fragment.

familial-EOAD-patient-specific (*PSEN1^{A246E}*) iPSC-derived neuron models, with the testing of the Aβ-peptide-lowering efficacy of the GSM, BPN-15606, and the GSI, semagacestat, enabling the simultaneous evaluation of the ability to attenuate Aβ peptide variant production and to modify the familial-EOAD-associated transcriptional state. Using EOAD-patient lineage *PSEN1^{A246E}* hiPSC-derived neurons, RNA-seq is used to characterize AD-associated endotypes, which in turn are used as a metric for the evaluation of two distinct gamma-secretase-targeted therapeutic approaches (GSIs and GSMs). This endotype-centric screening approach offers a new paradigm by which candidate AD therapeutic small molecules can be evaluated for their overall ability to reverse disease endotypes associated with familial EOAD.

8.5 Summary

Incorporation of familial EOAD patient-based iPSC-derived neuronal cell models into the AD drug discovery and preclinical development processes provides for a tremendous technological advance, with implications extending from a far more thorough preclinical, pharmacological evaluation, using human patient-derived cellular model systems to assess efficacy against established, clinically relevant disease-associated biomarkers, including the evaluation of the effects on disease-associated endotypes, to unveiling previously unknown pathologically relevant pathways and identifying new and potentially druggable therapeutic targets.

Acknowledgments

This work was supported by the Veterans Affairs RR&D 1I01RX002259, the Cure Alzheimer's Fund, the National Institute of Neurological Communicative Disorders and Stroke and the National Institute of Aging; NIH/NINDS Blue Print and NIA, U01 Grants NS 074501 and U01AG048986, R01AG055523, RO1AG054223, and RO1AG056061. We also acknowledge support from the DH Chen Foundation (R-86U55A). The contents do not represent the views of the U.S. Department of Veterans Affairs or the U.S. government.

References

1. Tanzi RE, Bertram L. Twenty years of the Alzheimer's disease amyloid hypothesis: a genetic perspective. *Cell* 2005; **120**: 545–55.

2. Coric V, van Dyck CH, Salloway S, et al. Safety and tolerability of the gamma-secretase inhibitor avagacestat in a phase 2 study of mild to moderate Alzheimer disease. *Arch Neurol* 2012; **69**: 1430–40.

3. Fleisher AS, Raman R, Siemers ER, et al. Phase 2 safety trial targeting amyloid beta production with a gamma-secretase inhibitor in Alzheimer disease. *Arch Neurol* 2008; **65**: 1031–8.

4. Miles LA, Crespi GA, Doughty L, Parker MW. Bapineuzumab captures the N-terminus of the Alzheimer's disease amyloid-beta peptide in a helical conformation. *Sci Rep* 2013; **3**: 1302.

5. Salloway S, Sperling R, Fox NC, et al. Two phase 3 trials of bapineuzumab in mild-to-moderate Alzheimer's disease. *N Engl J Med* 2014; **370**: 322–33.

6. Sevigny J, Chiao P, Bussière T, et al. The antibody aducanumab reduces Aβ plaques in Alzheimer's disease. *Nature* 2016; **537**: 50–6.

7. Iwatsubo T, Odaka A, Suzuki N, et al. Visualization of A beta 42(43)and A beta 40 in senile plaques with end-specific A beta monoclonals: evidence that an initially deposited species is A beta 42(43). *Neuron* 1994; **13**: 45–53.

8. Kumar-Singh S, Theuns J, Van Broeck B, et al. Mean age-of-onset of familial alzheimer disease caused by presenilin mutations correlates with both increased Abeta42 and decreased Abeta40. *Hum Mutat* 2006; **27**: 686–95.

9. Alzheimer's Association Expert Advisory Workgroup on NAPA. Workgroup on NAPA's scientific agenda for a national initiative on Alzheimer's disease. *Alzheimers Dement* 2012; **8**: 357–71.

10. Shi Y, Inoue H, Wu JC, Yamanaka S. Induced pluripotent stem cell technology: a decade of progress. *Nat Rev Drug Discov* 2017; **16**: 115–30.

11. Khurana V, Tardiff DF, Chung CY, Lindquist S. Toward stem cell-based phenotypic screens for neurodegenerative diseases. *Nat Rev Neurol* 2015; **11**: 339–50.

12. Yagi T, Ito D, Nihei Y, Ishihara T, Suzuki N. N88S seipin mutant transgenic mice develop features of seipinopathy/BSCL2-related motor neuron disease via endoplasmic reticulum stress. *Hum Mol Genet* 2011; **20**: 3831–40.

13. Liu Q, Waltz S, Woodruff G, et al. Effect of potent gamma-secretase modulator in human neurons derived from multiple presenilin 1-induced pluripotent stem cell mutant carriers. *JAMA Neurol* 2014; **71**: 1481–9.

14. Kounnas MZ, Danks AM, Cheng S, et al. Modulation of gamma-secretase reduces beta-amyloid deposition in a transgenic mouse model of Alzheimer's disease. *Neuron* 2010; **67**: 769–80.

15. van der Kant R, Langness VF, Herrera CM, et al. Cholesterol metabolism is a druggable axis that independently regulates tau and amyloid-β in iPSC-derived Alzheimer's disease neurons. *Cell Stem Cell* 2019; **24**: 363–75.e9.

16. Israel MA, Yuan SH, Bardy C, et al. Probing sporadic and familial Alzheimer's disease using induced pluripotent stem cells. *Nature* 2012; **482**: 216–20.

17. Kondo T, Imamura K, Funayama M, et al. iPSC-based compound screening and in vitro trials identify a synergistic anti-amyloid β combination for Alzheimer's disease. *Cell Rep* 2017; **21**: 2304–12.

18. Shi Y, Kirwan P, Smith J, et al. A human stem cell model of early Alzheimer's disease pathology in Down syndrome. *Sci Transl Med* 2012; **4**: 124ra29.

19. Brownjohn PW, Smith J, Portelius E, et al. Phenotypic screening identifies modulators of amyloid precursor protein processing in human stem cell models of Alzheimer's disease. *Stem Cell Rep* 2017; **8**: 870–82.

20. Kukar TL, Ladd TB, Bann MA, et al. Substrate-targeting γ-secretase modulators. *Nature* 2008; **453**: 925–9.

21. Weggen S, Eriksen JL, Das P, et al. A subset of NSAIDs lower amyloidogenic Abeta42 independently of cyclooxygenase activity. *Nature* 2001; **414**: 212–16.

22. Crump CJ, Johnson DS, Li Y-M. Development and mechanism of γ-secretase modulators for Alzheimer's disease. *Biochemistry* 2013; **52**: 3197–216.

23. Wagner SL, Rynearson KD, Duddy SK, et al. Pharmacological and toxicological properties of the potent oral gamma-secretase modulator BPN-15606. *J Pharmacol Exp Ther* 2017; **362**: 31–44.

24. Wagner SL, Zhang C, Cheng S, et al. Soluble gamma-secretase modulators selectively inhibit the production of the 42-amino acid amyloid beta peptide variant and augment the production of multiple carboxy-truncated amyloid beta species. *Biochemistry* 2014; **53**: 702–13.

25. Rynearson KD, Buckle RN, Herr RJ, et al. Design and synthesis of novel methoxypyridine-derived gamma-secretase modulators. *Bioorg Med Chem* 2020; **28**: 115734.

26. Rynearson KD, Buckle RN, Barnes KD, et al. Design and synthesis of aminothiazole modulators of the gamma-secretase enzyme. *Bioorg Med Chem Lett* 2016; **26**: 3928–37.

27. Sunderland T, Linker G, Mirza N, et al. Decreased beta-amyloid1–42 and increased tau levels in cerebrospinal fluid of patients with Alzheimer disease. *JAMA* 2003; **289**: 2094–103.

28. Hardy JA, Higgins GA. Alzheimer's disease: the amyloid cascade hypothesis. *Science* 1992; **256**: 184–5.

29. Gilman S, Koller M, Black RS, et al. Clinical effects of Abeta immunization (AN1792) in patients with AD in an interrupted trial. *Neurology* 2005; **64**: 1553–62.

30. Wagner SL, Tanzi RE, Mobley WC, Galasko D. Potential use of gamma-secretase modulators in the treatment of Alzheimer disease. *Arch Neurol* 2012; **69**: 1255–8.

31. Potter R, Patterson BW, Elbert DL, et al. Increased in vivo amyloid-beta42 production, exchange, and loss in presenilin mutation carriers. *Sci Transl Med* 2013; **5**: 189ra77.

32. Kretner B, Fukumori A, Gutsmiedl A, et al. Attenuated Aβ_{42} responses to low potency γ-secretase modulators can be overcome by many pathogenic presenilin mutants by second-generation compounds. *J Biol Chem* 2011; **286**: 15240–51.

33. Koch P, Tamboli IY, Mertens J, et al. Presenilin-1 L166P mutant human pluripotent stem cell-derived neurons exhibit partial loss of γ-secretase activity in endogenous amyloid-β generation. *Am J Pathol* 2012; **180**: 2404–16.

34. Yuan SH, Martin J, Elia J, et al. Cell-surface marker signatures for the isolation of neural stem cells, glia and neurons derived from human pluripotent stem cells. *PLoS One* 2011; **6**: e17540.

35. Rynearson KD, Ponnusamym M, Prikhodko O, et al. Preclinical validation of a potent γ-secretase modulator for Alzheimer's disease prevention. *J Exp Med* 2021; **218**: e20202560.

36. Caldwell AB, Liu Q, Schroth GP, et al. Dedifferentiation and neuronal repression define familial Alzheimer's disease. *Sci Adv* 2020; **6**: eaba5933.

37. Antonell A, Lladó A, Altirriba J, et al. A preliminary study of the whole-genome expression profile of sporadic and monogenic early-onset Alzheimer's disease. *Neurobiol Aging* 2013; **34**: 1772–8.

Preclinical Longitudinal In Vivo Biomarker Platform for Alzheimer's Disease Drug Discovery

Min Su Kang, Eduardo R. Zimmer, Julie Ottoy, Monica Shin, Marcel Seungsu Woo, Arturo Aliaga, Gassan Massarweh, A. Claudio Cuello, Serge Gauthier, and Pedro Rosa-Neto

9.1   Introduction

Alzheimer's disease (AD) has been reconceptualized as a pathophysiological process that is characterized by the progressive accumulation of amyloid-beta (Aβ) and tau aggregates and downstream neurodegeneration. While protein aggregation dominates the presymptomatic phase of the disease, the significant neurodegeneration taking place during the symptomatic phase highlights the importance of disease-modifying approaches. The use of genetically modified animals, carriers of disease pathology, played an important role in the early development of AD disease-modifying therapeutics. In this chapter, we will focus on innovative methods for preclinical AD drug discovery. First, we will cover new developments in the animal models, and how choosing the appropriate model to test a new drug for specific endpoints improves the translational value from the preclinical to clinical trials. Second, we will discuss the advantages of using a longitudinal study design and the same in vivo biomarkers to evaluate novel disease-modifying interventions at early development stages. Last, we propose the same level of rigor and standardization as human AD clinical trials for the preclinical evaluation of the drug discovery.

9.2   Preclinical Rodent Models for AD

AD is a complex disorder with multiple pathophysiological processes that simultaneously or even synergistically occur in the brain as the disease progresses over time. Among others, Aβ and tau pathologies, neuroinflammation, oxidative stress, and neurodegeneration are among the key features that are invariably present in AD [1]. Interventions targeting specific AD pathophysiological processes

can be tested using animal models carrying these specific features of AD. Here, we will discuss how various rodent models, as they are the most commonly used model organism for AD drug discovery, have served to advance the understanding of the individual pathological events and their consequential cognitive decline.

Multiple AD-like rodent models have been developed in the past decades [2]. Chemical models – induced by the cerebral injection of Aβ, okadaic acid, streptozotocin, and others – have been instrumental in the early days for understanding neurotoxicity features associated with AD [3–5]. Indeed, these models present a certain degree of neurodegeneration and cognitive abnormalities but do not replicate the full Aβ and tau pathologies that define human AD. More specifically, murine forms of Aβ and tau do not form mature insoluble Aβ plaques and tau tangles, respectively. To overcome this major limitation, several transgenic models harboring human gene mutations have been developed [2]. These transgenic models have played an invaluable role to investigate the cascade of events elicited by the individual pathological effects, which is not possible in humans. For example, there are mouse models harboring human amyloid precursor protein (APP), presenilin 1, and presenilin 2 mutations, which display AD-like Aβ pathology and are still by far the most used. These models develop a progressive accumulation of Aβ plaques and subsequent tau hyperphosphorylation, mild neurodegeneration, neuroinflammation, and cognitive abnormalities but do not develop tau tangles (neurofibrillary tangles). Therefore, the AD-like Aβ animal models have allowed the investigation of the Aβ as the hypothesized etiopathology of the disease and progression over time, isolated from the effects of tau tangles. In addition, many efforts have been put into model tau pathology. For example, microtubule-associated protein tau (*MAPT*) gene mutations found in individuals with frontotemporal degeneration and parkinsonism (FTDP-17) have been used for developing transgenic tau mouse models. These animals progressively accumulate tau tangles, yielding a pattern of tau pathology spreading associated with heavy neurodegeneration and behavior abnormalities [6, 7]. However, they do not develop Aβ plaques. Collective perspective from the Aβ and tau transgenic mouse models shows strong evidence that Aβ pathology precedes tau abnormality in AD and supports the "Aβ cascade hypothesis" [8]. This has been one of the greatest motivations for the greater investment in anti-amyloid therapies compared to anti-tau therapies.

Recently, a few AD transgenic rat models have been developed. There are models genetically engineered for developing Aβ pathology (the McGill-R-Thy1-APP [9] and the TgF344-AD [10]) and for mimicking tau pathology (the R962-hTau [11]). Transgenic rat models of AD have been more challenging to produce compared to mice due to the more arduous transfection process during the embryonic stage [12]. However, rats may be a superior model organism than mice when evaluating a new therapy for AD [12, 13]. Rats are bigger than mice, and this brings a great benefit. Rats can provide more frequent longitudinal blood and cerebrospinal fluid (CSF) collections based on a simpler and less invasive procedure than mice [12]. Also, the bigger brain size of rats provides higher-resolution neuroimaging data and can be linked to richer behavior outcomes (Figure 9.1) [12, 13]. Moreover, rats are evolutionarily closer to humans than mice [12]. Considering all of the preclinical studies of anti-amyloid immunotherapies that have been conducted in mice, evaluating a novel drug target engagement, therapeutic efficacy, and safety profile in transgenic rats may provide richer information that may have been missed in mice.

However, a major drawback of the aforementioned models is the overexpression of mutated human genes. Such variants may generate gene expression above physiological levels, which may introduce artificial changes not seen in human pathology [14]. In order to address such a void, researchers generated human APP knock-in (KI) models. The idea here was to have animals overproducing Aβ but with no overexpression of human mutations. After several years of research, KI models have been developed and they recapitulate age-dependent Aβ pathology [15]. More recently, the field has been redefined toward the development of models that better resemble sporadic, non-familial AD. A major initiative, called Model Organism Development and Evaluation for Late-Onset AD (MODEL-AD, www.model-ad.org), is currently underway. Thus, the next generation of AD rodent models are promising to better resemble sporadic human pathology. A full list of AD models currently available can be found at www.alzforum.org/research-models.

9.3 In Vivo Biomarkers in Preclinical Animal Models of AD

The discovery and validation of in vivo biomarkers for AD pathophysiology have led to a paradigm shift in the clinical diagnostic guidelines, research criteria, and clinical trial enrichment toward a biomarker-based approach. Yet, the initial preclinical evaluation of the latest five major anti-amyloid immunotherapies (bapineuzumab [16], solanezumab [17], gantenerumab [18], lecanemab (BAN2401) [19], and aducanumab [20]), which have completed or reached Phase 3 of the clinical trials, was conducted in APP mice models based on the biochemical in vitro assays that are cross-sectional in nature with different sensitivity, specificity, and noise level compared to the in vivo biomarkers used in the clinical trials. Interestingly, these assays supported the effectiveness of the drug in animal models. However, a systematic analysis of AD trials from 2002 to 2012 (a total of 413) revealed a success rate of 0.4% [21]. As such, the preclinical studies so far have provided limited predictive information on the direct effect size of the therapeutic target engagement from the individual's baseline condition. Furthermore, the therapeutic efficacy (i.e., improved neurodegenerative biomarkers) and safety profile due to the treatment were not evaluated accurately relative to the prior condition either. By adapting the same in vivo biomarker methodologies and longitudinal study design used in AD clinical trials, the preclinical studies of AD drug discovery can provide a direct and accurate measure of the effect size in the target engagement, therapeutic efficacy, and safety profile, which are the main outcomes investigated in the clinical trials (Figure 9.2).

107

AD animal models: mice and rats

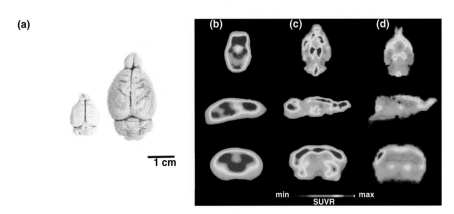

Behavior/memory test: Morris water maze

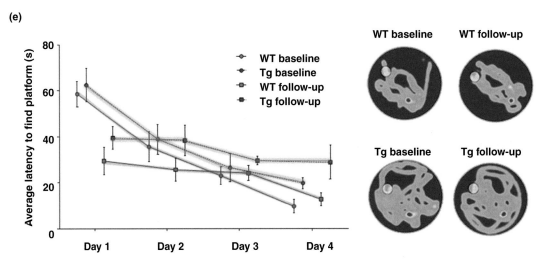

Figure 9.1 (a) The size of a mouse and a rat brain, and an [^{18}F]FDG PET SUVR image from (b) a wild-type (WT) mouse, (c) rat, and (d) a McGill-R-Thy1-APP transgenic rat brain. This shows a significant improvement in the image resolution due to the bigger brain size in rats compared to mice, therefore, it provides richer data to investigate the group differences. (e) A Morris water maze latency plot over time and average swimming paths to find the hidden platform, demonstrating significant memory loss in the transgenic (Tg) rats.

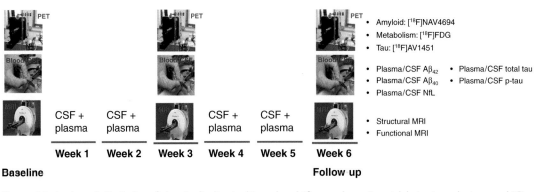

Figure 9.2 A schematic illustration of a longitudinal in vivo biomarker platform and experimental design to evaluate a novel AD drug discovery.

The in vivo biomarker-based AD clinical diagnosis and research framework focuses on Aβ (A), tau (T), and neurodegeneration (N), where A/T defines AD based on the presence of biological and pathological aggregates of Aβ/tau proteins, and N defines the disease stages/severity [22]. Investigating the preclinical animal models of AD using the same in vivo biomarkers in parallel with human studies has also accelerated the discovery and validation of novel biomarkers, longitudinal pathophysiological processes, and consequent dysfunction in the behaviors and cognition. Such a complementary and dynamic process between the bench-to-bedside and bedside-to-bench (reverse-translation) will advance our understanding of the disease mechanisms, enable the discovery of new therapeutic targets, and bring us one step closer to finding a cure in precision/personalized medicine. We will now discuss and summarize the evidence reported in the preclinical animal models of AD to support the use of A/T/(N) biomarkers in evaluating preclinical trial outcomes based on neuroimaging and fluid biomarkers in parallel with human studies. Also, we will discuss important methodological considerations that can improve the effective use of the biomarkers to accelerate the AD drug discovery.

9.4 Positron Emission Tomography Imaging in Rodents

Positron emission tomography (PET) imaging has been dominating in the AD biomarkers field [23]. Indeed, PET versatility allows for the quantification of Aβ, tau, and neurodegeneration in living individuals. Thus, an individual can be binarized (i.e., positive or negative) in the A/T/(N) system by using multi-tracer PET imaging. In the last years, multiple studies have used PET imaging to investigate A/T/(N) biomarkers in AD rodent models [13].

9.4.1 Aβ PET Imaging in Rodents

There are various Aβ tracers currently available, including ¹¹C-Pittsburgh compound B ([¹¹C]PiB), [¹⁸F]AV45 ([¹⁸F]florbetapir), [¹⁸F]florbetaben, [¹⁸F]flutemetamol, and [¹⁸F]NAV4694 [24]. Multiple studies have demonstrated that [¹¹C]PiB is capable of detecting Aβ plaques in the APP23 mouse model. Indeed, a longitudinal assessment demonstrates that the APP23 mouse model seems highly suitable for evaluating progressive Aβ accumulation [25–29]. By contrast, studies using

the Tg2576 mouse model usually fail to detect Aβ accumulation [27, 29–31]. In an interesting series of studies, Snellman and colleagues confirmed that [¹¹C]PiB and [¹⁸F]flutemetamol retention were highly dependent on the AD mouse model [27, 29]. Specifically, it seems that the conformation of Aβ plaques developed by the mouse model is crucial for having positive outcomes. For example, Aβ plaques failing to develop human-like binding pockets (or with low availability of binding pockets) will intuitively have no specific binding. Age-dependent amyloid-load has also been detected with [¹⁸F]florbetapir in the APP/presenilin 1 (PS1)-21 mouse model [32]. A study testing four transgenic models suggested that the APP/presenilin 2 (PS2) mouse model scanned with [¹⁸F]florbetaben captured a progressive Aβ deposition in the brain [33]. Additionally, a longitudinal interventional study, using a beta-site amyloid precursor protein cleaving enzyme (BACE1) inhibitor, has demonstrated the feasibility of using [¹⁸F]florbetaben to monitor drug effects on Aβ deposition in the APP/PS2 mice model [34]. A longitudinal Aβ PET study using [¹⁸F]NAV4694 also has been conducted in the McGill-R-Thy1-APP transgenic rat model, in which age-dependent accumulation of Aβ has been observed [35] (Figure 9.3a).

In summary, it is possible to visualize Aβ plaques in vivo in animal models harboring human APP mutations. One should have in mind that the concentration and conformation of Aβ plaques are highly variable among animal models; thus, animal models and radiopharmaceuticals should be carefully defined.

9.4.2 Tau PET Imaging in Rodents

Multiple imaging agents targeting tau pathology have been developed in the past years [36, 37]. The first generation of tau tracers includes the THK family [¹⁸F]THK523, [¹⁸F]THK5117, [¹⁸F]THK5317, and [¹⁸F]THK5351), [¹⁸F]AV-1451 ([¹⁸F]flortaucipir), and [¹¹C]PBB3, while the second generation includes [¹⁸F]MK-6240, [¹⁸F]RO-948, [¹⁸F]PI-2620, and [¹⁸F]PM-PBB3. Earlier this year, the US Food and Drug Administration (FDA) approved [¹⁸F]flortaucipir as the first radiopharmaceutical used to non-invasively visualize tau pathology in the brain (www.fda.gov/news-events/press-announcements/fda-approves-first-drug-image-tau-pathology-patients-being-evaluated-alzheimers-disease). It is important to mention that tau pathology is a feature common to a collective of neurodegenerative disorders called

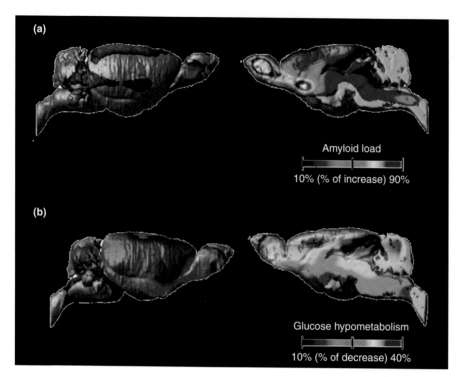

Figure 9.3 (a) Percent increase in [^{18}F]NAV4694 non-displaceable binding potential from age 9–11 months to 16–19 months in the McGill-R-Thy1-APP transgenic rats. (b) Percent decrease in [^{18}F]FDG SUVR from age 9–11 months to 16–19 months in the McGill-R-Thy1-APP transgenic rats.

tauopathies. Thus, the potential in the clinical utility of the tau PET imaging goes beyond AD.

Some of these tracers have already been tested in transgenic tau models. Early studies have demonstrated that [^{18}F]THK523 and [^{11}C]PBB3 are capable of detecting tau tangles in rTg4510 and PS19 mice models, respectively [38, 39]. Two additional studies using [^{11}C]PBB3 identified tau pathology in the rTg4510 mice [40, 41]. Brendel and colleagues also identified tau tangles with [^{18}F]flortaucipir and [^{18}F]THK5117 in a series of longitudinal micro-PET scanning using the P301S mouse model [42]. They also found positive [^{18}F]THK5117 binding using the biGT mouse model (a bigenic glycogen synthase kinase-3β [GSK-3β] × tau-P301L model).

In summary, it is possible to visualize tau tangles in vivo in animal models harboring *MAPT* gene mutations. Moreover, some critical points are the conformation and concentration of tau tangles, which can strongly vary among animal models. It is important to emphasize that the tau transgenic models currently available are developed using *MAPT* gene mutations found in FTDP-17 patients. Thus, tau tangle binding-site availability may vary among tauopathies, which should be carefully

evaluated in terms of AD preclinical studies aiming at translation to clinics.

9.4.3 Fluorodeoxyglucose PET Imaging in Rodents

The glucose analog ^{18}F-fluorodeoxyglucose ([^{18}F]FDG) is the most widely used radiopharmaceutical. Biochemically speaking, a [^{18}F]FDG signal indicates tissue hexokinase activity, a rate-limiting step of glucose metabolism [43]. The biological interpretation of [^{18}F]FDG PET data indicates that its signal is proportional to synaptic activity (sensitive to neuronal and astrocyte metabolism) [44, 45]. The current clinical research framework adopts [^{18}F]FDG hypometabolism as a biomarker of neurodegeneration [22]. Indeed, the brain [^{18}F]FDG PET has provided invaluable contributions to basic and clinical research [46]. An [^{18}F]FDG PET metabolic signature, which includes hypometabolism in the parietal, temporal, and posterior cingulate cortices, is highly conserved in AD patients and has been used to increase diagnosis accuracy in clinical settings [47–49].

As glucose is the mammalian brain's main energy fuel, [^{18}F]FDG PET is directly applicable to rodents. However, AD-like models do not precisely recapitulate human disease signatures since the degree of neurodegeneration varies among models. For example, the Tg2576 model presents hypermetabolism at 7 months of age but normal metabolism at subsequent ages (9, 13, and 15 months) [31, 50, 51]. The APP23 mouse presents normal [^{18}F]FDG PET metabolism at 13 months [52]. One could argue that mild neurodegeneration observed in APP models may be responsible for these discrepancies. By contrast, APP/PS1 mouse models show [^{18}F]FDG hypermetabolism in the early stages of Aβ plaque deposition [53]. These peculiar changes may be associated with compensatory mechanisms, which could be associated with glial abnormalities. A longitudinal [^{18}F]FDG PET study has reported mild [^{18}F]FDG PET hypometabolism in the McGill-R-Thy1-APP transgenic rat model (Figure 9.3b) [35]. Also, [^{18}F]FDG PET has been used for monitoring drug efficacy in AD mouse models [54].

In summary, AD animal models do not present a clear "hypometabolic signature" as seen in human AD. Brain metabolism changes in these models are not precisely explained by the degree of Aβ or tau pathologies. It seems that additional pathological mechanisms – such as microglial activation or astrocyte reactivity – may play an important role in rodent [^{18}F]FDG PET imaging. In addition, there are many sources of potential bias in metabolic studies: (1) handling: stressful handling and immobilization may increase the acute release of corticosteroids, consequently affecting brain glucose metabolism [55]; (2) anesthesia: central anesthetics suppress synaptic activity, which may decrease brain glucose metabolism [56]. Thus, the interpretation of [^{18}F]FDG micro-PET should be carefully conducted, taking into consideration sources of bias. As a recommendation to increase reproducibility in [^{18}F]FDG PET studies in rodents models of AD, one should first conduct the uptake phase in fasting awake animals; then the scanning phase (10–20 minutes) should follow under anesthesia with continuous monitoring/documenting of physiological conditions (temperature, heart rate, and blood pressure).

9.4.4 Critical Considerations and Validation Parameters in Micro-PET Studies

More elaborated research focusing on in vivo A/T/(N) gold-standard quantification using micro-PET constitutes a challenging task. In mouse models, the need for repeated blood samples for estimation of plasma concentrations of radiopharmaceuticals is a major limitation. In rats, the larger body mass and blood volume permit proper estimation of plasma input function necessary for quantitative assessments using kinetic modeling, which are necessary to validate simplified methods such as standardized uptake value (SUV) and SUV ratio (SUVR). Also, rats' bigger brains are more suited for the resolution of micro-PET scanners currently available [13]. Additionally, the reference region needs to be critically defined and validated. While the cerebellar gray- and white-matter regions are widely used as a reference region to quantify Aβ in humans, different rodent models may need to adapt their reference region due to the presence of Aβ in either the cerebellar gray- or relatively small white-matter region [10, 57, 58].

9.5 Magnetic Resonance Imaging

MRI is one of the most widely utilized in vivo imaging techniques in both preclinical and clinical stages of AD research. MRI is sufficiently powerful to be able to characterize and quantify a diverse array of physiological measurements at various scales. For example, MRI can provide structural measurements such as brain volume or gray-matter density to assess brain atrophy as well as functional measurements such as blood-oxygen-level-dependent (BOLD) signals that indirectly measure the neurovascular coupling to represent a functional brain network [22, 59]. This is possible due to the underlying principle of MRI signal acquisition, which is to create a magnetic field at various strengths and frequencies where an object or a tissue is magnetized inside the scanner and consequently send a radio frequency signal to be detected. Given the compositions of the brain or physiological properties for neuronal activities (i.e., neurovascular coupling), a unique set of signals is then reconstructed into a physiologically meaningful metric called a biomarker. Importantly, the evolutionarily conserved compositions of the brain (i.e., gray matter and white matter) and properties of neuronal activities allow MRI to reverse-translationally characterize the animal models of AD based on the same biomarkers used to evaluate human AD clinical trials [60]. Therefore, in vivo neuroimaging techniques such as MRI are ideal to establish the disease pathophysiological processes and relate to the behavioral outcomes in parallel across the species, and create a unique platform for preclinical evaluation of novel therapeutics. Such a platform will likely increase the potential to translate the findings from the bench to the bedside. Here, we will discuss major biomarkers used in AD research based on MRI.

Although neurodegeneration itself is not specific to AD, it can define different stages of AD and is closely linked to the disease progression and cognition compared to the pathological hallmarks of AD [22]. Notably, the hippocampal volume based on structural MRI has been reported to be significantly associated with neurofibrillary tangles and cognitions, and it is able to predict mild cognitive impairment (MCI) to AD conversion in humans [61–64]. In parallel, the hippocampal volume is also significantly decreased in various AD transgenic animal models recapitulating AD pathological hallmarks, $A\beta$ plaques or neurofibrillary tangles. For example, Parent et al. revealed a modest but significant decline in hippocampal volume in the McGill-R-Thy1-APP rat model displaying AD-like $A\beta$ pathology compared to wild-type animals (Figure 9.4) [35]. When the number of neurons was examined at histological sections, Heggland et al. showed a significant reduction only in the subiculum, suggesting that the hippocampal volumetric changes may not only reflect cell death but also synaptic reduction [35, 65]. Concurrently, more commonly used transgenic mice models of AD also all showed a significant reduction in hippocampal volume [66–68]. Supporting the growing body of literature in human AD studies, rodent models of AD expressing tau pathology also demonstrate a greater degree of neurodegeneration compared to $A\beta$ transgenic models.

Voxel-based morphometry (VBM) is a computational technique that measures volumetric changes at every voxel without any bias from different parcellation schemes. As such, VBM is ideal to provide comprehensive local neurodegenerative processes with topographical information from different species even without having a complete pairing of homologous or complementary brain regions. One particular study led by Kang et al. has capitalized on this aspect of the VBM technique to validate a putative fluid biomarker for neurodegeneration in AD called neurofilament light chain (NfL) [69]. By associating NfL and VBM, Kang et al. revealed a significant inverse relationship between NfL and gray-matter density within AD-related regions such

as the parietal associative cortex and medial temporal cortex only in the transgenic animals, replicating the human findings – a substantial inverse association between NfL and gray-matter density within AD-related regions only in $A\beta$-positive MCI and AD [69]. Amid a multitude of evidence showing NfL in plasma or CSF as a sensitive biomarker for neurodegeneration, the topographical association between NfL and gray-matter density at a whole-brain level in the context of $A\beta$ pathology was elucidated. Therefore, both genetically modified and controlled experiments from animal and human data provide strong evidence that the biomarkers based on structural MRI (i.e., hippocampal volume and VBM) can be a valuable biomarker to evaluate a novel therapeutic efficacy.

Resting-state functional MRI (rs-fMRI) is another neuroimaging modality that has been widely used to characterize various functional networks in the brain. It can measure BOLD signals that reflect the changes in blood flow and deoxyhemoglobin due to brain activities – a process called neurovascular coupling. This process seems to be conserved among the majority of animal models of AD used to evaluate novel therapeutics, enabling the application of fMRI across the species [60]. Furthermore, analytical methods for BOLD signals such as hypothesis-driven seed-based connectivity or data-driven independent component analysis (ICA) add an additional factor allowing translation of the findings between the species (Figure 9.5). For example, since the identification of the default mode network (DMN), which is thought to be a large-scale brain organization that is unique to humans due to its role in conceptual processing, mind-wandering, and sustenance for consciousness, the DMN has been demonstrated also in anesthetized macaques, chimpanzees, and rodent brains based on both seed-based connectivity and ICA analyses [36, 70, 71]. Thus, the intrinsically connected regions defining the DMN appear to be fundamental in mammalian brains. In AD, a remarkable overlap in the topographical distribution of $A\beta$, hypometabolism, and neurodegeneration within the regions forming DMN regions has been demonstrated by Buckner et al. in 2005 [59]. Since then, a myriad of studies has shown converging evidence that the intrinsic connectivity in the DMN is altered in AD, and supported DMN alteration as an early biomarker of AD [72–74]. Notably, aberrant increased hippocampal activities in the DMN were associated with $A\beta$ during

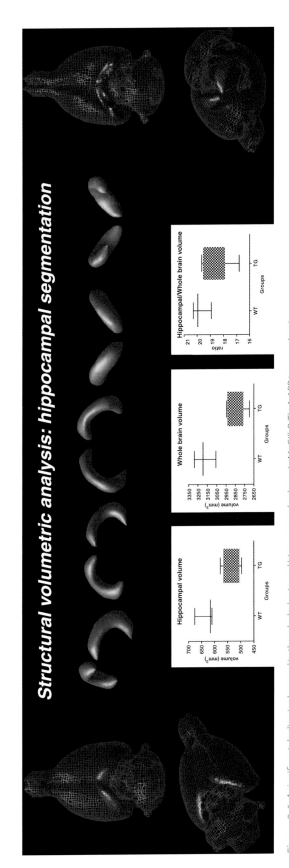

Figure 9.4 A significant decline is observed in the whole-brain and hippocampal volume in McGill-R-Thy1-APP transgenic rats.

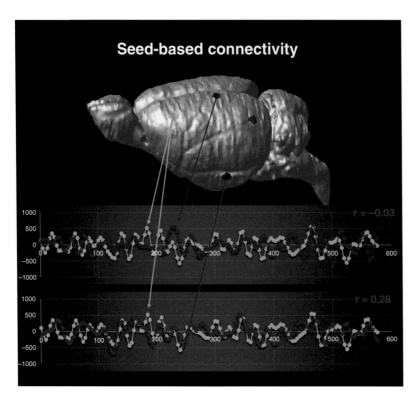

Figure 9.5 An illustration of seed-based connectivity patterns, representing the temporal correlation between fluctuation in BOLD signals of the seed (green) and target (red, purple) regions in the rat brain. This shows that the target region in red (correlation factor $r = 0.91$) functionally connected to the seed region compared to the target region in purple ($r = -0.56$).

the preclinical stage of AD while reduced DMN activities were associated with more advanced AD pathology or stage [75, 76]. Similarly, the McGill-R-Thy1-APP transgenic rat model displaying AD-like Aβ pathology recapitulated the aberrant increased connectivity from the hippocampus within the DMN at early stages (9–11 months old) and reduced connectivity at later stages (16–19 months old) [35]. Therefore, rs-fMRI can serve as an early AD biomarker in preclinical models of AD to detect individuals who are on their path to more advanced stages of AD.

In June 2021, aducanumab (Aduhelm™) was conditionally approved under the accelerated approval pathway by the US FDA although its clinical benefit is still uncertain. While the search for a disease-modifying therapeutic is still ongoing, the recent reports of the anti-amyloid immunotherapy trials have highlighted the importance of safety issues related to amyloid-related imaging abnormalities (ARIA) edema (ARIA-E) or micro-hemorrhages (ARIA-H), which is thought to be associated with the removal of Aβ found in vessel walls [20, 77, 78]. The ARIA is suggested to occur

in a dose-dependent manner and is reported in all of the anti-amyloid immunotherapy trials, especially at the highest dose group and in apolipoprotein E ε4 (*APOE-4*) carriers. Therefore, evaluating potential ARIA at the preclinical assessment of AD therapeutics would provide valuable information on the safety concerns. ARIA are typically detected using MRI T2*-weighted imaging, and the same technique can be applied to different species. For example, Luo et al. reported that T2*-weighted imaging protocol reliably detected incidents of ARIA-H due to the monoclonal antibody treatment in the APP transgenic mice model of AD when compared to the histological evidence of ARIA-H [79].

9.6 Motion Tracking

So far, we have discussed how MRI and PET, the two most widely used neuroimaging techniques in AD research, can be utilized to bridge the translation of preclinical assessments of novel therapeutics in AD. Despite the many advantages that we have discussed, one of the greatest limitations in preclinical neuroimaging studies is the use of anesthesia. The current neuroimaging platform in animal research inevitably uses anesthesia to scan animals without any motions. However, the effect of anesthesia on physiology cannot be ignored as it changes neuronal activity, blood flow, heart rate, physiological temperature, and more. In this section, we will briefly discuss the effects of anesthesia and new developments in the effort to conduct neuroimaging studies in animal research to eliminate the greatest confounding factor, anesthesia.

In the previous section, we have discussed how fMRI, particularly rs-fMRI, is an important early biomarker for AD. However, most of the preclinical animal models require anesthesia to circumvent any motions during the data acquisition. Although anesthesia is necessary, it leads to various confounding effects in the data and subsequent analysis. First, the condition under anesthesia does not reflect the true "resting-state" or normal awake condition, in which neuronal activity is measured [80]. Second, it affects physiological variables such as blood flow, body temperature, heart rate, and metabolism, in which such physiological variables affect BOLD fluctuations [80]. Altogether, it has been well established that rs-fMRI acquired under anesthesia does not replicate the awake condition in the same fashion. For example, the most commonly used anesthesia in preclinical imaging, isoflurane, is reported to show significantly reduced BOLD fluctuation and amplitude, effectively reducing the power of the BOLD signals while significantly increasing the regional correlation coefficients [81–83]. To be able to interpret the preclinical fMRI data without anesthetic effects relative to the human rs-fMRI findings, various awake rs-fMRI preclinical platforms have been developed; most of them focus on rodent imaging and have created a restrainer and acclimation protocol [84]. While the details within different protocols vary in their training, a general protocol follows about a week of training by mimicking the real scanning environment settings such as the rs-fMRI sequence noises and installation within a restrainer following light anesthesia. Within about a week of training, the stress-level hormone, cortisol, becomes as close as normal to physiological concentration, and rodents are able to endure a full rs-fMRI protocol completely awake [81, 85]. On the other hand, a recent study investigating the effect of a short-restraint awake rs-fMRI training

(≤ 3 days) revealed a heightened activation in the amygdala related to nociceptive stimuli [86]. Thus, it is imperative to design an awake rs-fMRI protocol that will not rewire the brain connectivity in question. With an awake fMRI protocol in rodent imaging, the rs-fMRI biomarkers from preclinical research are able to substantiate human findings and interpret without the confounding effects of anesthesia.

Similarly, PET is not exempted from the confounding effects of anesthesia. To accurately quantify the distribution of PET tracer, it is imperative to keep the normal physiological parameters such as blood flow, temperature, and heart rate. Notably, the effect of anesthesia in PET quantification depends on the anesthesia, tracer, and tissues. For example, the most commonly used anesthesia, isoflurane, showed a substantial increase in the $[^{18}F]$ FDG uptake, while the ketamine/xylazine mixture decreased the uptake in the heart [56]. With regard to the brain, the $[^{18}F]FDG$ uptake was significantly lower in both isoflurane and ketamine/xylazine mixture compared to the awake condition [87, 88]. Furthermore, for a tracer targeting dopamine D1 receptor, $[^{11}C]SCH23390$, the binding potential is significantly increased in the striatum in rodents under chloral hydrate and ketamine anesthesia and decreased under pentobarbital anesthesia compared to awake animals [89]. To circumvent the use of anesthesia, there have been different micro-PET methodologies developed in the past decade as well. Similar to awake rs-fMRI, there have been restraining devices used to scan awake animals, while motion-tracking equipment based on a fiducial tracker and even miniature PET equipment have been created [87, 90, 91]. Although the majority of the protocols need a surgical installation on the animals or additional tracking equipment on top of the rodent head, Miranda et al. reported a motion-tracking system based on a few fiducial points that do not require any surgery or additional equipment to track the motion [92, 93]. By pasting a few fiducial points produced from salts emitting $[^{18}F]$ radioisotope activity on the animal's head, motion can be tracked and corrected during a list-mode reconstruction without impeding the animal's behavior or physical stress. In addition, this method allows the acquisition of PET data from awake and freely interacting animals (Figure 9.6). This creates an unprecedented opportunity to investigate social interactions at neurochemical levels.

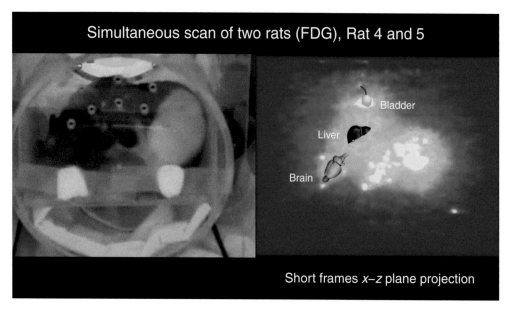

Figure 9.6 Simultaneous awake [¹⁸F]FDG PET imaging of two rats interacting together in a PET scanner. This imaging platform can track motion and associate behavioral measurements, representing social interaction and brain metabolism or neurotransmitters measured by PET.

9.7 Fluid Biomarkers

In clinics, more commonly used in vivo biomarkers are based on fluid platforms such as the plasma or CSF. With the advent of novel methodologies that accurately detect the hallmarks of AD proteins in plasma, the integration of the fluid biomarkers in evaluating clinical trial enrichment, target engagements, and efficacy will substantially reduce the cost associated with PET or MRI while making the screening process widely available [94, 95]. As such, the characterization and validation of the fluid biomarkers in preclinical animal models of AD are imperative.

Although there is evidence of Aβ in the brains of some animals, the AD hallmarks of abnormal aggregates of both Aβ and hyperphosphorylated tau (p-tau) proteins do not naturally occur in the current preclinical animal models of AD (www.alzforum.org/webinars/alzheimers-disease-uniquely-human-disorder). Therefore, genetic manipulation introducing human forms of Aβ and/or tau genes to initiate the AD pathophysiological processes is necessary. Consequently, this allows the same methodologies in detecting Aβ and/or tau in plasma or CSF to be applied in the preclinical animal models of AD. For example, it is well established that the CSF $A\beta_{42}$ concentration is inversely associated with the Aβ deposition in the

brain [96]. Furthermore, longitudinal studies have reported the ratio between $A\beta_{42}$ and $A\beta_{40}$ declines significantly over time with reduced variability compared to $A\beta_{42}$ alone [97]. Based on the same enzyme-linked immunosorbent assay (ELISA) technique, Parent et al. have replicated the same characteristic of CSF $A\beta_{42}$ decline in the McGill-R-Thy1-APP rat model [35]. In addition, for the first time, a longitudinal CSF $A\beta_{42}/A\beta_{40}$ progression was characterized in an AD rat model based on the single-molecule-array (Simoa®) technique, replicating the human findings (Figure 9.7a) [69]. On the other hand, CSF total tau and p-tau concentrations are significantly increased as the neurofibrillary tangles deposit in the brain in AD and this is also replicated in the tau mice model [98, 99]. Barten et al. reported an age-dependent increase in CSF tau in various transgenic tau mice models using their novel technique in collecting CSF from mice [98]. Furthermore, the P301L tau mouse model showed a significant increase in total tau and p-tau in both serum and CSF corresponding to the tau pathological progression reported in human serum and CSF [99].

Besides the core AD pathological biomarkers, neurodegeneration can be measured in the blood and CSF as well. The NfL has gained myriads of strong evidence recently as a putative plasma and CSF biomarker of neurodegeneration in AD. For

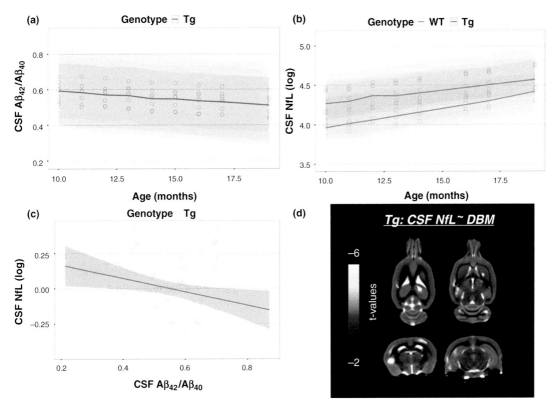

Figure 9.7 A longitudinal progression of (a) CSF $A\beta_{42}/A\beta_{40}$ in the McGill-R-Thy1-APP transgenic rat model and (b) NfL in a wild-type and a McGill-R-Thy1-APP transgenic rat model with the shadows representing a 95% confidence interval per animal. (c) A significant association is shown between CSF $A\beta_{42}/A\beta_{40}$ and NfL concentration, while in (d) there is a significant voxel-based association between the CSF NfL and deformation-based morphometry (DBM) only in the McGill-R-Thy1-APP transgenic rat model. This figure has been adapted from Kang et al. [69].

example, the NfL increased significantly over the disease progression and its rate of change was able to discriminate the familial-AD mutation carriers from non-carriers decades before the expected onset of symptoms [100]. However, such targets in the preclinical animal models of AD are endogenous to the animals. While the same assay applied in human AD was applicable for detecting Aβ and tau in the animals, the same assay targeting the endogenous animals' NfL will not work properly. As a result, a new assay that is specific to the species must be developed and validated. For murine NfL assays, various groups have replicated the characteristic of NfL profile in the plasma and CSF as the human AD, and they demonstrated that the NfL can be used to evaluate a novel AD therapeutic efficacy. For example, the McGill-R-Thy1-APP rat model demonstrated a longitudinal increase in the CSF NfL that is inversely associated with CSF Aβ, replicating the human findings [69] (Figure 9.7b–d). Similarly, various proteopathic mice models

(alpha-synuclein, tau, and Aβ) revealed a significant age-dependent increase in plasma and CSF NfL, and BACE1 inhibitor treatment in APP/PS1 mice substantially reduced the NfL concentration in CSF compared to the control APP/PS1 mice [101].

9.8 Study Design: Rigor and Reproducibility in Animal Model Studies

Over the past years, hundreds of clinical trials testing potential neuroprotective drugs have not been successful in widespread regulatory and clinical use despite showing efficacy in preclinical studies [21]. Besides the greater translational value related to the in vivo methodologies that we have described so far, there are other important technical aspects to consider. As we discussed above, animal models do not precisely mimic full-blown AD, but rather each animal model focuses on one or a few aspects of AD pathophysiology of interest. Therefore,

AD-like Aβ and tau pathology models are ideal to evaluate the target engagement in reducing Aβ and tau and its efficacy to mitigate neurodegeneration. However, all of the Phase 3 anti-amyloid clinical trials have always considered a cognitive benefit as the primary endpoint beyond the therapeutic target engagement. Although many of the anti-amyloid drugs tested in the animals also showed some cognitive benefit in addition to the target engagement, the link between Aβ and cognition in AD is weak [63]. Furthermore, myriads of pathophysiological mechanisms bridging the Aβ pathology and cognition in AD are not completely replicated in an AD-like Aβ pathology rodent model. For example, they do not develop neurofibrillary tangles, which are considered to impose greater toxic insults leading to neurodegeneration in AD. Moreover, preclinical studies lack the same rigor in their study design and reproducibility principles. In general, blinding and randomization are usually neglected by basic researchers. Another important issue is the lack of multicentric studies, as most drugs are tested in a single institution and/or a single animal model. Finally, there is a lack of drug testing studies publishing negative outcomes. All these issues certainly have undermined studies and their reproducibility.

9.9 Past, Present, and Future AD Drug Development: Toward In Vivo Biomarker Preclinical Platform

Considering the role of in vivo biomarkers and the previous limitations discussed above, there are a few strategies for closing this gap, as recently demonstrated by Kang et al. [102]. The use of in vivo biomarkers may hold the key for improving the translational power in preclinical drug pipelines in AD. First, longitudinal studies in AD models with imaging and fluid biomarkers for assessing the A/T/(N) and linking to the cognition and behavior provide an excellent strategy for drug target engagement and monitoring drug efficacy. Second, the AD animal model needs to be cleverly defined. For example, if your primary outcome is reducing Aβ pathology, an APP model seems ideal. However, if cognitive benefit based on the therapeutic target engagement is the primary outcome, then you may need a model combining APP and tau mutations with the understanding of the pathophysiological processes between the pathology and cognition.

Last, the predefinition of endpoints and sample size with appropriate statistical power analysis is very much needed. Study preregistration, which is a mandatory measure in clinical trials, would be very helpful in this regard. There are interesting initiatives in this respect, such as the implementation of critical incident reporting, which has become widely used in clinical medicine [103].

9.10 Take-Home Messages

1. Biomarkers for human and animal models can provide the same biological information.
2. In contrast with traditional histological methods, animal models allied to in vivo biomarkers allow for preclinical drug discovery using longitudinal designs.
3. Animal models allow us to assess the effects of therapies targeting specific disease processes while removing the bias of co-pathologies present in human AD.
4. Biomarkers allow the incorporation of good practices from human research to early drug development.
5. Sample size calculations for human research can be better extrapolated from biomarkers rather than traditional histological outcomes.

References

1. Polanco JC, Li C, Bodea LG, et al. Amyloid-beta and tau complexity: towards improved biomarkers and targeted therapies. *Nat Rev Neurol* 2018; **14**: 22–39.

2. Gotz J, Bodea LG, Goedert M. Rodent models for Alzheimer disease. *Nat Rev Neurosci* 2018; **19**: 583–98.

3. Grieb P. Intracerebroventricular streptozotocin injections as a model of Alzheimer's disease: in search of a relevant mechanism. *Mol Neurobiol* 2016; **53**: 1741–52.

4. Kamat PK, Rai S, Nath C. Okadaic acid induced neurotoxicity: an emerging tool to study Alzheimer's disease pathology. *Neurotoxicology* 2013; **37**: 163–72.

5. Kim HY, Lee DK, Chung BR, Kim HV, Kim Y. Intracerebroventricular injection of amyloid-beta peptides in normal mice to acutely induce Alzheimer-like cognitive deficits. *J Vis Exp* 2016; **109**: 53308.

6. de Calignon A, Polydoro M, Suarez-Calvet M, et al. Propagation of tau pathology in a model of early Alzheimer's disease. *Neuron* 2012; **73**: 685–97.

7. Braak H, Braak E. Neuropathological stageing of Alzheimer-related changes. *Acta Neuropathol* 1991; **82**: 239–59.

8. Hardy J, Selkoe DJ. The amyloid hypothesis of Alzheimer's disease: progress and problems on the road to therapeutics. *Science* 2002; **297**: 353–6.

9. Leon WC, Canneva F, Partridge V, et al. A novel transgenic rat model with a full Alzheimer's-like amyloid pathology displays pre-plaque intracellular amyloid-beta-associated cognitive impairment. *J Alzheimers Dis* 2010; **20**: 113–26.

10. Cohen RM, Rezai-Zadeh K, Weitz TM, et al. A transgenic Alzheimer rat with plaques, tau pathology, behavioral impairment, oligomeric Abeta, and frank neuronal loss. *J Neurosci* 2013; **33**: 6245–56.

11. Malcolm JC, Breuillaud L, Do Carmo S, et al. Neuropathological changes and cognitive deficits in rats transgenic for human mutant tau recapitulate human tauopathy. *Neurobiol Dis* 2019; **127**: 323–38.

12. Do Carmo S, Cuello AC. Modeling Alzheimer's disease in transgenic rats. *Mol Neurodegener* 2013; **8**: 37.

13. Zimmer ER, Parent MJ, Cuello AC, Gauthier S, Rosa-Neto P. MicroPET imaging and transgenic models: a blueprint for Alzheimer's disease clinical research. *Trends Neurosci* 2014; **37**: 629–41.

14. Kuang E, Wan Q, Li X, et al. ER stress triggers apoptosis induced by Nogo-B/ASY overexpression. *Exp Cell Res* 2006; **312**: 1983–8.

15. Saito T, Matsuba Y, Mihira N, et al. Single APP knock-in mouse models of Alzheimer's disease. *Nat Neurosci* 2014; **17**: 661–3.

16. Bard F, Cannon C, Barbour R, et al. Peripherally administered antibodies against amyloid beta-peptide enter the central nervous system and reduce pathology in a mouse model of Alzheimer disease. *Nat Med* 2000; **6**: 916–19.

17. DeMattos RB, Bales KR, Cummins DJ, et al. Peripheral anti-A beta antibody alters CNS and plasma A beta clearance and decreases brain Abeta burden in a mouse model of Alzheimer's disease. *Proc Natl Acad Sci USA* 2001; **98**: 8850–5.

18. Bohrmann B, Baumann K, Benz J, et al. Gantenerumab: a novel human anti-A beta antibody demonstrates sustained cerebral amyloid-beta binding and elicits cell-mediated removal of human amyloid-beta. *J Alzheimers Dis* 2012; **28**: 49–69.

19. Lord A, Gumucio A, Englund H, et al. An amyloid-beta protofibril-selective antibody prevents amyloid formation in a mouse model of Alzheimer's disease. *Neurobiol Dis* 2009; **36**: 425–34.

20. Sevigny J, Chiao P, Bussiere T, et al. The antibody aducanumab reduces Abeta plaques in Alzheimer's disease. *Nature* 2016; **537**: 50–6.

21. Cummings JL, Morstorf T, Zhong K. Alzheimer's disease drug-development pipeline: few candidates, frequent failures. *Alzheimers Res Ther* 2014; **6**: 37.

22. Jack CR Jr., Bennett DA, Blennow K, et al. NIA-AA Research Framework: toward a biological definition of Alzheimer's disease. *Alzheimers Dement* 2018; **14**: 535–62.

23. Alzheimer's Association. 2019 Alzheimer's disease facts and figures. *Alzheimers Dement* 2019; **15**: 321–87.

24. Amadoru S, Dore V, McLean CA, et al. Comparison of amyloid PET measured in centiloid units with neuropathological findings in Alzheimer's disease. *Alzheimers Res Ther* 2020; **12**: 22.

25. Maeda J, Ji B, Irie T, et al. Longitudinal, quantitative assessment of amyloid, neuroinflammation, and anti-amyloid treatment in a living mouse model of Alzheimer's disease enabled by positron emission tomography. *J Neurosci* 2007; **27**: 10957–68.

26. Maeda J, Zhang MR, Okauchi T, et al. In vivo positron emission tomographic imaging of glial responses to amyloid-beta and tau pathologies in mouse models of Alzheimer's disease and related disorders. *J Neurosci* 2011; **31**: 4720–30.

27. Snellman A, Lopez-Picon FR, Rokka J, et al. Longitudinal amyloid imaging in mouse brain with ^{11}C-PIB: comparison of APP23, Tg2576, and APPswe-PS1dE9 mouse models of Alzheimer disease. *J Nucl Med* 2013; **54**: 1434–41.

28. Snellman A, Rokka J, Lopez-Picon FR, et al. Applicability of [(11)C]PiB micro-PET imaging for in vivo follow-up of anti-amyloid treatment effects in APP23 mouse model. *Neurobiol Aging* 2017; **57**: 84–94.

29. Snellman A, Rokka J, Lopez-Picon FR, et al. In vivo PET imaging of beta-amyloid deposition in mouse models of Alzheimer's disease with a high specific activity PET imaging agent [(18)F]flutemetamol. *EJNMMI Res* 2014; **4**: 37.

30. Toyama H, Ye D, Ichise M, et al. PET imaging of brain with the beta-amyloid probe, ^{11}C]6-OH-BTA-1, in a transgenic mouse model of Alzheimer's disease. *Eur J Nucl Med Mol Imaging* 2005; **32**: 593–600.

31. Kuntner C, Kesner AL, Bauer M, et al. Limitations of small animal PET imaging with ^{18}F]FDDNP and FDG for quantitative studies in a transgenic mouse model of Alzheimer's disease. *Mol Imaging Biol* 2009; **11**: 236–40.

32. Poisnel G, Dhilly M, Moustie O, et al. PET imaging with [18 F]AV-45 in an APP/PS1-21 murine model of amyloid plaque deposition. *Neurobiol Aging* 2012; **33**: 2561–71.

119

33. Brendel M, Jaworska A, Griessinger E, et al. Cross-sectional comparison of small animal [18F]-florbetaben amyloid-PET between transgenic AD mouse models. *PLoS One* 2015; **10**: e0116678.

34. Brendel M, Jaworska A, Overhoff F, et al. Efficacy of chronic BACE1 inhibition in PS2APP mice depends on the regional Abeta deposition rate and plaque burden at treatment initiation. *Theranostics* 2018; **8**: 4957–68.

35. Parent MJ, Zimmer ER, Shin M, et al. Multimodal imaging in rat model recapitulates Alzheimer's disease biomarkers abnormalities. *J Neurosci* 2017; **37**: 12263–71.

36. Zimmer ER, Leuzy A, Gauthier S, Rosa-Neto P. Developments in tau PET imaging. *Can J Neurol Sci* 2014; **41**: 547–53.

37. Leuzy A, Chiotis K, Lemoine L, et al. Tau PET imaging in neurodegenerative tauopathies: still a challenge. *Mol Psychiatry* 2019; **24**: 1112–34.

38. Fodero-Tavoletti MT, Okamura N, Furumoto S, et al. 18F-THK523: a novel in vivo tau imaging ligand for Alzheimer's disease. *Brain* 2011; **134**: 1089–100.

39. Maruyama M, Shimada H, Suhara T, et al. Imaging of tau pathology in a tauopathy mouse model and in Alzheimer patients compared to normal controls. *Neuron* 2013; **79**: 1094–108.

40. Ishikawa A, Tokunaga M, Maeda J, et al. In vivo visualization of tau accumulation, microglial activation, and brain atrophy in a mouse model of tauopathy rTg4510. *J Alzheimers Dis* 2018; **61**: 1037–52.

41. Ni R, Ji B, Ono M, et al. Comparative in vitro and in vivo quantifications of pathologic tau deposits and their association with neurodegeneration in tauopathy mouse models. *J Nucl Med* 2018; **59**: 960–6.

42. Brendel M, Yousefi BH, Blume T, et al. Comparison of (18)F-T807 and (18)F-THK5117 PET in a mouse model of tau pathology. *Front Aging Neurosci* 2018; **10**: 174.

43. Hattori N, Huang SC, Wu HM, et al. Acute changes in regional cerebral (18)F-FDG kinetics in patients with traumatic brain injury. *J Nucl Med* 2004; **45**: 775–83.

44. Zimmer ER, Parent MJ, Souza DG, et al. [(18)F]FDG PET signal is driven by astroglial glutamate transport. *Nat Neurosci* 2017; **20**: 393–5.

45. Stoessl AJ. Glucose utilization: still in the synapse. *Nat Neurosci* 2017; **20**: 382–4.

46. Silverman DH. Brain 18F-FDG PET in the diagnosis of neurodegenerative dementias: comparison with perfusion SPECT and with clinical evaluations lacking nuclear imaging. *J Nucl Med* 2004; **45**: 594–607.

47. Bohnen NI, Djang DS, Herholz K, Anzai Y, Minoshima S. Effectiveness and safety of 18F-FDG PET in the evaluation of dementia: a review of the recent literature. *J Nucl Med* 2012; **53**: 59–71.

48. Mosconi L, Tsui WH, Herholz K, et al. Multicenter standardized 18F-FDG PET diagnosis of mild cognitive impairment, Alzheimer's disease, and other dementias. *J Nucl Med* 2008; **49**: 390–8.

49. Chételat G, Arbizu J, Barthel H, et al. Amyloid-PET and 18F-FDG-PET in the diagnostic investigation of Alzheimer's disease and other dementias. *Lancet Neurol* 2020; **19**: 951–62.

50. Luo F, Rustay NR, Ebert U, et al. Characterization of 7- and 19-month-old Tg2576 mice using multimodal in vivo imaging: limitations as a translatable model of Alzheimer's disease. *Neurobiol Aging* 2012; **33**: 933–44.

51. Martin-Moreno AM, Brera B, Spuch C, et al. Prolonged oral cannabinoid administration prevents neuroinflammation, lowers beta-amyloid levels and improves cognitive performance in Tg APP 2576 mice. *J Neuroinflamm* 2012; **9**: 8.

52. Heneka MT, Ramanathan M, Jacobs AH, et al. Locus ceruleus degeneration promotes Alzheimer pathogenesis in amyloid precursor protein 23 transgenic mice. *J Neurosci* 2006; **26**: 1343–54.

53. Poisnel G, Herard AS, El Tannir El Tayara N, et al. Increased regional cerebral glucose uptake in an APP/PS1 model of Alzheimer's disease. *Neurobiol Aging* 2012; **33**: 1995–2005.

54. Lu XY, Huang S, Chen QB, et al. Metformin ameliorates Abeta pathology by insulin-degrading enzyme in a transgenic mouse model of Alzheimer's disease. *Oxid Med Cell Longev* 2020; **2020**: 2315106.

55. Sung KK, Jang DP, Lee S, et al. Neural responses in rat brain during acute immobilization stress: a [F-18]FDG micro PET imaging study. *Neuroimage* 2009; **44**: 1074–80.

56. Toyama H, Ichise M, Liow J-S, et al. Evaluation of anesthesia effects on [18F]FDG uptake in mouse brain and heart using small animal PET. *Nucl Med Biol* 2004; **31**: 251–6.

57. Ottoy J, Verhaeghe J, Niemantsverdriet E, et al. Validation of the semiquantitative static SUVR method for (18)F-AV45 PET by pharmacokinetic modeling with an arterial input function. *J Nucl Med* 2017; **58**: 1483–9.

58. Price JC, Klunk WE, Lopresti BJ, et al. Kinetic modeling of amyloid binding in humans using PET imaging and Pittsburgh Compound-B. *J Cereb Blood Flow Metab* 2005; **25**: 1528–47.

59. Buckner RL, Snyder AZ, Shannon BJ, et al. Molecular, structural, and functional characterization of Alzheimer's disease: evidence for a relationship between default activity, amyloid, and memory. *J Neurosci* 2005; **25**: 7709–17.

60. Lu H, Zou Q, Gu H, et al. Rat brains also have a default mode network. *Proc Natl Acad Sci USA* 2012; **109**: 3979–84.

61. Jack CR Jr., Wiste HJ, Vemuri P, et al. Brain beta-amyloid measures and magnetic resonance imaging atrophy both predict time-to-progression from mild cognitive impairment to Alzheimer's disease. *Brain* 2010; **133**: 3336–48.

62. Terry RD, Masliah E, Salmon DP, et al. Physical basis of cognitive alterations in Alzheimer's disease: synapse loss is the major correlate of cognitive impairment. *Ann Neurol* 1991; **30**: 572–80.

63. Jagust W. Imaging the evolution and pathophysiology of Alzheimer disease. *Nat Rev Neurosci* 2018; **19**: 687–700.

64. Ottoy J, Niemantsverdriet E, Verhaeghe J, et al. Association of short-term cognitive decline and MCI-to-AD dementia conversion with CSF, MRI, amyloid- and (18)F-FDG-PET imaging. *Neuroimage Clin* 2019; **22**: 101771.

65. Heggland I, Storkaas IS, Soligard HT, Kobro-Flatmoen A, Witter MP. Stereological estimation of neuron number and plaque load in the hippocampal region of a transgenic rat model of Alzheimer's disease. *Eur J Neurosci* 2015; **41**: 1245–62.

66. Macdonald IR, DeBay DR, Reid GA, et al. Early detection of cerebral glucose uptake changes in the 5×FAD mouse. *Curr Alzheimer Res* 2014; **11**: 450–60.

67. Yoshiyama Y, Higuchi M, Zhang B, et al. Synapse loss and microglial activation precede tangles in a P301S tauopathy mouse model. *Neuron* 2007; **53**: 337–51.

68. Chiquita S, Ribeiro M, Castelhano J, et al. A longitudinal multimodal in vivo molecular imaging study of the 3×Tg-AD mouse model shows progressive early hippocampal and taurine loss. *Hum Mol Genet* 2019; **28**: 2174–88.

69. Kang MS, Aliaga AA, Shin M, et al. Amyloid-beta modulates the association between neurofilament light chain and brain atrophy in Alzheimer's disease. *Mol Psychiatry* 2020;https://doi.org/10.1038/s41380-020-0818-1.

70. Vincent JL, Patel GH, Fox MD, et al. Intrinsic functional architecture in the anaesthetized monkey brain. *Nature* 2007; **447**: 83–6.

71. Rilling JK, Barks SK, Parr LA, et al. A comparison of resting-state brain activity in humans and chimpanzees. *Proc Natl Acad Sci USA* 2007; **104**: 17146–51.

72. Greicius MD, Srivastava G, Reiss AL, Menon V. Default-mode network activity distinguishes Alzheimer's disease from healthy aging: evidence from functional MRI. *Proc Natl Acad Sci USA* 2004; **101**: 4637–42.

73. Buckner RL, Sepulcre J, Talukdar T, et al. Cortical hubs revealed by intrinsic functional connectivity: mapping, assessment of stability, and relation to Alzheimer's disease. *J Neurosci* 2009; **29**: 1860–73.

74. Sheline YI, Raichle ME. Resting state functional connectivity in preclinical Alzheimer's disease. *Biol Psychiatry* 2013; **74**: 340–7.

75. Wang L, Zang Y, He Y, et al. Changes in hippocampal connectivity in the early stages of Alzheimer's disease: evidence from resting state fMRI. *Neuroimage* 2006; **31**: 496–504.

76. Huijbers W, Mormino EC, Schultz AP, et al. Amyloid-beta deposition in mild cognitive impairment is associated with increased hippocampal activity, atrophy and clinical progression. *Brain* 2015; **138**: 1023–35.

77. Salloway S, Sperling R, Gilman S, et al. A Phase 2 multiple ascending dose trial of bapineuzumab in mild to moderate Alzheimer disease. *Neurology* 2009; **73**: 2061–70.

78. Sperling RA, Jack CR Jr., Black SE, et al. Amyloid-related imaging abnormalities in amyloid-modifying therapeutic trials: recommendations from the Alzheimer's Association Research Roundtable Workgroup. *Alzheimers Dement* 2011; **7**: 367–85.

79. Luo F, Rustay NR, Seifert T, et al. Magnetic resonance imaging detection and time course of cerebral microhemorrhages during passive immunotherapy in living amyloid precursor protein transgenic mice. *J Pharmacol Exp Ther* 2010; **335**: 580–8.

80. Constantinides C, Murphy K. Molecular and integrative physiological effects of isoflurane anesthesia: the paradigm of cardiovascular studies in rodents using magnetic resonance imaging. *Front Cardiovasc Med* 2016; **3**: 23.

81. Stenroos P, Paasonen J, Salo RA, et al. Awake rat brain functional magnetic resonance imaging using standard radio frequency coils and a 3D printed restraint kit. *Front Neurosci* 2018; **12**: 548.

82. Paasonen J, Stenroos P, Salo RA, Kiviniemi V, Grohn O. Functional connectivity under six anesthesia protocols and the awake condition in rat brain. *Neuroimage* 2018; **172**: 9–20.

83. Wu TL, Mishra A, Wang F, et al. Effects of isoflurane anesthesia on resting-state fMRI signals and functional connectivity within primary somatosensory cortex of monkeys. *Brain Behav* 2016; **6**: e00591.

84. Ferris CF, Smerkers B, Kulkarni P, et al. Functional magnetic resonance imaging in awake animals. *Rev Neurosci* 2011; **22**: 665–74.

85. Dopfel D, Zhang N. Mapping stress networks using functional magnetic resonance imaging in awake animals. *Neurobiol Stress* 2018; **9**: 251–63.

86. Low LA, Bauer LC, Pitcher MH, Bushnell MC. Restraint training for awake functional brain scanning of rodents can cause long-lasting changes in pain and stress responses. *Pain* 2016; **157**: 1761–72.

87. Mizuma H, Shukuri M, Hayashi T, Watanabe Y, Onoe H. Establishment of in vivo brain imaging method in conscious mice. *J Nucl Med* 2010; **51**: 1068–75.

88. Alstrup AK, Smith DF. Anaesthesia for positron emission tomography scanning of animal brains. *Lab Anim* 2013; **47**: 12–18.

89. Momosaki S, Hatano K, Kawasumi Y, et al. Rat-PET study without anesthesia: anesthetics modify the dopamine D1 receptor binding in rat brain. *Synapse* 2004; **54**: 207–13.

90. Kyme AZ, Zhou VW, Meikle SR, Fulton RR. Real-time 3D motion tracking for small animal brain PET. *Phys Med Biol* 2008; **53**: 2651–66.

91. Schulz D, Southekal S, Junnarkar SS, et al. Simultaneous assessment of rodent behavior and neurochemistry using a miniature positron emission tomograph. *Nat Methods* 2011; **8**: 347–52.

92. Miranda A, Kang MS, Blinder S, et al. PET imaging of freely moving interacting rats. *Neuroimage* 2019; **191**: 560–7.

93. Miranda A, Staelens S, Stroobants S, Verhaeghe J. Fast and accurate rat head motion tracking with point sources for awake brain PET. *IEEE Trans Med Imaging* 2017; **36**: 1573–82.

94. Nakamura A, Kaneko N, Villemagne VL, et al. High performance plasma amyloid-beta biomarkers for Alzheimer's disease. *Nature* 2018; **554**: 249–54.

95. Janelidze S, Mattsson N, Palmqvist S, et al. Plasma p-tau181 in Alzheimer's disease: relationship to other biomarkers, differential diagnosis, neuropathology and longitudinal progression to Alzheimer's dementia. *Nat Med* 2020; **26**: 379–86.

96. Niemantsverdriet E, Ottoy J, Somers C, et al. The cerebrospinal fluid Abeta1-42/Abeta1-40 ratio improves concordance with amyloid-PET for diagnosing Alzheimer's disease in a clinical setting. *J Alzheimers Dis* 2017; **60**: 561–76.

97. Hansson O, Zetterberg H, Buchhave P, et al. Prediction of Alzheimer's disease using the CSF Abeta42/Abeta40 ratio in patients with mild cognitive impairment. *Dement Geriatr Cogn Disord* 2007; **23**: 316–20.

98. Barten DM, Cadelina GW, Hoque N, et al. Tau transgenic mice as models for cerebrospinal fluid tau biomarkers. *J Alzheimers Dis* 2011; **24**: 127–41.

99. Acker CM, Forest SK, Zinkowski R, Davies P, d'Abramo C. Sensitive quantitative assays for tau and phospho-tau in transgenic mouse models. *Neurobiol Aging* 2013; **34**: 338–50.

100. Preische O, Schultz SA, Apel A, et al. Serum neurofilament dynamics predicts neurodegeneration and clinical progression in presymptomatic Alzheimer's disease. *Nat Med* 2019; **25**: 277–83.

101. Bacioglu M, Maia LF, Preische O, et al. Neurofilament light chain in blood and CSF as marker of disease progression in mouse models and in neurodegenerative diseases. *Neuron* 2016; **91**: 56–66.

102. Kang MS, Shin M, Ottoy J, et al. Preclinical in vivo longitudinal assessment of KG207-M as a disease-modifying Alzheimer's disease therapeutic. *J Cereb Blood Flow Metab* August 2021; doi: 10.1177/0271678X211035625.

103. Dirnagl U, Przesdzing I, Kurreck C, Major S. A laboratory critical incident and error reporting system for experimental biomedicine. *PLoS Biol* 2016; **14**: e2000705.

Biobanking and Biomarkers in the Alzheimer's Disease Drug-Development Ecosystem

Jefferson Kinney and Arnold Salazar

10.1 Introduction

Alzheimer's disease (AD) is a multifaceted, neurological disease characterized by the progressive degeneration of memory and cognitive functions, and subsequent death. It is a major health problem that significantly impacts the global societies and economies. Since it was first described by Dr. Alois Alzheimer in 1906, a tremendous amount of information from scientific research has been generated that provides a much better understanding of the disease. However, at present, there is still no known cure for AD.

Biobanks and biomarker discovery workflows have played a fundamental role in understanding AD, and have also become central features of drug development in the testing of novel therapeutics. The first clinical trials of novel therapeutics for AD relied on biobanking for storage and future examination of tissues, largely for safety and tolerability biomarker evaluations. As the investigations of the underlying biology of AD have advanced, so too has the development of assays and techniques to identify biomarkers in AD. These biomarkers have provided the opportunity to better diagnose AD, but also for the evaluation of treatment efficacy that have evolved into endpoint measures in AD clinical trials. In the sections below, we highlight some of the basic features and requirements of biobanks and biomarker discovery workflow, as well as how these approaches have been utilized in AD drug discovery and clinical trials. While the number of biomarkers that serve a central role in AD clinical trials have been increasing, there is still tremendous room for growth in the next several years. To highlight the tremendous potential of biomarker work in AD clinical trials we have also included several of the emerging approaches that show promise in AD and will soon serve as endpoint measures in clinical trials.

10.2 Biobanks

A biobank is a long-term repository of biological specimens collected, stored, and managed mainly for research and/or clinical purposes. It may include a complete organization with employees, programs, protocols for processing specimens, database management, and research/clinical studies [1]. Maintaining high-quality samples and stream-lined data management are some of the most important functions of a biobank, thus regulations and standards must be established by governing institutions. Below are some of the best practices that are being implemented or used as guidelines in the establishment of biobanks [1–5].

10.2.1 Material Collection, Processing, and Handling

Important information must be collected and recorded upon arrival of all samples at the facility. The entire biobanking and biomarker discovery workflow requires exceptional accuracy of sample details as well as stringent rules and protocols for storing and processing samples. All events or observations should be noted prior to sample processing. The first necessary step is the use of integrated sample identification, typically consisting of barcodes that allow for the entire chain of custody of samples to be clearly available. This includes steps to ensure that samples are scanned at each step of the process from collection through storage and specific assays being performed. This detailed approach in conjunction with establishing a robust database system that associates the unique identification number assigned on the bar code to patient information and chain of custody is necessary. A reliable database is essential for traceability and reliability of specimens. Depending on the intended use of the sample, a suitable procedure should be identified and strictly followed to ensure consistency. A standard protocol appropriate for the collection and processing is needed to maintain the stability and high quality of the specimen. Various automations have been in practice for large biorepositories, such as barcoding, automated sample extraction or isolation and aliquoting, and automated freezers.

10.2.2   Storage and Security

Proper storage conditions may vary based on the type and requirements of the samples. Appropriate durable vessels and labels/barcodes should be able to withstand the duration of the storage condition, including an inventory system that will provide information of the exact locations of the specimen. For security purposes, specimens should be aliquoted and stored in at least two different storage containers that may be in separate locations within the same building or a different building. Installation of automated alarm systems (fire and freezer-temperature monitor) to allow appropriate response in a timely manner is needed. Further, backup freezers and liquid nitrogen freezers are recommended.

10.2.3   Quality Assurance/Control and Management

Critical in the success of a biobank is the set of written documents detailing the standard operating procedures (SOPs) that the facility strictly implements. Additional sets of procedures are also needed to evaluate the performance of the biobank based on the established SOPs. International standards have been developed and adopted as a quality system for international biobanking collaborations. Included in these standards are efforts to ensure reproducibility of data in all experimental approaches. This can be difficult given the variability across patients; however, it is necessary to have regular replications of data sets for consistency.

10.2.4   Data Collection and Management

As biobanks collect and process specimens using multiple procedures, appropriate annotations are crucial in the overall utility of the samples. Methodologies and the results of studies conducted on biobank specimens constitute relevant information that can increase the usefulness of the biobank samples. This should be done with consent and necessary privacy policies.

10.2.5   Specimen Shipment

Significant to the maintenance and assurance of high-quality specimens during shipment is the establishment of rules and regulations that must be strictly followed. Shipment time, shipment temperature, and delivery tracking are some of the relevant considerations. Further, a signed material transfer agreement should provide all formal documentations that are relevant to the recipient/user and the biobank administrator.

10.3   Biomarkers

Biobank specimens have been used for a variety of purposes that include, but are not limited to, target discovery and validation, early detection, genetic studies, epidemiological analyses, and drug development. They increasingly play fundamental roles in biomarker discovery and in the development of therapeutics for a wide variety of human diseases such as AD. As the available knowledge about the pathological hallmarks of AD has advanced, the inclusion of biomarker examinations in clinical research has grown. The availability of numerous techniques, coupled with better characterization of AD pathology, now provides the opportunity for biomarkers to serve as necessary entry- and end-points of clinical trials. Over the last 20 years, drug discovery in AD has begun to highlight the need for better characterization of patient populations, as well as better understanding of variance among patients to interpret clinical data. The availability of consistent disease-state specific biomarkers now serves as vital inclusion and exclusion criteria for the selection of patients in clinical trial research. In addition, as the number of available biomarkers that capture AD-specific changes in pathology have increased, several biomarkers are now advancing to endpoint measures in clinical trials, as well as part of the go/no-go decision process between progressive phases of trials and/or the decision to submit to the US Food and Drug Administration (FDA) for an indication.

Biomarkers are among the 121 agents that are being evaluated in the AD drug-development pipeline [6]. They are distributed among Phase 1, Phase 2, and Phase 3 trials and are being used to identify patients and evaluate results. Biomarkers of AD are essential to detect associated functional changes involved in cognitive impairment and to predict time to dementia [7, 8]. In some cases, the very same biomarkers used to characterize a disease can be targets of novel treatment regimens and serve as measures of success. Additionally, biomarkers can be used as indicators of drug activity and efficacy. However, there are still a high number of clinical trials that are not including biomarkers for diagnostic confirmation, target engagement, support of disease modification, and monitor for safety [6, 7]. One of the most intriguing features as well as being one of the most difficult aspects of biomarker discovery is the pace at which techniques have been advancing to better evaluate samples for disease-specific biomarkers. The rapid advancements have made possible the examination of samples beyond the cerebrospinal fluid (CSF), as well as the use of novel and emerging approaches. We highlight below details on specific samples that can be evaluated, as well as some of the approaches that are demonstrating promise in AD drug discovery.

10.4 Emerging Candidate Biomarker Samples Employed in Clinical Trial Research

As we uncover more information on the pathology and diagnosis of human diseases and conditions, the variety of specimens considered for safe-keeping in biorepositories should equally expand to provide for easy access for research and clinical purposes. Below are some of the most common samples that are collected and managed in biobanks. We also present some interesting biological samples together with emerging discoveries and their importance in the field of AD-related investigations.

10.4.1 Blood, Serum, Plasma, and CSF

Blood, serum, plasma, and CSF are some of the most commonly collected and studied biological samples in AD research; as such, the progressions in biomarker discovery and drug development are mostly attributed to these biofluids. Their composition provides a milieu that allows for a complex scrutiny of indicators of health and disease conditions. Fluid-based biomarkers have been some of the most promising and at time contentious biomarkers in the understanding of AD, as well as the evaluation of novel therapeutics efficacy. The most prevalent and widely adopted biomarker in AD drug discovery is certainly the isolation of DNA from blood samples for determination of the presence of specific genetic risk factors (e.g., the apolipoprotein-E ε4 gene [*APOE-4*]). Direct measures

of amyloid beta (Aβ) and tau have been very promising in CSF samples; however, the difficulty in collecting CSF and the ability to stage the severity of AD based on levels of Aβ and hyperphosphorylated tau (p-tau) complicates the process. Blood-based (serum and plasma) biomarkers have considerable appeal due to the ease of collection and processing. However, until recently there were mixed results at evaluating amyloid or tau levels in peripheral blood supply. Recent advancements (see below) show considerable promise in blood-based biomarkers in diagnoses, as well as serving as primary or secondary outcome measures in clinical trials. Many of these CSF and blood-based markers are downstream of the accumulation of Aβ, p-tau, or neurodegeneration as secondary measures of core AD pathology. These includes recent promising targets such as neurofilament light chain [9–15], neurogranin [16–19], sortilin-related receptor 1 [20–26], visin-like protein 1 [27–29], and numerous markers of inflammation [30]. The continuous discovery of new and promising biomarkers from CSF, blood, plasma, and serum proves the versatility and utility of these primary biofluids in advancing our knowledge toward finding effective and efficient therapeutics for AD. Several promising current biomarkers are being used in the evaluation of novel therapeutics, primarily as secondary measures.

10.4.2 Urine

Examining urine is not new in the medical field. Urine is a significant source of metabolites, proteins, and DNA. Collecting urine for biobanks has been gaining momentum as evidence arises on its utility for the diagnosis and prognosis of several diseases [31]. Its potential for early biomarker discovery and drug development or drug effectivity studies presents a significant advancement in AD research. Compared to other biofluids, urine is easy to collect and highly non-invasive. A recent study evaluated the utility of urine for developing a new approach for AD risk assessment. Early AD and healthy patient urine samples were examined for levels of lipid peroxidation compounds using a previously validated analytical method, and data were analyzed using linear and nonlinear regression models. A set of new lipid peroxidation biomarkers for early AD risk assessment was determined which include 15-keto-15-F2 t-IsoP, 4(*RS*)-F4 t-NeuroP, 1a,1b-dihomo-PGF2α, ent-7(*RS*)-7-F2 t-dihomo-IsoP, and 17-epi-17-F2 t-dihomo-IsoP, although their AD specificity still needs further evaluation [32]. Another study explored the potential of urine as a source of early biomarkers for AD. Yao et al. reported the first differentially expressed proteins in urine of AD patients. The group examined 15 differentially expressed genes in the urine samples of healthy controls and AD patients using isobaric tags for relative and absolute quantitation, after employing computational methods to analyze the brain-tissue-based gene expression data of AD. Further validation revealed three proteins in the urine of AD patients that are variably expressed, namely SPP1 (osteopontin), GSN (gelsolin), and IGFBP7 (insulin growth factor binding protein 7) [33], which are potential AD biomarkers.

10.4.3 Saliva

While work on saliva biomarkers for AD is in its infancy, efforts toward standardization of saliva collection, handling, and storage should be undertaken soon to avoid inconsistencies. The identification of patients with AD through saliva has been increasingly gaining attention over the last years. This is partly because saliva samples are easily accessible, and collection is non-invasive and inexpensive. The levels of enzymes and proteins in saliva are being investigated to provide better staging assays for early detection of AD. Acetylcholinesterase [34, 35], $A\beta_{42}$ [36–38], tau [39], and antimicrobial peptide lactoferrin [40] are some of the few targets that showed promise in detecting AD. However, further investigation is still needed on the applicability and reliability of these potential saliva biomarkers for AD detection.

10.4.4 Cells

In 2006, Takahashi and Yamanaka reported their work on inducing pluripotent stem cells from mouse fibroblasts through the introduction of four transcription factors [41]. The group found that combinations of Oct4 (also known as Pou5f1), Sox2, Krüppel-like factor 4 (Klf4), and c-Myc are sufficient to reprogram the fibroblast into a new state that expresses endogenous pluripotent genes [42]. Further refinement of the protocol ensued and paved the way to the utilization of induced pluripotent stem cell (iPSC) technology in several studies including neurodegenerative diseases. iPSC technology uses a patient's somatic cells to generate a new population of cells that have the capacity for unlimited self-renewal and differentiation into several cell types, and with colony morphology, growth characteristics, and gene expressions generally identical to embryonic stem cells [41, 43, 44]. In 2011, a human AD-iPSC related study successfully generated forebrain neurons for anti-Aβ drug evaluation [45]. Yahata et al. further indicated that the neuronal cells showed Aβ production and secretion into the media in the presence of their own amyloid precursor protein (APP), and functional beta- and gamma-secretases. Administration of secretase inhibitors and modulators further revealed a reduction in Aβ production. In the same year, neuronal cells were generated from iPSCs derived from fibroblasts of familial-AD patients with mutations in the presenilin 1 and 2 genes (*PSEN1* and *PSEN2*), with the aim of characterizing the stages of differentiation [46]. Yagi et al. found increased Aβ secretions in the patient-derived neurons, recapitulating the mechanism of familial AD with *PSEN1* and *PSEN2* mutations. In 2015, Hossini et al. employed iPSC technology to generate neuronal cells from dermal fibroblasts of an 82-year-old female patient with sporadic AD [47]. The group detected the expression of p-tau and glycogen synthase kinase-3β in the neuronal cells. In addition, the treatment of gamma-secretase inhibitor resulted in the down-regulation of p-tau. These works in AD-related iPSCs have demonstrated the potential utilization and benefits of the technology, not only to better understand cellular mechanisms but also to biomarker discovery and drug development. AD iPSC-based studies have been conducted to elucidate the mechanisms of the disease (through AD modeling), proof of principle, and to develop/test therapeutic strategies [48, 49]. Defining AD subgroups with iPSC technology presents an excellent opportunity for a truly personalized approach to the treatment of the disease [42]. AD models that represent the real human disease and associated unique physiological attributes, and which can be created in laboratory settings, can become invaluable in the success of drug discovery and development efforts [50], serving as preclinical tools for screening [48]. They can also circumvent the inefficiencies tied to the translation of animal research for human use [51]. The technology is not without limitations. Donor-to-donor variability and intercellular heterogeneity are obstacles to fully understanding the mechanism of AD across patient population [52, 53], as well as the high susceptibility of the disease-related cells to develop AD pathology in cell culture that do not arise in patients' brains, insertional mutagenesis. It may take a while to fully realize the application of iPSCs in AD; thus, storing these precious resources should be done to provide for a consistent and reliable supply in future preclinical and clinical endeavors. Currently, iPSCs are being explored for cell replacement therapy of neurodegenerative diseases. The transplantation of neural progenitor cells may find utility not only in providing direct cell replacement but also for delivering potential therapeutic agents [49].

10.4.5 Intestine/Gut Microbiota

Several studies have explored the potential role of the gut microbiota in AD pathology. This concept is linked to the fact that the intestinal microflora can influence brain activity and its functions though the existence of the microbiota–gut–brain axis (MGBA), a bidirectional interaction between the gut and the brain [54–56]. In addition, the link between gut microbiota and AD is related to the central role of inflammation in AD development and progression [57, 58], as well as aging and metabolic disorders. Several communication pathways between the gut and the brain have been proposed and investigated that include the autosomal nervous system, enteric nervous system, immune system and neuroimmunity, enteroendocrine signaling, neurotransmitters, branched-chain amino acids, bile acids, short-chain fatty acids, spinal mechanisms, hypothalamic–pituitary–adrenal axis, and peptidoglycans [54, 59].

Studies on AD patients and animal models demonstrated the significant changes in the composition of gut microbiota when compared to control groups [60]. Generally, the population/ frequency of beneficial microorganisms are found reduced while those involved in pro-inflammatory processes are increased, which also correlate with cognitive impairment and exacerbation of AD pathology (increased $A\beta$ production, neuroinflammation, and neurofibrillary tangles [NFTs]) [60–62]. This change in the equilibrium is known as gut dysbiosis. This condition was further investigated and proven by the administration of several interventions in both AD patients and animal models that include fecal transfer, bacterial inoculation, probiotic and plant metabolite treatments, pharmacological agents, and dietary restrictions, which resulted in the improvement of AD pathology (reduced $A\beta$ deposition, neuroinflammation, and NFTs) and cognition deficits [59, 61]. There is

now growing evidence that strengthens the relationship between gut microbiota and AD pathology. It has been demonstrated that the MGBA can significantly impact neurodegenerative diseases [54–56]. Several agents included in AD clinical trials target specific aspects of the disease. However, it is interesting to note that these agents and their target mechanisms may seem to be related, in one way or another, to the MGBA as they are involved in inflammation, immune response, metabolism, behavior, cognition, synaptic plasticity, and metabolism. In China, an agent named GV-971 (sodium oligomannate) has been approved for the treatment of AD [63]. It is an orally administered mixture of acidic linear oligosaccharides derived from marine brown algae that affects the dysbiosis of the gut microbiome [64]. GV-971 reduces the secretion of phenylalanine and isoleucine that stimulate the proliferation of T-helper cells that cross the blood–brain barrier and eventually contribute to neuroinflammation [64]. To date, there is one agent in the 2020 AD drug pipeline that specifically targets the gut microbiome. Fecal microbiome transplantation is in a Phase 1 clinical trial with the aim of improving gut microbiota and reducing AD pathology [6].

Gut microbiota will find significant utilities in biomarker discovery and drug-development initiatives. Thus, collecting and storing fecal samples, post-mortem tissues of the intestines, and tissue biopsies are essential for current and future preclinical and clinical explorations. The discovery of early biomarkers using these biological samples will greatly advance AD-based research. Gut microbiota may serve as entry criteria and/or outcome measures for drug trials.

10.4.6 Brain

Biobanks may store brain samples of patients who succumb to their disorders or of normal controls who die of non-central-nervous-system disorders. These precious samples provide insight into disease processes and into the effects of therapy. The tissues are also examined to identify biomarkers altered in the course of clinal trials.

Trials of the active vaccine AN1792 were the first attempt to provide immunotherapy for AD. When 6% of patients in the trial exhibited encephalitis, the trial was terminated [65]. Of 14 patients with AD receiving the active agent and who came to autopsy there was evidence of plaque removal (very extensive removal = 5, intermediate = 4, very limited = 3, no removal = 2). Two patients with AD who died 14 years after immunization had only very sparse or no detectable plaques in all regions examined. There was a significant inverse correlation between post-vaccination peripheral blood anti-AN1792 antibody titers and post-mortem plaque scores [66]. These observations were critical as an impetus to pursue immunotherapy as a potential treatment for AD and led to the current repertoire of monoclonal antibodies and second-generation vaccines that are potential therapies for AD.

Post-mortem studies of patients treated with nerve growth hormone delivered by an adenovirus vector showed that the treatment had inadequate penetration to targeted areas of the brain, likely contributing to the observed lack of benefit of therapy [67]. These observations will lead to adjustments in delivery mechanisms.

The role of inflammation in AD has become increasingly central to understanding of the disease. Autopsy studies designed to elucidate the effects of anti-inflammatory therapies showed that non-steroidal anti-inflammatory drugs (NSAIDs) had no detectable effect on inflammation in AD [68], while patients on steroids showed reduced neuritic plaques and NFTs compared to an untreated control group and a comparison group who had received NSAIDs [69].

Preliminary clinical data suggest that statins are associated with improved cognition function [70]. The potential benefit of statins was supported by post-mortem examinations showing a reduced burden of NFTs in patients receiving statins compared to those without anti-hypercholesterolemia therapy [71].

Cummings et al. examined the relationship between scores on clinical trial instruments and neuropathological changes in patients who had come to autopsy. They found strong ($p < 0.001$) correlations between most clinical measures and both neuritic plaque burden and NFT counts. The amount of variance in the instrument attributable to the assessed pathology was relatively modest (13–40%), suggesting that other neuropathological and biological features contributed importantly to scores [72].

Autopsy studies have had a vital role in confirming that biomarkers are accurately reporting on the pathology of AD. The relationship between Aβ positron emission tomography (PET) and autopsy-based neuritic plaque counts have been shown for all FDA-approved amyloid ligands including [^{18}F]florbetapir [73], [^{18}F]florbetaben [74], and [^{18}F]flutemetamol [75]. Autopsy studies with [^{18}F]flortaucipir PET have substantiated the relationship between the flortaucipir signal and the NFT burden [76]. Studies with 7-tesla MRI demonstrated significant correlations with Braak stage, NFT burden, and neuritic plaque burden at autopsy [77]. Reduced CSF levels of Aβ$_{42}$ correlate with an increased neuritic plaque burden in the neocortex and hippocampus [78], supporting the posited relationship between increasing brain plaque and decreasing spinal fluid levels of the monomeric form of Aβ. Autopsy studies have supported the discriminative power of Aβ, total tau, and p-tau between AD and controls, and between AD and other dementias [79].

These studies show the value of post-mortem examination for establishing the relationship of therapy to changes in the brain and the association of biomarker measures to autopsy findings.

10.5 Emerging Approaches to Biomarker Discovery and Drug Development in AD

The advent of new technologies provides improved and novel methodologies in uncovering and further understanding potential AD biomarkers. Biomarkers play a significant role in the advancement of drug development in AD [7]. The advances in "omic" technologies offer researchers a holistic view of the genes, messenger RNA, proteins, metabolites [80], lipids [81], and extracellular environment [82] that make up a cell, tissue, or organism in a non-targeted and non-biased approach. Examining the multiple-omic levels concurrently can provide a more comprehensive and integrated understanding of the complexity of AD for the development of well-focused/targeted therapeutics. Several of these technologies are being used extensively in the search of new and/or improved AD biomarkers. We highlight below some of the emerging approaches in AD biomarker discovery.

10.5.1 Genomics

The high heritability of AD (~58–79%) demonstrated on twin-based research [83, 84] has presented a great challenge on geneticists to elucidate the genetic landscape of the disease. Genetic factors associated with the risk of developing AD are continuously being examined as new information becomes available from biobanks. One approach that has been employed is genome-wide association studies (GWAS). In GWAS, millions of common coding and non-coding genetic variants across the genome are examined for involvement with a trait [85]. The discovery power of GWAS is largely dependent on the study design. Also, the large sample size of genotyped individuals and the availability of biomarkers are ideal to increase the statistical and prediction power during an association analysis, which are now available in large biobanks. In 2007, the first two reports on GWAS for AD employed a small sample size and revealed the *APOE* locus as a major risk factor of late-onset AD in the human genome [86, 87]. Thereafter, several genes such as *ABCA7, BIN1, CD2AP, CD33, CLU, CR1, EPHA1, MSA4A, PICALM,* and *XOC3L2/MARK4/BLOC1S3* were also reported to be associated with AD [88], as well as *TREM2* [89, 90]. With ever increasing GWAS data sets, additional candidate genes have been identified and continue to expand.

10.5.2 Transcriptomics

Analyzing the whole transcript population of a cell, tissue, or organ in the disease and normal state is a valid course of action to evaluate for potential biomarkers of AD. This approach has shown large potential in elucidating pathogenesis of complex diseases such as AD [91]. Transcriptomic technologies are largely used in tandem with other procedures. The large advances in transcriptomics is mostly attributed with the introduction of next generation sequencing (NGS) [92]. RNA sequencing has been used in several AD-related studies [93–98].

10.5.3 Exosome-Based Approach

Exosomes are extracellular membrane vesicles, generated through the endocytic cellular pathway, secreted via exocytosis [99, 100], and perform a variety of functions [101]. They have a diameter range of 30–100 nm, in contrast to microvesicles that have a diameter range of 100 nm to 1 μm [102, 103]. Exosomes and microvesicles carry distinct protein products and lipid composition [103–105]. Studies have presented the role of exosomes in relation to neurodegenerative diseases [101, 104, 106–109].

10.5.4 Metabolomics

Metabolomics is a systems biology approach to identify, quantify, and characterize the global population of small-molecular-mass metabolites in cells, tissues, or biological fluids [110]. It embodies the relationship of internal biological regulation and external environmental influences on disease [111–118].

To examine the serum metabolomic profiles associated with the progression from mild cognitive impairment to AD, Orešič et al. employed two analytical platforms for metabolomics – ultrahigh-performance liquid chromatography (UPLC) mass spectroscopy and two-dimensional gas chromatography and time-of-flight mass spectrometry (TOF MS). The results showed that 2,4-dihydroxybutanoic acid is a predictive biomarker of progression to AD [119].

To discover biomarkers for early metabolic changes in AD, Cui et al. employed UPLC–quadrupole TOF MS and examined the serum and urine metabolome from AD patients and non-AD controls. Disordered amino acid and phospholipid metabolism and dysregulated palmitic amide are observed in AD patients [120]. Further validation using independent samples revealed a decrease in lysophosphatidylcholine in serum, and an increase in 5-L-glutamylglycine in urine is observed in AD patients.

Using targeted mass spectrometry, Zhou et al. quantified potential biomarkers using AD, non-AD cognitive impairment, and control brain-derived CSF, and showed three metabolism-related protein products (pyruvate kinase muscle isozyme, fatty acid binding protein 3, and fructose-bisphosphate aldolase/aldolase A [ALDOA]) that have low coefficients of variation. Further analyses revealed that ALDOA, a key enzyme in the fourth step of glycolysis, is a biomarker candidate that can best discriminate between individuals with AD and non-AD cognitive impairment [121].

In addition to brain, CSF, serum, and plasma, saliva and urine are now being used for metabolomic studies to explore potential AD biomarkers [122]. Using saliva samples, sphinganine-1-phosphate, ornithine, and phenyllactic acid are found potential predictors for early AD diagnosis [123].

10.6 Concluding Remarks

The importance and necessity of biobanking and biomarker discovery in the AD therapeutic pipeline has grown tremendously from an initial approach to evaluate tolerability and toxicity of candidate therapeutics to an approach that now requires the demonstration of changes in specific biomarkers in order for a candidate to move through discreet phases. As highlighted

129

above, the specific samples and approaches are constantly evolving. Further, given the pace at which new technologies are advancing, the use of several novel biomarkers as diagnostic criteria, as a method of determination of the disease severity, and as a measure of a treatment efficacy will continue to expand in the AD drug-development ecosystem.

References

1. Hallmans G, Vaught JB. Best practices for establishing a biobank. In *Methods in Biobanking*, Dillner J (ed.). New York: Humana Press; 2011: 241–60.

2. Betsou F, Lehmann S, Ashton G, et al. Standard preanalytical coding for biospecimens: defining the sample preanalytical code. *Cancer Epidemiol Prev Biomark* 2010; **19**: 1004–11.

3. Dillner J (ed.). *Methods in Biobanking*. New York: Humana Press; 2011.

4. Lehmann S, Guadagni F, Mooreet H, et al. Standard preanalytical coding for biospecimens: review and implementation of the Sample PREanalytical Code (SPREC). *Biopreserv Biobank* 2012; **10**: 366–74.

5. McQueen MJ, Keys JL, Bamford K, Hall K. The challenge of establishing, growing and sustaining a large biobank: a personal perspective. *Clin Biochem* 2014; **47**: 239–44.

6. Cummings J, Lee G, Ritter A, Sabbagh M, Zhong K. Alzheimer's disease drug development pipeline: 2020. *Alzheimers Dement (N Y)* 2020; **6**: e12050.

7. Cummings J. The role of biomarkers in Alzheimer's disease drug development. In *Reviews on Biomarker Studies in Psychiatric and Neurodegenerative Disorders*, Guest PC (ed.). New York: Springer; 2019: 29–61.

8. Jack CR, Vemuri P, Wistet HJ, et al. Evidence for ordering of Alzheimer's disease biomarkers. *Arch Neurol* 2011; **68**: 1526–35.

9. Ashton NJ, Leuzy A, Lim YM, et al. Increased plasma neurofilament light chain concentration correlates with severity of post-mortem neurofibrillary tangle pathology and neurodegeneration. *Acta Neuropathol Commun* 2019; **7**: 5.

10. Mattsson N, Andreasson U, Zetterberg H, Blennow K. Association of plasma neurofilament light with neurodegeneration in patients with Alzheimer disease. *JAMA Neurol* 2017; **74**: 557–66.

11. Mattsson N, Cullen NC, Andreasson U, Zetterberg H, Blennow, K. Association between longitudinal plasma neurofilament light and neurodegeneration in patients with Alzheimer disease. *JAMA Neurol* 2019; **76**: 791–9.

12. Pereira JB, Westman E, Hansson O. Association between cerebrospinal fluid and plasma neurodegeneration biomarkers with brain atrophy in Alzheimer's disease. *Neurobiol Aging* 2017; **58**: 14–29.

13. Preische O, Schultz SA, Apel A, et al. Serum neurofilament dynamics predicts neurodegeneration and clinical progression in presymptomatic Alzheimer's disease. *Nat Med* 2019; **25**: 277–83.

14. Rojas JC, Karydas A, Bang J, et al. Plasma neurofilament light chain predicts progression in progressive supranuclear palsy. *Ann Clin Transl Neurol* 2016; **3**: 216–25.

15. Sánchez-Valle R, Heslegrave A, Foiani MS, et al. Serum neurofilament light levels correlate with severity measures and neurodegeneration markers in autosomal dominant Alzheimer's disease. *Alzheimers Res Ther* 2018; **10**: 113.

16. Janelidze S, Hertze J, Zetterberg H, et al. Cerebrospinal fluid neurogranin and YKL-40 as biomarkers of Alzheimer's disease. *Ann Clin Transl Neurol* 2015; **3**: 12–20.

17. Liu W, Lin H, He X, et al. Neurogranin as a cognitive biomarker in cerebrospinal fluid and blood exosomes for Alzheimer's disease and mild cognitive impairment. *Transl Psychiatry* 2020; **10**: 1–9.

18. Portelius E, Olsson B, Hoglund K, et al. Cerebrospinal fluid neurogranin concentration in neurodegeneration: relation to clinical phenotypes and neuropathology. *Acta Neuropathol* 2018; **136**: 363–76.

19. Wellington H, Paterson RW, Portelius E, et al. Increased CSF neurogranin concentration is specific to Alzheimer disease. *Neurology* 2016; **86**: 829–35.

20. Liu G, Sun J-Y, Xu M, Yang X-Y, Sun B-L. *SORL1* variants show different association with early-onset and late-onset Alzheimer's disease risk. *J Alzheimers Dis* 2017; **58**: 1121–8.

21. Nicolas G, Charbonnier C, Wallon D, et al. *SORL1* rare variants: a major risk factor for familial early-onset Alzheimer's disease. *Mol Psychiatry* 2016; **21**: 831–6.

22. Pottier C, Hannequin D, Coutant S, et al. High frequency of potentially pathogenic *SORL1* mutations in autosomal dominant early-onset Alzheimer disease. *Mol Psychiatry* 2012; **17**: 875–9.

23. Rogaeva E, Meng Y, Lee JH, et al. The neuronal sortilin-related receptor SORL1 is genetically associated with Alzheimer's disease. *Nat Genet* 2007; **39**: 168–77.

24. Thonberg H, Chiang H-H, Lilius L, Forsell, C. Identification and description of three families with familial Alzheimer disease that segregate

variants in the *SORL1* gene. *Acta Neuropathol Commun* 2017; **5**: 43.

25. Verheijen J, Van den Bossche T, van der Zee J, et al. A comprehensive study of the genetic impact of rare variants in *SORL1* in European early-onset Alzheimer's disease. *Acta Neuropathol* 2016; **132**: 213–24.

26. Wen Y, Miyashita A, Kitamura N, et al. *SORL1* is genetically associated with neuropathologically characterized late-onset Alzheimer's disease. *J Alzheimers Dis* 2013; **35**: 387–94.

27. Kester MI, Teunissen CE, Sutphen C, et al. Cerebrospinal fluid VILIP-1 and YKL-40, candidate biomarkers to diagnose, predict and monitor Alzheimer's disease in a memory clinic cohort. *Alzheimers Res Ther* 2015; **7**: 59.

28. Lee J, Blennow K, Andreasen N, et al. The brain injury biomarker VLP-1 is increased in the cerebrospinal fluid of Alzheimer disease patients. *Clin Chem* 2008; **54**: 1617–23.

29. Tarawneh R, D'Angelo G, Macy E, et al. Visinin-like protein-1: diagnostic and prognostic biomarker in Alzheimer disease. *Ann Neurol* 2011; **70**: 274–85.

30. Kinney JW, Bemiller SM, Murtishaw AS, et al. Inflammation as a central mechanism in Alzheimer's disease. *Alzheimers Dement Transl Res Clin Interv* 2018; **4**: 575–90.

31. Moatamed NA. Biobanking of urine samples. In *Biobanking: Methods and Protocols*, Yong WH (ed.). New York: Springer; 2019: 115–24.

32. Peña-Bautista C, Vigor C, Galano J-M, et al. New screening approach for Alzheimer's disease risk assessment from urine lipid peroxidation compounds. *Sci Rep* 2019; **9**: 14244.

33. Yao F, Hong X, Li S, et al. Urine-based biomarkers for Alzheimer's disease identified through coupling computational and experimental methods. *J Alzheimers Dis* 2018; **65**: 421–31.

34. Boston PF, Gopalkaje K, Manning L, Middleton L, Loxley M. Developing a simple laboratory test for Alzheimer's disease: measuring acetylcholinesterase in saliva: a pilot study. *Int J Geriatr Psychiatry* 2008; **23**: 439–40.

35. Sayer R, Law E, Connelly PJ, Breen KC. Association of a salivary acetylcholinesterase with Alzheimer's disease and response to cholinesterase inhibitors. *Clin Biochem* 2004; **37**: 98–104.

36. Bermejo-Pareja F, Antequera D, Vargas T, Molina JA, Carro E. Saliva levels of Abeta1–42 as potential biomarker of Alzheimer's disease: a pilot study. *BMC Neurol* 2010; **10**: 108.

37. Lee M, Guo JP, Kennedy K, McGeer EG, McGeer PL. A method for diagnosing Alzheimer's disease based on salivary amyloid-β protein 42 levels. *J Alzheimers Dis* 2017; **55**: 1175–82.

38. Tsuruoka M, Hara J, Hirayama A, et al. Capillary electrophoresis-mass spectrometry-based metabolome analysis of serum and saliva from neurodegenerative dementia patients. *Electrophoresis* 2013; **34**: 2865–72.

39. Shi M, Sui Y-T, Peskind ER, et al. Salivary tau species are potential biomarkers of Alzheimer disease. *J. Alzheimers Dis* 2011; **27**: 299–305.

40. Carro E, Bartolomé F, Bermejo-Pareja F, et al. Early diagnosis of mild cognitive impairment and Alzheimer's disease based on salivary lactoferrin. *Alzheimers Dement Diagn Assess Dis Monit* 2017; **8**: 131–8.

41. Takahashi K, Yamanaka S. Induction of pluripotent stem cells from mouse embryonic and adult fibroblast cultures by defined factors. *Cell* 2006; **126**: 663–76.

42. Ooi L, Sidhu K, Poljak A, et al. Induced pluripotent stem cells as tools for disease modelling and drug discovery in Alzheimer's disease. *J. Neural Transm (Vienna)* 2013; **120**: 103–11.

43. Takahashi K, Tanabe K, Ohnuki M, *et al.* Induction of pluripotent stem cells from adult human fibroblasts by defined factors. *Cell* 2007; **131**: 861–72.

44. Yu J, Vodyanik MA, Smuga-Otto K, et al. Induced pluripotent stem cell lines derived from human somatic cells. *Science* 2007; **318**: 1917–20.

45. Yahata N, Asai M, Kitaoka S, et al. Anti-Aβ drug screening platform using human iPS cell-derived neurons for the treatment of Alzheimer's disease. *PLoS One* 2011; **6**: e25788.

46. Yagi T, Ito D, Okada Y, et al. Modeling familial Alzheimer's disease with induced pluripotent stem cells. *Hum Mol Genet* 2011; **20**: 4530–9.

47. Hossini AM, Megges M, Prigione A, et al. Induced pluripotent stem cell-derived neuronal cells from a sporadic Alzheimer's disease donor as a model for investigating AD-associated gene regulatory networks. *BMC Genomics* 2015; **16**: 84.

48. Majolo F, Marinowic DR, Machado DC, Da Costa JC. Important advances in Alzheimer's disease from the use of induced pluripotent stem cells. *J Biomed Sci* 2019; **26**: 15.

49. Yang J, Li S, He X-B, Cheng C, Le W. Induced pluripotent stem cells in Alzheimer's disease: applications for disease modeling and cell-replacement therapy. *Mol Neurodegener* 2016; **11**: 39

50. Zhang R, Zhang L, Xie X. iPSCs and small molecules: a reciprocal effort towards better approaches for drug discovery. *Acta Pharmacol Sin* 2013; **34**: 765–76.

51. Dragunow M. The adult human brain in preclinical drug development. *Nat Rev Drug Discov* 2008; **7**: 659–66.

131

52. Israel MA, Yuan SH, Bardy C, et al. Probing sporadic and familial Alzheimer's disease using induced pluripotent stem cells. *Nature* 2012; **482**: 216–20.

53. Kondo T, Asai M, Tsukita K, et al. Modeling Alzheimer's disease with iPSCs reveals stress phenotypes associated with intracellular Aβ and differential drug responsiveness. *Cell Stem Cell* 2013; **12**: 487–96.

54. Cryan JF, O'Riordan KJ, Cowan CSM, et al. The microbiota-gut–brain axis. *Physiol Rev* 2019; **99**: 1877–2013.

55. Gareau MG. Microbiota–gut–brain axis and cognitive function. In *Microbial Endocrinology: The Microbiota–Gut–Brain Axis in Health and Disease*, Lyte M, Cryan JF (eds.). New York: Springer; 2014: 357–71.

56. Quigley EMM. Microbiota–brain–gut axis and neurodegenerative diseases. *Curr Neurol Neurosci Rep* 2017; **17**: 94.

57. Calsolaro V, Edison P. Neuroinflammation in Alzheimer's disease: current evidence and future directions. *Alzheimers Dement* 2016; **12**: 719–32.

58. Jia W, Rajani C, Kaddurah-Daouk R, Li H. Expert insights: the potential role of the gut microbiome-bile acid–brain axis in the development and progression of Alzheimer's disease and hepatic encephalopathy. *Med Res Rev* 2020; **40**: 1496–507.

59. Angelucci F, Cechova K, Amlerov J, Hort J. Antibiotics, gut microbiota, and Alzheimer's disease. *J Neuroinflamm* 2019; **16**: 108.

60. Liu S, Gao J, Zhu M, Liu K, Zhang H-L. Gut microbiota and dysbiosis in Alzheimer's disease: implications for pathogenesis and treatment. *Mol Neurobiol* 2020; **57**: 5026–43.

61. He Y, Li B, Sun D, Chen S. Gut microbiota: implications in Alzheimer's disease. *J Clin Med* 2020; **9**: 2042.

62. Seo D-O, Holtzman DM. Gut microbiota: from the forgotten organ to a potential key player in the pathology of Alzheimer's disease. *J Gerontol Ser A* 2020; **75**: 1232–41.

63. Syed YY. Sodium oligomannate: first approval. *Drugs* 2020; **80**: 441–4.

64. Wang X, Sun G, Geng M, et al. Sodium oligomannate therapeutically remodels gut microbiota and suppresses gut bacterial amino acids: shaped neuroinflammation to inhibit Alzheimer's disease progression. *Cell Res* 2019; **29**: 787–803.

65. Gilman S, Koller M, Black RS, et al. Clinical effects of Abeta immunization (AN1792) in patients with AD in an interrupted trial. *Neurology* 2005; **64**: 1553–62.

66. Nicoll JAR, Buckland GR, Harrison CH, et al. Persistent neuropathological effects 14 years following amyloid-β immunization in Alzheimer's disease. *Brain J Neurol* 2019; **142**: 2113–26.

67. Castle MJ, Baltanás FC, Kovacs I, et al. Postmortem analysis in a clinical trial of AAV2-NGF gene therapy for Alzheimer's disease identifies a need for improved vector delivery. *Hum Gene Ther* 2020; **31**: 415–22.

68. Halliday GM, Shepherd CE, McCann H, et al. Effect of anti-inflammatory medications on neuropathological findings in Alzheimer disease. *Arch Neurol* 2000; **57**: 831–6.

69. Beeri MS, Schmeidler J, Lesser GT, et al. Corticosteroids, but not NSAIDs, are associated with less Alzheimer neuropathology. *Neurobiol Aging* 2012; **33**: 1258–64.

70. Sparks DL, Sabbagh M, Connor D, et al. Statin therapy in Alzheimer's disease. *Acta Neurol Scand Suppl* 2006; **185**: 78–86.

71. Li G, Larson EB, Sonnen JA, et al. Statin therapy is associated with reduced neuropathologic changes of Alzheimer disease. *Neurology* 2007; **69**: 878–85.

72. Cummings JL, Ringman J, Vinters HV. Neuropathologic correlates of trial-related instruments for Alzheimer's disease. *Am J Neurodegener Dis* 2014; **3**: 45–9.

73. Clark CM, Pontecorvo MJ, Beach TG, et al. Cerebral PET with florbetapir compared with neuropathology at autopsy for detection of neuritic amyloid-β plaques: a prospective cohort study. *Lancet Neurol* 2012; **11**: 669–78.

74. Doré V, Bullich S, Rowe CC, et al. Comparison of ^{18}F-florbetaben quantification results using the standard Centiloid, MR-based, and MR-less CapAIBL® approaches: validation against histopathology. *Alzheimers Dement* 2019; **15**: 807–16.

75. Thal DR, Beach TG, Zanette M, et al. Estimation of amyloid distribution by [^{18}F]flutemetamol PET predicts the neuropathological phase of amyloid β-protein deposition. *Acta Neuropathol* 2018; **136**: 557–67.

76. Fleisher AS, Pontecorvo MJ, Devous MD, Sr., et al. Positron emission tomography imaging with [^{18}F]flortaucipir and postmortem assessment of Alzheimer disease neuropathologic changes. *JAMA Neurol* 2020; **77**: 829–39.

77. Apostolova LG, Zarow C, Biado K, et al. Relationship between hippocampal atrophy and neuropathology markers: a 7 T MRI validation study of the EADC-ADNI Harmonized Hippocampal Segmentation Protocol. *Alzheimers Dement* 2015; **11**: 139–50.

78. Strozyk D, Blennow K, White L, Launer LJ. CSF Aβ 42 levels correlate with amyloid-neuropathology in a population-based autopsy study. *Neurology* 2003; **60**: 652–6.

79. Seeburger JL, Holder DJ, Combrinck M, et al. Cerebrospinal fluid biomarkers distinguish postmortem-confirmed Alzheimer's disease from other dementias and healthy controls in the OPTIMA cohort. *J Alzheimers Dis* 2015; **44**: 525–39.

80. Horgan RP, Kenny LC. 'Omic' technologies: genomics, transcriptomics, proteomics and metabolomics. *Obstet Gynaecol* 2011; **13**: 189–95.

81. Wenk MR. The emerging field of lipidomics. *Nat Rev Drug Discov* 2005; **4**: 594.

82. Astarita G, Piomelli D. Towards a whole-body systems [multi-organ] lipidomics in Alzheimer's disease. *Prostaglandins Leukot Essent Fatty Acids* 2011; **85**: 197–203.

83. Gatz M, Pedersen NL, Berg S, et al. Heritability for Alzheimer's disease: the study of dementia in Swedish twins. *J Gerontol Ser A* 1997; **52**: M117–25.

84. Gatz M, Reynolds CA, Fratiglioni L, et al. Role of genes and environments for explaining Alzheimer disease. *Arch Gen Psychiatry* 2006; **63**: 168.

85. Andrews SJ, Fulton-Howard B, Goate A. Interpretation of risk loci from genome-wide association studies of Alzheimer's disease. *Lancet Neurol* 2020; **19**: 326–35.

86. Coon KD, Myers AJ, Craig DW, et al. A high-density whole-genome association study reveals that *APoE* is the major susceptibility gene for sporadic late-onset Alzheimer's disease. *J Clin Psychiatry* 2007; **68**: 613–18.

87. Grupe A, Abraham R, Li Y, et al. Evidence for novel susceptibility genes for late-onset Alzheimer's disease from a genome-wide association study of putative functional variants. *Hum Mol Genet* 2007; **16**: 865–73.

88. Raghavan N, Tosto G. Genetics of Alzheimer's disease: the importance of polygenic and epistatic components. *Curr Neurol Neurosci Rep* 2018; **17**: 78

89. Guerreiro R, Wojtas A, Bras J, et al. *TREM2* variants in Alzheimer's disease. *N Engl J Med* 2013; **368**: 117–27.

90. Jonsson T, Stefansson H, Steinberg S, et al. Variant of *TREM2* associated with the risk of Alzheimer's disease. *N Engl J Med* 2013; **368**: 107–16.

91. Courtney E, Kornfeld S, Janitz K, Janitz M. Transcriptome profiling in neurodegenerative disease. *J Neurosci Methods* 2010; **193**: 189–202.

92. Costa V, Angelini C, De Feis I, Ciccodicola A. Uncovering the complexity of transcriptomes with RNA-seq. *J Biomed Biotechnol* 2010; DOI: http://doi.org/10.1155/2010/853916.

93. Burgos K, Malenica I, Metpally R, et al. Profiles of extracellular miRNA in cerebrospinal fluid and serum from patients with Alzheimer's and Parkinson's diseases correlate with disease status

and features of pathology. *PLoS One* 2014; **9**: e94839.

94. Magistri M, Velmeshev D, Makhmutova M, Faghihi MA. Transcriptomics profiling of Alzheimer's disease reveal neurovascular defects, altered amyloid-β homeostasis, and deregulated expression of long noncoding RNAs. *J Alzheimers Dis* 2015; **48**: 647–65.

95. Mills JD, Nalpathamkalam T, Jacobs HIL, et al. RNA-seq analysis of the parietal cortex in Alzheimer's disease reveals alternatively spliced isoforms related to lipid metabolism. *Neurosci Lett* 2013; **536**: 90–5.

96. Mills JD, Janitz M. Alternative splicing of mRNA in the molecular pathology of neurodegenerative diseases. *Neurobiol Aging* 2012; **33**: 1012.e11–24.

97. Twine NA, Janitz K, Wilkins MR, Janitz M. Whole transcriptome sequencing reveals gene expression and splicing differences in brain regions affected by Alzheimer's disease. *PLoS One* 2011; **6**: e16266.

98. Wu Y, Xu J, Xu J, et al. Lower serum levels of miR-29c-3p and miR-19b-3p as biomarkers for Alzheimer's disease. *Tohoku J Exp Med* 2017; **242**: 129–36.

99. Qin J, Xu Q. Functions and application of exosomes. *Acta Pol Pharm* 2014; **71**: 537–43.

100. Yuyama K, Igarashi Y. Exosomes as carriers of Alzheimer's amyloid-ß. *Front Neurosci* 2017; **11**;DOI: http://doi.org/10.3389/fnins.2017.00229.

101. Vella LJ, Sharples RA, Nisbet RM, Cappai R, Hill AF. The role of exosomes in the processing of proteins associated with neurodegenerative diseases. *Eur Biophys J* 2008; **37**: 323–32.

102. Johnstone RM, Adam M, Hammond JR, Orr L, Turbide C. Vesicle formation during reticulocyte maturation. Association of plasma membrane activities with released vesicles (exosomes). *J Biol Chem* 1987; **262**: 9412–20.

103. Malm T, Loppi S, Kanninen KM. Exosomes in Alzheimer's disease. *Neurochem Int* 2016; **97**: 193–9.

104. Théry C, Ostrowski M, Segura E. Membrane vesicles as conveyors of immune responses. *Nat Rev Immunol* 2009; **9**: 581.

105. Joshi P, Turola E, Ruiz A, et al. Microglia convert aggregated amyloid-β into neurotoxic forms through the shedding of microvesicles. *Cell Death Differ* 2014; **21**: 582–93.

106. Chivet M, Hemming F, Pernet-Gallay K, Fraboulet S, Sadoul R. Emerging role of neuronal exosomes in the central nervous system. *Front Physiol* 2012; **3**: 145.

107. Colombo E, Borgiani B, Verderio C, Furlan R. Microvesicles: novel biomarkers for neurological disorders. *Front Physiol* 2012; **3**: 63.

133

108. Verderio C, Muzio L, Turola E, et al. Myeloid microvesicles are a marker and therapeutic target for neuroinflammation. *Ann Neurol* 2012; **72**: 610–24.

109. Raposo G, Stoorvogel W. Extracellular vesicles: exosomes, microvesicles, and friends. *J Cell Biol* 2013; **200**: 373–83.

110. Sato Y, Suzuki I, Nakamura T, et al. Identification of a new plasma biomarker of Alzheimer's disease using metabolomics technology. *J Lipid Res* 2012; **53**: 567–76.

111. Wilcoxen KM, Uehara T, Myint KT, Sato Y, Oda Y. Practical metabolomics in drug discovery. *Expert Opin Drug Discov* 2010; **5**: 249–63.

112. Graham SF, Chevallier OP, Elliott CT, et al. Untargeted metabolomic analysis of human plasma indicates differentially affected polyamine and L-arginine metabolism in mild cognitive impairment subjects converting to Alzheimer's disease. *PLoS One* 2015; **10**: https://doi.org/10.1371/journal.pone.0119452.

113. Kaddurah-Daouk R, Zhu H, Sharma S, et al. Alterations in metabolic pathways and networks in Alzheimer's disease. *Transl Psychiatry* 2013; **3**: e244.

114. Kori M, Aydın B, Unal S, Arga KY, Kazan D. Metabolic biomarkers and neurodegeneration: a pathway enrichment analysis of Alzheimer's disease, Parkinson's disease, and amyotrophic lateral sclerosis. *OMICS J Integr Biol* 2016; **20**: 645–61.

115. Mousavi M, Jonsson P, Antti H, et al. Serum metabolomic biomarkers of dementia. *Dement Geriatr Cogn Disord Extra* 2014; **4**: 252–62.

116. Toledo JB, Arnold M, Kastenmüller G, et al. Metabolic network failures in Alzheimer's disease: a biochemical road map. *Alzheimers Dement* 2017; **13**: 965–84.

117. Trushina E, Mielke MM. Recent advances in the application of metabolomics to Alzheimer's disease. *Biochim Biophys Acta* 2014; **1842**: 1232–9.

118. Voyle N, Kim M, Proitsi P, et al. Blood metabolite markers of neocortical amyloid-β burden: discovery and enrichment using candidate proteins. *Transl Psychiatry* 2016; **6**: e719.

119. Orešič M, Hyötyläinen T, Herukka S-K, et al. Metabolome in progression to Alzheimer's disease. *Transl Psychiatry* 2011; **1**: e57.

120. Cui Y, Liu X, Wang M, et al. Lysophosphatidylcholine and amide as metabolites for detecting Alzheimer disease using ultrahigh-performance liquid chromatography–quadrupole time-of-flight mass spectrometry–based metabonomics. *J Neuropathol Exp Neurol* 2014; **73**: 954–63.

121. Zhou M, Haque RU, Dammer EB, et al. Targeted mass spectrometry to quantify brain-derived cerebrospinal fluid biomarkers in Alzheimer's disease. *Clin Proteomics* 2020; **17**: 19.

122. Sapkota S, Huan T, Tran T, et al. Metabolomics analyses of salivary samples discriminate normal aging, mild cognitive impairment, and Alzheimer's disease groups and produce biomarkers predictive of neurocognitive performance. *Alzheimers Dement* 2015; **11**: P654.

123. Liang Q, Liu H, Zhang T, et al. Metabolomics-based screening of salivary biomarkers for early diagnosis of Alzheimer's disease. *RSC Adv* 2015; **5**: 96074–9.

Phase 1 Trials in Alzheimer's Disease Drug Development

Manfred Windisch

11.1   Introduction

There are years of work on drug discovery, series of in vitro and in vivo experiments to get the full information about the pharmacology of a new chemical entity. This process is accompanied by the development of scalable synthetic procedures, which should finally allow the production based on good manufacturing practice in a reproducible manner; and, most importantly, the developed compound should have many pharmaceutical properties to make it really druggable. Without being complete, this certainly includes acceptable stability and solubility in vehicles acceptable for clinical use; ideally, it should be well absorbed in the gastrointestinal tract and be able to penetrate the blood–brain barrier (BBB). This introduction already provides a summary of many obstacles even before such a program enters the preclinical regulatory phase of development, starting with genetic toxicology, toxicology, toxicokinetics, and a series of safety pharmacology studies. After years of hard, dedicated work there will be the decision to bring a well-selected new chemical entity to clinical trials in human subjects for the first time. This is a very special moment, in particular for smaller drug-development companies that experience for the first time their new compound suddenly becoming an investigational medicinal product (IMP). Now this new chemical entity or biological product needs to be proved safe and tolerable in human subjects in order to move forward into further stages of clinical development, to investigate whether the drug is safe enough to be finally tested for efficacy. There are no approved guidelines on how to perform Phase 1 trials, but of course all of the studies need to follow the International Conference on Harmonization (ICH) good clinical practice (GCP) guidelines as well as local medical law, and the design must consider the Declaration of Helsinki human rights. The studies need approval from ethical committees or institutional review boards (IRBs) and from the regulatory competent authority. Subjects involved in Phase 1 cannot expect any benefit from the participation, because these are non-therapeutic studies. No procedure involving human subjects is allowed without appropriate information being given to the subjects about the nature of the study and the potential involved risks, and an informed consent form (ICF) needs to be signed. All study subjects are informed that their participation in such an investigation is voluntary and that they can withdraw at any time, without any particular reason. It is important not to forget that Phase 1 has as the absolute main objective of documentating the drug safety and to identify the maximum tolerated dose (MTD), to obtain information about the human pharmacokinetics (PK) and, if possible, pharmacodynamics (PD). A Phase 1 trial is a transition into clinical pharmacology and, to allow safe conduct, in particular of the first-in-human (FIH) study, a multidisciplinary approach is required, with collaboration between toxicologists, pharmacologists, statisticians, and clinicians. Such studies need careful planning. One of the first important steps is the calculation of the maximum allowed starting dose, based on data from toxicology or pharmacology, to ensure the safety of the volunteers, and a strategy for dose escalation so that the MTD can be determined. A relatively high safety margin is particularly important for Alzheimer's disease (AD), because of the long-term chronic treatment of the patients. The collected data on safety and the PK will form the basis for the right dose selection in Phase 2.

11.2   Study Subjects

In particular for FIH trials, usually healthy young male and female volunteers are recruited. For the multiple ascending dose (MAD) tolerance studies study cohorts with elderly healthy subjects are sometimes added in order to explore the consequence of age-dependent metabolic changes on drug exposure to enable the selection of safe doses for the later trials in AD. But if treatments are under investigation, where the interaction with the IMP is directed to AD-specific pathology, as in the case with immunotherapy against amyloid-beta (Aβ) or tau proteins, it may be necessary to start FIH trials with patients, so as, on the one hand, not to expose healthy subjects to any avoidable risk and, on the other hand, to investigate any possible toxic reaction that could be the consequence of the drug/biological interaction with pathogenetically relevant structures. Independent from the trial population, young or elderly subjects and in some cases patients, the selection of the subjects should provide homogeneous cohorts.

My company, NeuroScios, usually collaborates either with pharmacology units of university hospitals or specialized Phase 1 contract research organizations. In both cases, they have a big database of healthy volunteers who are interested to take part, and the same is true for the healthy elderly subjects. The majority of the younger volunteers are students, but there are also some from the wider community who are interested in this type of research and may also be attracted by the renumeration they receive for their participation. We do not accept any persons suspected of having drug-related problems or who are homeless. This is because we need reliable participants who can fully comply with the study requirements. This is important for obtaining solid data and also for guaranteeing the safety of those people in long-term follow-up. Additional sources for recruitment are from advertising in different media, or referrals from other physicians. Usually the healthy subjects are aged between 19 and 45 years, and they need to be completely healthy according to their medical history, a physical examination, vital signs, and laboratory data, which are collected during a screening visit or are already on file. Any medical condition that requires chronic medication, any active infectious disease, or a history of cancer or auto-immune disease are exclusion criteria. Any prescriptive drugs and other over-the-counter medications are prohibited within 10 to 14 days before enrollment. The elderly subjects are usually aged between 55 and 80 years and in generally good health. As for the young volunteers, any person with an infectious disease within a certain time period before the first dosing will be excluded; depending on the investigated drug, some age-dependent diseases, such as diabetes or hypertension, can be accepted if they are well controlled and the medication is stable for at least 2 months before enrollment and during the Phase 1 clinical trial.

In the young and the elderly populations, women of child-bearing potential are excluded and of course a positive pregnancy test at screening would also prevent their enrollment. Female subjects are advised to practice contraception during the active study period, usually using double barrier methods.

11.3 Selection of Maximum Starting Dose and Dose Escalation

The primary concern of a Phase 1 trial is the safety of the participants [1, 2] and therefore a clear definition of a safe starting dose is extremely important. One of the most common methods is based on the no observed adverse event level (NOAEL) in the most sensitive and appropriate species used in toxicology. The most appropriate species should show drug metabolism as close as possible to humans, and it should also express the drug target. In AD, this is not always trivial and cannot be fully met because, in general, the toxicology species do not overexpress pathogenetically important markers, such as Aβ peptides or aggregated tau proteins, and do not develop AD brain pathology. In an ideal setting, the NOAEL is similar in the different species. First a conversion to a human-equivalent dose is needed [3], either based on drug dose per kilogram of body weight or calculated based on body surface area. In general, the body surface area calculations are the more conservative approach and provide a wider margin of safety. In any case, a safety factor is always applied to the human equivalent dose (HED) based on the NOAEL approach, and so the maximum recommended starting dose (MRSD) is usually about 10% of this value. This safety factor should also consider specific toxicity observed in the animal studies, which may translate into a clinically significant and relevant way to humans. For an appropriate choice of the MRSD the human pharmacologically active dose (PAD), derived from proof-of-concept studies in animal models, should be considered. If the human-equivalent PAD is lower than the MRSD, this is an immediate signal to decrease the clinical starting dose! In particular, when the NOAEL approach gives divergent results, depending on the species used for the calculation, alternative approaches should be considered; for instance, starting with a minimum anticipated biological effect level (MABEL) [4, 5], which is always recommended when there are risk factors associated with the mode of action or the nature of the target. A safety factor needs to be applied and if the NOAEL and the MABEL calculations end up with similar values, the lower starting dose should be selected. Depending on the specific risks of a new compound or a biological product, additional considerations for deciding on the MRSD are needed, such as comparing data with data from compounds in a similar class, or supporting the dose selection by a PK/PD modeling approach.

The next crucial point is deciding on the dose escalation steps and here again the preclinical toxicology data need careful consideration. If we can expect a wide margin of safety and the PAD in humans is far above the MRSD, the initial escalation may allow bigger steps, but it must be always kept in mind that escalations can lead to sudden unexpected adverse reactions, and this should obviously be avoided. In most of the studies I am involved with, I use an escalation factor of two or three. If the MRSD is far below the expected PAD, a wider escalation is possible. This usually keeps the number of steps needed low, and studies can be finished after four to five cohorts at most. For safety, the subjects are under permanent observation in the clinical unit and, if needed, continuous cardiac monitoring; at the very least, careful ECG recordings are made several times after drug application. If there are any indications of organ-specific toxicity derived from the animal studies, this needs to be most carefully monitored. A full clinical safety laboratory analysis, including blood biochemistry and hematology, is routine in such a study. For central nervous sytem (CNS)-active drugs, measuring the influence on suicidal ideation should be also included, by using appropriate scales. Because even in the most careful preparation of the FIH studies, unexpected adverse events may occur, it is a must that the Phase 1 unit is closely connected to intensive care units and the study team has sufficient experience and current training in emergency situations. I routinely recommend the establishment of a drug safety monitoring board (DSMB) that gives an independent consultation in the case of adverse events or serious adverse events. These boards usually also help to decide about further escalation steps. One goal of such a study is the determination of the MTD, which is defined as the dose expected to produce some degree of medically unacceptable dose-limiting toxicity in a specified proportion of patients, defining the target toxicity level (TTL) [6]. But this means that some patients would experience dose-limiting toxicity, and the dose level below is then considered as the MTD. A clinical trial design to directly titrate the MTD is considered as unethical [7] according to new guidelines for safety in clinical trials. An alternative is the use of a statistical model to estimate the relationship between dose and the risk of dose-limiting toxicity, and a maximum dose should be defined before start of the FIH trial. The most well-known model-based design is the continual reassessment method (CRM) [8], which combines all available trial data to estimate the MTD. A CRM is only one approach for an improved modeling; in terms of patients' safety, the current opinion is that it is preferable to define a clinically driven maximum dosing, not an endpoint defined by toxicity. So an estimate of the therapeutic dose or dose range is a key factor, maybe similar to the definition of the starting dose using the MABEL; then, of course, an upper safety margin should be added. If PD effects can be measured, the adequate monitoring of the "therapeutic dose range" is easier. This could for example be the investigation of a gamma-secretase inhibitor and its dose-dependent effect on plasma or cerebrospinal fluid (CSF) Aβ peptides. Unfortunately, for many AD drugs there are no such biomarkers defined, in particular not for sporadic AD, when the real effect only develops over a longer treatment period. Also, the BBB may play an important role, because concentrations of the drug in the target organ may differ substantially from plasma levels. For a safe assessment of the maximum used dose drug–drug interaction, the substance accumulation, receptor saturation, and non-target toxicity need to be part of the considerations.

To learn about human PK is another essential part of Phase 1 studies. Therefore, a plasma sampling schedule derived from the animal PK data is needed to allow the calculation of all important PD outcome variables. It is essential to have a relatively tight sampling schedule around the expected time of the maximum drug concentration (T_{max}) to allow a most accurate assessment of this readout. The results from the single ascending dose (SAD) tolerance study will then help to guide the PK assessments in the subsequent Phase 1 trials. In drug development for AD, these initial studies are of course critical to move into efficacy testing, but they might not allow any assumptions to be made about the expected efficacy in the target indication, in particular if no appropriate biomarkers/PD efficacy variables can be measured. Phase 1 is certainly important for the risk reduction in further drug development, but it is the experience of drug developers that it is quite difficult to raise money for these investigations, because most of the time the outcome does not afford conclusions about the potential efficacy. Still, I recommend focusing, in early trials, on PK, safety, and tolerability. Of course, if specific drugs allow monitoring of readouts that can be in direct correlation with the expected therapeutic effect, it should be included in the trial design. Solid data from Phase 1 will then allow an educated selection of safe doses for Phase 2 and Phase 3 studies.

11.4 SAD Tolerance Studies

The FIH clinical trial is usually the so-called SAD tolerance study, where the IMP is applied in single doses and there is a continuous increase in doses until the pre-specified maximum dose is reached, or safety and tolerability concerns force an early termination of the study. There are no specific regulations that such a study needs to be placebo-controlled or blinded. Of course the placebo control will allow some monitoring of procedure-dependent adverse events in comparison to drug-related events and may help in a more unbiased interpretation of the safety outcome. The same is true for a blinding process because unblinding of the study personnel may bias the interpretation of the study data. So, there is the choice of single blinding and double blinding and even more complex blinding procedures versus an open-label trial.

The basis of a SAD study is a clinical trial protocol based on ICH GCP guidelines and all relevant international and local guidelines, which needs to be approved by competent authority and ethical committees/IRBs. Due to the fact that nowadays such protocols are usually quite complex – because different parts of Phase 1 are often integrated into one document, such as a food interaction study, the MAD tolerance study, and eventually even other investigations into one document – I will only focus on the single dose study. But in fact some of the principles will apply for all other Phase 1 trials. It is important that the study subjects are informed that this is a non-therapeutic study and they are not expected to have any benefit, and they need to be completely informed about all eventual risks. The informed consent form, which needs to be signed before any study-specific procedure is initiated, also requires approval by the ethical committee.

A very important decision now is whether healthy subjects or patient subjects should be selected for a study. Healthy subjects allow an easy and fast recruitment and the interpretation of data might be easier because there is no confounding pathology and no concomitant medications; another advantage is that data might be applicable for other indications of this IMP. Healthy subjects are usually quite uniform and so the whole trial may profit from high internal validity. Of course, there could be a problem with missing or limited target-related PD biomarker data, which is also due to the fact that some targets might not be available in sufficient concentration. If a target-related toxicity is expected, it may be that such data cannot be obtained from healthy cohorts. Depending on the age of the subjects, and already based on the fact that they are healthy, the PK could be different from real patients. So, for several reasons there might be a justification for enrolling patient subjects. But in this case there could be a problem in selecting a sufficient number of subjects and the control of variability, which is influenced by the apolipoprotein-E genotype, disease severity, concomitant diseases, and concomitant medication. So, patient subject studies will take much longer and they will be more expensive. However, this is the only way to test target-specific toxicity and to get relevant PD biomarker data (whether or not the investigated IMP is influencing such markers). Data derived from patient subjects can potentially not be used to draw conclusions about safety in other disease indications because of different underlying pathology. In AD, we are dealing with a vulnerable population and in most countries the majority of diagnosed patients are already on treatment with standard of care, so fully placebo-controlled studies might be problematic, even for a short time. In a first trial, the cohorts are usually relatively small, with the aim of exposing as few subjects as possible to a risk, but still allowing reliable safety conclusions for the next steps. So usually we use eight to ten subjects per cohort, and two per cohort receive placebo.

Furthermore, we have different possibilities, such as the sequential group design, where each cohort is assigned only to one dose of active drug and maybe, as mentioned before, two get placebo. More subjects are needed but, because there is no need for washout periods, the study can run relatively quickly, as long as there are no safety concerns. The advantage of sequential cohorts is the prevention of any carry-over effects and can be applied even for compounds with a long half-life ($T_{1/2}$). In any case, the step to the next dose can be done only after completing one cohort, getting all the data, including PK, and, as we do at NeuroScios, getting a recommendation from the DSMB about the next escalation step. A cross-over design saves a lot of subjects and may even reduce variability because every subject is its own control, but still within-subject and between-subject differences can be evaluated. The issue is certainly the possibility of carry-over effects and an increased risk because every subject is exposed to multiple doses of the drug. A compromise is the sequential cross-over study, where doses are escalated within a cohort, but in every cohort each subject receives only two or three verum applications and two subjects get the placebo. The second cohort gets then the next two or three escalated doses. A variation is a cross-over design with alternating cohorts, which allows longer breaks between the different doses and is therefore suitable for long washout periods. Whenever the IMP with an unknown and potentially high risk is investigated, at NeuroScios we use sentinels in our study. This is the case when a completely new target is addressed, when there is a first-in-class compound (i.e., a completely new chemical entity), when there are compounds with a relatively steep dose response, as known from animal experiments, and several other reasons. For the sake of safety, the first dose is applied only to one subject and, in parallel, another is treated with placebo. These sentinels usually remain for a prolonged period (depending on the expected $T_{1/2}$) under close monitoring to assess eventual delayed adverse reactions. Only when all the data of this sentinel group are available, the principal investigator together with the DSMB and the sponsor decide to include the next subjects, but usually in relatively small groups to reduce risk. It is also essential to decide how the drug will be applied. An intravenous application allows the highest degree of flexibility. In case of emergent adverse events during infusion, the treatment can be stopped immediately. It is also useful as a benchmark to assess oral bioavailability in later studies. In most of our cases we use oral application because this will be the way the drugs will be applied in clinical practice for AD. In most cases a full formulation development is not performed at this early trial stage and so we use frequently filled capsules without excipients, if this is possible. Depending on the chemical properties of a compound, in particular its solubility, a minimum of formulation development is required before the study is started. The selection of the maximum allowed starting dose has already been discussed in general terms, as well as the escalation steps, but the protocol is usually written in a way that allows flexibility in dose adaptation, if needed, because, for example even at low dose levels, unexpected tolerability issues occur. The protocol should also allow adaptation for the group of cohorts. A very important issue is certainly the planning of the blood sampling for assessment of PK data, and this can be only estimated from the preclinical data. In particular, until the expected T_{max} is reached, sampling should be quite tight. But the data from the SAD study will then be used to optimize the sampling protocol in MAD studies. Ideally, even during SAD studies some fine-tuning should be possible, if the initial analysis shows that the PK in humans is extremely different from the animal PK.

The Phase 1 trial with desoxypeganine [9] is one of the few with a very simple design, only addressing single dosing in a cross-over design with 18 male and female subjects. At that time, no biomarkers were added and the study objective was the determination of safety, defining 150 mg of the compound once per day as the MTD, forming the basis of the next series of trials. To my knowledge, the Phase 1 program was completed, but due to a lack of funding the development was stopped in spite that the combination of acetylcholinesterase inhibition and the inhibition of monoamine oxidase A is an interesting concept; a similar compound, ladostigil, entered Phase 2 clinical trials [10].

For the orthosteric muscarinic M1 agonist NGX267 (AF267B) [11] a parallel-group design was used for an adaptive dose titration study. Only healthy young subjects were used. Initially, only two in each cohort were dosed with increasing doses of the compound until signs of toxicity were shown. Then, the next lower dose was investigated. Every subject only received one dose of the drug. But the design allowed a rapid performance of the study and an enrollment of more subjects in a dose range around the MTD. Further data at lower dosages were not explored, to allow a more precise estimate of MTD in the higher dose range. The study was mainly driven by clinical observation and PK. No biomarker signals were included in the trial.

For an FIH trial of the orally available antiprionic compound PRI-002 a team from NeuroScios used a randomized placebo-controlled, parallel-group design; based on the fact that this was a first-in-class compound with a completely novel mechanism of action, dose titration was done carefully, including sentinels at each escalation step, and the readouts were focused on safety, tolerability, and PK [12]. The SAD data supported moving to further clinical trials. In order to determine the safe dose range in a fast and economic way in the SAD study, no biomarker data were collected to speed up the enrollment of subjects, which could have been much more difficult if lumbar puncture had been included as one of the procedures. So the principle was followed to avoid invasive measures and focus on clinical, biochemical, and hematological variables.

The sigma-2 receptor complex allosteric antagonist CT1812 [13] used a complex study protocol and the SAD study was conducted in seven cohorts of healthy human subjects aged below 65 years. The SAD part was utilized to define a safe dosing range for the multiple dosing studies, which will be discussed later.

For the gamma-secretase modulator PF-06648671 [14] a Phase 1 program with three distinct studies was performed. In the FIH trial, a placebo-controlled cross-over design, with alternating cohorts, was used with five to eight subjects per dose to determine the PK, safety, tolerability, and plasma biomarkers. The investigators then moved to a single-dose, parallel-group, placebo-controlled study with lumbar catheterization for serial CSF sampling. Only two cohorts were investigated, and CSF samples were used to learn about the time course of biomarker effects. This study design already allows modeling of the PK and PD, and the selected biomarker, changes in $A\beta_{42}$ and $A\beta_{40}$ levels support the mode of action. It could be demonstrated, in spite of high variability, that $A\beta_{42}$ decreased in a dose-dependent way up to 36 hours after the dosing. But it was also found that there is a delay between T_{max} and the maximum PD effect. So, in two single-dose studies, substantial information was collected for multiple dosing.

To determine the relative bioavailability of lanabecestat, a beta-site amyloid precursor protein cleaving enzyme (BACE1) inhibitor [15], an open-label, randomized, three-period cross-over study in healthy male and non-fertile female subjects was used to determine the effects of two different formulations and an oral solution. It was also determined that a single dose of the drug was well tolerated, regardless of the form of application. The strategy for FIH studies is quite similar in immunotherapy trials. For aducanumab [16], the FIH trial was a sequential, randomized, double-blind,

placebo-controlled SAD study. In this first trial the primary outcome was safety and tolerability, but with a prolonged observation period due to the relatively long $T_{1/2}$ of antibodies. In the next Phase 1 trial, biomarker readouts, cognition, and function were included. In my opinion, a very interesting SAD study was done for the glutaminyl cyclase inhibitor PQ912 [17]. Here, a randomized, sequential, double-blind, placebo-controlled study design was used, combining safety, PK, and PD, first in young and then also in elderly subjects. But for the SAD study, three cohorts with cross-over arms were incorporated, so that information could be obtained in parallel on the effect of food and the formulation. The drug concentration was investigated not only in the plasma, but in the CSF to get information about BBB penetration, with the finding that CSF–plasma area-under-the-curve (AUC) ratios were independent of the dose. Measuring the activity of the target enzyme glutaminyl cyclase allowed the study of PK–PD relationship and also demonstrated that the PD active concentration of the compound was achieved in the CSF.

11.5 MAD Tolerance Studies

The next important step in the drug-development process is multiple dosing, which means that every single trial subject receives several doses of the new IMP. Dosing continues until a steady state is reached, and of course the aim of the study is to determine the safety of continuous treatment and to see differences in the PK after a single dose and at the end of the study, when a steady state has been reached. This allows us to get information about the potential accumulation of the drug and its metabolites, and to learn about dose proportionality; after multiple dosing, the MTD should be determined. A safe starting dose is selected based on the SAD data, and the single-dose PK will help to estimate the time to the steady state. These studies are of particular importance in a disease condition like AD, where a safe dose that can be applied over years needs to be found. Usually, cohorts of 10 to 16 subjects are recruited, and they are allocated to either verum or placebo. Again, the main objective of such a study is safety and tolerability, and therefore careful planning is needed. Very often the MTD is part of the initial protocol, but based on the SAD results, adaptations are now needed to determine first the investigated dose levels and the dosing intervals, which means the time between single doses. The time points for PK sample collection can be optimized using the SAD results, and the use of biomarkers becomes even more important because, with the length of treatment, some of the effects might be less variable and more pronounced to allow later PK/PD modeling. In principle, similar designs as already described above for SAD studies can be used, but in most of the cases a sequential group design was used. Since the tragic accident that happened during the early clinical trials of BIA 10–2474 developed by Bial [18], additional safety precautions are usually taken. This compound that inhibited a fatty acid hydrolase to enhance endogenous endocannabinoid concentrations suddenly produced unexpected severe adverse events in the third-escalation cohort after 5 days of administration. Therefore, MAD studies are performed only with the use of sentinels. That means that first one placebo- and one verum-treated subject is dosed, to minimize risks of adverse events to multiple subjects, and they are thoroughly monitored and controlled, usually over an extended observation period to address possible delayed reactions. Full PK data were collected from the first subjects to get an estimate of potential drug accumulation over time and to make sure that the initial protocol can be followed and assess whether appropriate adaptations need to be made. The MTD again needs to be predefined and will not be titrated, and so starting from one preselected SAD dose there is a maximum escalation up to the MTD of the SAD study. Usually this requires three to five cohorts. Every single cohort starts with a sentinel and after each cohort there is first a blinded analysis of adverse events; then the DSMB receives unblinded PK data, and they will give the recommendation about the next escalation step or stop the trial. In order to save time and expose less subjects to a risk, a titration type of study is very often performed. In short, the first MAD cohort receives 75% of the SAD MTD. If this is well tolerated, the full MTD dose is given. If this dose also does not produce any intolerable adverse events, and safety is comparable to the placebo group, it can be concluded that the MTD after single and multiple dosing is equal and a safe dose for the later clinical trials has been defined. If the SAD MTD produces adverse events, the 75% MTD is defined as the safe dose and the study can be stopped because it can justifiably be assumed that every dose below this value will also be safe. Coming back to the first step, if the 75% MTD is considered to be unsafe, the dose can be reduced to 50%, and again depending on the results, this will then be the new MAD MTD. If there are the slightest safety concerns, a further down-titration will be needed, and in that cohort more subjects will be investigated in order to obtain sufficient information on the tolerability. This approach was recently used in the MAD study of a new antiprionic compound for treatment of AD [12]. All these investigations are usually run on healthy younger subjects; a decreased drug metabolism can be assumed in elderly people. Therefore we usually study one cohort of elderly subjects using 75% of the MAD MTD dose level. The results will show differences in exposure, if any, and will deliver information about different safety signals in such an elderly population, which might be much closer to AD patients for Phase 2 trials. The translation from healthy elderly subjects to the diseased population can still be problematic, because usually AD patients are already exposed to several drugs and have multimorbidity. So data from the elderly cohorts need to be carefully considered to select a safe dose range for Phase 2. The MAD study will also allow us to learn more about the distribution of the IMP in the body, so it can be seen if there is a non-compartmental distribution or if the drug follows some multiple-compartment kinetics, which will then have consequences for final dosing decisions. The potential of accumulation is another quite important factor and, if possible, PD effects should be also followed over the whole time course because in some rare cases PD effects may last longer than the elimination; a good example of this is irreversible inhibitors. As we learned from the development of the irreversible acetylcholinesterase inhibitor metrifonate [19], the initial SAD and MAD studies in a patient population could not predict the rare side effects that finally stopped the development in Phase 3 in spite of consistent cognitive and functional improvement [20]. It is essential to find out about dose proportionality in SAD and MAD studies. In an ideal world, doses show a linear proportionality, which makes it very easy to estimate drug exposure after different doses, but depending on absorption, metabolic characteristics, excretion, saturation of transport systems, etc., the PK often does not show full proportionality, which requires additional safety considerations, because further dose escalation may induce an unexpectedly high increase in exposure.

There are of course many examples of MAD studies in AD, with new chemical entities, biologics, and active vaccinations. In early studies, the inhibition of acetylcholinesterase in red blood cells was used as a PD biomarker, which allowed some conclusions about the potential therapeutic efficacy. Of particular interest is a study with eptastigmine [21], which was shown to be tolerated up to 20 mg given three times a day. With these results an additional investigation was done in a few subjects, raising the dose every day by 4 mg three times a day to titrate the MTD. It was determined that 48 mg dosing three times a day resulted in sufficient inhibition of acetylcholinesterase and an acceptable tolerability. It is interesting that almost 20 years later a similar approach was taken to examine the safety of methanesulfonyl fluoride, an irreversible acetylcholinesterase inhibitor [22]. The special design involved the subjects initially receiving only a single dose, followed by 1 week washout, then the drug was applied three times per week to the subjects. The long intervals were chosen because of the irreversible inhibition. A relationship between the dose and acetylcholinesterase inhibition was established, from which clinical usefulness, enhancing cognitive function, was concluded. A similar combination of SAD and MAD design can also be used to compare safety, tolerability, and PK of prodrugs to the parent compound as it was done with ZT-1, a prodrug of the acetylcholinesterase inhibitor huperzine A [23]. For lecozotan, a competitive selective 5-hydroxytryptamine (5-HT) 1A receptor agonist [24], a MAD study was directly used to compare safety and PK between young and elderly subjects. In contrast to the SAD study, where the maximum well-tolerated dose was 10 mg, in the MAD study the safe dose was determined to be 5 mg lecozotan in both healthy and elderly subjects. The Phase 1 program for the selective 5-HT 6 receptor antagonist SUVN-502 was quite complex, combining single and multiple oral dosing and a fed and fasted crossover design in the SAD study [25]. The MAD study was performed for 7 days with a maximum dose of 130 mg once a day, and for 14 days in both healthy and elderly with 100 mg once a day. There was not much influence seen for food and gender, but an important result was that the exposure shown by the AUC ratio and C_{max}, the maximum plasma concentration of an IMP after application, was almost three times higher in the elderly. This study resulted in the selection of 50 and 100 mg once a day for further development. In another study on the histamine H3 receptor antagonist ABT-288, healthy young and elderly subjects were compared [26], showing similar safety and tolerability in both populations.

The AUC ratio was proportional over the evaluated dose ranges. A steady state was reached after 10 days of once-daily dosing, but with an accumulation of 3.4- to 4.2-fold. Based on these findings, 1 and 3 mg once-daily doses were selected for further clinical trials. Also worthy of note is the Phase 1 studies with the antiprionic compound PRI-002, in particular because the above-mentioned titration design based on 75% of the SAD MTD [12] was used to quickly determine the upper maximum well-tolerated dose and to get sufficient information on the PK. In the report about the sigma-2 receptor allosteric antagonist CT1812 combining SAD and MAD studies [13] into one protocol, different well-tolerated doses were determined in both SAD and MAD studies in healthy young and healthy elderly cohorts. It is important to note that in this study the plasma drug concentrations were compared to CSF concentrations on at least 2 days. Cognitive testing was also used as a functional readout in the MAD study, but did not show treatment-dependent differences in the healthy cohort, as expected from previous preclinical findings. Also, for the glutaminyl cyclase inhibitor PQ912, it was shown in a MAD study that exposure to the drug in elderly subjects is almost double compared to the young but, as discussed before, it was a very informative study because in the CSF not only the drug IMP concentration, but also the PD readout of inhibition of glutaminyl cyclase, could be related to the dose [17]. This is an important proof of target engagement. Several Phase 1 clinical studies on ALZ-801, an orally available prodrug of tramiprosate [27], have been published. Here the multiple dosing studies were interesting because they were also used to relate the safety and PK of the parent compound to the prodrug and an ALZ-801 dose could be determined that showed the exposure of a certain active tramiprosate dosing, reproducing positive cognitive effects in earlier trials. Several Phase 1 trials on gamma- and beta-secretase inhibitors have been published, including MAD studies. A quite intense program was done with AZD3293, which investigated different treatment schedules including once-daily and once-weekly administration [28], and the effects on plasma and CSF biomarkers. It turned out that this was the only BACE1 inhibitor with prolonged suppression of plasma Aβ and up to more than 70% of a reduction. The combined application of cromolyn and ibuprofen increases the challenges because safety limits and PK must be established for single-, as well as double-dose administration. The eventual differences in PK must also be considered for such a development [29]. Just as an example from immunotherapy, I want to mention the Phase 1b clinical trial with aducanumab [30], which is quite different from chemical entities. Due to the long $T_{1/2}$ of antibodies, the study was extended to 1 year in contrast to usually 7- to 14-day MAD studies. The trial was more like a Phase 2 clinical study, including several PD measures, such as the successful demonstration of brain Aβ reduction by Aβ positron emission microscopy (PET) and the proof of slowing clinical decline by cognitive (Mini-Mental State Examination) and functional (Clinical Dementia Rating [CDR]) examination. Of course this was done with a seamless safety documentation. For active vaccinations, the approach is again different because here it can be expected that the first administration of the antigen already triggers a long-lasting immune response. For example, the first active vaccine clinical trial against tau protein with the antigen AADvac1 started with a 12-week randomized, double-blinded, placebo-controlled parallel-group design followed by another 12 weeks of an open-label study [31, 32]. In this phase, every subject received three doses of the vaccine, and vaccination continued during the open-label phase. Here, besides all relevant safety measures, there is focus on the induction of antibodies to show a stable immunogenicity of the preparation.

11.6 Outcome Variables

In accordance with the fact that safety is the main objective of Phase 1, every adverse event that occurs from the time point of first drug intake is recorded. First, there is an assessment about the nature of adverse events, without judging the relationship with treatment. An adverse event is any medical occurrence in a trial subject that received a dose of the IMP. This needs to be differentiated from a serious adverse event, which causes hospitalization or a prolongation of hospitalization, or results in a persistent or significant disability. Finally, there are the suspected unexpected adverse reactions; that is, any adverse reaction that is not consistent with the reference safety information. Then there is a rating of every single adverse event to describe the severeness, ranging from mild to severe, where mild is considered if symptoms are only transient and do not interfere with the subject's daily activities, severe means an unacceptable interference with daily activities. And of course every adverse event will be considered in relation to the study

drug [33]. A definite adverse event shows a plausible temporal sequence in relation to the drug administration or to tissue and blood concentration levels: the nature of the adverse event matches with the known adverse reaction scheme for the IMP and it cannot be explained by the occurrence of a concomitant disease, or the intake of other drugs or chemicals. Also, when the drug is withdrawn, there should be an observed clinical improvement. If the adverse event occurs again after a re-challenge, this will underline the definite relationship.

Probable adverse events also occur in some temporal relationship to drug intake; the difference between a possible and a definite adverse event is the lack of re-exposure to complete the definition. Possible adverse events have a similar definition, but they may be due to the patient's clinical condition or the intake of other treatments. Usually there is no information about withdrawal. Any clinical events, including abnormalities in laboratory tests that are not in a causal relationship to drug intake, are rated as unlikely, and they can also be explained by other conditions. All adverse events need to be followed up and, according to GCP or local medical law, reported to the ethical committee and the health authorities. All adverse events are coded according to the current MEDDRA version (the medical dictionary for regulatory activities), which is a product of the ICH [2] as a clinically validated international terminology dictionary–thesaurus, including the adverse event classification dictionary. This coding ensures a uniform classification and description of adverse events. During the study the subjects are interviewed on a regular basis in a standardized way about their condition. The most commonly reported adverse events include headache, gastrointestinal discomfort, and dizziness and similar symptoms. As already mentioned, every clinically relevant and significant change in blood biochemistry, hematology, or urine analysis is classified as an adverse event. The blood biochemistry is usually a complete standard safety laboratory and may include specific determinations, if any specific changes are known and expected from preclinical data. Usually, special attention is given to all markers of liver or kidney damage. Any abnormality that is rated as relevant by the principal investigator usually results in the withdrawal of the study medication and then laboratory readouts are followed until normalization. A very important part is the recording of vital signs and, in particular, the documentation of cardiac safety. A 12-lead ECG recording is done at baseline and then at different time points after drug intake to document the relationship between the PK and drug concentration. In order to assess a potential arrhythmic property of an IMP, a careful investigation of the QTc interval is most relevant. Any significant increase or decrease of this readout may increase the risk of developing malignant arrhythmias and even sudden cardiac death. It must be considered that there are different formulas for the QTc correction and in early drug-development regulators suggest the use of the Fridericia method; however, the choice of method will depend on the nature of the IMP and experience with the drug class. There are recommendations by the US Food and Drug Administration (FDA) and the European Medicines Agency (EMA) to define an upper limit of normal of 450 ms irrespective of gender. This applies for early clinical trials, but alternatively cut-off values of > 450 ms for males and > 460 ms for females are considered as relevant thresholds. Any drug-dependent increase of more than 10 ms needs further investigation, and of course every new IMP should be carefully investigated for cardiac side effects in a so-called thorough QT trial [34].

The second important part of the Phase 1 trial is the assessment of PK properties of the drug: the absorption, distribution, metabolism, and finally elimination of the IMP from the body. If there is a comparison of the PK after intravenous versus parenteral application, this opens the possibility of calculating the absolute bioavailability, showing how much of the applied drug is absorbed and distributed in the body. This knowledge is essential for comparing different formulations and forms of application. Important PK characteristics include C_{max}, T_{max}, and the AUC. The C_{max} and T_{max} characterize the absorption phase. T_{max} is the most critical characteristic, because this depends on the appropriate planning of the plasma sampling. A precise estimate may need some adaptation of the sampling time points around the expected T_{max} during ongoing trials. Finally, the AUC shows the complete IMP exposure to the subject and it also includes the elimination phase. There are different commonly used AUC estimates, such as calculating the exposure from the application time point to the time of the last observed concentration, or until the time of the last sampling point. Complete modeling also needs an assessment of the elimination rate constants and the calculation of $T_{1/2}$. Here

we have to differentiate between the elimination half-life, which is the time it takes for the drug reaching the system to decline by 50%; it is different from the distribution or plasma $T_{1/2}$, which only considers the plasma concentration, a value caused by distribution and excretion. Knowing $T_{1/2}$ is important for dosing considerations in order to avoid drug accumulations up to toxic levels during multiple dosing. Another important parameter is the clearance, which describes a defined volume of plasma that is completely cleared of the drug within a time period. This gives an estimate of the total elimination. The volume of distribution indicates the potential accumulation of the drug from distribution into other body tissues, so-called compartments, than the plasma, for example adipose tissue. The PK values also allow conclusions to be drawn on metabolism to assess if there is a linear relationship between the drug concentration and the metabolic rate or if there are other more complex relationships, which will finally influence the system drug availability. The same is true for the distribution kinetics, which could follow a simple non-compartmental distribution or could have complex two- or multi-compartment distributions. Finally, a comparison of all PK parameters, in particular C_{max}, $T_{1/2}$, and AUC in relation to the applied dose, will give data on dose proportionality. The most desirable result is a linear relationship to allow a prediction of exposure depending on the applied dose in a safe and reliable way. Due to the saturation of transport systems, metabolic pathways, or excretion, super- or supra-proportionality can also occur, making the dose calculations more complex. For AD and other CNS disorders in particular, it is of interest to plan for PK assessment of the CSF, to get an idea about the available active drug that reaches the target organ. Again the relationship of the drug with the plasma PK is highly relevant. The above gives only a short overview of the complexity of the PK assessments, a deeper analysis is beyond the scope of this chapter.

Additional readouts that could be implemented in Phase 1 are of course all plasma and CSF biomarkers, such as enzyme inhibition, concentration of different marker proteins, and changes in pro-inflammatory cytokines, together with measures of receptor occupancy, measures of brain load of Aβ and tau/hyperphosphorylated tau (p-tau) using PET and many other options, depending on the mode of action of a new IMP. Electrophysiological and functional measures can also be implemented.

I cannot overstate the fact that all of these readouts need extremely careful interpretation in Phase 1, because these small studies are not powered for the detection of efficacy. The numbers of participants are much too low for conclusive efficacy data.

To conclude, all adverse reactions, the severity of these reactions, and all biomarker readouts can be investigated under consideration of PK parameters, and of course compared to placebo. Only a few possibilities should be highlighted. Are adverse events more frequent around T_{max}? Does their occurrence depend more on complete body exposure (AUC)? Is influence on some PD readouts correlated to the plasma or CSF concentration of a compound, or do these effects have different kinetics? Very often PD readouts can still be shown after a drug has been already completely eliminated, in particular when intracellular pathways are triggered by the IMP. Such findings require PD assessment to find $T_{1/2}$ values. This needs specific consideration in order to choose the right dosing and the right dosing regimen. If all these data are considered together, the most appropriate doses for Phase 2 and Phase 3 trials can be chosen. These doses should of course be within the range of the expected PD active dose in humans and it should leave a wide safety margin, particularly considering the need for long chronic dosing in conditions like AD. The next step is to choose the most appropriate therapeutic doses in early Phase 2.

11.7 Special Measures in Phase 1 Studies

In Phase 1 clinical trials in healthy volunteers there are very few reports about the use of cognitive testing because, in general, it is believed that cognitive function can not really be improved in a healthy population. In the MAD study with CT1812 cognitive testing was performed in the elderly cohort at baseline and after 14 days of treatment using the AD Assessment Scale – cognitive subscale and an additional cognitive battery, but as expected there were no demonstrable effects [13]. Of course the use of sensitive computerized testing batteries, such as the Cogstate, CDR, or Cambridge Neuropsychological Test Automated Battery, could be used to detect subtle changes, for example in reaction time. This could be indicative of potential therapeutic effects in AD trials but certainly can not be considered as a real proof of concept. In a small experimental trial it was shown that spatial

learning and memory using a very novel paradigm was impaired by the cholinergic antagonist scopolamine, and treatment with donepezil [35] could restore the cognitive function. Although this was not a real Phase 1 study, a similar paradigm was used previously in the development of cholinergic drugs. I believe that in the very near future the use of continuous surveillance with wearable devices could highlight the influence of a novel IMP on functional readouts, even in Phase 1 studies. This has so far not been widely implemented, but initial data are promising.

In my opinion, up to now, cognitive and functional improvements, or the slowing down of progression, have only been proven in the Phase 1b clinical trial with aducanumab [30], in this case leading directly to a Phase 3 trial; but then unfortunately there was a controversial outcome in two different studies, which was explained by differences in total drug exposure, delaying the approval of this immunotherapy. But in June 2021 FDA finally approved aducanumab, as the first disease-modifying treatment

In AD research, there is now an increasing interest in the use of quantitative EEG and event-related potentials, such as the P300 wave and similar readouts. The use of EEG needs very careful consideration because there are so many different data and calculated ratios that there is a high probability of finding some statistical differences by chance. Therefore, such studies need extremely careful planning in the prospective definition of primary and secondary outcome variables, and the studies should follow the methodology that is recommended by guidelines of the International Pharmaco-EEG Society [36]. In spite of careful planning and experience in the field, the variability of most readouts is extremely high and so in small Phase 1 trials it is a challenge to find conclusive results. If it is known that a drug already showed electrophysiological results in preclinical studies, EEG should be considered as a part of the assessments. But besides direct effects on the different EEG frequency bands, the calculation of ratios, such as the alpha slow-wave index, blotting the effects on alpha-frequency bands vs. the slow-frequency bands, should be implemented. It is important to consider in advance the probability that a drug acts in a way that indicates a positive influence on neuronal function. Here, there is much previous experience with cholinergic drugs, because there seems to be a consistent decrease

145

in alpha- and beta-frequency bands during aging and development of AD [37] and an increase in delta and/or theta frequencies. For cholinergic drugs, the scopolamine challenge seems interesting because it produces a frequency change similar to that seen in AD [38, 39]. Acetylcholinesterase inhibitors are able to counteract these antagonistic effects, decreasing the slow-wave activities and increasing alpha- and beta-frequency bands [40, 41]. Donepezil in healthy volunteers had opposite effects because it increased slow-wave activity and decreased the alpha power [42]. Also, MK-7622, an M1-positive allosteric modulator, used quantitative EEG analysis in healthy volunteers but, interestingly, increased delta and theta power, no effect on alpha bands, but an increase in beta01 frequency were found [43]. In fact, such investigations could be also of interest for compounds that interact with amyloid metabolism because it was shown that AD-specific CSF $A\beta_{42}$ patterns significantly correlate with increased slow-wave frequencies [44], and in contrast increased p-tau and tau CSF values decreased the high-frequency bands significantly. I believe that with more refined analysis techniques and the implementation of artificial intelligence [45] to analyze complex frequency changes that can give information on brain connectivity, it may be possible to deliver further important data for understanding drug effects in Phase 1 trials.

The use of different AD-specific biomarkers as readout in Phase 1 has been discussed above, in particular when drugs directly interfere with pathogenetically important pathways, involving amyloid precursor or tau proteins. Nowadays, these investigations can be more widely applied due to the availability of reliable methods to measure these proteins in plasma; CSF sampling is also an option, in particular in MAD studies. The use of continuous sampling via a spinal catheter needs to consider influence of the procedure on the concentration of these biomarkers because such influences may be considerable, depending on the sampling frequency [46].

11.8 How Does Phase 1 Fit into the Ecosystem of AD Drug Development?

The priority of every drug-development program is to reach the phase of clinical investigations, and of course to successfully finalize a Phase 3 study, in order to achieve a marketing authorization by any health authority worldwide. Phase 1 clinical trials are the entrance to human research, and the outcome of such studies will finally support a decision to move into more progressed studies in patients or, in the worst case, to move back to preclinical research or even discard the program altogether. The good news is that about 70% of the investigated IMPs show sufficient safety and tolerability to be promoted to Phase 2. In disease areas like AD particularly, it is often extremely difficult to obtain sufficient information on the useful therapeutic dosing range. Just to show sufficient safety over a certain, but always relatively short, time period of perhaps 28 days will not be sufficient because the investigated doses should clearly cover the pharmacologically active dose in humans, and should leave a sufficient safety margin, in particular because these drugs will be used for years of treatment in a vulnerable population that shows multimorbidity and usually polypharmacy for treatment of concomitant diseases. By doing careful modeling based on all preclinical efficacy and safety findings, and relating this to the findings of the Phase 1 studies, including all the PK readouts, a dose range for Phase 2 can be chosen, which is still primarily focused on safety in patients, but may then allow the first proof-of-concept data. With increasing knowledge of disease mechanisms and related biomarkers, the Phase 1 study may already support the therapeutic concept sufficiently. It is important to first do a check for safety in healthy subjects, which is fast and relatively inexpensive, and then focus more on safety and efficacy in patients in Phase 2a; or Phase 1 trials may be started in a diseased population.

Without doubt these data are all sensitive for future decisions and therefore it is essential that well-established protocols are used and followed. For reliable data it is crucial to work with experienced Phase 1 units, regardless of whether they are commercial entities, academic institutions, or hospital-based units. For our clients, NeuroScios mainly runs clinical trials in specialized clinical pharmacology departments of university clinics. Here, we can guarantee sufficient experience and training of every single team member, and most importantly also their skills to handle emergency situations, if, which fortunately seldom happens, unexpected and severe adverse reactions occur. It is a must that they have up-to-date training in resuscitation and that intensive care units are available in close vicinity, ideally even within the unit.

Using the experience of the team members, particular protocols have been developed, with a particular focus on the specific drug and its mode of action; then we do sufficient team training to make sure that everybody understands each single step of the protocol. Surveillance of the unit pharmacy, a check of all necessary equipment, including for example appropriate sample storage in safe places with continuous temperature monitoring, are also important elements of the study preparation. As NeuroScios is a relatively small company, but focused on neurodegenerative diseases, our typical clients are small drug-development companies and university spin-offs that do not have the internal experience for Phase 1 trials and who need support for the regulatory preparation. We are flexible and work quickly to collect all information from the clients on their compound and their future development plans, in order to compile all the regulatory documents. As a European company, NeuroScios is focused on the EMA regulatory environment. So, the essential study documents, besides the protocol and the informed consent forms and the case report forms, are the IMP dossier summarizing chemistry and manufacturing and control of the IMP and then the Investigator's Brochure, which is practically identical to FDA requirements. All these documents can be easily translated to any regulatory environment. We make our clients also familiar with the team of the Phase 1 unit and try to keep them involved as closely as possible. This is of course a very exciting time, in particular for the small companies that build everything on a single platform or even one compound, because the outcome may determine the future of the whole team. For these companies it is essential to get Phase 1 data that support their proposed therapeutic concept. There should be low toxicity, wide safety margins, predictable PK properties and, if available, data about BBB penetration (indirect via PK measures in CSF) and signs of target engagement supported by biomarker readouts, measures of enzyme inhibition, or receptor occupancy. Usually, these data sets are important for the next essential financing rounds to create enough financial support to run the much more expensive Phase 2 program. For most of them it is extremely difficult to get funding for the Phase 1 studies, because at entry to Phase 1 there is not enough risk reduction for most of the big pharmaceutical companies to partner or license such programs. Therefore, different organizations, such as the Alzheimer's Drug Discovery Foundation or the Alzheimer's Association or local funding agencies (National Institutes of Health, National Institute on Aging, European funding programs) are other sources for raising money for the early clinical trials. Very often companies forget that as well as the pure trial costs there is also considerable financial need for good manufacturing practice synthesis, formulation, and quality control of the IMP. Consistent Phase 1 data are opening the way for investments, in particular if the data fulfil all the above-mentioned criteria. But still, big partners may hesitate because of the lack of a firm proof of concept. Solid Phase 1 studies and a robust data set are the basis for further success; however, particularly in the field of neurodegenerative disorders, these are by no means a guarantee for ultimate success.

References

1. Zhou Y. Choice of designs and doses for early phase trials. *Fundam Clin Pharmacol* 2004; **18**: 373–8.

2. Lindstrom-Gommers L, Mullin T. International Conference on Harmonization: recent reforms as a driver of global regulatory harmonization and innovation in medical products. *Clin Pharmacol Ther* 2019; **105**: 926–31.

3. Nair AB, Jacob S. A simple practice guide for dose conversion between animals and humans. *J Basic Clin Pharm* 2016; **7**: 27–31.

4. Muller PY, Milton M, Lloyd P, Sims J, Brennan FR. The minimum anticipated biological effect level (MABEL) for selection of first human dose in clinical trials with monoclonal antibodies. *Curr Opin Biotechnol* 2009; **20**: 722–9.

5. Agoram BM. Use of pharmacokinetic/pharmacodynamic modelling for starting dose selection in first-in-human trials of high-risk biologics. *Br J Clin Pharmacol* 2009; **67**: 153–60.

6. Wheeler GM, Mander AP, Bedding A, et al. How to design a dose-finding study using the continual reassessment method. *BMC Med Res Methodol* 2019; **19**: 18.

7. Dekker M, Bouvy JC, O'Rourke D, et al. Alignment of European regulatory and health technology assessments: a review of licensed products for Alzheimer's disease. *Front Med (Lausanne)* 2019; **6**: 73.

8. Jaki T, Clive S, Weir CJ. Principles of dose finding studies in cancer: a comparison of trial designs. *Cancer Chemother Pharmacol* 2013; **71**: 1107–14.

9. Algorta J, Pena MA, Maraschiello C, et al. Phase I clinical trial with desoxypeganine, a new cholinesterase and selective MAO-A inhibitor: tolerance and pharmacokinetics study of escalating

single oral doses. *Methods Find Exp Clin Pharmacol* 2008; **30**: 141–7.

10. Schneider LS, Geffen Y, Rabinowitz J, et al. Low-dose ladostigil for mild cognitive impairment: a Phase 2 placebo-controlled clinical trial. *Neurology* 2019; **93**: e1474–84.

11. Ivanova A, Murphy M. An adaptive first in man dose-escalation study of NGX267: statistical, clinical, and operational considerations. *J Biopharm Stat* 2009; **19**: 247–55.

12. Kutzsche J, Jurgens D, Willuweit A, et al. Safety and pharmacokinetics of the orally available antiprionic compound PRI-002: a single and multiple ascending dose phase I study. *Alzheimers Dement (N Y)* 2020; **6**: e12001.

13. Grundman M, Morgan R, Lickliter JD, et al. A Phase 1 clinical trial of the sigma-2 receptor complex allosteric antagonist CT1812, a novel therapeutic candidate for Alzheimer's disease. *Alzheimers Dement (N Y)* 2019; **5**: 20–6.

14. Ahn JE, Carrieri C, Dela Cruz F, et al. Pharmacokinetic and pharmacodynamic effects of a gamma-secretase modulator, PF-06648671, on CSF amyloid-beta peptides in randomized Phase I studies. *Clin Pharmacol Ther* 2020; **107**: 211–20.

15. Ye N, Monk SA, Daga P, et al. Clinical bioavailability of the novel BACE1 inhibitor lanabecestat (AZD3293): assessment of tablet formulations versus an oral solution and the impact of gastric pH on pharmacokinetics. *Clin Pharmacol Drug Dev* 2018; **7**: 233–43.

16. Ferrero J, Williams L, Stella H, et al. First-in-human, double-blind, placebo-controlled, single-dose escalation study of aducanumab (BIIB037) in mild-to-moderate Alzheimer's disease. *Alzheimers Dement (N Y)* 2016; **2**: 169–76.

17. Lues I, Weber F, Meyer A, et al. A Phase 1 study to evaluate the safety and pharmacokinetics of PQ912, a glutaminyl cyclase inhibitor, in healthy subjects. *Alzheimers Dement (N Y)* 2015; **1**: 182–95.

18. Kerbrat A, Ferre JC, Fillatre P, et al. Acute neurologic disorder from an inhibitor of fatty acid amide hydrolase. *N Engl J Med* 2016; **375**: 1717–25.

19. Cutler NR, Jhee SS, Cyrus P, et al. Safety and tolerability of metrifonate in patients with Alzheimer's disease: results of a maximum tolerated dose study. *Life Sci* 1998; **62**: 1433–41.

20. Lopez-Arrieta JM, Schneider L. Metrifonate for Alzheimer's disease. *Cochrane Database Syst Rev* 2006; **2**: CD003155.

21. Sramek JJ, Block GA, Reines SA, et al. A multiple-dose safety trial of eptastigmine in Alzheimer's disease, with pharmacodynamic observations of red blood cell cholinesterase. *Life Sci* 1995; **56**: 319–26.

22. Moss DE, Fariello RG, Sahlmann J, et al. A randomized Phase I study of methanesulfonyl fluoride, an irreversible cholinesterase inhibitor, for the treatment of Alzheimer's disease. *Br J Clin Pharmacol* 2013; **75**: 1231–9.

23. Jia JY, Zhao QH, Liu Y, et al. Phase I study on the pharmacokinetics and tolerance of ZT-1, a prodrug of huperzine A, for the treatment of Alzheimer's disease. *Acta Pharmacol Sin* 2013; **34**: 976–82.

24. Patat A, Parks V, Raje S, et al. Safety, tolerability, pharmacokinetics and pharmacodynamics of ascending single and multiple doses of lecozotan in healthy young and elderly subjects. *Br J Clin Pharmacol* 2009; **67**: 299–308.

25. Nirogi R, Mudigonda K, Bhyrapuneni G, et al. Safety, tolerability and pharmacokinetics of the serotonin 5-HT6 receptor antagonist, SUVN-502, in healthy young adults and elderly subjects. *Clin Drug Investig* 2018; **38**: 401–15.

26. Othman AA, Haig G, Florian H, et al. Safety, tolerability and pharmacokinetics of the histamine H3 receptor antagonist, ABT-288, in healthy young adults and elderly volunteers. *Br J Clin Pharmacol* 2013; **75**: 1299–311.

27. Hey JA, Yu JY, Versavel M, et al. Clinical pharmacokinetics and safety of ALZ-801, a novel prodrug of tramiprosate in development for the treatment of Alzheimer's disease. *Clin Pharmacokinet* 2018; **57**: 315–33.

28. Cebers G, Alexander RC, Haeberlein SB, et al. AZD3293: pharmacokinetic and pharmacodynamic effects in healthy subjects and patients with Alzheimer's disease. *J Alzheimers Dis* 2017; **55**: 1039–53.

29. Brazier D, Perry R, Keane J, Barrett K, Elmaleh DR. Pharmacokinetics of cromolyn and ibuprofen in healthy elderly volunteers. *Clin Drug Investig* 2017; **37**: 1025–34.

30. Sevigny J, Chiao P, Bussiere T, et al. The antibody aducanumab reduces Abeta plaques in Alzheimer's disease. *Nature* 2016; **537**: 50–6.

31. Novak P, Schmidt R, Kontsekova E, et al. Safety and immunogenicity of the tau vaccine AADvac1 in patients with Alzheimer's disease: a randomised, double-blind, placebo-controlled, phase 1 trial. *Lancet Neurol* 2017; **16**: 123–34.

32. Novak P, Schmidt R, Kontsekova E, et al. FUNDAMANT: an interventional 72-week phase 1 follow-up study of AADvac1, an active immunotherapy against tau protein pathology in Alzheimer's disease. *Alzheimers Res Ther* 2018; **10**: 108.

33. Karch FE, Lasagna L. Toward the operational identification of adverse drug reactions. *Clin Pharmacol Ther* 1977; **21**: 247–54.

34. Timmers M, Sinha V, Darpo B, et al. Evaluating potential QT effects of JNJ-54861911, a BACE inhibitor in single- and multiple-ascending dose studies, and a thorough QT trial with additional retrospective confirmation, using concentration-QTc analysis. *J Clin Pharmacol* 2018; **58**: 952–64.

35. Laczo J, Markova H, Lobellova V, et al. Scopolamine disrupts place navigation in rats and humans: a translational validation of the Hidden Goal Task in the Morris water maze and a real maze for humans. *Psychopharmacology (Ber)* 2017; **234**: 535–47.

36. Jobert M, Wilson FJ, Ruigt GS, et al. Guidelines for the recording and evaluation of pharmaco-EEG data in man: the International Pharmaco-EEG Society (IPEG). *Neuropsychobiology* 2012; **66**: 201–20.

37. Tsolaki A, Kazis D, Kompatsiaris I, Kosmidou V, Tsolaki M. Electroencephalogram and Alzheimer's disease: clinical and research approaches. *Int J Alzheimers Dis* 2014; **2014**: 349249.

38. Liem-Moolenaar M, de Boer P, Timmers M, et al. Pharmacokinetic–pharmacodynamic relationships of central nervous system effects of scopolamine in healthy subjects. *Br J Clin Pharmacol* 2011; **71**: 886–98.

39. Ebert U, Kirch W. Scopolamine model of dementia: electroencephalogram findings and cognitive performance. *Eur J Clin Invest* 1998; **28**: 944–9.

40. Adler G, Brassen S. Short-term rivastigmine treatment reduces EEG slow-wave power in Alzheimer patients. *Neuropsychobiology* 2001; **43**: 273–6.

41. Adler G, Brassen S, Chwalek K, Dieter B, Teufel M. Prediction of treatment response to rivastigmine in Alzheimer's dementia. *J Neurol Neurosurg Psychiatry* 2004; **75**: 292–4.

42. Balsters JH, O'Connell RG, Martin MP, et al. Donepezil impairs memory in healthy older subjects: behavioural, EEG and simultaneous EEG/fMRI biomarkers. *PLoS One* 2011; **6**: e24126.

43. Uslaner JM, Kuduk SD, Wittmann M, et al. Preclinical to human translational pharmacology of the novel M1 positive allosteric modulator MK-7622. *J Pharmacol Exp Ther* 2018; **365**: 556–66.

44. Smailovic U, Koenig T, Kareholt I, et al. Quantitative EEG power and synchronization correlate with Alzheimer's disease CSF biomarkers. *Neurobiol Aging* 2018; **63**: 88–95.

45. Simpraga S, Alvarez-Jimenez R, Mansvelder HD, et al. EEG machine learning for accurate detection of cholinergic intervention and Alzheimer's disease. *Sci Rep* 2017; **7**: 5775.

46. Van Broeck B, Timmers M, Ramael S, et al. Impact of frequent cerebrospinal fluid sampling on Abeta levels: systematic approach to elucidate influencing factors. *Alzheimers Res Ther* 2016; **8**: 21.

Chapter 12

The Importance of Phase 2 in Drug Development for Alzheimer's Disease

Philip Scheltens, Willem de Haan, Roos J. Jutten, Everhard Vijverberg, Arno de Wilde, and Niels Prins

12.1   Introduction

Clinical trials in drug development are commonly divided into three phases. The first phase aims to find the range of doses of potential clinical use, usually by identifying the maximum tolerated dose, usually in healthy volunteers, occasionally also in the target population. The second phase aims to find doses that demonstrate promising efficacy with acceptable safety in the target population. The third phase aims to confirm the benefit previously found in the second phase using clinically meaningful endpoints and to demonstrate safety more definitively, tested in the population for which the drug is ultimately meant and that will end up being listed on the label.

Among the goals of Phase 2 are:

- finding the right dose by exploring safety and tolerability related to the dose;
- establishing target engagement by use of biomarkers;
- looking for early efficacy signals, either by biomarkers or clinically testing several outcome measures.

In short: efficacy, dose, and side effects. Dose-finding trials – studies conducted to identify the most promising doses or doses to use in later studies – are a key part of this second phase and are intended to answer the dual questions of whether future development is warranted and what dose or doses should be used. If too high a dose is chosen, adverse effects in later confirmatory Phase 3 trials may threaten the development program. If too low a dose is chosen, the treatment effect may be too small to yield a positive confirmatory trial and may cause the program to fail. In the recent past in the dementia field, we have seen examples of both. A well-designed dose-finding trial is able to establish the optimal dose of a medication and facilitate the decision to proceed with a Phase 3 trial. The ultimate decision to go or not go with the compound under study should be made after a carefully designed Phase 2 trial, in which all the questions above have been answered.

This chapter deals with the importance of conducting a Phase 2 study in the course of developing drugs for Alzheimer's disease (AD). Its role cannot be overestimated nor the importance overrated. As we will demonstrate in this chapter, carrying out a good Phase 2 trial will set the stage for developing a successful Phase 3 study.

12.2   Planning

Before an AD clinical program can proceed to Phase 2 studies, the trials performed in Phase 1, also referred to as first-in-human (FIH) trials, at a minimum must have demonstrated that the candidate compound is safe for use in humans. Often, the study population of Phase 1 trials consists of healthy volunteers, although sometimes in AD drug-development programs one may choose to perform the Phase 1 trial in patients ("first-in-patient" trials). A reason for the latter may be when particular side effects can be expected that arise only in the interaction between the drug and specific components of the AD pathophysiological process. An example is the occurrence of amyloid-related imaging abnormalities (ARIA) in monoclonal antibody or vaccine trials against amyloid beta, which will only be seen in trial participants who are amyloid positive. Besides safety, Phase 1 trials should have identified the maximum tolerated dose (MTD) and the dose-limiting toxicities (DLTs) associated with the drug. Together with the pharmacokinetic profile, insight into the pharmacodynamics, and possibly an early indication of efficacy of the candidate compound, this information can be used to decide whether or not a candidate drug can proceed to Phase 2, and what doses should be further examined [1].

Phase 2 of the clinical development of AD drugs usually includes multiple studies in different stages, among them are a proof-of-concept (POC) study (Phase 2a) and a dose-finding (DF), or dose-ranging study (Phase 2b) [2]. The LipiDiDiet and safety data from Phase 1 can be used in Phase 2 to establish doses that are high enough to establish systemic drug concentrations that may have a positive impact on AD pathophysiology and/or disease symptoms, and that are low enough to stay below the MTD. POC studies (Phase 2a) are usually conducted to demonstrate clinical efficacy with a small to moderate number of patients. Typically, POC studies use two treatment groups in a placebo-controlled, parallel design, with either a clinical measure or surrogate markers as the efficacy endpoint. If the POC study provides proof of efficacy, a DF study is often conducted to assess the efficacy as well as safety with a relatively larger number of patients to find the optimal dose(s) for Phase 3 confirmatory trials, where the primary efficacy endpoint is assessed at a later time point, post dosing [3]. DF studies are mostly placebo-controlled with parallel dose groups. The maximal duration of treatment is limited by animal toxicity coverage. Many doses of the investigational drug are used to explore a range of efficacious doses.

The study population in Phase 2 trials consists of participants who have the condition that the drug is affecting. In primary prevention AD trials, the population will consist of participants at risk of developing AD pathology, whereas in secondary-prevention trials the target population consists of people with AD pathology at risk of developing clinical symptoms. Symptomatic AD drug trials or tertiary prevention trials will target patients with mild cognitive impairment (MCI) or dementia due to AD. In order to increase the chance of a positive result if the drug is effective, one should aim for a homogenic study population using strict in- and exclusion criteria. Such a population will limit the noise that may obscure a positive signal. The number of participants in Phase 2 AD trials is typically between 100 and 300.

Biomarkers are increasingly used in Phase 2 to support decision making for development programs. First, biomarkers are used for inclusion of the right participants by confirming the diagnosis of AD, in line with the recently published diagnostic framework that states that the diagnosis of AD is a biological one [4]. In the not-so-distant past, clinical trials have been carried out in which the clinical diagnosis of AD proved not to be substantiated by biomarkers of amyloid and tau in more than 25% of the cases, indicating these patients did not have the pathobiology of AD; hence, in hindsight they are not suitable to be treated by treatments directed against this pathology. Based on what we now know using these biomarkers, 50% of the patients who were included on the basis of the diagnosis of MCI did not have AD pathology [3]. Secondly, biomarkers in Phase 2 AD trials can be used as surrogate outcome measures, by showing target engagement as well as downstream therapeutic effects. Over the last couple of years this use in Phase 2 trials has become of paramount importance, which is highlighted by the inclusion of this use in the denomination of the five rights of drug development [5].

In classical drug development, development phases are clearly separated, and Phase 3 trials are initiated to confirm the efficacy and safety findings from the completed Phase 2 trials. An alternative approach is the so-called seamless, or adaptive, Phase 2–3 design. In this design, the objective is to combine dose selection, efficacy, and safety confirmation in one trial. In the first stage, patients are enrolled into the trial and, based on interim safety and surrogate marker data, the optimal dose of the study drug is selected. In the second stage, enrollment continues only in the selected dose arm and the placebo arm. All data from the selected and placebo arm are used in the final analyses, using novel statistical methods for combining evidence from the first and second stage of the trial to control for false positive error rate and to maintain the integrity of the trial [6].

With regard to the sample size needed in Phase 2 trials, several statistical concepts are important in general to take into consideration. These are the estimated effect size, level of significance, and power. Sample-size estimation needs an adjustment in accommodating interim analysis, and an adjustment for covariates. To make educated guesses on the required sample size, especially in trials in which target engagement is tested with biomarkers, the natural course of these biomarkers needs to be known, as well as the estimated effect the drug could have on the marker. Very often these data are not exactly known and one needs to adapt the dosing and length of the study to the results at various time points. This shows that Phase 2 design needs to be flexible to a certain extent, and not bound to perceived rules set by regulators or others.

151

The goal of Phase 2 is to learn as much as there can be learned about the effect of the drug, before an expensive and large Phase 3 study is started.

12.3 Design

Choosing the right primary outcome(s), secondary outcomes, and exploratory outcomes is crucial for any Phase 2 study and there needs to be careful consideration of the mode of action of the drug (and possible learnings from Phase 1) on the one hand and the availability of markers and outcome measures that can answer the questions that need to be addressed in Phase 2, as detailed above. Following this, there is no fixed mandatory design for a Phase 2 trial; it needs to be a tailormade program, fit for the drug, the population, and it will be dependent on resources and expertise as well as taking into account the patient burden. As stated above, Phase 2 is the phase in which one can experiment still and can feel free to add measures that may not be used later in Phase 3. The danger, however, is that some protocols look like Christmas trees, with too many balls in it. There needs to be a balance between all these aspects for a protocol to be feasible and acceptable to institutional review board (IRBs), sites, and patients.

In the following we will detail imaging, fluid, and cognitive markers that are of particular relevance to the design of a Phase 2 study.

12.3.1 Fluid Biomarkers

Fluid biomarkers are objective measures of a biological or pathological process that can be used for AD diagnosis and to evaluate disease progression/monitor therapeutic interventions in AD. Cerebrospinal fluid (CSF) is in direct contact with the extracellular space of the brain and offers direct measurements of AD-related proteins, whereas plasma/serum is on the other side of the blood–brain barrier, hence concentrations are lower. Both fluid biomarkers are an optimal source for the variety of goals in Phase 2 clinical trials.

Biomarkers for the inclusion of AD participants in Phase 2 trials are mainly based on the National Institute on Aging (NIA)–Alzheimer's Association (AA) Research Framework criteria [4], also named biomarker-based participant selection. Currently, biomarker classification relies on the presence of amyloid (A) and tau pathology

(T) and neurodegeneration (N). A designation of A+T+ or A+T− is sufficient to include AD patients in secondary-prevention trials or symptomatic treatment trials. With regard to fluid biomarkers, CSF amyloid beta ($A\beta$) accounts for A status, CSF hyperphosphorylated tau protein (specific phosphorylation at threonine 181 [p-tau$_{181}$]) accounts for T status, and for N, CSF total tau (t-tau) is used. This approach is to confirm that the target pathology or targets in the cascade of AD are present in the patients that are included in the trial. In the NIA–AA Research Framework criteria and in current clinical trial design, blood biomarkers such as plasma $A\beta_{40}$ or $A\beta_{42}$ and plasma p-tau$_{181}$ or p-tau$_{217}$ are not yet included as inclusion criteria; however, the rapid and substantial research in this field will speed up the implementation of these solid fluid AD biomarkers [7].

Fluid biomarkers are the future in Phase 2 clinical trials with disease-modifying therapies that aim to confirm biological/pharmacodynamic effect. In recent years, numerous publications have described novel CSF and blood biomarkers beyond the markers $A\beta$ and tau. A recent comprehensive overview has been published [8]. Almost in every target class using the Common Alzheimer's and Related Dementias Research Ontology (CADRO) [9] a potential outcome measurement can be selected for biological effect. CSF biomarkers, more than blood biomarkers, provide information that the investigational medical product has an effect on specific pathogenic processes directly in patients with AD.

Fluid biomarkers can also be used as safety-monitoring markers: an increase in inflammation (CSF cell count, immunoglobin G (IgG)/immunoglobin M (IgM) index, oligoclonal bands), the integrity of the blood–brain barrier (CSF/serum albumin ratio), or an increase in neurodegeneration (neurofilament light chain [NfL]). Using CSF as a surrogate for CNS exposure for drugs given orally or intravenously is not recommended due to the difference in barriers between the blood–CSF barrier and the blood–brain-barrier.

It is beyond the scope of this chapter to discuss the individual CSF/blood biomarkers in the field (see Table 12.1 for a short overview of current candidate CSF/blood biomarkers for amyloid, tau, inflammation, synapses, and neurodegeneration). An update on the current use of biomarkers in Phase 2 trials can be found in Cummings et al. [10].

Table 12.1 CSF/blood biomarkers in Phase 2 trials

Target class	Fluid	Biomarker
Amyloid		
	CSF/blood	$A\beta_{42}$, $A\beta_{40}$, $A\beta_{42}/A\beta_{40}$ ratio
Tau		
	CSF/blood	t-tau
		p-tau$_{181}$
		p-tau$_{217}$
		Other p-tau epitopes
Inflammation		
	CSF	Glial fibrillary acidic protein (GFAP)
		YKL40
	CSF/blood	Interleukin (IL)-1B, IL-2, IL-6, IL-8, IL-10, interferon gamma, and tumor necrosis factor alpha
Synapses		
	CSF/blood	Neurogranin
	CSF	Synaptotagmin
	CSF	Synaptosomal-associated protein 25 (SNAP-25)
	CSF	Growth associated protein 43 (GAP-43)
Neurodegeneration		
	CSF/blood	NfL
	CSF	Visinin-like protein-1 (VLP-1)

12.3.2 Neuroimaging Biomarkers

Neuroimaging in Phase 2 AD trials can be used for the selection of AD participants, as well as a pharmacodynamic marker or for safety monitoring. These biomarkers can be divided into structural imaging (MRI of the brain) and molecular imaging. Structural imaging is used for measuring neural loss or damage over time, inflammation, or other structural lesions such as edema or micro-hemorrhages. Molecular imaging represents the accumulation of neuropathological load, synaptic loss, or inflammation.

Theoretically, the selection of the correct AD population in a Phase 2 trial can solely be based on neuroimaging, since neuroimaging is well imbedded in the NIA–AA Research Framework criteria. As mentioned above in the fluid biomarker section, classification of the diagnosis of AD is based on the presence of amyloid (A+) and tau pathology (T+). For imaging, amyloid status can be measured by $A\beta$ positron emission microscopy (PET) imaging and T status by tau PET imaging. The N status can be ascertained by structural MRI (i.e., hippocampal volume, whole brain volume, or cortical thickness) or by using fluordeoxyglucose (FDG) PET. Choosing an imaging biomarker or a fluid biomarker is dependent on many external factors, such as costs, availability, number of patients, country, level of expertise, etc. In general, fluid and imaging biomarkers are interchangeable when it comes to the diagnostic performance, although discrepancies exist [11]. Especially when targeting very early $A\beta$ pathology there is some discussion surrounding which marker (CSF $A\beta$ or $A\beta$ PET) signifies the earliest changes [12].

Molecular imaging in Phase 2 studies is increasingly used when trying to confirm the biological effects of a therapeutic agent. The decision as to which PET ligand to include as the outcome strongly depends on the mechanism of action of the investigated medical product. As an example, measuring the effects of an anti-$A\beta$ therapy is probably best done by using an $A\beta$ PET ligand, as is seen in the elegant Phase 1b aducanumab study, in which a dose-dependent $A\beta$-lowering effect was seen on PET [13]. If the target is p-tau, a tau PET ligand is most suitable to be included as an outcome measure, although discussions around the exact way to measure changes over time are ongoing [14]. In addition, tau PET may be more informative than CSF p-tau in this respect because of the regional information, which may pertain to the mode of action [15]. Upcoming new PET ligands may be used in the near future to image other proteinopathies (TAR DNA-binding protein 43 [TDP-43] or alpha-synuclein), synaptic density (e.g., ^{11}C-UCB-J PET tracer), or for detecting microglial activation (translocator protein 18 KDa [TPSO] PET tracer).

Choosing FDG PET-scan or volume-based MRI measurements to measure neurodegeneration depends heavily on the perceived mechanism of action of the tested compound. FDG PET suffers from a lack of sensitivity to change over the period of time usually applied in Phase 2 [16]. MRI measurements have the great advantage of being a relatively standard procedure now, and may show changes much earlier than cognitive measures, which increases the power and reduces the number of patients needed to show an effect. In addition, MRI may yield regional information that can be informative on the mechanism of action of the compound tested, for instance when rate of hippocampal atrophy is selectively affected over whole brain atrophy, as in the LipiDiDiet study [17].

To monitor safety, MRI of the brain and/or spinal cord is used to find structural abnormalities or detect adverse events caused by the investigated medical product. As an example, in anti-Aβ monoclonal antibody trials, ARIA are observed and monitored and have proven to be the single most important side effect of the class of monoclonal anti-Aβ antibodies. In earlier trials using Aβ immunotherapy, MRI showed greater atrophy rates in the treated versus the placebo group and signs of active inflammation, causing great concern around this type of intervention. These examples underscore the significance for using MRI as a safety outcome.

Given the great interest and potential of antisense oligonucleotide therapies in AD, which need to be administered intrathecally, MRI of the brain and spine may be needed to study the anatomy beforehand and to measure CSF volume non-invasively, for pharmacokinetic purposes [18].

12.3.3 Electroencephalography

Although in previous decades EEG proved to be a sensitive technique for detecting effects of cholinergic treatment in AD patients, up until now it has not been employed often in amyloid-targeting pharmacotherapeutic trials [19]. This is surprising, since Aβ (oligomer) toxicity leads to neurophysiological changes such as hyperexcitability, synaptic failure, and neural circuit malfunction, before structural pathology such as neurodegeneration and plaque deposition become apparent [20, 21]. Ideally, one would be able to measure these early, direct functional changes, and the technique would be sensitive to quick, successful target engagement and restoration of neuronal activity. Neurophysiological techniques, with a more direct assessment of neuronal activity and a temporal resolution far superior to functional MRI, are therefore in principle the most appropriate. However, an important limit of human scalp EEG is its spatial resolution, which is confined to

capturing regional activity (±6 cm^2 per electrode in a routine set-up). EEG is therefore a macroscale assessment of neuronal circuit integrity, not of activity patterns of individual neurons or circuits (which can be recorded with invasive electrodes). However, for clinical purposes the performance of larger and anatomically distant neuronal assemblies is actually more important than the contribution of individual neurons or synapses. A second technical limit of EEG is that deeper sources like the hippocampus are very challenging to record reliably. Magnetoencephalography is able to do so, but does not have the obvious advantages of EEG in being very cost-effective and widely available [22]. Fortunately, as oscillatory disruption of the cortex in early AD is increasingly recognized, EEG is a suitable instrument for clinical trials in AD [23]. A further argument for using EEG is the relatively short time span of clinical trials (especially in Phase 2), in which substantial structural changes might not be expected, but functional neurophysiological changes as a response to treatment can happen within days to weeks, as we know from the classical cholinesterase studies. Commonly used quantitative EEG measures of resting-state data are sufficient to detect relevant therapeutic change in AD (see also Chapter 36 for a more detailed discussion of the use of EEG in AD drug trials). At present, an increase in relative theta (4–8 Hz) spectral power is regarded as the most sensitive oscillatory activity marker in the earliest stages of AD [24]. Besides regional activity patterns, long-range connectivity between cortical regions can be assessed. This is relevant because cognitive processing is heavily dependent on brain-wide communication, and so-called "functional connectivity" measures have been shown to be related both to cognitive performance and to AD pathophysiology [25]. Whether EEG connectivity measures can become powerful therapeutic markers, as well as enhance our understanding of cognitive failure in AD, is not yet clear, but is being investigated at the moment. An example of a recent Phase 2 study in which EEG was successfully employed is shown in Box 12.1.

The example in Box 12.1 is one of many Phase 2 trials employing EEG and it illustrates that straightforward quantitative EEG techniques can provide a direct, sensitive early marker of treatment effects targeting neuronal cortico-cortical disconnection. This makes it a promising instrument for Phase 2a trials in AD.

Box 12.1

A good example of the potential of EEG is the SAPHIR trial with the anti-oligomer drug PQ912 [26]. PQ912 blocks the production of pyro-glutamyl Aβ through inhibition of the quality control enzyme and this specific type of Aβ has been shown to effectively induce neurotoxicity, mediated by disrupting *N*-methyl-D-aspartic acid and calcium-channel function. The Phase 2a study that was conducted to provide biological support for the hypothesized PQ912 efficacy in counteracting cortico-cortical disconnection in prodromal to mild AD had an EEG resting-state assessment at baseline and at 12 weeks follow-up. *Stabilization* of relative theta power was found in the PQ912 treatment arm, whereas it *increased* in the placebo arm (see Figure 12.1). At 12 weeks, the power in the placebo group at slower frequencies (especially the theta frequency band)

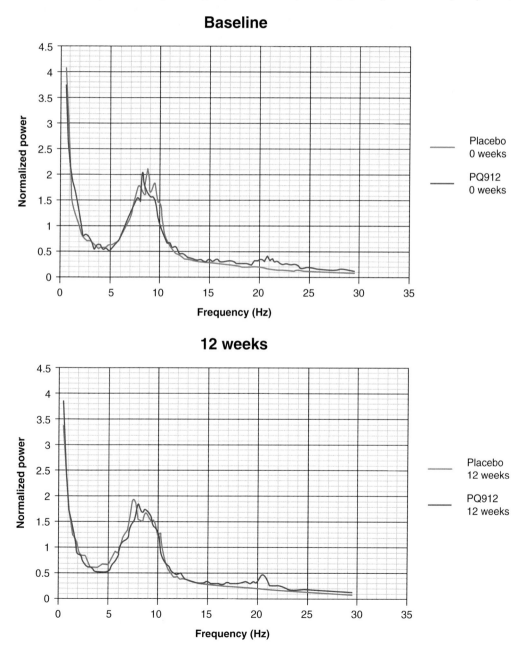

Figure 12.1 Average power spectra at baseline and after 12 weeks of PQ912 treatment.

Box 12.1 (cont.)

was higher compared to the PQ912 group, and the peak frequency had decreased. In contrast, the power spectrum of the PQ912 group remained stable. This indicates that pathological slowing of brain oscillatory activity, reflecting disease progression, occurred during the 12-week study period, and that within this short time span a beneficial treatment effect could be detected. Coupled with the significant reduction in glutaminyl cyclase activity, an average target occupancy of > 90%, and a significant improvement in a cognitive (executive function) test, this was a promising result, establishing that target engagement and efficacy conform with the perceived mechanism of action. Moreover, subsequent functional connectivity analysis showed a significant improvement of "healthy" alpha-band (8–10 Hz) connectivity patterns, which has not been shown before. Additional analyses that focused on "functional connectivity," namely interregional neuronal communication (for more detail see also Chapter 36), illustrated relevant improvements in the treatment group, indicating a novel way to track potentially beneficial effects on neuronal (and synaptic) function [27]. The size of the effect may appear to be modest, but it is important to realize that the only previous reporting of an improvement of brain activity patterns was in the clinical responder group of previous cholinesterase trials in the 1990s. Currently, a Phase 2b study is underway to evaluate the long-term effect of PQ912 by investigating persistent differences in theta power after the cessation of the treatment period. EEG markers are incorporated as a secondary endpoint in this Phase 2b study.

12.4 Clinical Outcomes

Slowing, halting, or possibly reversing cognitive decline is typically the key clinical endpoint in AD trials, hence outcome measures of cognition and daily functioning are used to explore clinical efficacy in Phase 2 trials [28]. Common guidance for the selection of clinical measurement instruments holds that selected measures should be reliable, valid, and ideally free from range restrictions in scoring (i.e., floor or ceiling effects) [29]. The optimal selection of measure(s) will also depend on the target population, as the nature as well as the rapidity of cognitive decline differs by clinical stage of AD [30]. Further, it is of crucial importance that outcome measures are chosen to match the mechanism of action, meaning the selection of cognitive and functional tests one would theoretically expect to decline as a result of the disease process (in the absence of a treatment effect).

Historically, the traditional clinical instrumentation for AD trials includes paper-and-pencil cognitive tests such as the Mini-Mental State Examination (MMSE) developed in 1975 [31], and the Alzheimer's Disease Assessment Scale – cognitive subscale (ADAS-cog) developed in 1984 [32], study-partner-based questionnaires assessing activities of daily living (ADL) functioning such as the Alzheimer's Disease Cooperative Study – ADL scale developed in 1997 [33], and global scales including elements of both cognitive and functional performance, such as the Clinical Global Impression of Change (CGIC) published in 1976 [34] or modified versions such as the more recently developed Clinical Dementia Rating – sum of boxes (CDR-sb) scale [35]. However, a challenge when employing these measures is the limited rate of change over time observed in individuals with the very earliest manifestations of AD, especially when the follow-up time interval is relatively short [36], which is usually the case in Phase 2 trials. For a more elaborate discussion the reader is referred to the chapter of Prof Harrison in this book (Chapter 24).

Moreover, the recent shift of the field toward secondary prevention has further urged the need for refined outcome measures capturing the more subtle cognitive changes that occur prior to overt dementia onset. Several endeavors have been undertaken to improve the measurement of clinical changes in early AD, particularly the design of composite measures such as the Preclinical Alzheimer Cognitive Composite [37], the Alzheimer's Prevention Cognitive Composite [38] for preclinical AD, and the Alzheimer's Disease Composite Score [39] and the Cognitive-Functional Composite [40] for prodromal to mild AD. Each of these composites combine multiple tests across cognitive domains that are relevant in early AD, which increase signal-to-noise ratio and thereby improve the detection of change over time. Still, a limitation of most of these measures is that decline is only observable at annual in-clinic testing [30] and the fact that large sample sizes are required to detect subtle cognitive decline, thereby requiring lengthy and large Phase 2 trials in order to provide accurate information about potential directional clinical effects.

Computerized cognitive testing has the potential to capture more fine-grained performance information with improved sensitivity than paper-and-pencil measures. Digital scoring software can capture accuracy and speed simultaneously as well as reduce administration and scoring errors, and thereby further increase the signal-to-noise ratio over repeated measurements [41]. Also, by applying computerized adaptive algorithms, everyday functioning questionnaires can be personalized, only asking the questions relevant to the individuals' level of functioning [42, 43]. An additional advantage of computerized testing is that it allows for remote assessment (i.e., at an individual's home), enabling more frequent and rapid assessments (i.e., daily/monthly instead of yearly) while reducing participant and rater burden by avoiding lengthy in-clinic assessments [44], and facilitating the inclusion and monitoring of larger samples in a cost-effective manner. Several studies have already indicated the feasibility and utility of computerized test batteries for clinical trials of AD [45–48]. Validation of these novel techniques against current gold-standard measures and biomarkers of AD pathology is crucial to moving these potentially more efficient and cost-effective measures from research to clinical trials.

In sum, time has not stood still in the development of new ways of monitoring clinical outcomes, which outperform the classic ADAS-cog, as the new techniques are more sensitive to cognitive changes observed in the earlier phase of the disease. These new methods offer better psychometric properties as well as covering a broader spectrum of cognitive abilities that may individually be targeted by an intervention.

12.5 The Role of Phase 2 Trials in the AD Drug-Development Ecosystem

As mentioned above, well-conducted Phase 2 studies are an essential element in drug development for AD and provide several crucial pieces of information: target engagement, dose–response range, and downstream biological effects [5]. However, the importance of an early indication of a clinical effect should not be underestimated. A principal factor in the failure of Phase 3 trials in patients with mild-to-moderate AD in the past 15–20 years is the lack of Phase 2 clinical data prior to entering Phase 3, as biomarker results alone were commonly relied upon [49]. Regularly, sponsors tended to initiate a full Phase 3 program based solely on evidence of target engagement in small Phase 2 studies. The imperfect association observed to date between biomarkers and clinical effects in Phase 3 clinical trials renders this a very high-risk approach [49]. As such, AD trial experts are increasingly aware that there should be hints, or consistent signals, of efficacy that are in concordance with the biomarker signals, before a Phase 3 trial can be initiated.

The very low rates of agents successfully passing Phase 2 and 3 clinical trials have caused the biopharmaceutical industry to be somewhat hesitant to invest in AD (clinical) programs. This hesitant attitude has been further maintained by a lack of drug diversity. Historically, the Phase 2 pipeline predominantly contained either disease-modifying agents targeting amyloid pathology or cognitive-enhancing agents. However, learnings from the past drug failures, increased global recognition of the AD pandemic by governments and the public, and the exponential growth of scientific knowledge in AD over the last two decades (~3,300 AD-related publications in PubMed in 2000, ~6,900 in 2010, and ~13,700 in 2020), further fueled by increased funding from the NIA in the United States, have culminated in an expanded and radically diversified AD drug pipeline.

This positive development is very well captured by the current Phase 2 pipeline. For example, the number of agents in Phase 2 clinical trials has increased by 44%, from 45 in 2016 to 65 in 2020 [10, 50]. Further, the proportion of disease-modifying agents increased from 30/45 (67%) to 55/65 (85%). Even more important, the proportion of disease-modifying agents targeting amyloid pathology decreased from 43% to 15% during this period, as these are being replaced by agents targeting novel biological pathways that play a role in the AD pathophysiology. The Phase 2 pipeline has further benefitted from technological advances in other diseases, exemplified by the development of a tau-targeting antisense therapy by Ionis Pharmaceuticals and Biogen, the first of its kind in AD. We expect a further translation of antisense and other gene therapies in the near future to Alzheimer's, as these therapies have proven to be successful in several other (neurological) diseases [18].

As a result of the growth and diversification of the number of clinical AD agents, and the development of novel therapies that are increasingly applied in AD, the AD drug-development pipeline nowadays looks very promising and represents significant value [51]. Consequently, the AD field is increasingly attractive for the biopharmaceutical industry, as demonstrated by several recent multibillion deals, such as the $2.37 billion licensing agreement between Biogen and Sangamo that allows Biogen to develop Sangamo's novel gene therapy for AD and other tauopathies, and Eli Lilly's $1.04 billion acquisition of gene-therapy player Prevail Therapeutics, developing therapies for AD and other neurodegenerative diseases.

12.6 Lessons Learned by Phase 2 Programs for AD Drug Development

Every failed trial, or even a successful trial, provides learnings for the future development of drugs for AD. Many of the issues in drug development and trial learnings have been extensively studied in Cummings et al. [3]. With respect to Phase 2 clinical trials in AD and the issues discussed in this chapter, a few lessons can be summarized as follows.

- **AD diagnosis should be supported by biomarkers**. Especially in Phase 2 where numbers of patients are often small, all patients should have the underlying pathology that the drug needs to act on. A+ T+ from the ATN framework secures that the patients have AD pathology. Further to that, one is at liberty to add cognitive measures to narrow down the severity spectrum, or to make sure a level of cognitive decline is present (and that there is an increased likelihood of decline over a shorter period). Or one may add certain MRI, EEG, or biofluid biomarkers measures to pre-specify certain characteristics of the group (certain ratings of medial temporal lobe atrophy, presence of alpha slowing, p-tau levels); in fact, the availability of all the possibilities mentioned in this chapter allows an adequate grouping of patients to be studied with a specific compound according to its mechanism of action. In Phase 2 there is no such thing as "one size fits all."
- **Ensure target engagement**. As seen in the example in Box 12.1, it is possible even in a short time period of 3 months to assert target engagement on a biomarker level (reduction of the targeted enzyme in the CSF), EEG level (as an indication that synaptic function indeed changed a function of the intervention), and

even cognitive level (using very sensitive attention and memory tasks, related to synaptic function and completely in line with the expected mechanism of action). This was enough for the "go" decision, and in absence would have argued strongly for a "no-go" decision. Results of Phase 2b trials are awaited to further strengthen the signals obtained in Phase 2a.

- **Small steps; do not skip proper Phase 2**. Finding a final dose, establishing a proper dose response, and evidencing target engagement are all within the scope of Phase 2, and are needed to advance to Phase 3. To quote Cummings [3] "drug formulation decisions should be completed in Phase 2 prior to Phase 3." An example of this lesson can be seen in the development program of aducanumab. In the Phase 1b study, a small sample (166) of patients were offered placebo and four different dosages (1, 3, 6, and 10 mg/kg) [13]. A nice dose–response relationship (target engagement) was noted on Aβ PET, but not very convincingly on CDR-sb. A logical next step would have been to design a Phase 2 study, with two–three times the number of patients, a selection of two dosages, adapted to apolipoprotein-E ε4 (*APOE-4*) carriership, selection of sensitive cognitive outcomes, gathering safety data related to dose and *APOE-4* status, etc. However, this phase was skipped and two large Phase 3 studies were started with, yet unpublished, but reportedly different outcomes cognitively and functionally, while target engagement was again established. The latter was the reason for accelerated approval by the FDA on June 7, 2021, under the condition that clinical effects need to be proven in additional trials. Partially failed expensive Phase 3 programs and the need for additional trials could perhaps have been prevented by taking the time to conduct a proper Phase 2. An expensive learning.
- **There is more in life than ADAS and MMSE**. The new classes of drugs that have been developed and tested, including monoclonal antibodies, gamma-secretase modulators, gamma-secretase inhibitors, beta-site amyloid precursor protein cleaving enzyme (BACE) inhibitors, receptor for advanced glycation end products (RAGE) inhibitors, nicotinic agonists, 5-hydroxytryptamine 6 (5HT6)

antagonists, and others, have all used the ADAS-cog as the primary scale to determine efficacy, leading to failure in most programs. Despite numerous advances in cognitive testing as detailed above, it is striking to see how many sponsors stick to these old tests, as if they were the gold standard in testing outcomes, even in very mildly affected individuals. A frequently heard argument is that "these are required by registration authorities." Nothing is less true. The FDA put out a new position statement in 2018 informing the field on possible considerations for demonstrating efficacy to open the path for approval. For a review and discussion on this topic see Sabbagh et al. [52]. All the examples they indicate are mentioned above in this chapter for further guidance. Especially in Phase 2, one needs to adapt the testing and outcome measures to the mechanism of action and the perceived target! As mentioned earlier, there is no size that fits all, and this holds true especially for cognitive tests.

12.7 Conclusion

Well-conducted Phase 2 studies are an essential element in drug development for AD and provide several crucial pieces of information: target engagement, dose–response range, downstream biological effects, and hints or proof of a clinical effect. A proper Phase 2 trial is the foundation for a successful Phase 3 program. The future for drug development in AD looks bright, since all the instruments to conduct a meaningful Phase 2 program are in place, while funding and research output is steadily increasing and appetite from the investment community is on the rise as well. The five rights for drug development [5] can be used as a "cookbook" and are especially relevant for designing and conducting Phase 2 programs. As long as sponsors are willing to abide to the rights and also are able to kill drugs that do not survive Phase 2, there is a chance that new drugs for AD will come to the market in the next decade.

References

1. Blass BE. *Basic Principles of Drug Discovery and Development*. Boston, MA: Academic Press; 2015.

2. Yuan J, Pang H, Tong T, et al. Seamless Phase IIa/IIb and enhanced dose-finding adaptive design. *J Biopharm Stat* 2016; **26**: 912–23.

3. Cummings J, Ritter A, Zhong K. Clinical trials for disease-modifying therapies in Alzheimer's disease: a primer, lessons learned, and a blueprint for the future. *J Alzheimers Dis* 2018; **64**: S3–22.

4. Jack CR Jr., Bennett DA, Blennow K, et al. NIA–AA Research Framework: toward a biological definition of Alzheimer's disease. *Alzheimers Dement* 2018; **14**: 535–62.

5. Cummings J, Feldman HH, Scheltens P. The "rights" of precision drug development for Alzheimer's disease. *Alzheimers Res Ther* 2019; **11**: 76.

6. Bauer P, Kieser M. Combining different phases in the development of medical treatments within a single trial. *Stat Med* 1999; **18**: 1833–48.

7. Scheltens P, De Strooper B, Kivipelto M, et al. Alzheimer's disease. *Lancet* 2021; **397**: 1577–90.

8. Molinuevo JL, Ayton S, Batrla R, et al. Current state of Alzheimer's fluid biomarkers. *Acta Neuropathol* 2018; **136**: 821–53.

9. National Institute on Aging, Alzheimer's Association. *International Alzheimer's and Related Dementias Research Portfolio: Common Alzheimer's and Related Dementias Research Ontology (CADRO)*. Bethesda, MD: National Institutes of Health; 2020.

10. Cummings J, Lee G, Ritter A, Sabbagh M, Zhong K. Alzheimer's disease drug development pipeline: 2020. *Alzheimers Dement (N Y)* 2020; **6**: e12050.

11. de Wilde A, Reimand J, Teunissen CE, et al. Discordant amyloid-β PET and CSF biomarkers and its clinical consequences. *Alzheimers Res Ther* 2019; **11**: 78–84.

12. Reimand J, Boon BDC, Collij LE, et al. Amyloid-β PET and CSF in an autopsy-confirmed cohort. *Ann Clin Transl Neurol* 2020; **7**: 2150–60.

13. Sevigny J, Chiao P, Bussière T, et al. The antibody aducanumab reduces Aβ plaques in Alzheimer's disease. *Nature* 2016; **537**: 50–6.

14. Golla SS, Wolters EE, Timmers T, et al. Parametric methods for ^{18}[F]flortaucipir PET. *J Cereb Blood Flow Metab* 2020; **40**: 365–73.

15. Wolters EE, Ossenkoppele R, Verfaillie SCJ, et al. Regional ^{18}[F]flortaucipir PET is more closely associated with disease severity than CSF p-tau in Alzheimer's disease. *Eur J Nucl Med Mol Imaging* 2020; **47**: 2866–78.

16. Scheltens NME, Briels CT, Yaqub M, et al. Exploring effects of souvenaid on cerebral glucose metabolism in Alzheimer's disease. *Alzheimers Dement (N Y)* 2019; **5**: 492–500.

17. Soininen H, Solomon A, Visser PJ, et al. 36-month LipiDiDiet multinutrient clinical trial in prodromal Alzheimer's disease. *Alzheimers Dement* 2021; **17**: 29–40.

159

18. Bennet CF, Krainer AR, Cleveland DW. Antisense oligonucleotide therapies for neurodegenerative diseases. *Annu Rev Neurosci* 2019; **42**: 385–406.

19. Babiloni C, Blinowska K, Bonanni L, et al. What electrophysiology tells us about Alzheimer's disease: a window into the synchronization and connectivity of brain neurons. *Neurobiol Aging* 2020; **85**: 58–73.

20. Busche MA, Chen X, Henning AH, et al. Critical role of soluble amyloid-β for early hippocampal hyperactivity in a mouse model of Alzheimer's disease. *Proc Natl Acad Sci USA* 2012; **109**: 8740–5.

21. Palop JJ, Mucke L. Network abnormalities and interneuron dysfunction in Alzheimer disease. *Nat Rev Neurosci* 2016; **17**: 777–92.

22. Engels M, Hillebrand A, van der Flier WM, et al. Slowing of hippocampal activity correlates with cognitive decline in early onset Alzheimer's disease. An MEG study with virtual electrodes. *Front Hum Neurosci* 2016; **10**: 238.

23. van Straaten EC, Scheltens P, Gouw AA, Stam CJ. Eyes-closed task-free electroencephalography in clinical trials for Alzheimer's disease: an emerging method based upon brain dynamics. *Alzheimers Res Ther* 2014; **6**: 86–92.

24. Gouw AA, Alsema AM, Tijms BM, et al. EEG spectral analysis as a putative early prognostic biomarker in nondemented, amyloid positive subjects. *Neurobiol Aging* 2017; **57**: 133–42.

25. Rossini PM, Di Iorio R, Vecchio F, et al. Early diagnosis of Alzheimer's disease: the role of biomarkers including advanced EEG signal analysis. Report from the IFCN-sponsored panel of experts. *Clin Neurophysiol* 2020; **131**: 1287–310.

26. Scheltens P, Hallikainen M, Grimmer T, et al. Safety, tolerability and efficacy of the glutaminyl cyclase inhibitor PQ912 in Alzheimer's disease: results of a randomized, double-blind, placebo-controlled Phase 2a study. *Alzheimers Res Ther* 2018; **10**: 107–12.

27. Briels CT, Stam CJ, Scheltens P, et al. In pursuit of a sensitive EEG functional connectivity outcome measure for clinical trials in Alzheimer's disease. *Clin Neurophysiol* 2020; **131**: 88–95.

28. Food and Drug Administration. *Early Alzheimer's Disease: Developing Drugs for Treatment. Guidance for Industry*. US Department of Health and Human Services Food and Drug Administration Center for Drug Evaluation and Research (CDER) Center for Biologics Evaluation and Research (CBER); 2018.

29. Prinsen CA, Vohra S, Rose MR, et al. How to select outcome measurement instruments for outcomes included in a "core outcome set": a practical guideline. *Trials* 2016; **17**: 449.

30. Jutten RJ, Sikkes SAM, Amariglio RE, et al. Identifying sensitive measures of cognitive decline at different clinical stages of Alzheimer's disease. *J Int Neuropsychol Soc* 2020; **27**: 1–13.

31. Folstein MF, Folstein SE, McHugh PR. "Mini-mental state". A practical method for grading the cognitive state of patients for the clinician. *J Psychiatr Res* 1975; **12**: 189–98.

32. Rosen WG, Mohs RC, Davis KL. A new rating scale for Alzheimer's disease. *Am J Psychiatry* 1984; **141**: 1356–64.

33. Galasko D, Bennett D, Sano M, et al. An inventory to assess activities of daily living for clinical trials in Alzheimer's disease. *Alzheimer Dis Assoc Disord* 1997; **11**: S33–9.

34. Guy W. *Clinical Global Impressions. ECDEU Assessment Manual for Psychopharmacology – Revised*. Rockville, MD: US Department of Health, Education, and Welfare, Public Health Service, Alcohol, Drug Abuse, and Mental Health Administration, National Institute of Mental Health, Psychopharmacology Research Branch, Division of Extramural Research Programs; 1976: 218–22.

35. Williams MM, Storandt M, Roe CM, Morris JC. Progression of Alzheimer's disease as measured by Clinical Dementia Rating Sum of Boxes scores. *Alzheimers Dement* 2013; **9**: S39–44.

36. Evans S, McRae-McKee K, Wong MM, et al. The importance of endpoint selection: How effective does a drug need to be for success in a clinical trial of a possible Alzheimer's disease treatment? *Eur J Epidemiol* 2018; **33**: 635–44.

37. Donohue MC, Sperling RA, Salmon DP, et al. The Preclinical Alzheimer Cognitive Composite: measuring amyloid-related decline. *JAMA Neurol* 2014; **71**: 961–70.

38. Langbaum JB, Hendrix SB, Ayutyanont N, et al. An empirically derived composite cognitive test score with improved power to track and evaluate treatments for preclinical Alzheimer's disease. *Alzheimers Dement* 2014; **10**: 666–74.

39. Wang J, Logovinsky V, Hendrix SB, et al. ADCOMS: a composite clinical outcome for prodromal Alzheimer's disease trials. *J Neurol Neurosurg Psychiatry* 2016; **87**: 993–9.

40. Jutten RJ, Harrison JE, Brunner AJ, et al. The cognitive-functional composite is sensitive to clinical progression in early dementia: longitudinal findings from the Catch-Cog study cohort. *Alzheimers Dement (N Y)* 2020; **6**: e12020.

41. Reimers S, Stewart N. Presentation and response timing accuracy in Adobe Flash and HTML5/JavaScript web experiments. *Behav Res Methods* 2015; **47**: 309–27.

42. Bilder RM, Reise SP. Neuropsychological tests of the future: how do we get there from here? *Clin Neuropsychologist* 2019; **33**: 220–45.

43. Sikkes SA, Knol DL, Pijnenburg YA, et al. Validation of the Amsterdam IADL Questionnaire©, a new tool to measure instrumental activities of daily living in dementia. *Neuroepidemiology* 2013; **41**: 35–41.

44. Gold M, Amatniek J, Carrillo MC, et al. Digital technologies as biomarkers, clinical outcomes assessment, and recruitment tools in Alzheimer's disease clinical trials. *Alzheimers Dement (N Y)* 2018; **4**: 234–42.

45. Buckley RF, Sparks KP, Papp KV, et al. Computerized cognitive testing for use in clinical trials: a comparison of the NIH toolbox and Cogstate C3 batteries. *J Prev Alzheimers Dis* 2017; **4**: 3–11.

46. Rentz DM, Dekhtyar M, Sherman J, et al. The feasibility of at-home iPad cognitive testing for use in clinical trials. *J Prev Alzheimers Dis* 2016; **3**: 8–12.

47. Koo BM, Vizer LM. Mobile technology for cognitive assessment of older adults: a scoping review. *Innov Aging* 2019; **3**: igy038.

48. Sliwinski MJ, Mogle JA, Hyun J, et al. Reliability and validity of ambulatory cognitive assessments. *Assessment* 2018; **25**: 14–30.

49. Gray JA, Fleet D, Winblad B. The need for thorough Phase II studies in medicines development for Alzheimer's disease. *Alzheimers Res Ther* 2015; **7**: 67.

50. Cummings J, Morstorf T, Lee G. Alzheimer's drug-development pipeline: 2016. *Alzheimers Dement (N Y)* 2016; **2**: 222–32.

51. Cole MA, Seabrook GR. On the horizon: the value and promise of the global pipeline of Alzheimer's disease therapeutics. *Alzheimers Dement (N Y)* 2020; **6**: 1–9.

52. Sabbagh M, Hendrix S, Harrison JE. FDA position statement "early Alzheimer disease: developing drugs for treatment, guidance for industry". *Alzheimers Dement (N Y)* 2019; **5**: 13–19.

Alzheimer's Disease Drug Development in Pharmaceutical Companies

Eric Siemers, Robert A. Dean, James E. Senetar, Janice M. Hitchcock, and Russell L. Barton

13.1 Introduction

The development of disease-modifying treatments for Alzheimer's disease (AD) has clearly been a challenge for all stakeholders in AD [1, 2]. These stakeholders include patients and caregivers most importantly, and also a variety of researchers trying to advance the science of AD in order to develop better treatments. Researchers in AD can be broadly divided into four categories – researchers in university settings, researchers in government settings, researchers in non-profit organizations, and researchers in the pharmaceutical industry. Each of these groups brings specific strengths and areas of expertise, yet it is increasingly clear that only with broad collaboration between these groups can meaningful advances be realized. This chapter focuses on efforts of the pharmaceutical industry, with the realization that all of these stakeholders, including patients and caregivers, play a crucial role in ultimate successes.

Within the pharmaceutical industry, efforts to discover and develop novel treatments for AD are being made by organizations ranging from small virtual biotech organizations to large multinational pharmaceutical companies [3]. Within this spectrum of pharmaceutical drug developers, an interplay exists that is not dissimilar to the interplay between university-based, government-based, and non-profit-based organizations with large pharmaceutical companies. Regarding small biotech companies, an important inflection point occurs when sufficient data on a drug candidate are generated that a large multinational pharmaceutical company might express interest in partnering or acquiring it. Large pharmaceutical companies may have drug-development resources that smaller biotech companies do not have; however, true innovation may occur in even the smallest of biotech companies. Some biotech companies take an alternate route and continue development of their drug candidate independently, through additional external investment or filing an initial public offering. Large pharmaceutical companies have their own drug discovery efforts within the company, which can provide early drug candidates for the company in a way similar to the role of biotech companies and universities, which can also generate drug candidates. In fact, many universities now spin out small biotech companies to play just such a role.

13.2 Drug Development and Clinical Trials in Pharmaceutical Companies

13.2.1 Drug-Development Strategy and Process

Drug development is a long and complex process that involves many individuals and, frequently, many organizations. The starting point is often a novel idea for a new target that might be "druggable." After generating positive in vitro or in vivo animal model data based on the hypothesis, a nascent lead molecule (small molecule or biologic) can be identified. The lead molecule may have potency only in the micromolar range, but then must be optimized to nanomolar or even picomolar potency as well as selectivity for its biological target. Non-clinical safety then must be demonstrated, ultimately in toxicology studies that are compliant with good laboratory practice (GLP). Based on pharmacokinetic/pharmacodynamic studies, GLP toxicology studies, and margin of safety calculations, an Investigational New Drug (IND) submission can be made to the US Food and Drug Administration (FDA) (for a proposed clinical trial in the USA) or other regulatory authority (for a proposed clinical trial in another country).

After the FDA allows an IND to go into effect in the United States, or other approvals outside the United States, a Phase 1 trial can be undertaken. A Phase 1 "first-in-human" (FIH) study must emphasize safety as the primary outcome. For AD drugs, especially monoclonal antibodies, increasingly patients rather than healthy volunteers are included in FIH studies, and biological target engagement measures are often utilized. Usually, these FIH studies will include single ascending dose (SAD) and multiple ascending dose (MAD) components. Following a Phase 1 study demonstrating safety and evidence of target engagement, Phase 2, Phase 3, or adaptive Phase 2/3 studies can be considered.

For AD and other neurodegenerative diseases, the design of a traditional Phase 2 study has been problematic. Clinical efficacy measures for AD and other neurodegenerative diseases generally require several hundred subjects per arm to achieve statistical powering, with studies generally lasting 18 months or longer. The size, cost, and conduct of such studies is historically consistent with Phase 3 registration trials. Given these challenges, novel Phase 2 and Phase 3 designs have been suggested, including Phase 2/3 seamless adaptive designs. Considerations for designs of Phase 2 and 3 studies are discussed further below.

13.2.2 Requirements of Large Pharmaceutical Companies Doing Due Diligence

When projects originated at a small biotech company are being considered for partnering or acquisition by a large pharmaceutical company, a key point in this transition is aligning on the answer to "What amount of data is enough?" to justify the investment. Not surprisingly, frequently there is a disconnect between what a small biotech company or university may think is "enough" and the large pharma expectation. In the vast majority of cases, large pharmaceutical companies are publicly traded on stock exchanges, meaning that the companies have a fiduciary obligation to shareholders in addition to their mission to advance science in a way that will ultimately be beneficial to patients. Thus, the large pharmaceutical companies are obligated to perform complex estimations of probabilities of success, and weigh those against development costs and potential future revenue. A small change in probability of success at the beginning of a development plan can make large changes in probabilized future revenues. Thus, a large pharmaceutical company will greatly value data from a small biotech company that will increase the

ultimate probability of success, but they will also need to discount value when data packages are deemed insufficient for the phase of development of the asset.

13.2.3 Operational Considerations in Drug Development

Operational considerations are also important in the transition from university/biotech/small-pharma to large-pharma development. Large pharmaceutical companies may have internal resources to perform Phase 2 and large Phase 3 studies, but these operational responsibilities are increasingly being outsourced to contract research organizations (CROs). CROs may be as large as some large pharmaceutical companies, and as such have considerable resources to implement clinical trials. Regardless of whether a large pharmaceutical company works with a CRO or implements trials with internal resources, the ability of a large pharmaceutical company to implement Phase 2 and large Phase 3 trials is an important component of drug development.

An important alternative to the model of a large pharmaceutical company working with a large CRO is the possibility of a pharmaceutical company working with non-profit or university-based organizations that may provide many of the capabilities of large CROs. Typically, these research organizations focus on a particular disease state. Although the possibility to utilize these research organizations for Phase 3 studies should be acknowledged, these organizations have proven their value in implementing exploratory Phase 2 studies. Examples of such research organizations for neurodegenerative diseases include the Alzheimer's Therapeutic Research Institute, Alzheimer's Disease Cooperative Study, Parkinson Study Group, and the Huntington Study Group.

13.2.4 The Role of Data Safety Monitoring Boards in Drug Development

Data safety monitoring boards (DSMBs, aka data monitoring committees and other similar names) play an important role in any clinical trial, but their importance in Phase 2 and especially Phase 3 trials has increased. A DSMB is a group of independent experts who are not employees of the sponsor of the trial. Monitoring safety has always been the core function of a DSMB; in some cases, the DSMB has access to unblinded safety data but no efficacy data. This situation is particularly likely for Phase 1 and Phase 2 studies.

163

For Phase 3 trials that a pharmaceutical company may be implementing, the DSMB has increasingly been given multiple responsibilities, which may involve evaluation of efficacy data. First, the DSMB may be charged with a determination of futility for a clinical trial that has not yet reached completion. A broad consensus for the statistical definition of futility has not been reached, and thus trials may be stopped for futility only to later find that further review of efficacy data supported a positive drug effect. A recent, much-debated example of this situation eventually resulted in an FDA accelerated approval of the first novel treatment for AD in more than a decade [4, 5] (see also Section 13.2.5). Futility analyses are sometimes desired by sponsors since a declaration of futility could reduce the costs and duration of a study that is not likely to succeed, could decrease participant exposure to a drug that may not be efficacious, and does not require a statistical penalty (an "alpha spend") in the analysis. Nevertheless, the value of futility analyses has been debated, in part given that while they can be defined for individual sponsors and studies, there is not a general consensus on statistical criteria for futility. Conversely, a DSMB may be given responsibility for an interim analysis that could be used to stop a study for overwhelming efficacy, thus saving time in development and potentially bringing an efficacious treatment to patients sooner. However, such an interim analysis does require an "alpha spend," which means that if overwhelming efficacy is not demonstrated, a higher statistical hurdle for efficacy (beyond the traditional $p < 0.05$) will be necessary to declare that the study is positive at the conclusion of the trial. Another major potential limitation of an interim analysis that stops a study for efficacy is that a smaller amount of safety and efficacy data is obtained than if the trial had been completed. In addition, a false-positive interim result could occur, meaning that a drug without efficacy could be declared efficacious.

Taken together, these developments mean that a DSMB may be required not only to play a traditional role in evaluating safety, but could also be called into the evaluation of outcomes more closely linked to important drug-development decisions. If a trial is declared futile, or is declared overwhelmingly positive based on an interim analysis, most sponsors will unblind a small number of people in senior management to review the recommendations of the DSMB. Thus, the role of the DSMB has evolved so that it not only ensures safety of the study participants but also may provide recommendations for a study that are likely of financial interest to the sponsor.

13.2.5 Regulatory Considerations in AD Drug Development

Regulatory strategy and interactions with regulators play key roles in AD drug development by pharmaceutical companies, large or small. Advice from regulators regarding a drug-development plan is typically sought by pharmaceutical companies at multiple times throughout a drug's life cycle: prior to the initial clinical trial, when important clinical results become available, when development issues arise, prior to pivotal clinical trials to support registration, and prior to submission of a marketing application. Until the recent FDA accelerated approval of aducanumab for the treatment of AD, the development of drugs that target underlying AD pathophysiology and thus may affect the disease course (potential disease-modifying drugs) brought regulatory challenges in part because of the lack of regulatory precedent for approval of such treatments. Regulators addressed some of these challenges by issuing or updating guidelines on AD drug development. Guidelines and recommendations from the FDA [6], European Medicines Agency (EMA) [7], and Japan's Ministry of Health, Labour, and Welfare (MHLW)/Pharmaceuticals and Medical Devices Agency (PMDA) [8] are not fully aligned with each other, but share many similarities [9]. They provide clear advice to be considered as a pharmaceutical company develops its AD drug registration strategy, including decisions on when to approach regulators with proposals that may not be endorsed specifically in the guidance. Regulatory guidelines from all three regions encourage the development of novel clinical measures for early stages of AD, although novel measures have not yet been used as primary endpoints in pivotal registration trials. Regulators have been open to novel design features for AD trials, including platform trials that assess more than one drug, adaptive trials that use interim analyses to adjust parameters such as dose levels, or delayed-start trials, which compare drug effects in groups that start active drug treatment at the beginning or later in the trial. Definition of the trial population (especially early AD stages) and the associated primary endpoint measure to demonstrate a clinically meaningful effect in that population are key considerations that require discussion and negotiation with regulators prior to conducting the large, lengthy trials needed to support registration of a potential disease-modifying treatment for AD.

The recent controversial FDA approval of aducanumab has opened a potential regulatory pathway not previously used for AD drugs. Aducanumab was approved under the accelerated approval pathway, in which a drug that addresses an unmet medical need in a serious disease is approved based on a surrogate marker that is reasonably likely to predict clinical benefit [10]. This pathway allows earlier access to the drug for patients and, importantly, requires a post-marketing confirmatory trial to verify the clinical benefit. The FDA can withdraw the approval if a clinical benefit is not demonstrated. The FDA's accelerated approval of aducanumab was based on reduction of brain amyloid plaque as a surrogate marker; the FDA acknowledged uncertainty regarding the clinical benefit. Clinical outcomes, both positive and negative, as well as additional biomarkers, were considered in the decision [11]. Based on this precedent, both positive surrogate biomarker data and supportive clinical data would likely be needed for a sponsor to propose accelerated approval of an AD treatment. The FDA's guidance on expedited regulatory pathways [10] recommends that sponsors considering the accelerated approval pathway for any disease indication consult with the FDA regarding the proposed endpoints and data package for submission.

Discussion of the scientific and regulatory implications of the aducanumab accelerated approval continues in the AD research field. Importantly, regulators are also part of the AD research community, and participate in AD scientific conferences with academic and industry researchers and patient/caregiver advocacy groups to discuss scientific advances and regulatory policies that affect AD drug development.

13.2.6 The Role of "Key Opinion Leaders"

"Key opinion leaders" (KOLs) are frequently but not always university-based researchers, who provide advice on a variety of topics to pharmaceutical companies. An important role for KOLs is acting as an "outside set of eyes" to review drug-development plans within a pharmaceutical company. Within a pharmaceutical company or any other organization, the possibility of "groupthink" is real, and a review by a group of KOLs can help mitigate this possible risk. KOLs may have input at many stages of drug development. An early point when KOLs can be utilized is to review non-clinical data on a drug candidate and the strategy before entering the clinic. KOLs may provide more specific input into clinical trial design and protocol development. A group of KOLs who remain blinded to treatment assignment may provide operational input to the conduct of a clinical trial, especially if the trial is large and multinational. Finally, KOLs may provide advice prior to the launch of a new drug on how the drug could be best utilized in clinical practice based on its safety and efficacy.

The topic of data sharing is beyond the scope of this chapter since it applies not only to pharmaceutical clinical trial data but also to many other data sets. Increasingly, KOLs are utilized to provide independent or collaborative analyses of large clinical trial data sets with the pharmaceutical sponsor. Such independent or collaborative analyses can play an important role in the presentation of results at scientific conferences and in the writing of scientific manuscripts for publication.

13.3 Commercialization Activities in Pharmaceutical Companies

13.3.1 Preparing for Launch and Marketing Strategies

Preparing for the launch of a new drug and formulating the marketing strategy to be employed is a large body of work that can only be summarized here. The marketing strategy is largely related to specifics regarding the drug; this includes the realization that a drug requiring administration by specialists will be very different than the strategy for a drug intended to be prescribed by primary care physicians. Given that several monoclonal antibodies are in development for AD currently, these provide examples of some of the complexities involved in developing launch strategies. While the need for intravenous infusions and infusion clinics is common in oncology, and has developed for patients with multiple sclerosis, a broad infrastructure for infusions does not yet exist for patients with AD and other neurodegenerative diseases. Given such a situation, early adopters of a new monoclonal antibody given by intravenous infusion are likely to be top-tier KOLs (generally university-based neurologists) at tertiary referral centers with access to existing infusion facilities. Regional KOLs (either university-based or practiced-based) might subsequently have sufficient interest to establish an infusion clinic. Given the clinical utility of the antibody, large neurology practices might then establish infusion clinics. For general neurologists and certainly for primary care physicians, establishment of infusion clinics is unlikely. In this case, establishing referral systems from general neurologists and primary care physicians to organizations that have incorporated infusion clinics will be important.

Most monoclonal antibodies in development target individuals with mild cognitive impairment or mild dementia due to AD, and these early stages of the disease are likely to be underdiagnosed. Therefore, a rapidly evolving area of research is how to identify and diagnose patients earlier in the disease. Cognitive screening might be combined with blood-based biomarkers to determine the need for positron emission tomography (PET) studies or cerebrospinal fluid (CSF) analyses to assess for the presence of amyloid pathology. Ultimately, PET or CSF data are likely to be needed to begin treatment with monoclonal antibodies, but given that PET and CSF are expensive or invasive, cognitive screening and blood biomarkers would be useful to enrich the sample of people with suspected AD pathology prior to PET or CSF testing.

13.3.2   Payer Relationships

As noted above, payer relationships are important for a company launching a drug to be able to realize maximum value of the asset for the company. Payer perspectives vary by country, but some general themes are present.

In the United States, many payers are present in the form of insurance companies, although for those over 65 years of age who are Medicare recipients, the system in the United States is similar to other countries with government funding for healthcare costs. In the United States, the Centers for Medicare and Medicaid Services (CMS) determines national guidelines for reimbursement, which are provided to regional CMS centers. An example of the importance of CMS policy decisions for AD is related to reimbursement of amyloid PET scans. In 2013, the CMS determined that amyloid PET scans (in this case specifically for the first

FDA-approved ligand, florbetapir) did not meet the criteria for CMS reimbursement and needed further study to investigate how the results of the test contribute to the determination of patient treatment [12]. That CMS decision led to limited use of florbetapir PET scans in practice, given the out-of-pocket payments which would be required. CMS is likely to again evaluate amyloid PET scans for reimbursement now that a disease-modifying AD treatment has received accelerated approval, as PET scans may be needed to identify patients most likely to benefit from the treatment. While the reimbursement decision for florbetapir PET scanning was related to a diagnostic agent, similar considerations and decisions could be related to an AD therapeutic.

Countries with nationalized health services typically have agencies which evaluate the cost/benefit of new drugs. For example, in the United Kingdom, the National Institute for Health and Care Excellence provides guidance on reimbursement for healthcare which is generally accepted by the National Health Service. Similar government organizations exist in France (Transparency Committee), Germany (Institute for Quality and Economics in Healthcare), and many other countries. The fact that in the European Union the EMA provides approval of a drug, but each individual country determines pricing, is important to note. Because drug-approval decisions are based on medical science without regard to pricing considerations, in many countries the agencies to determine reimbursement are separate from the regulatory agencies responsible for drug approval. Thus, the topic of payer relationships in a global development program is extremely complex.

13.3.3   Advertising by Pharmaceutical Companies

Advertising by pharmaceutical companies is a controversial topic, with different opinions held by different stakeholders. Direct-to-consumer advertising is forbidden in most countries. Various targeted audiences may be sought, including prescribers and consumers.

Advertising to prescribers is not dissimilar to sales representatives detailing to prescribers, although the activities involved differ substantially. In the past, most advertising to potential prescribers took the form of print advertisements in medical journals. With journals now increasingly online, this model may need to change somewhat. Detailing to potential prescribers by sales representatives who are employees of a pharmaceutical company has changed in recent years, and likely will continue to change. Many university-based clinics no longer see sales representatives at all. Potential prescribers in private practice may still see sales representatives, although these interactions are highly regulated. All information discussed must be contained in the package insert label, and anything provided by the sales representative of value (e.g., lunch) must be disclosed in the United States as provided in the Sunshine Act of 2010.

Direct-to-consumer advertising regarding specific drugs is permitted in only two countries, the United States and New Zealand. While most individuals are familiar with the reading of a long list of potential adverse events required by the FDA in advertising in the United States, these commercials are used extensively and, barring major changes in regulatory requirements, may continue.

The use of websites to market a particular drug is relatively new but increasingly common. These websites typically have an area for healthcare professionals (which generally contains the package insert) as well as an area for the general public. Claims made on websites are subject to regulatory review.

13.3.4 Meetings and Symposia

Meetings and symposia are generally administered by the medical organization within a pharmaceutical company, and thus are not considered advertising. Especially for a drug with a relatively recent launch, these meetings and symposia may increase awareness of the drug's safety and efficacy by potential prescribers. If thoughtfully organized around a specific scientific topic or question, meetings and symposia may provide important scientific information and discussions.

13.3.5 Role of Scientific Liaisons

The scientific-liaison position has been used increasingly by the pharmaceutical industry, and some important differences between scientific liaisons and sales representatives should be noted. Scientific liaisons are typically part of the medical rather than sales organizations. As their focus is on medical and scientific data, they are permitted to discuss both on-label and off-label use of a drug with a clinician. Frequently, scientific liaisons are most utilized for newly launched drugs, and they may play a role in developing Phase 4 studies that address scientific questions not answered at the time of launch.

13.4 Intellectual Capital: Where Do Pharmaceutical Personnel Come from and How Are They Identified?

An important consideration in drug development broadly is where does the human intellectual capital arise. Undergraduate or graduate degrees in various components of drug development (e.g., pharmacology, toxicology, medicinal chemistry) do exist, but comprehensive knowledge of drug development, including clinical trial design, is typically gained through experience. Senior positions in large pharmaceutical companies can be filled through internal promotion or by recruitment of senior individuals in university-based positions or government positions (e.g., the National Institutes of Health). Some mid-career individuals in university-based programs have also entered pharma. Less common is an individual who has completed medical training and moves directly to a pharmaceutical company.

There are numerous positions within pharmaceutical companies that require a terminal degree, including positions for individuals with medical training (MDs) and for those with basic science training (PhDs). Individuals with PhDs more commonly enter the pharmaceutical sector directly, while individuals with MDs more frequently initially have university positions or are in clinical practice.

An important consideration with regard to intellectual capital is that a very large skill set is required to take a novel idea for a therapeutic, then generate fundamental basic science supporting the hypothesis, then find lead molecules that can be optimized, then optimize those drugs for safety and efficacy, then translate the non-clinical data to clinical trial designs, then design early-phase clinical studies focused initially on safety, then cross the Phase 2 abyss, and then finally conclude a successful Phase 3 study. Few, if any, individuals on the planet incorporate all those skills, which means that joining together intellectual capital is a necessity for successful drug development, especially in the field of AD.

167

13.5 Conclusions: The Role of Pharmaceutical Companies in the Ecosystem of AD Drug Development

As noted elsewhere, the ecosystem of drug development for AD is a system of interacting organizations that broadly can be considered as based in universities, government agencies, non-profit organizations, and pharmaceutical companies. Pharmaceutical companies are diverse, especially considering that the size of the company may range from a small biotech to a large multinational corporation. Each of these types of organizations may play important roles in the long pathway from the initial concept of a new drug mechanism to a marketed treatment for AD becoming available to patients. The role of each type of organization is influenced in part by the incentives for each type of organization. For example, lead optimization, pharmacokinetic analyses, and toxicology studies are very important aspects leading up to the introduction of a drug in clinical trials. These types of studies, however, are not frequently published in the scientific literature (although perhaps they should be), making university-based researchers less likely to pursue these areas of research. University-based researchers and government agencies can provide essential conceptual advances that are readily published. Non-profit organizations, assuming sufficient funding, can also play a critical role in filling in gaps in research that advance the field in important aspects, and thus provide value to their donors.

Although not strictly linear, a frequent scenario is that a concept for a new drug may arise from a pharmaceutical company discovery research group, a university-based researcher, a government agency, or a small biotech company. If from the latter three, at some point the development program is often partnered with a large pharmaceutical company and progressed through an IND application to the FDA and Phase 1 and perhaps Phase 2 trials. With later clinical development in Phase 2 and Phase 3 trials, university-based researchers may again become more involved, usually in their roles as KOLs. In addition to the substantial funding of clinical trials by large pharma, non-profit organizations and government agencies may provide funding for clinical trials conducted by small biotechs. Thus, successful drug development is likely to take not just a village, but a vibrant city composed of a variety of organizations and individuals all working to the same goal of better treatments for AD.

References

1. Siemers E. Drug development in AD: point of view from the industry. *J Prev Alzheimers Dis* 2015; **2**: 216–18.

2. Cummings J, Ritter A, Zhong K. Clinical trials for disease-modifying therapies in Alzheimer's disease: a primer, lessons learned, and a blueprint for the future. *J Alzheimers Dis* 2018; **64**: S3–22.

3. Rinaldi A. Setbacks and promises for drugs against Alzheimer's disease: as pharmaceutical companies are retreating from drug development for Alzheimer's, new approaches are being tested in academia and biotech companies. *EMBO Rep* 2018; **19**: e46714.

4. Biogen. Biogen plans regulatory filing for aducanumab in Alzheimer's disease based on new analysis of larger dataset from Phase 3 studies. *Investor Relations* 2019; Oct. 22. Available at: https://investors.biogen.com/news-releases/news-release-details/biogen-plans-regulatory-filing-aducanumab-alzheimers-disease (accessed January 2021).

5. Food and Drug Administration. FDA's decision to approve new treatment for Alzheimer's disease. Available at: www.fda.gov/drugs/news-events-human-drugs/fdas-decision-approve-new-treatment-alzheimers-disease (accessed June 2021).

6. Food and Drug Administration. *Early Alzheimer's Disease: Developing Drugs for Treatment Guidance for Industry*. US Department of Health and Human Services Food and Drug Administration Center for Drug Evaluation and Research (CDER) Center for Biologics Evaluation and Research (CBER); 2018.

7. European Medicines Agency. Clinical investigation of medicines for the treatment of Alzheimer's disease: CPMP/EWP/553/1995. Available at: www.ema.europa.eu/en/documents/scientific-guideline/guideline-clinical-investigation-medicines-treatment-alzheimers-disease-revision-2_en.pdf (accessed January 2021).

8. Pharmaceuticals and Medical Devices Agency (PMDA). Project to promote the development of innovative pharmaceuticals, medical devices, and regenerative medical products (Ministry of Health, Labour, and Welfare) regulatory science research for the establishment of criteria for clinical evaluation of drugs for Alzheimer's disease. Available at: www.pmda.go.jp/files/000221585.pdf (accessed January 2021).

9. Morant AV, Vestergaard HT, Lassen AB, Navikas V. US, EU, and Japanese regulatory guidelines for development of drugs for treatment of Alzheimer's disease: implications for global drug development. *Clin Transl Sci* 2020; **13**: 652–64.

10. Food and Drug Administration. Expedited programs for serious conditions: drugs and biologics, May 2014. Available at: www.fda.gov/regulatory-information/search-fda-guidance-documents/expedited-programs-serious-conditions-drugs-and-biologics (accessed June 2021).

11. Food and Drug Administration. Summary memorandum. Available at: www.accessdata.fda.gov/drugsatfda_docs/nda/2021/Aducanumab_BLA761178_Dunn_2021_06_07.pdf (accessed June 2021).

12. Centers for Medicare and Medicaid Services. Decision memo for beta amyloid positron emission tomography in dementia and neurodegenerative disease (CAG-00431N). Available at: www.cms.gov/medicare-coverage-database/details/nca-decision-memo.aspx?NCAId=265 (accessed January 2021).

Chapter 14

Trial Site Infrastructure and Management: Importance to Alzheimer's Disease Drug Development

Marwan Sabbagh, Jiong Shi, Philip Scheltens, and Niels Prins

14.1   Introduction

Novel drugs are urgently needed for the clinical treatment of Alzheimer's disease (AD). Over 30 have failed in Phase 3 in the past two decades [1] but over 75 are still in development [2]. Most drug discovery and development, either in commercial or academic organizations, moves from the laboratory, to the preclinical safety and toxicology studies, to the investigational new drug (IND) filing, to clinical trials in human subjects. With over 5 million Americans affected and over 50 million worldwide [3], the need for drugs that have a meaningful impact on AD symptoms, quality of life, and disease trajectory will continue to grow. Each phase of a clinical trial (Phases 1–3) has different demands from a regulatory standpoint, but also from a trial-site perspective. In fact, there is a sub-specialization of site activities. Phase 1 sites, geared for first-in-human studies and safety studies because of their focus on healthy volunteers and generic services, are not suited for Phase 3 AD studies that require access to AD patients and specialistic knowledge of the disease. Drug development does follow a prescribed path even if the mechanism of action differs from drug to drug.

14.2   Contribution of Sites to AD Drug Development

As explained below, there is a prescribed structure with the sponsor, contract research organization (CRO), and the performance site. Depending on the "DNA" and focus of the trial site, its staff may contribute to the design, protocol, or regulatory documents. At a minimum, sites provide feedback on processes to the sponsor or CRO. Therefore, the contribution of performance sites to drug development should not be understated. These sites are responsible for (1) hiring, training, and retaining high-quality personnel; (2) recruiting qualified participants into the clinical trials; (3) following the institutional review board (IRB) approved protocols, completing any trial-specific training, performing study visits and prescribed assessments, and capturing and entering high-quality data into the electronic data capture systems; and (4) quality control measures, performed in conjunction with an independent monitor. Without the sites providing high-quality data gathered from subjects and meeting the specified criteria, there is little chance of success. This might be a contributing factor to the poor success rate of drugs developed for AD.

This chapter emphasizes both public and private aspects of AD drug development, since federal funding in the United States drives much early-stage AD drug discovery, and private funding and biopharmaceutical companies drive much of the late-stage development and commercialization of compounds.

14.3   Trial Sites

The execution of a clinical trial takes place at the trial site. The trial site is the central place where trial participants go, often accompanied by their study partners, to undergo their trial visits. During each visit, a number of assessments take place as defined by the trial protocol. In a single-center trial, all trial participants are from the same trial site. In a multi-center trial, the trial data are collected from participants from multiple trial sites. A large global multi-center AD trial typically recruits patients from over a hundred different trial sites, each having their unique site number and own principal investigator (PI). Trial sites may be situated within an academic hospital or may be private institutions. They may stand alone or as part of a trial-site network.

14.3.1 Types of Trial Sites: Academic Hospitals Versus Independent Commercial Sites

Different types of trial sites exist. Some trial sites may be located within larger institutions such as academic hospitals and memory clinics. Other sites are independent commercial organizations. Sites that are situated within a large academic hospital have the advantage of access to the existing infrastructure of the hospital: treatment rooms, imaging facilities, laboratory, pharmacy, and electronic health record systems. In case of a calamity, the hospital provides access to a crash team and high care or intensive care unit. With regard to patient recruitment, these sites may recruit trial participants from their own patient flow and databases because most academic hospitals have large medical and neurological practices with hundreds of patients with AD and other dementias to draw from.

A potential challenge for trial sites within hospitals is that running trials is not the main function of a hospital organization. Hospitals are organized primarily around patient care and academic research that is investigator initiated and usually government funded. Commercial clinical trials, sponsored by pharmaceutical or biotech companies, are not the primary focus of academia, which could lead to potential inefficiencies that may become apparent during the phase of budget and contract negotiations, recruitment, and trial management. Further, investigators are not rewarded with advancement or promotion when they are investigators on pharma-sponsored randomized controlled trials (RCTs), thereby providing a disincentive for participation of physician faculty. Further compounding physician/investigator engagement is the second disincentive – compensation. Almost all physicians in academic centers are on salary. Thus, they do not receive additional compensation of clinical trial activity, since such activity is considered within the scope of practice and work. Another drawback may be the mix of roles as treating physician and trialist, which may be confusing for both the patient and the clinician.

When situated within a large hospital, many different departments are involved in budget and contract processes, thus potentially negatively impacting turnaround times. Academic medical centers tend to have protracted negotiation and IRB times. Also, clinical tasks of members of the trial team that compete with the trial work may distract from patient recruitment, which, in turn, may lead to a lower number of screenings and randomizations.

Independent commercial trial sites are specifically organized for the function of effective trial management and aggressive recruitment. Since trial management is their core business, their people, processes, and systems are tailored to running clinical trials. For these sites, owning and maintaining trial infrastructure is relatively expensive, and they may therefore choose to subcontract external parties for part of the trial infrastructure (e.g., imaging, laboratory, and pharmacy facilities). Participants may be recruited by referral to the site by surrounding memory clinics, or the site may use direct-to-participant recruitment strategies. Commercial sites tend to rely heavily on advertisement. Trial sites not affiliated with (independent) memory clinics and unable to tap into existing patient flow may face an additional challenge, as they are dependent on outside referrals. The dependence on advertisement and referrals has an inherent disadvantage. If a commercial trial site is not the treating physician provider, then the site is dependent on the records provided to determine eligibility and appropriateness. Further, many clinical trial sites perform several different types of clinical trials and may lack the expertise for neurological diseases such as AD and other dementias. In addition, the financial incentive may overshadow quality, resulting in high screen failure rates.

14.4 Organization

AD clinical trials are complex projects that come with a large amount of interactions between the trial site and different stakeholders (participants, sponsors, CROs, vendors, hospital departments, etc.). Therefore, trial sites require a clear and effective organizational structure in order to run the trials successfully. Various organizational aspects can be identified and summarized into three pillars: processes, people (staff), and systems.

14.4.1 Processes

A distinction can be made between the primary and secondary processes of a clinical trial. The primary process consists of study start-up, participant recruitment, prescreening, screening, randomization, study visits, and end of study. In the paragraphs below, we will describe the primary processes of AD trials in more detail.

In addition to the primary process, secondary, or support, processes are needed. These are human resource management, ICT, finance, legal, and marketing/communication. The support processes can be regarded as overhead. Depending on the level of organization of the site, each process is as clearly described as possible, and roles and responsibilities are defined. Depending on whether the site is part of a larger institution or an independent organization, the support processes of the institution can be used, or support needs can be organized independently.

Processes are essential in the identification and selection of trials. In many cases, CROs keep lists of performance sites. When a sponsor contracts with a CRO, the CRO provides the sponsor with a list of performance sites for the sponsor to review. Once the sites list is finalized, the CRO reaches out to the sites to complete a site qualification visit (SQV). At the SQV, the CRO reviews the site capabilities, infrastructure, access to ancillary services, and the experience of the investigator.

Processes are also important from the site, particularly in identifying trials and assessing trial feasibility. Investigator experience is a key factor of these two components of a trial. Sites that have successfully enrolled in previous studies are contacted by the CROs repeatedly. Those who have met their contracted targets, had few protocol deviations/violations, and have adequately addressed monitor queries are generally of particularly high interest. The investigator, when identifying the suitability of a study, should consider: (1) Is the science behind the compound of high quality? (2) Is the study feasible to perform? (3) Does the study cover the costs of the staff? (4) Is the relationship with the sponsor or consortium important? (5) Does the investigator have access to the subjects required to complete the study? The last consideration is of particular relevance, because the investigator might have the target population but lack the infrastructure (space, lumbar punctures, imaging) to complete the study successfully.

Interacting with CROs is an essential component in site selection, which is the responsibility of CROs. They contact the sites to complete the SQV, which then certifies that a site is eligible, appropriate, and experienced in conducting the proposed study. The CRO surveys the qualifications and experience of the investigator and the infrastructure to complete the study visits. CROs rely on monitor reports from previous studies to determine whether the sites are likely to be successful. We would argue that the central or the local PI has an important responsibility as well, since he/she knows the field better and may know all of the investigators personally.

Another responsibility of the CRO is to review the personnel at the performance site. The CRO determines whether the site personnel have adequate training and certification and what additional training would be necessary to complete the protocol under consideration. In many cases, additional training is required. Experience and training of the site personnel is of the utmost importance.

14.4.2 Staff

The study team is the core of the trial site organization and is responsible for the primary process of the trial. This team consists of a PI, sub-investigator (sub-I), clinical research coordinator (CRC), and clinical raters. The PI is a medical doctor who heads the clinical team and is, from a good clinical practice perspective, responsible for the trial projects. In AD clinical trials, often the PI is a "key opinion leader" (KOL) in the dementia field and often has a background in neurology, geriatrics, or psychiatry, although this expertise is not a prerequisite. He or she fulfills the PI task, often assisted by a sub-I, a medical doctor to whom some of the PI tasks can be delegated and who often fulfills the day-to-day medical tasks in the trial, such as performing the physical and neurological examination and initial reviewing of medical tests results and adverse events (AEs) and serious adverse events (SAEs). Most protocols require that two physicians are on the study. One reviews AEs and SAEs and the other serves as a backup and carries out some of the required physician-focused examinations.

Another important role in the study team is fulfilled by the CRC. The CRC can be a registered nurse or another healthcare professional with the relevant skill set, training, and credentials. The CRC is responsible for the day-to-day activities of each study or trial. She/he is the linchpin between the PI and sub-I and the trial participants as well as representatives from the sponsor or CRO side, such as the clinical research assistant who performs the monitoring. The coordinator reviews the protocol for the schedule of visits, schedules participants for the study visits, consents participants with the supervision of the PI or sub-I, and conducts study related activities, including vitals, ECG, lab draws etc. The CRC also meets with the monitors, collects source documents, ensures electronic case report forms (CRFs) are filled, responds to the study, and ensures all training and certifications of the investigative team are current and documented.

In AD trials, clinical raters are also important members of the trial team, since they are responsible for rating the neuropsychological tests and other rating scales. Raters can be broken into two categories. One group comprises the global raters for the Clinical Dementia Rating (CDR) [4], Clinical Global Impression of Change (CGIC) [5], Clinician Interview-Based Impression of Change (CIBIC) [6], or activities of daily living (ADL) scales. Another group performs the psychometric tests: the Alzheimer's Disease Assessment Scale – cognitive subscale (ADAS-cog) [7], Dementia Rating Scale [8], Severe Impairment Battery (SIB) [9], or other cognitive tests required according to the protocol.

In addition to the core staff mentioned above, other staff members also play an important role. First is the site manager, who is responsible for interacting with the sponsor and CRO, completing the site qualification surveys, and receiving and processing the study package from the sponsor and CRO. They are also responsible for getting the protocol and informed consent form (ICF) to the regulatory coordinator for IRB submission and for overseeing the budget negotiations. They are also responsible for ensuring that the site is reimbursed for services that are complete and for reviewing the budget.

The regulatory coordinator is responsible for the IRB submission. Their responsibilities include filling out the IRB application, ensuring the protocol and ICF are complete for submission, ensuring the regulatory documents such as the US Food and Drug Administration (FDA) form 1572 are current and logged, and responding to the IRB. They are also responsible for filing regular reports to the IRB and for the submission of the study closeout. They interact with the sponsor and CRO about regulatory issues and IRB-generated queries.

Another possible position that can support a robust clinical trials program is a recruitment coordinator. Although it is not one of the core positions, it is very helpful. The recruitment coordinator is the first point of contact between the participant, the investigator, and the rest of the staff.

The recruitment coordinator can provide the ICF to the subject, schedule a screening visit, and notify the coordinator of a potential enrollee. The recruitment coordinator will be the contact when there is an advertisement or announcement regarding the trial. He/she can work with the PI, sponsor, and CRO on the advertisements to maximize return on investment. The recruitment coordinator can also mine databases of existing patients for eligibility and review the potential eligible participants with the PI for suitability.

14.4.3 Systems

Clinical trials do not occur in vacuums and are unlikely to be successful in an individual physician's office unless they have access to the personnel summarized in this chapter, the experience in dementia to identify and select potential participants, and the trial resources that are often required, such as MRI, positron emission tomography (PET), lumbar puncture, lab draws, etc. If the physician needs to subcontract lumbar punctures and imaging, the radiology center needs to be covered by the same IRB and certified in the study procedures. It is more advantageous to have the trial resources within the institution.

Current clinical trials have significant use of radiological services, such as PET and MRI. MRI can be used for three elements: screening for eligibility to rule out mass, cerebrovascular accidents, or normal pressure hydrocephalus; volumetric assessments as outcome measures; AE monitoring (e.g., amyloid-related imaging abnormalities). Current MRI protocols often require a phantom scan that is read centrally. PET scans can be used for amyloid imaging, fluorodeoxyglucose (FDG) PET, or tau PET, depending on the protocol for eligibility of target pathology and for proxy measures of efficacy. All imaging in clinical trials is exported for central processing, reading, and AE monitoring.

14.5 Study Start-Up

After the contract is signed, the IRB is approved, the staff have been trained, the imaging center has completed the qualification imaging, and the investigator meeting has taken place, the CRO can initiate a site by a site initiation visit. At this visit, the monitor reviews the protocol with the staff and activates the site. Then, screening and enrollment can begin.

173

14.5.1 Participant Recruitment

Participant recruitment is vital to the success of any RCT. Many academic medical centers have large medical and neurological practices that can be queried for potential eligible subjects as part of the prescreening process.

Other options include direct-to-physician letters, bulletins in local Alzheimer's Association newsletters, email blasts to physician communities, print advertisement, site management organizations (SMOs), or registries. Usually, the yield of expense to enrolled subject is low. SMOs are contracted by CROs to do national campaigns (website, call center, social media, etc.) that can screen eligible participants calling a central number and directing eligible participants to sites nearby the subject. Earned media (news articles and press releases) often have far higher yields of potential participants than paid media.

In recent times, registries have emerged as potential recruitment tools. These include healthybrains.org, https://hersenonderzoek.nl/, brainhealthregistry.org, and www.endalznow.org. Their advantage is that after the initial investment, they can be powerful tools to increase awareness and screen potential participants for studies with the ability to complete intake and notify study staff. They have been successful for many recent prevention and treatment trials.

14.5.2 Prescreening

Prescreening can start with the recruitment coordinator (if one is available) or the coordinator. The staff will select a few core inclusion/exclusion criteria (target condition: AD, mild cognitive impairment, normal control, etc.), age, and health conditions to identify potential subjects that might be suitable. One of the most common exclusions is pacemakers because of MRI incompatibility. After the prescreening list is culled and potential subjects are identified, the coordinator can review the list with the PI or sub-I for suitability. The coordinator or recruitment coordinator calls the potential participant and informs them of the study. In many cases, they have been notified about research or the particular study in advance. If the participant continues to express interest, they are scheduled for a screening visit.

14.5.3 Screening

Informed consent is usually provided to the participant in advance of the screening visit. During the screening visit, the ICF is reviewed with the coordinator and PI so that questions can be answered. Many studies require the participant to have a legally authorized representative (LAR) to sign with the study subject. Prior to signing the ICF, the study staff member explains all the study procedures, the risks and benefits, and alternatives to the study. Once the ICF is signed by the subject and LAR, screening can continue. This process includes screening for eligibility according to the inclusion/exclusion criteria, screening using the Mini-Mental State Examination or Montreal Cognitive Assessment, ascertainment of concomitant medications, review of medical history and medical records, and a screening medical examination. If there are laboratory tests to be drawn or imaging to be acquired, they are scheduled or completed during the screening phase.

14.5.4 Randomization

Randomization occurs at the baseline visit. By that time, the subject has completed all procedures from the screening visit and continues to meet eligibility. The protocol usually dictates that baseline cognitive testing (e.g., ADAS-cog, etc.) and global assessments (e.g., CDR, CGIC, etc.) are completed, and the study drug is usually dispensed at this visit. If the participant receives an infusion protocol (e.g., monoclonal antibodies against amyloid or tau), then the first infusion is performed at the baseline visit. Randomization is prescribed by the protocol (1:1, 2:1, etc.). Investigators and study staff are blinded to the treatment assignment.

14.5.5 Study Visits

Study visits are performed per protocol. Some are for AE monitoring, drug dispensing, concomitant medication surveillance, and examination of the participant. Some are for an assessment of outcome measures. Every protocol is different and follows a schedule of visits. Some study visits involve the investigator, coordinator, and rater but some involve the coordinator only. Most are in person, but some safety visits can be conducted telephonically per protocol.

The conduct of the protocol includes trial monitoring. Independent monitors from the sponsor or CRO visit the sites regularly and will review the CRF documentation and source documents from the study visits for completeness and in compliance with guidelines. The monitor will pose queries to the site regarding the monitor visits. Sites are required to respond to queries and file reports with the IRB on a regular basis.

Assessment and data capture (paper or electronic) are provided by the sponsor. Currently, many of the data are captured during the visit on tablet versions of the CRFs so that they can be transmitted and quality controlled immediately after the visit.

AE monitoring is one of the most important responsibilities of the study staff and is a requirement of all clinical trials. All trials create detailed procedures to monitor for AEs and SAEs. An SAE is hospitalization or death. All SAEs are required to be reported to the sponsor, CRO, and IRB within 24 hours. AEs can be quite broad and varied, and investigators are asked to attribute severity or causality to the investigational product. AEs are expected to be followed to resolution.

14.5.6   End of Study

The end-of-study visit can occur in two ways. First, the all-study visits are completed according to the schedule of visits. At the end-of-study visit, subjects usually undergo final cognitive and global assessments. Second, an end-of-study visit might be triggered by subject withdrawal. This can occur for three reasons, including an SAE that prompted the investigator to withdraw the subject, the subject or LAR withdraws consent, or the subject is lost to follow-up. After the end of study is completed, the coordinator should ensure that all electronic CRFs are completed and all queries for the monitor are addressed.

14.6   Site Contribution to the AD Drug-Development Ecosystem

The AD drug-development ecosystem is vast and complex. The individual site is the backbone of clinical trials because subjects and data are derived from enrolled participants at the sites. Ascertainment of quality data is critical to the success in determining the efficacy of drugs and devices. At face value, each site may contribute little to the drug development. However, as a whole, they can provide important feedback through sharing of best practices.

Clinical trials come to investigators through either industry or CROs or by federally funded academic trials. Academic trials may or may not have patent protection of the intellectual property

but might serve the public interest even without a clear path to profitability. Individual investigators can take either industry or academic trials, but most academic trials tend to take place at academic medical centers.

To boost recruitment and efficiency, trial networks have been created. These networks include the Alzheimer's Clinical Trials Consortium, the Alzheimer's Disease Cooperative Study, the European Prevention of Alzheimer Dementia, the Global Alzheimer's Platform, and the Dominantly Inherited Alzheimer's Network. They can offer RCTs to sites or provide sites to sponsors, National Institutes of Health, and other funding bodies and the CROs or can act as a CRO themselves.

14.7   Lessons Learned for AD Drug Development from the Site Perspective

The current structure of clinical trials is regimented with very little feedback from the sites to the sponsors, networks, or CROs. Individual sites face several challenges. First, clinical trials and clinical trial volumes ebb and flow, financially straining individual sites to maintain staff, especially if they are idle during down times. One solution is to create pools of qualified staff (like locum tenens) that are certified by the sponsor to complete study visits.

Second, a saying exists in clinical trials that 70% of enrollment comes from 30% of sites. CROs and trial networks should drop chronically underperforming sites (per monitor reports) and invest more in higher-performing sites. Quality will consequently improve, and, by not investing in sites or investigators that cannot enroll sufficient qualified subjects, efficiency might improve as well. The third challenge is cultural. Commercial sites are incentivized by profitability, which motivates them to enroll more participants. Academic medical centers do not have similar motivations. Compounding this challenge, academic medical centers do not reward investigators that do clinical trials as scholarly activity unless trials are investigator initiated, providing no incentive for academic clinicians to perform clinical trials. The remedy must be within the academic departments. One solution could be to house a commercial site organization inside an academic or general hospital, drawing on the advantages of both types of organization.

175

The fourth challenge is the need for reducing the redundancy of training and certification without compromising on data quality. This issue is serious and should be resolved by a joint effort of the networks mentioned above, sponsors, and CROs.

The fifth challenge is that centralized monitoring of raters and ratings is necessary to minimize variability and improve the homogeneity of data quality. Vendors such as MedAvante and Signant are specialized in meeting this need, and benefits have been shown. Not all investigators are satisfied with this process, but in our view it is essential to increase data quality.

The sixth challenge is related to the COVID-19 pandemic. Sites are required to postpone or prioritize clinical trials in order to provide more safety and social distance to subjects, especially healthy controls. Given the arrival of vaccination programs, hopefully COVID-19 will be under control soon. This challenge also provides us with an opportunity to boost tele-medicine. Remote digital assessment is urgently needed to facilitate AD trials.

References

1. Oxford AE, Stewart ES, Rohn TT. Clinical trials in Alzheimer's disease: a hurdle in the path of remedy. *Int J Alzheimers Dis* 2020; **2020**: 5380346.

2. Cummings J, Lee G, Ritter A, Sabbagh M, Zhong K. Alzheimer's disease drug-development pipeline: 2020. *Alzheimer Dement (N Y)* 2020; **6**: e12050.

3. Alzheimer's Association. 2020 Alzheimer's disease facts and figures. *Alzheimers Dement* 2020; **16**: 391–460.

4. Morris J. Clinical Dementia Rating: a reliable and valid diagnostic and staging measure for dementia of the Alzheimer type. *Int Psychogeriatr* 1997; **9**: 173–6.

5. Schneider LS, Olin JT, Doody RS, et al. Validity and reliability of the Alzheimer's Disease Cooperative Study–Clinical Global Impression of Change. The Alzheimer's Disease Cooperative Study. *Alzheimer Dis Assoc Disord* 1997; **11**: S22–32.

6. Reisberg B, Ferris SH, de Leon MJ, Crook T. The global deterioration scale for assessment of primary degenerative dementia. *Am J Psychiatry* 1982; **139**: 1135–9.

7. Rosen WG, Mohs RC, Davis KL. A new rating scale for Alzheimer's disease. *Am J Psychiatry* 1984; **141**: 1356–64.

8. Monsch AU, Bondi MW, Salmon DP, et al. Clinical validity of the Mattis Dementia Rating Scale in detecting dementia of the Alzheimer type. A double cross-validation and application to a community-dwelling sample. *Arch Neurol* 1995; **52**: 899–904.

9. Panisset M, Roudier M, Saxton J, Boller F. Severe Impairment Battery. A neuropsychological test for severely demented patients. *Arch Neurol* 1994; **51**: 41–5.

Chapter 15

ATRI and ACTC: Academic Programs to Accelerate Alzheimer's Disease Drug Development

Paul S. Aisen, Rema Raman, Michael S. Rafii, Reisa A. Sperling, and Ronald C. Petersen

15.1 Background and History

The first small, problematic study suggesting that Alzheimer's disease (AD) is treatable was published in 1986 by investigators at the University of California Los Angeles [1]. A larger, much more robust academic multi-center trial of the same compound, tacrine, was published in 1992 [2]. The tacrine efforts utilized design elements, outcome measures, and a regulatory plan that arose from intense interest and commitment from university investigators, funders, and regulators to bring effective AD therapies into clinical use. This work demonstrated the feasibility of this aim and led to major commitments from the pharmaceutical industry to develop AD drugs. As a result, the concept of co-primary outcome measures to demonstrate benefit on the primary cognitive symptoms of disease and global or functional benefit to establish clinical meaningfulness was widely adopted, and the Alzheimer's Disease Assessment Scale – cognitive subscale (ADAS-cog) [3] proved to be a useful measure of the primary cognitive manifestations of the disease. Approval of modestly effective symptomatic drugs, cholinesterase inhibitors, and memantine occurred between 1997 and 2003. The value of academic innovation funded by the National Institutes of Health (NIH) and other agencies in driving this international effort was clear. The National Institute on Aging (NIA) built on this early success by funding the Alzheimer's Disease Cooperative Study (ADCS), a collaboration among 35 academic centers in the United States, to continue to innovate in AD trial science and test candidate therapies [4].

The mission of the ADCS was to design and conduct AD studies that would not otherwise be pursued by the pharmaceutical industry, focusing on therapeutics that were repurposed or not patent-protected. Over time, the ADCS broadened its scope to include partnerships with small and large pharmaceutical and biotechnology companies. The NIA encouraged public–private partnership arrangements to take advantage of academic innovation and trial sites in addition to the most promising therapeutics developed by industry. The ADCS pursued ideas based on epidemiology and on basic laboratory science, examining therapeutics including vitamins [5–8], anti-inflammatory drugs [9, 10], hormones [11], statins [12], non-pharmacological interventions [13] and new chemical entities [14] (Table 15.1). Major milestones accomplished included the development and refinement of outcome measures, design and completion of the first pre-dementia trial [8], and

Table 15.1 Selected therapeutic strategies evaluated in academic AD trials

Agent	Class
Prednisone	Anti-inflammatory
Rofecoxib	Anti-inflammatory
Naproxen	Anti-inflammatory
Estrogen	Endocrine
Vitamin E	Antioxidant
Donepezil and vitamin E in mild cognitive impairment	Cholinesterase inhibitor; supplement
Vitamin E in aging individuals with Down syndrome	Supplement
Simvastatin	Statin
B vitamins	Supplement targeting homocysteine reduction
Docosahexaenoic acid	Antioxidant
RAGE (receptor for advanced glycation end products) inhibition	Amyloid-targeted and anti-inflammatory
Intravenous immunoglobulin	Amyloid-targeted; polyclonal antibody

the incorporation of genetic and biomarker measures into trial designs [8]. For biomarker work, the ADCS collaborated closely with the Alzheimer's Disease Neuroimaging Initiative (ADNI) [15], another large NIA-funded collaboration (with substantial industry contributions) to optimize and standardize biomarker measures, and to share its deeply phenotyped data set widely in near real time. The ADCS and ADNI together played a central role in academic and industry efforts to move beyond the initial symptomatic drugs to find effective disease-slowing therapies for AD.

15.2 Alzheimer's Therapeutic Research Institute (ATRI)

In 2015, investigators who had been working together at the ADCS at the University of California San Diego started a new institute, called the Alzheimer's Therapeutic Research Institute (ATRI). Located in San Diego but part of the University of Southern California (USC) Keck School of Medicine, the mission of ATRI is to accelerate the development of effective therapies for AD. While building on the experience of the ADCS and ADNI, ATRI was designed to facilitate effective academic–industry collaborations with major administrative support from USC. Its structure is unique among USC institutes. With several senior faculty members and a large research staff committed to a single mission, ATRI can efficiently conduct international multi-center clinical trials with its own biomarker, biostatistics, clinical monitoring, clinical operations, finance, informatics, regulatory, recruitment, and safety teams, as well as an independent data and safety monitoring board. Embedded USC human resources and contracting representatives enable efficient large-scale operations.

15.2.1 Principles of ATRI

ATRI is committed to advancing the field of AD therapeutics through innovative methods and trials. Toward this aim, the institute aims for maximal collaboration and data sharing. ATRI collaborators include universities and companies around the world. Data sharing is a key component of each ATRI project, ranging from near real time (as in ADNI) to phased sharing of trial data according to the principles of the Collaboration on Alzheimer's Prevention [16]. Documents, procedures, and instruments are shared on request.

The biomarker section stores, processes, and shares biospecimens from ATRI studies. The informatics section shares software, including the ATRI EDC and TRC-PAD (see below). To the extent feasible, sharing is at no cost or minimal cost to the recipient.

15.2.2 Structure of ATRI

ATRI is an institute of USC; its director, who holds a faculty appointment in the Department of Neurology, reports to the Dean of the USC Keck School of Medicine. The institute is housed in the Sorrento Mesa section of San Diego, with a recently completed expansion for its rapidly growing biomarker section. At present, ATRI is home to eight faculty members and approximately 170 staff. The institute's faculty members, while pursuing their own independent research, are all actively involved in the institute's primary mission, and so constitute a well-aligned research team. ATRI has six main sections, each with its own director: administration (including finance, human resources, shared services, regulatory services, quality assurance, and recruitment teams), biostatistics, clinical operations (including project management and data management), safety (including site clinical monitoring), informatics (including software development and information technology), and the biofluid biomarker section.

While ATRI has the capabilities of a commercial drug-development company to launch and manage multi-center trials, it is an academic institute dedicated to advancing knowledge through innovation and collaboration, always seeking improvements and efficiencies to methods and operations. The clinical and biostatistical trialists work particularly closely, with the view that this arrangement yields the strongest study designs and analytical approaches. (Necessary firewalling is nonetheless maintained between unblinded statisticians and blinded statisticians for each ongoing interventional trial.) The informatics team meets with each of the other groups regularly to continuously improve the software infrastructure in support of efficient data management and trial operations.

15.2.3 Clinical Trials in Alzheimer's Disease (CTAD) Conference

While the field of AD research has many national and international scientific meetings across the calendar, there is one conference that is devoted to clinical trial methods and data: Clinical Trials in Alzheimer's Disease (CTAD, www.ctad-alzheimer .com). Started over a decade ago, this annual meeting is jointly organized by teams in Toulouse and Montpelier in France and ATRI. Now drawing close to a thousand participants each year, the meeting is a key venue for the presentation of major findings in AD therapeutic research. It is held in conjunction with the smaller European Union/US Task Force on AD Trials, which addresses the key challenges facing the field [17].

15.2.4 ATRI Projects

During its first year, ATRI assumed the oversight of several major projects, including multi-center trials and observational studies.

A4 Study. The Anti-Amyloid treatment in Asymptomatic Alzheimer's (A4) study [18, 19] is the first multi-center trial in sporadic preclinical AD. The idea for A4 arose from observations on ADNI data that supported the notion that amyloid elevation in the brain in clinically normal individuals is associated with subtle cognitive and biomarker evidence of decline [20].

Thus, "preclinical AD" may be the optimal stage at which to intervene with anti-amyloid therapies, with sensitive cognitive tests [21] as well as secondary biomarker measurements as outcomes to establish efficacy. A4 was initially funded as a project of the ADCS. Solanezumab [22, 23], a monoclonal antibody against monomeric amyloid peptide, was selected as the therapeutic, and a public–private partnership with Lilly and the NIA was established to carry out the trial, with additional funding contributed by philanthropic groups. The primary outcome measure is the Preclinical Alzheimer's Cognitive Composite (PACC) [21], and the treatment period is four and a half years. A4 transitioned to USC ATRI in 2015 and was fully enrolled with 1,169 randomized participants across 67 sites by the end of 2017 [18]. It will be completed near the end of 2022. In accordance with the data-sharing principles of the Collaboration on Alzheimer's Prevention [16], public sharing of A4 pre-randomization data, which provides the largest data set on amyloid accumulation in clinically normal individuals, was released 1 year after completion of enrollment (Table 15.2).

Table 15.2 A4 pre-randomization data (from Sperling et al. [18])

Demographic characteristics	Number (%) All PET participants	Not elevated (Aβ−)	Elevated (Aβ+)	*p*-value for Aβ− vs. Aβ+[a]
Number of participants	4,486	3,163	1,323	
Age, mean (SD), in years	71.29 (4.67)	70.95 (4.53)	72.10 (4.89)	<0.001
Education, mean (SD), in years	16.58 (2.84)	16.60 (2.85)	16.54 (2.81)	0.53
PET SUVR, mean (SD)	1.09 (0.19)	0.99 (0.07)	1.33 (0.18)	<0.001
Female sex	2,663 (59)	1,885 (60)	778 (59)	0.64
Racial categories				
American Indian/Alaskan Native	32 (1)	22 (1)	10 (1)	>0.99[b]
Asian	171 (4)	141 (4)	30 (2)	0.002[b]
Native Hawaiian/Pacific Islander	2 (0)	2 (0)	0 (0)	>0.99[b]
Black/African American	167 (4)	133 (4)	34 (3)	0.03[b]
White	4,116 (92)	2,866 (91)	1,250 (94)	<0.001[b]
Unknown/not reported	26 (1)	18 (1)	8 (1)	>0.99[b]
Ethnicity				
Hispanic or Latino	142 (3)	103 (3)	39 (3)	
Not Hispanic or Latino	4,309 (96)	3,040 (96)	1,269 (96)	0.19
Unknown	35 (1)	20 (1)	15 (1)	

179

Table 15.2 (cont.)

Demographic characteristics	Number (%) All PET participants	Not elevated (Aβ−)	Elevated (Aβ+)	p-value for Aβ− vs. Aβ+[a]
Marital status				
Married	3,166 (71)	2,223 (70)	943 (71)	
Divorced	628 (14)	438 (14)	190 (14)	
Widowed	426 (9)	304 (10)	122 (9)	0.66
Never married	183 (4)	135 (4)	48 (4)	
Unknown	83 (2)	63 (2)	20 (2)	
Participant retired	3,401 (76)	2,396 (76)	1,005 (76)	0.93
Family history of dementia	3,113 (69)	2,137 (68)	976 (74)	0.001
ApoE genotype				
ε2/ε2	25 (1)	23 (1)	2 (0)	0.03[b]
ε2/ε3	449 (10)	380 (12)	69 (5)	<0.001[b]
ε2/ε4	116 (3)	74 (2)	42 (3)	0.12[b]
ε3/ε3	2,417 (54)	1,936 (61)	481 (36)	<0.001[b]
ε3/ε4	1,295 (29)	684 (22)	611 (46)	<0.001[b]
ε4/ε4	139 (3)	34 (1)	105 (8)	<0.001[b]

Abbreviations: Aβ, amyloid beta; ApoE, apolipoprotein-E; PET, positron emission tomography; SD, standard deviation; SUVR, standardized uptake value ratio.
[a] Fisher exact test for categorical variables and two-sample t test with unequal variances were used for continuous variables.
[b] Comparisons across individual racial categories and APoE genotype subgroups were done using a Fisher exact test with a Holm adjustment to the p-value to account for multiple comparisons. Participants were allowed to select more than one category for race. For APoE, there are missing or incomplete genotype data for 45 of 4,486 participants (1.0%).

LEARN. The A4 program evaluated over 5,000 clinically normal individuals at least 65 years of age with amyloid PET scans to select participants for the trial; as expected, about 30% of those screened had elevated brain fibrillar amyloid. Of the thousands of screened individuals who did not have elevated amyloid, just over 500 were invited to participate in the Longitudinal Evaluation of Amyloid Risk and Neurodegeneration (LEARN) study funded by the Alzheimer's Association. LEARN participants follow a similar protocol to A4, for the same period of time using the same assessments. Analysis of LEARN data in comparison to the A4 placebo arm will provide a careful examination of the impact of amyloid elevation on cognition and biomarkers of neurodegeneration.

ADNI. ADNI was funded by the NIA plus contributions from pharmaceutical companies in 2004 to optimize biomarker assessments in support of AD therapeutic trials [15]. This multi-center project conducted across 60 sites studied three cohorts, cognitively normal individuals, those with mild cognitive impairment (MCI), and those with mild AD dementia, with MRI, lumbar puncture for spinal fluid analysis, and cognitive and clinical assessments longitudinally. Amyloid PET imaging was added to the ADNI protocol in 2005, and tau PET was added in 2015. Remarkably, ADNI shares all data collected as soon as it is quality controlled; this aggressive data sharing has resulted in over 2,000 peer-reviewed publications using ADNI data. The coordinating center for ADNI moved to USC ATRI in 2015. ADNI data have been instrumental to the design of many therapeutic trials in the field. The latest application to continue ADNI is now in preparation.

DoD–ADNI. ADNI investigators were awarded funding from the Department of Defense (DoD) to launch DoD–ADNI [24] in 2012; the coordinating center moved to ATRI in 2015. Based on the long-held view that head trauma is an important risk factor for sporadic AD, this study used ADNI procedures and investigated the impact of traumatic brain injury and post-traumatic stress disorder on

AD biomarkers in Vietnam War veterans. The project is now winding down, with primary results to be published in late 2021.

Insulin. There is significant evidence pointing to an important role of insulin signaling in the brain in AD pathophysiology; indeed, AD has been called by some "type 3 diabetes." Preliminary studies have shown a beneficial effect of systemic insulin treatment on cognition in individuals with cognitive impairment. In 2012, the NIA funded a multi-center study of intranasal insulin for the treatment of MCI; the coordinating center for this study moved to ATRI in 2015. The trial was completed in 2019. While the primary analysis was negative, data from the study suggested the possibility that insulin administration by a specific active delivery device may be beneficial [25].

Fyn. Another strategy for treating AD involves targeting cellular pathways that are involved in the neurodegenerative process. The Fyn tyrosine kinase has been linked to synaptic function as well as amyloid toxicity and tau mechanisms, and results in rodent models have been encouraging [26]. A Phase 2 trial of the Fyn kinase inhibitor saracatinib was funded by the National Center for Advancing Translational Sciences at the NIH to determine whether 1 year of treatment had a beneficial effect in mild AD dementia. The primary outcome measure utilized an innovative analytical approach to measurement of cerebral metabolism with fluorodeoxyglucose (FDG) PET. This study, managed at ATRI, beginning in 2015, did not demonstrate efficacy [27].

Nicotine. Nicotinic cholinergic receptors in the brain play an important role in cognitive function, and a pilot study of 6 months of transdermal nicotine in MCI showed improvement on the primary measure, a computerized test of cognitive performance [28]. To build on this encouraging finding, the NIA is supporting a multi-center trial of transdermal nicotine for 2 years in MCI. The study, being conducted at ATRI, is nearing completion of enrollment.

EARLY. ATRI partnered with Janssen to conduct an international Phase 3 trial of the beta-site amyloid precursor protein cleaving enzyme (BACE) inhibitor atabecestat in preclinical AD. Building on the experience with the A4 recruitment, the EARLY trial screened clinically normal individuals for amyloid elevation in brain, as indicated by amyloid PET or cerebrospinal fluid analysis. The use of a BACE inhibitor at the asymptomatic stage of AD would seem the optimal timing for a drug that markedly reduces the generation of the amyloid peptide by inhibiting a required amyloid precursor protein cleavage step. The EARLY trial was halted when evidence of hepatotoxicity from atabecestat arose. Subsequently, analysis of the study data indicated reversible, dose-related cognitive worsening due to the study drug [29]. Cognitive worsening has now been reported with multiple BACE inhibitors tested in AD [30], and further investigation of this approach will likely modify drug doses such that BACE inhibition is kept below 50%.

TRC-PAD. The experience with recruitment for A4 and EARLY demonstrated the feasibility of enrolling asymptomatic participants with amyloid elevation by screening individuals at risk on the basis of age alone (or, in people under 65, based on age and other risk factors such as family history or apolipoprotein-E [ApoE] genotype). These first trials also demonstrated that the recruitment process was too lengthy and expensive, and represented a major roadblock in early intervention trials. Strategies to substantially reduce the cost and time required are needed. The Trial-Ready Cohort for Preclinical/Prodromal Alzheimer's Disease (TRC-PAD) project [31] was funded in 2017 to address this challenge by creating a new infrastructure for recruitment of asymptomatic or mildly symptomatic individuals into AD trials. The ATRI plan for TRC-PAD, shown in Figure 15.1, involved the creation of multiple linked components of a recruitment system, including a web-based longitudinal observation study to engage individuals 50 years and older with a potential interest in trials, while collecting cognitive and symptomatic data to allow estimation of the risk of amyloid elevation. Those with elevated risk are invited to in-person evaluation at TRC-PAD sites, where conventional cognitive testing and ApoE genotyping are performed to refine the risk estimate. High-risk participants move forward with amyloid testing by PET scan or lumbar puncture; those with elevated amyloid are followed in the trial-ready cohort until screening for an appropriate trial is available, while the rest resume follow-up in the webstudy. In 2021, plasma assays will be introduced into TRC-PAD, which will serve to further validate these blood-based markers in the earlier stages of AD, and have the potential to substantially reduce the number of PET scans and lumbar punctures for future prevention trials.

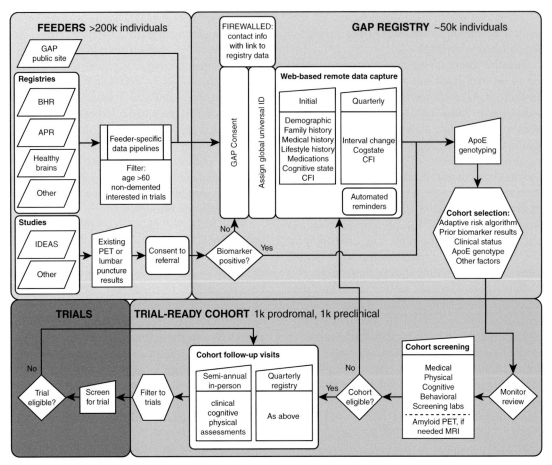

Figure 15.1 TRC-PAD organization. APR, Alzheimer's Prevention Registry; BHR, Brain Health Registry; CFI, cognitive function index; GAP, Global Alzheimer's Platform; IDEAS, Imaging Dementia – Evidence for Amyloid Scanning.

LEADS. ADNI has been widely credited with establishing foundational methods and data for therapeutic trials in AD. But ADNI has focused on the characterization of older individuals with sporadic AD. It has become evident that there exists a group of younger-onset persons (less than 65 years of age) with sporadic AD, featuring a prominent tauopathy with few confounding conditions that raises important opportunities for therapeutic research. The Longitudinal Early-Onset Alzheimer's Disease Study (LEADS) was funded in 2017, with its coordinating center established at ATRI, to apply ADNI-like methods to understand this population and guide the design of therapeutic trials. LEADS leverages data collected on this population through the NIA Alzheimer Disease Center/National Alzheimer's Coordinating Center programs, collects data on cognitive and clinical status, MRI and PET imaging, cerebrospinal fluid and plasma analysis, and genetics to provide the therapeutic research community with the tools in

anticipation of therapeutic trials for this unique AD population.

15.3 Alzheimer's Clinical Trials Consortium

As described above, the academic community has been pivotal in the launch and evolution of the field of AD therapeutic research, and as a result the NIA has remained committed to supporting such efforts. In 2016, the NIA released a funding opportunity announcement inviting applications for a new academic network called the Alzheimer's Clinical Trials Consortium (ACTC, actcinfo.org). The announcement incorporated many new ideas resulting from the decades of experience in the field, including the value of a central institutional review board, standing support for trial sites, and separation of project funding from the parent grant mechanism, among others. The first ACTC grant was awarded to a team of investigators at three institutions, USC, Harvard University, and the Mayo Clinic. The remainder of this chapter will focus on the first years of this new program.

15.3.1 Structure of the ACTC

The structure of the ACTC is shown in Figure 15.2. The leadership group consists of the three principal investigators, one from each of the primary institutions, plus the NIA program officer. This group of four meets regularly, assisted by the ACTC Program Administrator at ATRI, to oversee all meetings and communications, project proposal reviews, trials, data sharing, and other consortium activities.

Figure 15.2 shows each of the units that comprise the ACTC. The administrative, biostatistics, clinical operations, safety, informatics, and biomarker units comprise the ACTC coordinating center and are located at ATRI. The ACTC project administrator provides overall coordination, development of charters and procedures, management of meetings and communications, and the development and implementation of evaluation surveys. The ATRI and ACTC teams are closely aligned, but all ACTC activities follow the consortium procedures and decision-making paths.

The ACTC funding supports 35 primary academic trial sites across the United States (over 70 additional sites participate in ATRI and ACTC

trials). Each trial site has a site principal investigator (PI), associate PI, and site-liaison and trial staff, including study coordinators, raters, and recruitment personnel. The group of site PIs and unit leads form the ACTC steering committee, the principal advisory group to the leadership team. The steering committee and the unit leads must approve each project proposal that moves forward to an NIA application for consideration of funding.

ACTC Clinical Outcome Instruments Unit. This unit is responsible for guiding instrument selection during the protocol development process and overseeing the monitoring and quality-control procedures during trials. Academic teams have historically led the development of trial designs including cognitive/clinical assessments for various stages of AD [3, 32–41]. These include the key primary (PACC [21]) and secondary (cognitive function index [CFI] [42, 43]) outcomes currently used in preclinical studies such as A4, EARLY, and AHEAD 3–45 (discussed below). The primary cognitive performance tests in particular require meticulous attention to administration guidelines and scoring, with training and certification of raters and monitoring during the course of the trial (often with remote review of audio recordings of the test administration process).

Biostatistics. ATRI/ACTC biostatisticians have pursued novel methods for clinical trial

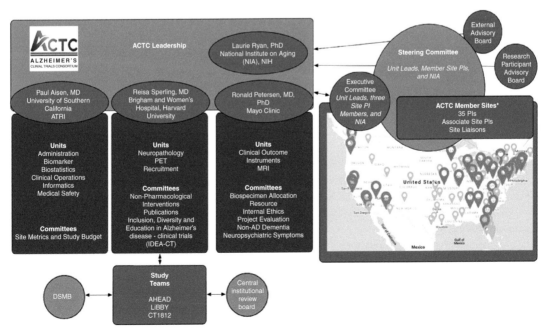

Figure 15.2 ACTC organization and sites.

design [20, 44, 45], assessment of outcomes [20, 21, 46–49], longitudinal data modeling [50–53], comparative analyses of various trial data analysis approaches [54–56], and assessment of robustness to pandemic-related disruptions of new analytical methods, in addition to providing the essential tasks of trial design, statistical analysis plans, safety reporting to the drug safety monitoring board (DSMB), risk-based monitoring of trial data, and activity and data analysis for ATRI/ACTC and external investigators.

Recruitment. Among the major challenges in AD drug development is the lack of diversity in trial populations. Testing drugs in groups that are not representative of the target clinical population creates uncertainty around the generalizability of the findings. Efforts to remedy this issue are growing, and ATRI and ACTC are committed to the goal of diverse study populations. Toward this aim, ACTC supports specific recruitment efforts for under-represented groups, and actively seeks diversity among faculty members and staff at the coordinating center and its collaborating sites. The Recruitment Unit funds and assesses targeted diversity efforts at selected sites and engages with external groups dedicated to addressing this challenge for each ACTC trial. The unit also works closely with all ACTC study PIs and the coordinating center in developing study-specific and inclusive recruitment strategies that are data-driven and evidence-based.

Education and Training. ATRI is also committed to the education and training of students, early-stage investigators, and established scientists, as well as clinical trial site and coordinating center staff. ATRI faculty members engage in educational activities through seminars and lectures, teaching at USC courses and conferences, activities at scientific meetings such as CTAD (see below), and through a major new training initiative of ACTC called IMPACT-AD (see below).

Clinical Operations. The Clinical Operations Unit is responsible for site start-up activities and the day-to-day coordination of all trial activities through study close-out. It includes both project management and data management teams that work together and collaborate closely with the Informatics, Biostatistics, Medical Safety, and Recruitment units.

Imaging. The ACTC MRI Unit is based at the Mayo Clinic, and the PET Unit is based at Harvard. Each of these teams is responsible for the incorporation of imaging modalities into trial design,

standardization of imaging procedures, and the oversight of image processing and analysis streams. In addition, these units guide the consortium image sharing activities.

Biomarkers. The ACTC Biomarker Unit participates in the planning of biofluid measures in trials, the standardization of fluid acquisition and processing at sites, the shipment of specimens, and the analysis and interpretation of findings. This unit maintains a large biorepository in San Diego, as well as the necessary equipment for major biochemical and genetic assay platforms. The team is involved in assay development and the translation of animal-model findings to human trials.

Safety, Risk-Based Monitoring, Site Monitoring. The safety team provides medical expertise to trial design and safety monitoring. These clinicians assist in the evaluation of medical issues during trial screening and trial conduct and DSMB reporting, and oversee remote and on-site monitoring of trial activities by the team of ATRI/ACTC clinical monitors. The ATRI/ACTC biostatistics team has created an innovative risk-based monitoring application to guide the efficient use of remote and on-site monitoring resources. The application provides visualization of compliance, safety, and outcome data through a dashboard and specific detail to highlight outliers and underperforming sites.

Informatics. Electronic data capture (EDC), data management, and data sharing are critical aspects of clinical trial operation. ATRI and ACTC have benefited from an informatics infrastructure created and continuously improved by its team of programmers. The informatics team addresses challenges faced by the various groups with customized adaptations to optimize efficiency, security, and access control. Working with the data management group, the programmers devise data transfer pipelines to connect external laboratories and analysts to the ACTC data sets.

Neuropathology. In order to best examine the impact of candidate therapeutics on AD-related processes in the brain, the acquisition of postmortem tissue from past trial participants is invaluable; this has been clearly demonstrated by the important lessons from the early anti-amyloid active vaccination trial of AN1792 [57]. ACTC has established a Neuropathology Unit to develop and implement protocols to facilitate autopsy and standardized neuropathological examination of trial participants.

Committees. The mandate of ACTC extends beyond AD trials of pharmacological interventions to other age-related cognitive disorders and to non-pharmacological therapies. The consortium therefore includes committees comprised of individuals with particular expertise necessary for a range of trials. As shown in Figure 15.2, these standing committees address non-pharmacological interventions, non-AD dementias, and neuropsychiatric symptoms; these committees join the review process and study teams for appropriate projects. Additional ACTC committees include the Internal Ethics Committee, overseeing conflict of interest disclosures and ethical issues in trial design; the Biospecimen Allocation Review Committee (BARC) to oversee the process of reviewing requests for specimens; the Site Metrics and Study Budget Committee to guide the evaluation and review process for ACTC sites and the development of site budgets for trials; the IDEA-CT Committee addressing diversity and inclusion issues in study design and consortium operations.

IMPACT-AD. The ACTC is strongly committed to the training of AD trialists. A new, week-long intensive course called the Institute on Methods and Protocols for Advancement of Clinical Trials in Alzheimer's and Related Dementias (IMPACT-AD, impact-ad.org) has been developed, and the initial session was conducted in 2020. A competitive application process selects enrollees for two tracks, one focused on training AD trial PIs, and the other aimed at a broader group including clinicians, study coordinators, psychometricians, and other study professionals. All costs of participation including travel and lodging are covered by the grant support from the NIA and the Alzheimer's Association.

Participant Advisory Group. The ACTC team is now engaging research participants at several levels, including the review of therapeutic strategies, recruitment approaches and trial designs, and discussing scientific advances in the field. An example of important guidance from this advisory group concerns the value to participants of return of research findings during the course of a study.

Project Selection. The selection of projects for the ACTC required the development of a staged review process to weigh feasibility and appropriateness, scientific merit, and practicality for ACTC sites, with feedback to applicants at each step. Approval by a majority of steering committee members and a majority of unit leads are required. Proposals that pass these reviews move to collaborative NIA application preparation among the applicants and ACTC units, yielding an R01 submission under the dedicated ACTC project funding opportunity announcement (https://grants.nih.gov/grants/guide/pa-files/par-18-513.html).

15.3.2 ACTC Projects

A45. The first ACTC project funded by the NIA was the A45 study. The goal of this project was to implement a tailored approach to amyloid removal in a preclinical AD population. In contrast to solanezumab, the therapeutic intervention in A4 that targets soluble monomeric amyloid-beta (Aβ) peptide, A45 employed a regimen that would remove fibrillar amyloid and maintain the normalized condition over a 4-year treatment period. A45 initially envisioned use of an antifibrillar antibody, followed by maintenance with a BACE inhibitor. Faced by the cognitive impairment seen with BACE inhibitors, A45 adopted two doses of the amyloid-reducing antibody BAN2401 [58] for induction and maintenance. In a public–private partnership with Eisai, the company developing BAN2401, the final design included A3 into a platform program with BAN2401 regimens tailored to intermediate or high initial amyloid levels. The active regimens are tailored to the initial amyloid level. In A45, enrolling individuals with elevated brain amyloid, after titration the high-dose treatment (10 mg/kg intravenously every 2 weeks) is continued for the duration of 2 years aiming to normalize the amyloid load, followed by maintenance with lower-dose treatment (10 mg/kg every 4 weeks) for an additional 2 years. A45 is the first study to evaluate fibrillar amyloid reduction to or toward normal in an asymptomatic population, and thus is a major test of the amyloid therapeutic hypothesis. The TRC-PAD program is a source of potential participants. The study team is also exploring the use of plasma biomarkers as prescreening tools prior to amyloid PET. A45 is a Phase 3 study; similar to A4, the primary outcome is a version of the PACC and the key secondary is the CFI.

A3. The Ante-Amyloid treatment in Alzheimer's (A3) trial enrolled individuals with intermediate levels of (sub-threshold) brain amyloid. The A3 trial has titration to a lower-dose regimen (10 mg/kg every 4 weeks) that is continued for the duration of 4 years. A3 is a Phase 2 study with the primary amyloid and tau PET measures (since cognitive decline is expected to be limited in this population). The A3 and A45 studies have a similar schedule of assessments, including a rich set of cognitive, imaging, and biofluid measures.

A45 and A3 are being conducted at the same sites and the same time, and share a common screening process. Together, these trials constitute the AHEAD platform study (aheadstudy.org), a public–private partnership with funding from the NIA, Eisai, and other funders.

CT1812. A prevalent view holds that diffusible oligomeric amyloid is the most toxic species and plays a critical role in driving AD neurodegeneration. CT1812, a novel small molecule developed by the company Cognition Therapeutics, interferes with Aβ oligomers interaction with the sigma-2 receptor, reducing toxicity and promoting clearance of oligomers. Having been approved at each stage of review by ACTC committees, a collaborative application to fund a Phase 2 study in early AD has been approved for funding. This will be a three-arm study enrolling a total of 540 individuals with biomarker-confirmed prodromal AD or mild AD dementia; the primary outcome is a change in the Clinical Dementia Rating scale – sum of boxes after 18 months of treatment, with an array of additional cognitive and biomarker assessments. This trial will be launched by the ACTC in 2022.

LiBBY. While disease-slowing drugs may be most promising at early stages of AD, the most devastating manifestations of disease for the families affected are usually the behavioral challenges at the end stage. Standard therapies have limited or no efficacy and a substantial risk of adverse effects. Cannabinoids have been proposed as candidate therapies for agitation and other disruptive and disturbing symptoms of dementia. The Life's End Benefits of Cannabidiol and Tetrahydrocannabinol (LiBBY) trial, an academic proposal that was approved at all stages of the ACTC project development process, submitted to the NIA and approved for funding, will test an oral regimen of tetrahydrocannabinol and cannabidiol for the treatment of behavioral disturbance in individuals with hospice-eligible dementia. The study will enroll 150 participants in the 12-week treatment trial; the primary outcome is change in behavior as measured by the Cohen Mansfield Agitation Inventory. LiBBY will begin in late 2021.

Affiliated Projects. The ACTC leadership and steering committee created an additional category for projects that utilize some consortium resources but have not been progressed through the entire ACTC project development process. Three projects, each funded prior to consideration by the ACTC, were approved for affiliated-project status by the steering committee and units. The A4 study, including an open-label extension funded by an additional NIA award, utilizes the ACTC recruitment, imaging, and biomarker unit resources. The A3 study, approved as an affiliated project, is being conducted in conjunction with A45 in the AHEAD platform as described above. The TRC-PAD project is utilizing the recruitment, imaging, and biomarker resources.

ACTS-DS and TRC-DS. Almost all individuals with Down syndrome (DS) accumulate brain amyloid in mid-life because they carry an extra copy of the amyloid precursor gene (on chromosome 21) leading to overproduction of Aβ. Alzheimer's dementia in DS usually occurs by the sixth decade of life. The NIH has been supporting longitudinal biomarker studies in the DS population in recent years [59, 60] and has now funded a trial-ready cohort program for DS that will lead to therapeutic trials in the coming years. The Alzheimer's Clinical Trial Consortium – Down Syndrome (ACTC-DS) (www.actc-ds.org) and the Trial Ready Cohort – Down Syndrome (TRC-DS) are being developed by ATRI and ACTC investigators and have been approved as ACTC-affiliated projects.

15.3.3 Future Plans for ATRI and the ACTC

Academic contributions to AD drug development will continue as the field moves closer to effective disease modification. Anti-amyloid, anti-tau, microglial, and ApoE-related interventions will require innovative trial designs, outcome measures, and use of biomarkers; academic contributions may accelerate these goals. ATRI and the ACTC will continue to pursue innovations in biostatistical analysis, informatics, data sharing, recruitment, and trial methodology, as well as new approaches to diversity, involvement of research participants, and return of research results. In particular, the ACTC is working to plan a tau platform "proof-of-concept" trial to allow evaluation of multiple anti-tau mechanistic approaches with biomarkers and tau PET imaging, and to accelerate the selection of the best candidates to move into Phase 3 trials.

Primary prevention of AD is a major goal that is coming within reach. Despite the painfully slow progress on bringing intervention to clinical use, understanding of the role of amyloid dysregulation in initiating AD pathology has grown, yielding a plausible path to primary prevention. Current sensitive plasma measures such as Aβ peptide ratios [61, 62] and hyperphosphorylated tau [63] may identify individuals at risk even before biomarker evidence of amyloid accumulation. Candidate therapeutics for prevention still include secretase inhibitors (specifically low-dose BACE inhibitors) and active anti-amyloid vaccines. Outreach programs such as TRC-PAD provide a vehicle for engaging the at-risk population before pathology begins. Academic investigation in these areas will bring the field closer to the critical but elusive goal of primary prevention of AD.

References

1. Summers WK, Majovski LV, Marsh GM, Tachiki K, Kling A. Oral tetrahydroaminoacridine in long-term treatment of senile dementia, Alzheimer type. *N Engl J Med* 1986; **315**: 1241–5.

2. Davis KL, Thal LJ, Gamzu ER, et al. A double-blind, placebo-controlled multicenter study of tacrine for Alzheimer's disease. The Tacrine Collaborative Study Group. *N Engl J Med* 1992; **327**: 1253–9.

3. Rosen WG, Mohs RC, Davis KL. A new rating scale for Alzheimer's disease. *Am J Psychiatry* 1984; **141**: 1356–64.

4. Thal LJ. The Alzheimer's Disease Cooperative Study in 2004. *Alzheimer Dis Assoc Disord* 2004; **18**: 183–5.

5. Sano M, Ernesto C, Thomas RG, et al. A controlled trial of selegiline, alpha-tocopherol, or both as treatment for Alzheimer's disease. The Alzheimer's Disease Cooperative Study. *N Engl J Med* 1997; **336**: 1216–22.

6. Aisen PS, Schneider LS, Sano M, et al. High-dose B vitamin supplementation and cognitive decline in Alzheimer disease: a randomized controlled trial. *JAMA* 2008; **300**: 1774–83.

7. Galasko DR, Peskind E, Clark CM, et al. Antioxidants for Alzheimer disease: a randomized clinical trial with cerebrospinal fluid biomarker measures. *Arch Neurol* 2012; **69**: 836–41.

8. Petersen RC, Thomas RG, Grundman M, et al. Vitamin E and donepezil for the treatment of mild cognitive impairment. *N Engl J Med* 2005; **352**: 2379–88.

9. Aisen PS, Davis KL, Berg JD, et al. A randomized controlled trial of prednisone in Alzheimer's disease. Alzheimer's Disease Cooperative Study. *Neurology* 2000; **54**: 588–93.

10. Aisen PS, Schafer KA, Grundman M, et al. Effects of rofecoxib or naproxen vs placebo on Alzheimer disease progression: a randomized controlled trial. *JAMA* 2003; **289**: 2819–26.

11. Mulnard RA, Cotman CW, Kawas C, et al. Estrogen replacement therapy for treatment of mild to moderate Alzheimer disease: a randomized controlled trial. Alzheimer's Disease Cooperative Study. *JAMA* 2000; **283**: 1007–15.

12. Sano M, Bell KL, Galasko D, et al. A randomized, double-blind, placebo-controlled trial of simvastatin to treat Alzheimer disease. *Neurology* 2011; **77**: 556–63.

13. Teri L, Logsdon RG, Peskind E, et al. Treatment of agitation in AD: a randomized, placebo-controlled clinical trial. *Neurology* 2000; **55**: 1271–8.

14. Grundman M, Farlow M, Peavy G, et al. A phase I study of AIT-082 in healthy elderly volunteers. *J Mol Neurosci* 2002; **18**: 283–93.

15. Petersen RC, Aisen PS, Beckett LA, et al. Alzheimer's Disease Neuroimaging Initiative (ADNI): clinical characterization. *Neurology* 2010; **74**: 201–9.

16. Weninger S, Carrillo MC, Dunn B, et al. Collaboration for Alzheimer's Prevention: principles to guide data and sample sharing in preclinical Alzheimer's disease trials. *Alzheimers Dement* 2016; **12**: 631–2.

17. Vellas B, Carrillo MC, Sampaio C, et al. Designing drug trials for Alzheimer's disease: what we have learned from the release of the Phase III antibody trials: a report from the EU/US/CTAD Task Force. *Alzheimers Dement* 2013; **9**: 438–44.

18. Sperling RA, Donohue MC, Raman R, et al. Association of factors with elevated amyloid burden in clinically normal older individuals. *JAMA Neurol* 2020; **77**: 735–45.

19. Sperling RA, Rentz DM, Johnson KA, et al. The A4 study: stopping AD before symptoms begin? *Sci Transl Med* 2014; **6**: 228fs13.

20. Donohue MC, Sperling RA, Petersen R, et al. Association between elevated brain amyloid and subsequent cognitive decline among cognitively normal persons. *JAMA* 2017; **317**: 2305–16.

21. Donohue MC, Sperling RA, Salmon DP, et al. The Preclinical Alzheimer Cognitive Composite: measuring amyloid-related decline. *JAMA Neurol* 2014; **71**: 961–70.

22. Siemers ER, Sundell KL, Carlson C, et al. Phase 3 solanezumab trials: secondary outcomes in mild Alzheimer's disease patients. *Alzheimers Dement* 2016; **12**: 110–20.

23. Doody RS, Thomas RG, Farlow M, et al. Phase 3 trials of solanezumab for mild-to-moderate

Alzheimer's disease. *N Engl J Med* 2014; **370**: 311–21.

24. Weiner MW, Harvey D, Hayes J, et al. Effects of traumatic brain injury and posttraumatic stress disorder on development of Alzheimer's disease in Vietnam Veterans using the Alzheimer's Disease Neuroimaging Initiative: preliminary report. *Alzheimers Dement (N Y)* 2017; **3**: 177–88.

25. Craft S, Raman R, Chow TW, et al. Safety, efficacy, and feasibility of intranasal insulin for the treatment of mild cognitive impairment and alzheimer disease dementia: a randomized clinical trial. *JAMA Neurol* 2020; **77**: 1099–109.

26. Kaufman AC, Salazar SV, Haas LT, et al. Fyn inhibition rescues established memory and synapse loss in Alzheimer mice. *Ann Neurol* 2015; **77**: 953–71.

27. van Dyck CH, Nygaard HB, Chen K, et al. Effect of AZD0530 on cerebral metabolic decline in Alzheimer disease: a randomized clinical trial. *JAMA Neurol* 2019; **76**: 1219–29.

28. Newhouse P, Kellar K, Aisen P, et al. Nicotine treatment of mild cognitive impairment: a 6-month double-blind pilot clinical trial. *Neurology* 2012; **78**: 91–101.

29. Henley D, Raghavan N, Sperling R, et al. Preliminary results of a trial of atabecestat in preclinical Alzheimer's disease. *N Engl J Med* 2019; **380**: 1483–5.

30. Egan MF, Kost J, Voss T, et al. Randomized trial of verubecestat for prodromal Alzheimer's disease. *N Engl J Med* 2019; **380**: 1408–20.

31. Aisen PS, Sperling RA, Cummings J, et al. The Trial-Ready Cohort for Preclinical/Prodromal Alzheimer's Disease (TRC-PAD) project: an overview. *J Prev Alzheimers Dis* 2020; **7**: 208–12.

32. Galasko D, Bennett DA, Sano M, et al. ADCS Prevention Instrument Project: assessment of instrumental activities of daily living for community-dwelling elderly individuals in dementia prevention clinical trials. *Alzheimer Dis Assoc Disord* 2006; **20**: S152–69.

33. Cummings JL, Raman R, Ernstrom K, Salmon D, Ferris SH, Alzheimer's Disease Cooperative Study Group. ADCS Prevention Instrument Project: behavioral measures in primary prevention trials. *Alzheimer Dis Assoc Disord* 2006; **20**: S147–51.

34. Schneider LS, Clark CM, Doody R, et al. ADCS Prevention Instrument Project: ADCS-clinicians' global impression of change scales (ADCS–CGIC), self-rated and study partner-rated versions. *Alzheimer Dis Assoc Disord* 2006; **20**: S124–38.

35. Ferris SH, Aisen PS, Cummings J, et al. ADCS Prevention Instrument Project: overview and initial results. *Alzheimer Dis Assoc Disord* 2006; **20**: S109–23.

36. Logsdon RG, Teri L, Weiner MF, et al. Assessment of agitation in Alzheimer's disease: the agitated behavior in dementia scale. Alzheimer's Disease Cooperative Study. *J Am Geriatr Soc* 1999; **47**: 1354–8.

37. Morris JC, Ernesto C, Schafer K, et al. Clinical dementia rating training and reliability in multicenter studies: the Alzheimer's Disease Cooperative Study experience. *Neurology* 1997; **48**: 1508–10.

38. Schmitt FA, Ashford W, Ernesto C, et al. The severe impairment battery: concurrent validity and the assessment of longitudinal change in Alzheimer's disease. The Alzheimer's Disease Cooperative Study. *Alzheimer Dis Assoc Disord* 1997; **11**: S51–6.

39. Galasko D, Bennett D, Sano M, et al. An inventory to assess activities of daily living for clinical trials in Alzheimer's disease. The Alzheimer's Disease Cooperative Study. *Alzheimer Dis Assoc Disord* 1997; **11**: S33–9.

40. Schneider LS, Olin JT, Doody RS, et al. Validity and reliability of the Alzheimer's Disease Cooperative Study–Clinical Global Impression of Change. The Alzheimer's Disease Cooperative Study. *Alzheimer Dis Assoc Disord* 1997; **11**: S22–32.

41. Ferris SH, Mackell JA, Mohs R, et al. A multicenter evaluation of new treatment efficacy instruments for Alzheimer's disease clinical trials: overview and general results. The Alzheimer's Disease Cooperative Study. *Alzheimer Dis Assoc Disord* 1997; **11**: S1–12.

42. Walsh SP, Raman R, Jones KB, Aisen PS, Alzheimer's Disease Cooperative Study Group. ADCS Prevention Instrument Project: the Mail-In Cognitive Function Screening Instrument (MCFSI). *Alzheimer Dis Assoc Disord* 2006; **20**: S170–8.

43. Amariglio RE, Donohue MC, Marshall GA, et al. Tracking early decline in cognitive function in older individuals at risk for Alzheimer disease dementia: the Alzheimer's Disease Cooperative Study Cognitive Function Instrument. *JAMA Neurol* 2015; **72**: 446–54.

44. Aisen PS, Andrieu S, Sampaio C, et al. Report of the task force on designing clinical trials in early (predementia) AD. *Neurology* 2011; **76**: 280–6.

45. Coley N, Raman R, Donohue MC, et al. Defining the optimal target population for trials of polyunsaturated fatty acid supplementation using the erythrocyte omega-3 index: a step towards personalized prevention of cognitive decline? *J Nutr Health Aging* 2018; **22**: 982–98.

46. Donohue MC, Sun CK, Raman R, et al. Cross-validation of optimized composites for preclinical Alzheimer's disease. *Alzheimers Dement (N Y)* 2017; **3**: 123–9.

47. Langford O, Raman R, Sperling RA, et al. Predicting amyloid burden to accelerate recruitment of secondary prevention clinical trials. *J Prev Alzheimers Dis* 2020; **7**: 213–18.

48. Papp KV, Rentz DM, Maruff P, et al. The Computerized Cognitive Composite (C3) in an Alzheimer's disease secondary prevention trial. *J Prev Alzheimers Dis* 2021; **8**: 59–67.

49. Sano M, Raman R, Emond J, et al. Adding delayed recall to the Alzheimer Disease Assessment Scale is useful in studies of mild cognitive impairment but not Alzheimer disease. *Alzheimer Dis Assoc Disord* 2011; **25**: 122–7.

50. Li D, Iddi S, Thompson WK, et al. Bayesian latent time joint mixed-effects model of progression in the Alzheimer's Disease Neuroimaging Initiative. *Alzheimers Dement (Amst)* 2018; **10**: 657–68.

51. Iddi S, Li D, Aisen PS, et al. Estimating the evolution of disease in the Parkinson's progression markers initiative. *Neurodegener Dis* 2018; **18**: 173–90.

52. Li D, Donohue MC. Disease progression models for dominantly-inherited Alzheimer's disease. *Brain* 2018; **141**: 1244–6.

53. Donohue MC, Jacqmin-Gadda H, Le Goff M, et al. Estimating long-term multivariate progression from short-term data. *Alzheimers Dement* 2014; **10**: S400–10.

54. Donohue MC, Aisen PS. Mixed model of repeated measures versus slope models in Alzheimer's disease clinical trials. *J Nutr Health Aging* 2012; **16**: 360–4.

55. Donohue MC, Gamst AC, Thomas RG, et al. The relative efficiency of time-to-threshold and rate of change in longitudinal data. *Contemp Clin Trials* 2011; **32**: 685–93.

56. Li D, Iddi S, Aisen PS, Thompson WK, Donohue MC. The relative efficiency of time-to-progression and continuous measures of cognition in presymptomatic Alzheimer's disease. *Alzheimers Dement (N Y)* 2019; **5**: 308–18.

57. Nicoll JA, Wilkinson D, Holmes C. Neuropathology of human Alzheimer disease after immunization with amyloid-beta peptide: a case report. *Nat Med* 2003; **9**: 448–52.

58. Satlin A, Wang J, Logovinsky V, et al. Design of a Bayesian adaptive phase 2 proof-of-concept trial for BAN2401, a putative disease-modifying monoclonal antibody for the treatment of Alzheimer's disease. *Alzheimers Dement (N Y)* 2016; **2**: 1–12.

59. Rafii MS, Zaman S, Handen BL. Integrating biomarker outcomes into clinical trials for Alzheimer's disease in Down syndrome. *J Prev Alzheimers Dis* 2021; **8**: 48–51.

60. Handen BL, Lott IT, Christian BT, et al. The Alzheimer's Biomarker Consortium – Down syndrome: rationale and methodology. *Alzheimers Dement (Amst)* 2020; **12**: e12065.

61. Ovod V, Ramsey KN, Mawuenyega KG, et al. Amyloid beta concentrations and stable isotope labeling kinetics of human plasma specific to central nervous system amyloidosis. *Alzheimers Dement* 2017; **13**: 841–9.

62. Nakamura A, Kaneko N, Villemagne VL, et al. High performance plasma amyloid-beta biomarkers for Alzheimer's disease. *Nature* 2018; **554**: 249–54.

63. Janelidze S, Berron D, Smith R, et al. Associations of plasma phospho-tau217 levels with tau positron emission tomography in early Alzheimer Disease. *JAMA Neurol* 2021; **78**: 149–56.

The European Prevention of Alzheimer's Disease Program: A Public–Private Partnership to Facilitate the Secondary Prevention of Alzheimer's Disease Dementia

Craig W. Ritchie, on behalf of the EPAD Consortium

16.1 Introduction

The European Prevention of Alzheimer's Dementia (EPAD) program was established in 2015 founded by funding from the European Union's Innovative Medicines Initiative (IMI). The IMI explicitly brings together the pharmaceutical industry (under the European Federation of the Pharmaceutical Industry and Associations [EFPIA]), academia, the third sector, and small and medium enterprises. The EPAD program was the winning response to a call put out by the IMI, called the European Proof of Concept for Alzheimer's Disease (IMI-EPOC-AD), with an initial award of €64 million.

The aim of EPAD was to assist in the development of interventions for the secondary prevention of Alzheimer's disease (AD). The objective therein was to develop a clinical trial platform that could test multiple interventions concurrently in scores of sites in Europe, which had access to highly phenotyped individuals eligible for secondary-prevention studies. These individuals would therefore be required to show evidence of AD but not be at the dementia stage of illness. The original focus of the IMI-EPOC-AD call had been on "preclinical" AD (evidence of Alzheimer's pathology but no clinical/cognitive symptoms) but in EPAD this was expanded to include people with prodromal AD (evidence of AD and cognitive/clinical symptoms present but insufficient to satisfy criteria for dementia). EPAD was to place itself within a portfolio of global initiatives with the specific purpose of Phase 2 trial delivery (Figure 16.1).

The driver for EPAD was the fact that no new pharmacological agent for AD had been developed in almost 15 years. The root cause, or causes, of this failure had been discussed at a meeting at

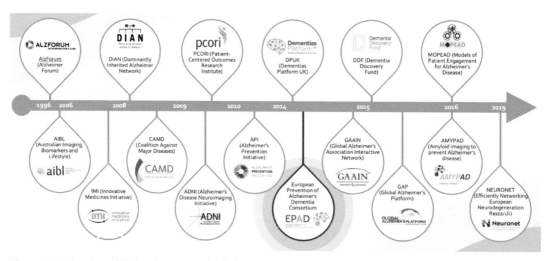

Figure 16.1 The place of EPAD within a series of globally important initiatives to better understand and treat AD.

the New York Academy of Sciences in 2013, which led to the emergence of IMI-EPOC-AD. The fundamental cause of failure was identified as the lack of knowledge gained in Phase 2 trials to help optimize design elements of Phase 3 programs. Phase 2 trials therefore needed to be more rewarding in terms of demonstrating proof of concept (POC), at the right dose and in the right population. In terms of the "right population," there was also consensus that the ability for an intervention to modify the course of disease required testing in people with very early stages of disease development, i.e., preclinical populations. There was also a recognition that the cost of clinical trials in AD was prohibitive, and efficiencies, both economic and scientific, would help ease access of more compounds into a robust testing environment. Therefore, a platform trial was proposed that would allow many linked aspects to be pre-established: (1) a single operational environment, (2) a single protocol for testing (to share placebo data), (3) a site network and community that conducted all three elements of research participant engagement (register, cohort, and trial) and, therefore, (4) a single sponsor to bind the whole program together under a single governance framework.

At the same time that EPAD was being established in Europe, the Global Alzheimer's Platform (GAP) was being developed in North America. From 2015 onwards, GAP–EPAD quarterly meetings took place and tracked the development of each other's protocols and developments. This led to much sharing of knowledge and information between two major international programs that shared a common aim.

In summary, EPAD (in the IMI period which ran from 2015 to 2020) was a 39-partner program which operated across 29 sites in 10 countries in Europe. To deliver on the aim, four key components were delivered (Figure 16.2):

1. A pan-European **register** from clinics and parent cohorts of several million individuals with an access system for data in this register (PrePAD) to identify the higher-risk population to enter the longitudinal cohort study (LCS).

2. A longitudinal **cohort** study to act as a readiness cohort for the EPAD POC trial.

3. The EPAD POC **trial** platform and protocol.

4. A trial delivery centre (TDC) **network** that accessed and delivered the above three components.

The objective of the register was to identify people likely to be eligible for a secondary-prevention trial for AD. These people may have been seen in clinics aligned to the TDCs or in existing cohorts established for other purposes. Non-disclosure of risk status was especially important when drawing from population-based cohorts and

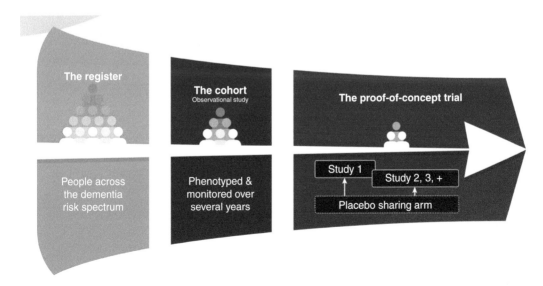

Figure 16.2 Schematic representation of the flow of research participants. It should be noted that research participants could be co-enrolled between the EPAD LCS and their parent cohort and that research participants completing their time in a POC trial could be re-entered into the EPAD LCS.

the mechanism for this using the PrePAD tool is described below.

The objective of the cohort was to undertake deep phenotyping research participants to determine their eligibility for a secondary-prevention POC trial. This would reduce screen failures when amyloid status, cognitive function, medical co-morbidities, and apolipoprotein-E (ApoE) status were all knowable prior to invitation to the POC trial.

The objective of the POC trial was to develop a platform and master protocol for a perpetual, Bayesian adaptive, POC trial for the secondary prevention of Alzheimer's dementia.

The objective of the TDC network was to establish a network and community of highly qualified, experienced sites across Europe, which would have access to their local instance of the register, undertake the cohort study, and thereafter the POC trial.

16.2 EPAD General Considerations

16.2.1 The EPAD Culture

In 2014, when academics across Europe were responding to the IMI-EPOC-AD call and EFPIA companies were being brought onboard the program, there remained an incredibly active portfolio of clinical trials in clinical development. In the 7 years since, however, none have shown convincing effectiveness and virtually all have ceased in development for their core indication. In essence the "problem statement" as articulated in 2013 at the New York Academy of Sciences remains as valid now as it did then.

It was recognized that to affect the direction of travel of the developmental pathway that paradoxically had yielded so little, there needed to be a fundamental and compelling reconsideration of each element of clinical trial delivery and design. This required a very large project that not only engaged but embedded innovative companies and individuals at the core of the program. With each innovative step to be taken came a series of downstream challenges. For instance when a decision is made to focus on preclinical patients then there is a downstream need to for example (1) address massive screen failure rates, (2) find reliable measures of an interventions impact (biomarker or cognitive) at such an early stage of disease, (3) develop sensitive ways to undertake risk disclosure, (4) adopt and adapt the regulatory framework, (5) find outcomes to furnish evolutionary analysis necessary in the Bayesian adaptive design, and (having done so) (6) convince or persuade intervention owners that placing their drug in this platform will yield more accurate and earlier decision making on the onward development of that drug in preclinical AD.

In essence, in EPAD a "revolutionary" culture was deliberately established whereby every primary and secondary element of drug development in AD was scrutinized and eligible for redesign [1]. It was thought by many involved that the scale of the problem and the scale of the program did represent a genuine opportunity to redirect drug development in AD. As will be discussed later, redirecting science and operational elements, though challenging, was more easily achieved than securing a willingness to innovate in legal, research governance, and institutional culture.

16.2.2 Organization and Overall Structure

From an operational perspective, EPAD was divided into eight work packages (WPs; see Box 16.1 and Figure 16.3). IMI projects are very

---

Box 16.1   The eight EPAD work packages

WP1:   Scientific development (divided into four scientific advisory groups)

WP2:   Data management and analysis (divided into a clinical trial and a disease modeling group)

WP3:   Registry development and delivery

WP4:   Cohort and POC design and delivery and TDC network

WP5:   Project management

WP6:   Communication

WP7:   Business sustainability

WP8:   Ethics, legal, and social implications

tightly managed and accountable to the funder through a series of annual reports and submissions of attainment of deliverables (all of which are publicly available on the EPAD website [www.ep-ad.org]). These work packages were complimented by transversal working groups and committees that dealt with specific needs at various stages of the programs development. For instance, rapid data flows were crucial in the operational delivery of the program. These were required to find and invite people from parent cohorts into the EPAD LCS, and to be able to look, in real time, at the balance across key variables within the LCS as recruitment proceeded and readjust the invitations to rebalance the LCS and ensure it had "readiness" for the POC (see Figure 16.2). The design of this data system took almost 2 years to establish with all the relevant partners contributing in the data oversight committee. Many of the elements of this (PrePAD and the Aridhia AgilityX analysis platform) have been taken forward into the core of the Alzheimer's Disease Data Interoperability (ADDI) platform. Moreover, from the outset it was recognized that the value of the data collected in the EPAD LCS (and

POC trial) would be at a breadth and scale to help facilitate great advancement in the understanding of disease models in the early phases of neurodegeneration. These data therefore must be open access and of the highest quality. Finally, rapid data flows and analysis would help inform trial design with reports on, for instance, changes in cognitive-test trajectories to mimic placebo-group declines to inform and then replace simulations.

The eight WPs were tightly bound by pre-set deliverables but were also designed such that adaptations could be made in order to to help achieve the aim of the program. This required substantial resources to be invested in project management (WP5) and (internal) communication (WP6).

The original IMI-EPOC-AD call had proposed seven work packages, but the EPAD Consortium's bid added an eighth, focused on ethics, legal, and social implications (ELSI), which early on and throughout the program yielded incredible outputs and advice about a range of relevant topics such as risk disclosure as well as overseeing and managing the research participants' panels [2]. The leadership on this work given by WP8 to the rest of

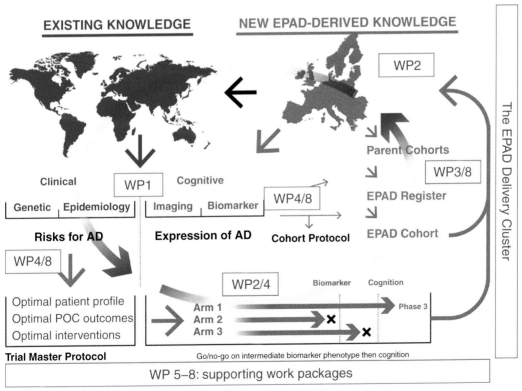

Figure 16.3 Overview of the eight EPAD work packages and their principal points of interaction with each other. The blue 360° circular arrow illustrates the flow of knowledge (and data), the perpetually refined understanding of disease mechanisms, trajectories of change in outcomes and their association with risk factors (e.g., genetics) as well as other subpopulations.

the program ensured that the research participants themselves became valued partners in the design, delivery, and outputs from the program.

16.2.3 Decision-Making Process

EPAD had a budget of €64 million, involved 39 partners, and (at its peak of activity) had 410 people from Europe and the United States receiving direct salary costs from the grant. It recruited over 2,000 research participants, generating several million data points and over 1 million aliquots of cerebrospinal fluid (CSF), plasma, serum, saliva, and urine. The research participant facing elements of the project were sponsored by the University of Edinburgh, supported by the clinical research organization IQVIA, who were a partner of the project. The program's governance was all developed *de novo*, and the initiation of the program. The IMI-EPAD-AD project was legally bound in a project agreement which was signed by all partners. The project agreement was a lengthy document that outlined the principles surrounding intellectual property (compliant with the framework set by IMI), data sharing, and sample access. This was complimented by the grant agreement, which covered the allocation of funds from the original grant to recipients (small and medium enterprises, third sector, and academic partners). EFPIA partners provided funding either in cash or as in-kind contributions (usually as staff).

The Governance of the EPAD program was provided by several official entities.

16.2.3.1 Program Coordinator (EFPIA Lead) and Associate Program Coordinator (Academic Lead)

The program coordinators took responsibility for the overall delivery of the program, signing all annual financial and scientific reports, and chairing the executive committee and project management office. The program coordinator was a senior employee of the lead partner of EPAD, Johnson & Johnson (J&J), and the associate program coordinator was a senior academic from the University of Edinburgh.

16.2.3.2 General Assembly

The main decision-making body for EPAD was the general assembly, which met annually. All representatives from each partner attended the general assembly, which typically ran over 3 days in May of each year of the project. This was attended by in excess of 200 academics, researchers, operational staff, and industry employees. These meetings included discussions on key design issues with the project as well as providing critical community-building activities maintain purpose and alignment to the original aims and vision of EPAD.

16.2.3.3 Executive Committee

The executive committee met on a monthly basis and was chaired by the program coordinator. They oversaw strategic developments of the project and provided senior support for the project management office. The executive committee had balanced representation from EFPIA (three representatives), academia (three representatives), and the project management office (one representative).

16.2.3.4 Project Management Office

The project management office oversaw the daily running of the project and was responsible for tracking budget allocations, financial reporting, completion of deliverables and organization of the general assembly. The project management office was jointly represented by J&J, the University of Edinburgh, and Sinapse (project management small and medium enterprise). The project management office met fortnightly and quarterly face to face.

16.2.3.5 Clinical Development Executive

The clinical development executive met every 2 months and was responsible for overseeing the delivery of the four key elements of the program, namely the register, the LCS, the POC trial, and the TDC network. Each work package sent at least one representative to clinical development executive, which was also attended by each of the partners providing data support, i.e., IXICO (neuroimaging partner), Aridhia (data management partner), and IQVIA (clinical research organization).

16.2.3.6 Other Long-Standing Committees

Each work package would also hold regular meetings to discuss their own deliverables and new developments. Moreover, EPAD established a balancing committee to meet monthly and review the "readiness" of the LCS in light of interventions in and on the POC pipeline, a data oversight committee, national and pan-European participants' panels, an EPAD Academy to support data usage and specifically the needs of early career researchers working in the program, and a national leads meeting of principal investigators from each of the countries represented with EPAD TDCs (France, Spain, the Netherlands, Scotland, England, Germany, Sweden, Switzerland, and Italy[1]). Finally, decisions on drugs being entered into the EPAD POC platform were overseen by the clinical candidate selection committee (CCSC). These committees are discussed in more detail below in specific sections of the chapter.

16.2.4   Industry Participation

The IMI was launched in 2009 with the aim of overcoming obstacles in drug development. As a consequence, calls are proposed by EFPIA partners and then discussed at one of a series of boards – in the case of EPAD, the Neuroscience Board, before being launched to receive applications from academic-led consortia. An EFPIA partner leads the call and will form a consortium of EFPIA partners with a shared interest in the topic; by gathering commitments (both in-kind and cash), the project budget is established with IMI matching the EFPIA contribution from public funds. The overarching objective of IMI and the leadership of the projects by industry highlight the core role of industry in this work. By responding to the call document, academics and their institutions align themselves to the objective and vision set out in the call. Fidelity to the call itself is maintained through the careful management of accountability for pre-agreed deliverables that are committed to, in the project and grant agreements. Within the neurodegenerative field, numerous projects have been undertaken but given each may have very different project partners and the calls themselves may be singularly focused on a small area of research, coordination between projects is not assured by any structural mechanism. To address this, IMI launched a "coordination action" in 2017, which led to the establishment of IMI-Neuronet (www.imi-neuronet.org), whose primary aim is to coordinate the activities of the other IMI projects focused on neurodegenerative diseases, to build a pan-European research community, and take practical steps to help projects work together more effectively and efficiently.

Within EPAD, the partnership between EFPIA and academia was achieved through all governance entities and work packages being jointly led by an EFPIA and an academic lead.

Given the aim of EPAD, it was vital to ensure that the readiness cohort, the POC master protocol, and all the necessary governance and data standards would attract a pharmaceutical or biotechnology company to place their compound into the trial platform. One of the key issues in this regard was the sponsorship of the cohort and the POC platform by the lead academic institution, namely the University of Edinburgh. IQVIA played a critical role in this assurance building work. The fact that funding for the clinical trial itself was not part of the IMI funding and that access to the platform was not limited to EPAD partners meant that substantial communication of the EPAD platform was required. In the first instance this was undertaken by the CCSC and latterly complimented by promotion through a major presence as an exhibitor at the Alzheimer's Association International Conference in Chicago (2018) and Los Angeles (2019). Post IMI, while the CCSC has (in effect) dissolved, access to research participants for clinical trials will still take place in partnership with GAP to help promote the EPAD site network and readiness cohort. This work was seriously hampered by the 2020/21 COVID-19 pandemic which curtailed the ability to set up new clinical trials or continue to follow up EPAD research participants.

The CCSC was jointly chaired by a senior EFPIA individual and the academic lead and also had membership from a further principal investigator and two independent experts from industry involved in drug development. The CCSC would review applications made by intervention owners (IOs) in a standardized format to gauge suitability for the EPAD platform and then (if approved) pass the IO to the POC operations team to work in partnership with the IO on developing their own appendix to the master protocol (Figure 16.4). This appendix writing group was led by the IO and tended to have substantial operational presence from the IO as well as from the sponsor and IQVIA.

Therefore, outside the core IMI–EPAD program, there was another level of partnership with industry collaborators who brought compounds into the platform. All this work was done under confidentiality agreements between the IO, University of Edinburgh, IQVIA, and the POC trial statisticians (Berry Consultants). Though necessary,

---

[1] Switzerland and Italy had a single representative, Germany was engaged at this level but was unable to open TDCs and TDCs were opened latterly in Greece and Belgium but were not directly represented at the national leads meeting. Scotland and England were split because of the large number of TDCs in each country.

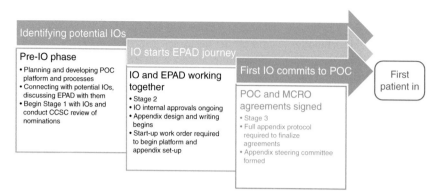

Figure 16.4 Overview of process by which an intervention owner (IO) places their compound into the EPAD POC Platform.

this often created some communication challenges in being able to share with the rest of the EPAD Consortium what stage discussions and developments were at with IOs, which would have had a substantial effect on motivation for recruitment and retention of individuals to and on the LCS.

16.2.5 Research Participants as "Partners"

All clinical research projects benefit from the insights which can be provided by research participants and/or those affected by the disease being targeted. Often, this patient and public engagement work will involve advocates and advocacy groups often previously established by third-sector organizations. In this regard, the EPAD program benefited greatly from Alzheimer's Europe as a partner. To compliment this, it was decided to establish a mechanism for direct engagement with research participants at a TDC, national, and pan-European level. This model was based on that undertaken in the PREVENT Dementia program [3]. One key aspect of both EPAD and PREVENT Dementia is that the research participants, by definition, are a healthy, dementia-free at-risk population, with their involvement more aligned to that of healthy volunteers. Their agency, however, was critical as ultimately the interventions being developed were to be for their benefit, and their insights and advice into study protocols were essential to ensure that the context was relevant for the population of interest.

Each individual TDC was at liberty to form their own network of research participants and provide research-participant-facing materials as they saw fit. This included local videos, pamphlets, and face-to-face public-engagement meetings. In Scotland, for instance, an annual joint meeting of

researchers, academics, and research participants took place, with workshops on key aspects of the program, and was attended by approximately 100 delegates. Research participants had the opportunity to network with their research and academic colleagues.

At a national level, the research participants were coordinated into national panels, who would discuss their experience of the LCS and help design communication materials. These national panels would also be asked to provide formal feedback on protocol amendments. By 2019, four national panels had been established, in Spain, the Netherlands, England, and Scotland, and each panel sent representation to the annual EPAD general assemblies.

As well as providing feedback and insights on the program, it was clear that researchers and academics from both EFPIA and academia gained much value from the joint working with research participants and, in particular, their attendance at the general assemblies, for all aspects of the work and social activities, helped in ensuring that the autonomy and agency of the research participants was evident consistently.

16.3 Register and TDC Network

16.3.1 The EPAD Register

The original target population for secondary-prevention studies was those individuals with preclinical AD. It was recognized that this population would not be known in large numbers to traditional memory clinics and that screening the general population for amyloid positivity would be restrictively time consuming and expensive and might also yield in those who were discovered to be amyloid positive a low prediction of progression to dementia [1]. The solution for this was to work in partnership with a range of cohort studies across Europe where data had originally been collected that would allow targeting of higher-risk populations. For instance in the cohort study, Generation Scotland (www.ed.ac.uk/generation-scotland), data were available on ApoE status, family history of dementia, age, and cognition and so, by applying an algorithm on these data, a high-risk individual could be identified who was, for example, an ApoE ε4 (*APOE-4*) homozygote, aged over 70 with a positive family history of dementia and cognitive test scores below 1 standard deviation of the population norm.

This theoretical capacity to identify people in existing cohorts was put into practice by WP3, led by VUMC and Pfizer (Figure 16.5). Building on the Café Variome tool developed by the University of Leicester through the IMI-EMIF program, data in parent cohorts were made visible to a new tool – PrePAD – that could be set to list people in the cohort with data within certain (adjustable) boundaries. The collaboration with parent cohorts was formalized through a contract that highlighted their value to the project and they were considered Associate Scientific Collaborators and invited to attend the EPAD general assembly.

As most parent cohorts had non-disclosure policies on, for example, ApoE status, the PrePAD tool would identify "cases" and then invite a random sample within disclosed parameters, such as age to match the cases. The parent cohorts would make the initial contact with the (potential) research participant using a derived ID (Derid) given to them by a group in EPAD called the algorithm running committee (ARC); the Derids had a one-way key that would allow the person in the

parent cohort to be identified though the parent cohort team would have no way of knowing if they were a case or a control. The ARC was split into two groups – one ran the algorithm to get a total number per query; then, once set, this was sent to the second group, which generated the Derids. This was because the first group included several people who worked at TDCs and therefore there was the potential for unblinding. As the project progressed it became clear that research participants with prodromal AD were required, so the program pivoted to focus on patients in clinics with mild cognitive impairment (MCI), often where amyloid status was known. This meant that TDCs were at liberty to work directly with their aligned memory clinics to invite people into the LCS with known/disclosed amyloid status; this system complemented the pre-existing system and was termed PrePAD-Velocity.

This system and the yield for each type of approach is summarized by Vermunt et al. [4], who highlight that the number needed to approach in population-based cohorts is incredibly high relative to directly working with clinics. The solution, moving forward, which is therefore being advocated for adoption in future programs of this nature is to develop high-quality, potentially federated, registers in clinics, which tools like PrePAD can work across. This approach was being developed through the Scottish Brain Health Register though this was compromised by the advent of COVID-19 in 2020, which meant that all clinical work became virtual. This will no doubt pick up again post COVID, and a similar approach may be adopted across other healthcare regions, mediated by initiatives like ADDI and the Davos Alzheimer's Collaborative.

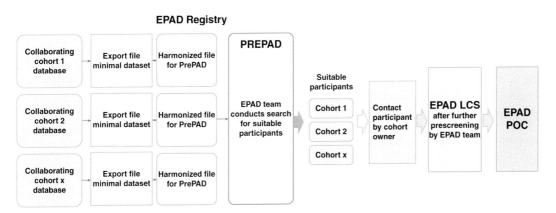

Figure 16.5 Schematic overview of participant and data flow in EPAD [4].

16.3.2 The Trial Delivery Center Network

The TDCs were aligned to the project either as EPAD partners or under a subcontract to the University of Edinburgh. The name "trial delivery center" was a slight misnomer, as the TDCs were in fact critical nodes in the entire pan-European EPAD community. The vast majority of early career researchers working on the project who formed the EPAD Academy were employed in TDCs and only a small part (if any) of their work was on delivering the LCS. In building this community, it was critical that subcontracted TDCs enjoyed the same privileges to data and sample access as "partner" TDCs and this was clearly articulated in their contract.

Given that, ultimately, these TDCs would be undertaking a POC study, their involvement with EPAD was only possible after they had successfully passed the EPAD TDC certification process. This was a very involved process run jointly by the sponsor (University of Edinburgh) and IQVIA, with input from the national lead under which the TDC and an EFPIA representative sat. This also created an opportunity for bringing researchers and academics at these TDCs onboard with the EPAD aims and culture noted previously. The first wave of TDC certifications were all done by face-to-face meetings that included the chief investigator but as numbers of TDCs rapidly increased toward the end of the IMI period this was no longer possible, and they were run by the clinical research associates of IQVIA with remote input from the sponsor.

It also emerged that laboratory procedures within EPAD were more complex than in other observational studies, so the sponsor then set up separate laboratory training for each TDC coordinated by the EPAD biobank principal investigator and her team.

The main aim of the TDC certification process was to build a tightly knit community of sites that were operating to the highest possible standard of assessment and delivery. These site set-ups were complemented at various points with national and pan-European principal investigator meetings, quarterly national lead meetings, and specific sessions at the EPAD general assembly.

This process was a deliverable in WP4 of EPAD and the documentation and knowledge gained was shared with colleagues in GAP as a very early and successful output of the GAP–EPAD collaboration in 2016. The GAP process informed the EPAD process and vice versa; therefore, the GAP and EPAD accreditation should give assurance for future potential sponsors of the quality of these sites which, in Europe, were almost exclusively academic sites based in public hospitals.

16.4 The EPAD Longitudinal Cohort Study

16.4.1 Background

The most substantial output from the IMI period of EPAD was the EPAD LCS. From May 2016 to the study closure in March 2020, 2,096 research participants were recruited, with a small proportion of the early recruits completing 3 years of follow-up and four study visits (baseline, month 6, month 12, month 24, and month 36) (Table 16.1). The data from the EPAD LCS have been released as V.IMI (V = version) and is now freely available to all researchers globally via the WizeHive application system (www.EP-AD.org/ERAP) (ERAP = EPAD research access process) and was the first full data set to be made available on the ADDI platform. Previous data releases are superseded by this one.

The cohort protocol has been published [5]. The main objective of the EPAD LCS was as a readiness cohort for the EPAD POC; as such, "readiness" was defined on two key parameters, namely amyloid status and Clinical Dementia Rating (CDR) score with scores >0.5 leading to exclusion at screening. Negative amyloid status was not an exclusion for both practical, ethical, and scientific reasons. From a practical perspective, batching and shipping of samples meant that from sampling to data being available could take up to 6 months as rapid testing of small batches or even individual samples would have been prohibitively expensive. From an ethical perspective, we followed a non-disclosure policy, as amyloid status and risk prediction at this severity of disease is not fully understood as yet and, from a scientific perspective, the secondary objective of disease modeling meant we needed a range of values of amyloid to inform modeling analyses. As it transpired, 37% of the sample were considered amyloid positive (CSF amyloid beta [Aβ] <1,000 pg/ml using the Roche Diagnostic Elecsys® System), with a large number of people fulfilling the original aim of the program to identify preclinical AD (n = 358) (Table 16.2).

Table 16.1 Number of completed research participant visits and availability of key assessment data at each visit.

	Visit 1 (baseline)	Visit 2 (6 months)	Visit 3 (1 year)	Visit 4 (2 years)	Visit 5 (3 years)
Actual number of participants visits	2,096	1,571	1,190	397	90
Number of participants with blood sample collected for ApoE[a]	2,007	0	0	0	0
Number of MRIs performed[b]	1,952	0	610	256	6
Number of lumbar punctures performed (includes "retest"[c])	1,806	0	350	204	8
Number of RBANS[d] tests	2,014	1,561	1,180	396	90
Number of CDR[e] tests	2,024	1,556	1,181	394	90

[a] Blood sample to measure ApoE is only collected at baseline visit as per protocol. [b] MRI scan is not performed at 6-month visit as per protocol. [c] Lumbar puncture is not performed at 6-month visit as per protocol. [d] Repeatable Battery for the Assessment of Neuropsychological Status. [e] Clinical Dementia Rating.

Table 16.2 Trial readiness as indexed by CDR and amyloid status. Overall, 34% of cohort were deemed trial "ready."

CDR global score	Amyloid status	Number of participants (*n*) (%)
0	Negative	904 (52.4%)
0	Positive	358 (20.7%) preclinical AD
0.5	Negative	234 (13.6%)
0.5	Positive	230 (13.3%) prodromal AD
		n = 1,726*

* This number is less than the 2,096 recruited as some samples were not collected as per protocol or were not available at the time of reporting due to shipment delays secondary to the COVID-19 lockdowns across Europe.

All research participants had at least one CSF sample. To complement this the protocol also focused heavily on neuroimaging with both a core and an advanced MRI sequence [6]. Blood was taken and both serum and plasma are available in the EPAD biobank and four projects are ongoing with these samples. Data from each of these projects will be returned to the main database after completing the necessary quality-control steps.

DNA was extracted from blood and ApoE status is known on all research participants and is in the V.IMI database. The global screening array for genome-wide data was made available in 2021.

Cognitive data were critical for indicating readiness as well as being able to provide pre-randomization "run-in" data for the POC trial. Repeated testing in the LCS also fully mitigated learning effects. As such, the primary cognitive outcome in the EPAD LCS had to be the same as the primary cognitive outcome in the EPAD POC. The Clinical and Cognitive Scientific Advisory Group deliberated on the choice of outcomes in an inclusive and thorough manner, involving experimental neuropsychologists, principal investigators, and experts in AD drug development from within the pharmaceutical industry. The process of these deliberations have been published [7] as well as the decision on the final battery [8]. This final battery included regulatory ready outcomes (RBANS and CDR) as well as more experimental measures believed to be more closely related to early hippocampal damages as a consequence of AD pathology. These included tests of visuospatial memory (allocentric and egocentric) and binding paradigms. The former already showing evidence of impairments associated with a high risk of dementia [9].

16.4.2 Research Participant Recruitment: Summary of the EPAD LCS

The EPAD LCS forms a valuable resource for disease modeling and fully characterized research

Table 16.3 Baseline characteristics of 1,843 non-screen failed participants in the EPAD LCS

Variable	Mean (SD)	Frequency (%)	Number currently unknown
Gender			
Female		1,035 (56.6%)	
Male		793 (43.4%)	
Age, years	65.7 (7.41)		
Age group			
Under 75 years old		1,612 (88.2%)	
75 years old and above		216 (11.8%)	
Years of formal education*	14.4 (3.70)		
Education			
Up to secondary		722 (39.5%)	
Beyond secondary to ordinary first degree		451 (24.7%)	
Postgraduate studies		655 (35.8%)	
Family history of AD?			
No		657 (35.9%)	
Yes		1,171 (64.1%)	
ApoE-4 genotype			57
No *APOE-4* alleles		1,077 (58.9%)	
One *APOE-4* allele		618 (33.8%)	
Two *APOE-4* alleles		76 (4.2%)	

*Years of education is country-specific.

participants for trial inclusion. The sample was predominantly female (56.6%), with a mean age of 65.7 (standard deviation [SD] = 7.41). Thirty-eight percent were ApoE+ (Table 16.3). Publication of the main variables in the V.IMI database of the EPAD LCS is anticipated and will be formatted in line with previous publication of earlier data sets (V500.0) [10]. Moreover, more detailed analysis of these data to describe the cohort in line with other classifications, such as the amyloid, tau, and neurodegeneration (A/T/N) criteria has occurred [11] and is anticipated to continue subsequent to the public release of the V.IMI data set.

16.4.3   Open-Access Data

It is expected that in the coming years, data analysis from numerous research groups will yield many important observations to be published and therein influence our collective knowledge of many biological and clinical aspects of AD. Moreover, further follow-up of research participants who were in the EPAD LCS will continue at both local and national levels under separate protocols and data can be linked back to the IMI data as well as across the new follow-up projects through designed-in data interoperability using e.g. the ADDI platform.

16.4.4   The EPAD Biobank

The EPAD LCS created a huge biobank of samples (CSF, blood, saliva, and urine), all stored in a single location under optimal conditions. Pre-analytical pathways were consistent using state of the art protocols and laboratory manuals which were monitored closely by the central lab in Edinburgh and IQVIA. Sample Access is governed through the Sample Access Committee, which makes recommendations to the Chief Investigator about sample release and/or analysis. EPAD works on the principle that samples should be used and not stored indefinitely for (potential) future use and also that access should not be prohibited by costly access requirements. In essence, access should only be affected by the quality of the scientific question and the willingness to share derived data back into the main EPAD database.

16.5   The EPAD Proof-of-Concept Platform

The primary objective of the IMI-EPAD-AD project was to develop a platform for the Phase 2 testing of interventions for the secondary prevention of AD dementia. While the platform was fully delivered, the project was unable to bring onboard a compound for testing before the end of the IMI period in 2020.

The clinical trial itself was to be a platform trial; a design that has proven hugely effective in drug development [12] in breast cancer, motor neuron disease, and COVID-19 trials. It remains disappointing that in a field with such great failure in drug development that a fully prepared platform formed by the leading companies, academics, and institutions working in AD supported by the European Union via the IMI was unable to persuade an intervention owner of the benefits of the approach at a scientific, methodological, and operational perspective. Future and ongoing trial failures will perhaps mediate a further reflection and rethinking at senior levels of companies to commit their compounds to a platform trial.

There were five primary components to the platform

(1) the readiness cohort;
(2) the site network;
(3) the master protocol;
(4) the appendix protocol; and
(5) the legal and governance framework.

The readiness cohort and site network have been described already.

16.5.1 Master Protocol and Appendices

The principles underpinning the master protocol were (1) that we would employ a Bayesian adaptive design with regular evolutionary analysis of the intervention's performance against placebo, (2) that placebo would be shareable between interventions, and (3) that we would position the trial in the learning space of Phase 2 whereby adaptations could be possible on effect on "intermediary" biomarker changes by dose or in subpopulations. The master protocol articulated general inclusion and exclusion criteria that all research participants would need to comply with. These were that they would be amyloid positive and have a CDR score of <1. More specific criteria on general co-morbidities and medical history were also included in the master protocol. More specific criteria relevant for a specific intervention were included in the tethered appendix (to the master protocol) (Figure 16.6).

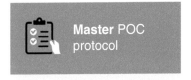

Master POC protocol

Description of common framework of the POC trial and minimum inclusion and exclusion criteria for all interventions

+

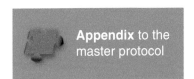

Appendix to the master protocol

Specifically for each intervention cohort
Will define the specific information and additional trial elements and inclusion/exclusion criteria

- Study population
- Maximum treatment duration – 4 years
- Randomization 3:1
- Minimum frequency of on-site visits
- Primary and secondary endpoints assessed every 6 months
- Statistical analyses including interim analyses
- Operational CRO platform

- Specific exclusions
- Subgroups enrolled
- Sample size and length of follow-up
  - Can be restricted numbers
- Randomization of sub-arms
- Biomarker analyses
- Additional endpoints/collection (+ default from master POC protocol)
- Additional analyses
  - More aggressive futility, specific subgroup analyses, decision triggers

Figure 16.6 Summary of key methodological elements in the master POC protocol expanded upon in each individual intervention's appendix protocol.

In the appendix protocol, specific exclusion criteria that related to a compound's safety profile could be added. Moreover, additional outcome measures and assessments could be added in the appendix protocol that were only undertaken in those patients who consented to that appendix of the platform trial. These could cover, for example, safety measures specific to the safety profile of the intervention or clinical or biomarker outcomes that were of specific relevance to the compound or the intervention owner. It was vital that new assessments or inclusion/exclusion criteria did not affect the ability to statistically and meaningfully pool placebo from across all the appendices.

The pooling of placebo was a critical benefit of the platform trial, it meant that more research participants would receive active drug and that the total sample size needing to be recruited was less than the total sample size available for analysis. A key aspect of the sharing of placebo was randomization. Non-random selection to one appendix or another would create a selection bias, which would detrimentally affect the ability to share placebo. For this reason, research participants would first be consented for inclusion in the master protocol once they had completed their screening assessments (which may include for instance checking there were no new medical problems since their last LCS visit); they would then be randomized to an appendix that they were eligible for. This random allocation was known to the investigator, participant, and sponsor. If a participant, for any reason, did not wish to enter a specific appendix, then they would not be put forward for consent to the master protocol. Information sharing as to the open appendices took place between TDC principal investigators and their LCS participants by way of a brochure of "open studies." The second-step randomization was concealed from all parties, and that was to active dose or placebo.

16.5.2 The Operational Readiness of the Platform

Operationally, all elements of the platform trial were in place with a single contract research organization (CRO) in place to support the sponsor (University of Edinburgh) and intervention owner via a contractual process that outlined the roles and responsibilities of each party – this was called the master CRO arrangement. The CRO was responsible for the management of the vendors working on the trial who were appointed through standard procurement routed by the sponsor. These vendors included laboratory services, imaging vendors, database systems, randomization systems, and cognitive test vendors. All these vendors were in place by 2019 and the legal framework for this was all completed. A master CRO arrangement was completed by each intervention owner and they could add vendors for specific purposes but they could not remove vendors or systems in place. The intervention owner paid for all activities in their appendix arm of the study, including investigator fees.

It can be seen that the governance of a platform trial like this needs to map onto the needs of the trial platform itself. The single operational system and data systems create vast efficiencies as does the sharing of placebo. Therefore, the offer from a platform is a single, well-designed, ready-for-use environment, in which interventions can come in and out with no disruption to the system (Figure 16.7). Accordingly, the single system required a single sponsor which needed to be experienced in trial sponsorship, adequately resourced, and neutral in terms of the outcomes from the trial, i.e., one pharmaceutical company could obviously not sponsor the trial of another company.

16.5.3 Statistical Approach and Evolutionary Analysis

The Bayesian adaptive design employed meant that a priori decisions on success and futility had to be articulated in the master protocol. These analyses were conducted on a limited number of variables by the independent data monitoring committee (IDMC), which was separate from the data and safety monitoring board (DSMB), which performed a more traditional role of looking at primarily safety outcomes from each appendix. There was to be one DSMB and one IDMC for all appendices that could look at all data.

It was agreed early in the course of the master protocol (and LCS) development that the RBANS would be the primary outcome used for evolutionary analysis.

Simulations of RBANS changes in different populations were made within WP2 and these simulations informed sample size calculations and duration for the Phase 2 trial (Figure 16.8). Intervention owners were at liberty to negotiate in their appendix specific sample sizes and durations,

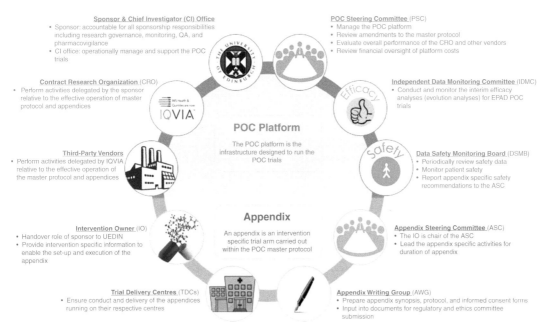

Figure 16.7 Overview of the key operational elements in place in the "plug and play" EPAD platform ecosystem.

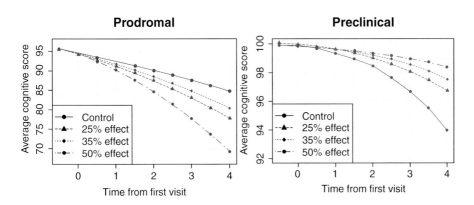

- A disease progression model for measuring the change in the rate of decline over time for a treatment compared to control arm (at least 50% at 1 year):
  - Success: if at any evolution analysis with a posterior probability of at least 85% of at least a 10% reduction in rate of cognitive slowing
  - Futility: if at any evolution analysis at least 90% probability of less than a 10% slowing in cognitive decline

Figure 16.8 Simulations of RBANS decline in preclinical and prodromal populations with indicative criteria for success and futility.

though the minimum duration was set at 2 years. Overly ambitious proposals for effect size were dealt with between the sponsor's appointed trial statistician (Berry Consultants) and the intervention owner.

The simulations were updated as the LCS data emerged, and assumptions confirmed or refuted and, over time, as POC data accumulated, the simulations would evolve into observed changes

in trajectories which were analyzed with reference to certain key parameters such as ApoE and tau status.

16.5.4   Summary of the EPAD POC Platform

In summary, the EPAD LCS POC was designed and set up in great detail to provide a high-quality testing environment guaranteeing low screen failure from the LCS where all necessary inclusion and exclusion criteria were known in a highly motivated participant population. The platform allowed for rapid set-up and incorporation in the EPAD ecosystem, with substantial cost savings from a "plug-and-play" approach with all vendors and sites prepared. Moreover, sharing placebo meant a 33% reduction in the total recruitment needed (assuming three appendices were running concurrently with 3:1 randomization ratio of active:placebo). However, trial sponsors, some of whom were EPAD partners who had invested much time and effort in establishing the platform, chose to use traditional trial methods and operations which have, over the last 20 years, demonstrated zero success. Time will tell whether those choices to continue engaging in an unsuccessful approach were the right ones.

16.6 The Role of EPAD in the AD Drug-Development Ecosystem

16.6.1 A (Slowly) Changing Landscape

The EPAD program was a well-resourced, multipartner effort to address a, still unresolved, issue around drug development for AD. All elements of the trial delivery process from an operational perspective were evaluated with a critical eye and adaptations made in the trial platform to address perceived shortcomings. The platform and program, however, were designed primarily for preclinical populations and at a time, as now, where clinical and regulatory leaders perceive the neurodegenerative disease as a cognitive disorder rather than a brain disease. As a result, as the program developed the original intent to look at preclinical populations and have much emphasis on biomarker readouts, it had to pivot (back) to engaging prodromal patients and retain emphasis on cognitive outcomes. This subtle change to the program had knock-on effects within the delivery as the program now sat within a more "competitive" environment in terms of ongoing trial programs. In 2021, the momentum behind "disease before dementia" is building, not least from the crystallization of thinking around "brain health," much of which emerged from the investigators within EPAD [13–15], perhaps facilitated by the existence of the close-knit EPAD community.

This reemergent thinking of AD as a brain disease underpins each new iteration of diagnostic criteria for AD in research use, where the emphasis on biomarkers as part of the diagnostic criteria gains increasing prominence [16]. The empirically based momentum behind this direction of travel will probably see biomarker criteria ascend above clinical symptoms, especially in early-disease populations, in the years ahead. At that point a program like EPAD could be highly sought after, where quicker-turn-around Phase 2 trials based on biomarker outcomes not as intermediaries but as primary outcomes will be of even greater advantage to the field and, therein, to patients with the earliest stages of AD, decades before the syndrome of dementia develops.

Until the point where the operational decision making catches up with the science, EPAD and the broader community can leverage the substantial assets developed. The EPAD LCS data and biobank are freely available and easily accessible via the ADDI platform and University of Edinburgh's Sample Access Committee, the TDC network is being incorporated into the truly global offering from GAP to trial sponsors for trial delivery, and the almost 100 early-career researchers who were part of the EPAD Academy will take forward their experience and learning from EPAD to the next stage of their careers. Through GAP, IMI-Neuronet, and follow-on funding from the Alzheimer's Association for the data and sample access systems, the EPAD assets will be maintained and, as and when sponsors seek a new platform trial to be established, the learnings from EPAD will ensure that this can be developed to be even more successful than this first pan-European attempt.

16.6.2 Lessons Learned

In true Bayesian fashion, had we known then what we know now, what would we do differently?

The truth is, very little. Perhaps, had EPAD looked more closely at the offering and maintained its focus in the preclinical space we would not have had downstream "competition" from existing disease programs. That was also the space where there was most uncertainty in disease models, forming a bridge between programs like the Dominantly Inherited Alzheimer Network (https://dian.wustl.edu/) (familial AD), the Alfa (www.barcelonabeta.org/en/alfa-study/study) and PREVENT studies (mid life), and the Alzheimer's Disease Neuroimaging Initiative (http://adni.loni.usc.edu/)

and the Australian Imaging, Biomarker and Lifestyle study (https://aibl.csiro.au/) (MCI, later life).

The management consultant guru, Peter Drucker, is famously quoted as saying that "culture eats strategy for breakfast," and whilst EPAD developed an amazing, internal "EPADista" culture, this was not broadly shared with key decision makers, especially outside of Europe. Whilst the collaboration and dialog with GAP was purposeful throughout, the GAP and EPAD programs evolved with different emphasis midway through the EPAD program, isolating the developments somewhat from global developments and culture. These two major programs are merging once more, which will be of huge benefit for all, under the umbrella of the Davos Alzheimer's Collaborative.

Finally, the legal and governance framework that EPAD existed within would not or could not change or flex to accommodate some of the more innovative aspects of the program. Intervention owners were being asked to place their lead assets for AD into a platform that was being governed by a third-party sponsor. There was no "proof of platform" to refer to, perhaps with a backup compound that would have mitigated concerns about this set-up for the ultimate decision makers in organizations which, in a historically unrewarding clinical area, may be risk averse. Had EPAD brought onboard some assets to test the system, perhaps drugs that could be repurposed, drugs that had failed Phase 2 (or 3) in mild AD dementia and prodromal AD, then we could have had real evidence as opposed to theoretical assurance that the system worked.

16.7   Final Thoughts

Billions of people worldwide will develop AD, and only by intervening early in preclinical disease can we make a fundamental difference to the rates of late-stage disease where clinical symptoms and societal burden manifest. The "problem statement" articulated in the New York Academy of Sciences in 2013 remains totally unchanged despite the passage of time and the €64 million of financial investment, and the time and toil invested by over 2,000 research participants and over 400 academics and researchers from 39 partners. The problem won't go away unless we take the outputs from huge programs like EPAD, learn, adapt, and keep going – confidently and collaboratively. Platform trials helped defeat COVID-19; from 2021 onwards they will be key to defeating the even greater killer which is AD.

References

1. Ritchie CW, Molinuevo JL, Satlin A, et al. The European Prevention of Alzheimer's Dementia (EPAD) Consortium: a platform to enable the secondary prevention of Alzheimer's dementia through improved proof of concept trials. *Lancet Psychiatry* 2016; **3**: 179–86.

2. Gregory S, Wells K, Forsyth K, et al. Research participants as collaborators: background, experience and policies from the PREVENT Dementia and EPAD programmes. *Dementia* 2018; **17**: 1045–54.

3. Ritchie K, Ritchie CW. The PREVENT study: a prospective cohort study to identify mid-life biomarkers of late-onset Alzheimer's disease. *BMJ Open* 2012; **2**: e001893.

4. Vermunt L, Veal CD, Ter Meulen L, et al. European Prevention of Alzheimer's Dementia Registry: recruitment and prescreening approach for a longitudinal cohort and prevention trials. *Alzheimers Dement* 2018; **14**: 837–42.

5. Solomon A, Kivipelto M, Molinuevoet JL, al. European Prevention of Alzheimer's Dementia Longitudinal Cohort Study (EPAD LCS): study protocol. *BMJ Open* 2018; **8**: e021017.

6. ten Kate M, Ingala S, Schwarz A, et al. Secondary prevention of Alzheimer's dementia: neuroimaging contributions. *Alzheimers Res Ther* 2018; **10**: 112.

7. Ritchie K, Ropacki M, Albala B, et al. Recommended cognitive outcomes in preclinical Alzheimer's disease: consensus statement from the European Prevention of Alzheimer's Dementia project. *Alzheimers Dement* 2017; **13**: 186–95.

8. Mortamais M, Ash J, Harrison J, et al. Detecting cognitive changes in preclinical Alzheimer's disease: a review of its feasibility. *Alzheimers Dement* 2017; **13**: 468–92.

9. Ritchie K, Carriere I, Howett D, et al. Allocentric and egocentric spatial processing in middle-aged adults at high risk of late-onset Alzheimer's disease: the PREVENT Dementia Study. *J Alzheimers Dis* 2018; **65**: 885–96.

10. Ritchie CW, Muniz-Terrera G, Kivipelto M, et al. The European Prevention of Alzheimer's Dementia (EPAD) longitudinal cohort study: baseline data release V500.0. *J Prev Alzheimers Dis* 2019; **7**: 8–13.

11. Ingala S, De Boer C, Masselink LA, the EPAD consortium. Application of the ATN classification scheme in a population without dementia: findings from the EPAD cohort. *Alzheimers Dement* 2021;DOI: http://doi.org/10.1002/alz.12292.

12. Angus D, Alexander B, Berry S, et al. Adaptive platform trials: definition, design, conduct, and reporting considerations. *Nat Rev Drug Discov* 2019; **18**: 797–807.

13. Frisoni G, Ritchie C, Carrera E, et al. Re-aligning scientific and lay narratives of Alzheimer's disease. *Lancet Neurol* 2019; **18**: 918–19.

14. Frisoni GB, Molinuevo JL, Altomare D, et al. Precision prevention of Alzheimer's and other dementias: anticipating future needs in the control of risk factors and implementation of disease-modifying therapies. *Alzheimers Dement* 2020; **16**: 1457–68.

15. Ritchie CW, Russ TC, Banerjee S, et al. The Edinburgh Consensus: preparing for the advent of disease-modifying therapies for Alzheimer's disease. *Alzheimers Res Ther* 2017; **9**: 85.

16. Jack CR Jr., Bennett DA, Blennow K, et al. NIA–AA Research Framework: toward a biological definition of Alzheimer's disease. *Alzheimers Dement* 2018; **14**: 535–62.

The Global Alzheimer's Platform Foundation®: Delivering New Medicines Faster by Accelerating Clinical Trials

Jason Bork, Cyndy Cordell, John Dwyer, Gabe Goldfeder, Debra R. Lappin, Richard Mohs, Julie Neild, Rona Schillinger, Jill Smith, Katy Smith, Leigh Zisko, and George Vradenburg

17.1 The Need for a Global Alzheimer's Disease Trial Network

The Global Alzheimer's Platform Foundation® (GAP) was created in response to the critical need to positively disrupt and improve the execution of Alzheimer's disease (AD) clinical trials. GAP's genesis was the product of collaboration between leaders from philanthropic organizations, research centers, the National Institutes of Health, and the pharmaceutical industry.

GAP was created in response to the passage of the National Alzheimer's Project Act (NAPA) in 2011. The National Plan to Address Alzheimer's Disease was subsequently released in 2012 and set a primary goal of preventing and effectively treating AD by 2025.

In 2013, UsAgainstAlzheimer's (UsA2) launched a series of global initiatives aimed at better understanding how to achieve the 2025 goal, and determined that a global clinical trial network was needed to improve the speed, efficiency, and quality of AD clinical trials. Following the first G8 Dementia Summit in December 2013, UsA2 and the Global CEO Initiative on AD (CEOi) identified the following top priority [1]:

> Priority One: Develop a global AD clinical trial platform to reduce the time, cost, and risk of drug testing; advance scientific understanding of disease pathogenesis; and increase the capacity and efficiency of the field to perform clinical trials. Such a platform, at the outset, should be considered for major markets (Europe, United States, Canada, Australia, Japan).

UsA2 formed a GAP Design Team in early 2014 that included both academic investigators and industry experts in AD drug development. The GAP Design Team recommended the following goals:

- the formation of a clinical trial network of academic (institution-based) and privately funded clinical trial sites, each with a proven level of quality and competence in AD trials, that would commit to standardized trial elements (e.g., a single institutional review board [IRB], a common contract, and rater certification);
- the development of biomarkers for earlier detection of disease pathology, trial enrichment, and ultimately as a surrogate endpoint; and
- the creation of a trial-ready cohort that would draw from registries of persons who have demonstrated an interest to be participants in a therapeutic clinical trial.

Initial funding for GAP was catalyzed during the 2015 global pharmaceutical annual meeting at Hever Castle in England. During that meeting, pharmaceutical leaders confirmed the need for better clinical trial infrastructure and execution of AD clinical trials. By early 2016, GAP received initial milestone-based commitments from seven pharmaceutical company sponsors and began to actively pursue its mission to reduce the duration and cost, and improve the effectiveness of AD clinical trials.

17.2 Overview of GAP Structure and Initiatives

The Global Alzheimer's Platform Foundation's site network (GAP-Net) – and GAP's partnership with the sites – is fundamental to enhancing participation in AD research and improving the performance of AD therapeutic trials.

17.2.1   GAP Site Network

Since 2016, GAP has pursued its mission in conjunction with a dedicated network of premier clinical trial sites that shared GAP's vision (GAP-Net). GAP-Net now comprises over 90 research centers (Figure 17.1). The site network includes academic and private sites to ensure that GAP's efforts address the needs of the whole clinical trial site ecosystem. GAP has established a Parkinson's disease (PD) site network to address unmet needs in other neurodegenerative disorders.

17.2.2   Streamlining AD Clinical Trial Processes

Streamlining clinical trial processes across the network is critical to improving clinical trial performance. GAP offers programs that benefit the entire network as well as trial-specific programs for sites participating in GAP-enabled trials.

- GAP offers concierge-level support for GAP-Net sites participating in GAP-enabled trials through the activation/start-up process. GAP's Study Start-Up (SSU) team helps sites activate efficiently by ensuring all trial requirements are met and approvals are expeditiously received. GAP also creates templated paper source documents to help GAP-Net sites avoid protocol deviations and save time and resources.

- GAP selected Advarra as its central IRB for all GAP-Net sites participating in GAP-enabled trials – a first-of-its-kind arrangement in AD clinical trials. Standardizing this process across the network saves time and reduces costs.

- The GAP Rater Certification program reengineers the traditional start-up process for cognitive scale raters by applying a comprehensive demonstration of mastery across the most-used cognitive scales. GAP, in collaboration with Cogstate, implemented a one-time process that ensures that raters at GAP-Net sites are qualified to administer scales according to procedures acceptable to scale developers and sponsors across multiple trials. GAP's Rater Certification program reduces the time and cost of initiating trials and greatly improves sites' opinions of a sponsor's trial.

- All GAP-Net sites are invited to participate in the annual GAP-Net Site Optimization Conference, the only operationally focused AD conference in the industry, now also including PD-related content. Sites benefit from networking and sharing best practices with trial sponsors, clinical research organizations (CROs), and other sites.

- GAP's Bio-Hermes study is designed to evaluate leading digital and blood-based biomarkers that are anticipated to accelerate enrollment,

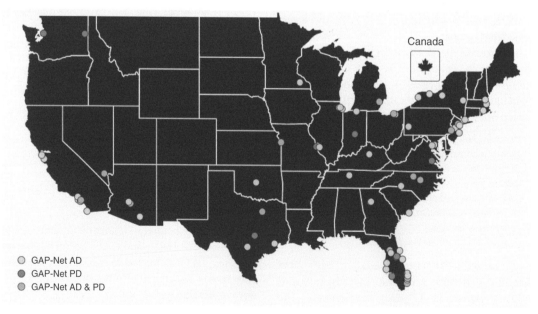

Figure 17.1 GAP-Net site locations in North America (includes expansion into a PD network described further in Section 17.6).

lower screen fail costs, and reduce variability when incorporated into therapeutic trials.

17.2.3 Enhancing Participation and Enrollment in AD Clinical Trials

Other GAP programs are designed to enhance participation and enrollment in clinical trials.

- The GAP Participant Services (GPS) program uses a team of clinical trialists to partner with sites on implementing customized recruitment and screening solutions that improve clinical trial performance. This high-touch approach delivers higher randomization rates than sites without the support of GPS.
- GAP works collaboratively in select markets with established community organizations who serve under-represented minority populations to provide information and education on AD clinical trials at nearby GAP-Net clinical research sites.
- GAP leverages communication channels in local Medicare Advantage (MA) plans to enable sites to better target both physicians needing additional education as well as beneficiaries who are seniors with new diagnoses or an interest in brain health.
- In partnership with Lyft, GAP's Clinical Trial Transportation program removes transportation as a barrier to participate in clinical trials. GAP-Net sites have access to transportation portals to schedule and monitor rides for their participants and study partners, with minimal administrative burden.
- GAP's Acti-v8 Your Brain program creates awareness of brain health as a risk mitigation strategy against cognitive decline and diseases such as AD. Acti-v8 Your Brain is unique as it is the only brain health program of its kind that includes a pillar promoting "get involved in research."
- The GAP Citizen Scientist Awards (CSAs) are the first-of-its-kind awards to celebrate AD and PD clinical trial participants and study partners. GAP-Net sites nominate Citizen Scientists and celebrate the nominees in local and regional events. Four selected honorees are recognized at a national event each year. The only way to find treatments and cures for AD and PD is through clinical trial research and these participants and study partners make that research possible.

17.3 How the GAP Network Functions

GAP's network of high-performing academic and private sites (GAP-Net) enables industry sponsors to complete clinical trials on a single, optimized trial platform. GAP-Net sites participating in GAP-enabled trials activate faster than non-GAP sites in the same trials by leveraging standardized programs including central IRB, common contract, and rater certification.

17.3.1 Benefits of a Site Network

GAP-Net consists of academic sites and private sites, which are all aligned with the GAP mission and are open to networking and learning from each other. Sites are identified through a variety of sources and complete a thorough qualification process which assesses several elements including staffing, equipment and facilities, clinical trial experience, and willingness and interest in positively disrupting clinical development. Upon signing the Definitive Network Agreement, sites can access GAP-Net services and begin to derive benefit from those services.

The sites within GAP-Net are willing to use a common central IRB and the GAP Rater Certification program. Sites also use a common contract which standardizes the legal language across multiple sponsor trials. GAP and GAP-Net sites collectively share their best practices through webinars and meetings, the MyGAP web portal, and the annual GAP-Net Site Optimization Conference. GAP-Net sites partner with GAP in GAP-enabled trials to accelerate therapeutic clinical trials. Additional benefits for sites include heightened reputation, enhanced community engagement, an opportunity to reshape clinical trials, and greater access to trials and emerging science.

17.3.2 GAP-Enabled Trials

When high-performing GAP-Net sites leverage GAP-Net services in GAP-enabled trials, clinical trial performance is improved. GAP selects trials based on several criteria:

- the ability to execute the protocol as written,
- the qualitative value to the trial participant/ study partner,
- the quality of the science and innovative approaches,
- the general potential to advance the field, and
- alignment with GAP's portfolio of ongoing GAP-enabled trials.

209

Trial selection may be completed in collaboration with the GAP Study Selection Advisory Board (SSAB). Principal investigators from both academic and private sites are part of the SSAB; they provide unique perspectives on operational efficiencies and protocol recommendations to optimize trial delivery.

GAP delivers both qualitative and quantitative benefits to GAP-enabled trial sponsors including the following:

- introducing new sites to trial sponsors;
- encouraging sites to leverage the central IRB;
- influencing sites to reconsider trials they initially declined; and
- activating sites more than 30% faster than non-GAP sites in the same trials when compared with Tufts benchmark data [2] (Table 17.1); GAP-Net sites activate 1.5 to nearly 3 months faster on average, thereby reducing the time and cost of clinical trials.

GAP delivers this acceleration through a high-touch concierge service that enables better communication (among sites, sponsors, vendors, and CROs) along with faster issue escalation and resolution. GAP's Rater Certification program leverages pre-certified raters and targeted training to reduce the time and cost of training raters during the study start-up.

17.4 Participant Recruitment: Addressing a Key Challenge in AD Clinical Trials

The GAP GPS program addresses recruitment challenges by developing and implementing site-specific outreach and recruitment strategies, leveraging existing MA channels of communication and education, and helping sites forge and/or nurture and develop minority community relationships. GAP-Net sites experience a faster screening rate, higher randomization rates, and fewer low/no randomizations per site compared with sites without the support of GPS.

17.4.1 Target Populations: Challenges with Recruiting Participants with Preclinical, Prodromal, and Mild Cognitive Impairment AD

The neuropathological process of AD occurs long before the presentation of clinical symptoms. To thwart AD clinical symptom onset or progression, current research primarily focuses on participants who are preclinical, prodromal, or mildly cognitively impaired and are positive for AD biomarkers. Barriers to finding eligible trial participants include the lack of a clear diagnostic pathway (e.g., no single test or biomarker), lack of time or interest in cognitive assessments during primary care visits, and the stigma associated with AD that prevents patients and families from reporting concerns. These barriers have resulted in undiagnosed dementia in approximately 40% of adults with probable dementia; 19% of adults are also unaware of their AD diagnosis [3]. The inability to identify eligible trial participants using participant self-reports or existing medical records requires screening large numbers of potential participants. For example, using only internet solicitation tactics would require screening millions of participants to meet enrollment targets (Figure 17.2).

Table 17.1 GAP impact on study start-up cycle times compared with non-GAP sites and industry benchmarks

Head-to-head trial comparison: GAP vs. non-GAP sites (April 2020)				Benchmark comparison: GAP vs. Tufts Center for CNS/ neuroscience (central nervous system) therapeutic area (April 2020)			
Study start-up	Duration (months)	Acceleration (months)	Improvement	First draft CTA to FPI	Duration (months)	Acceleration (months)	Improvement
All GAP-Net sites	4.8			All GAP-Net sites	5.9	2.8	32%
Academic	6.1	1.4	19%	Academic	7.2	2.6	27%
Private	3.5	1.7	32%	Private	4.4	2.1	32%

Abbreviations: CTA, clinical trial agreement; FPI, first patient in.

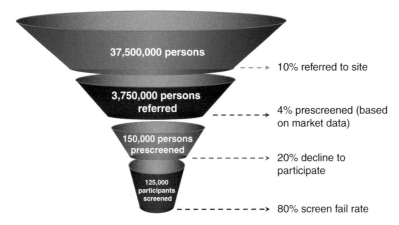

Figure 17.2 Challenges of recruiting for AD clinical research using digital recruitment strategies. Over 37 million persons may need to be contacted to recruit the estimated 25,000 participants needed for a range of oncoming Phase 2 and Phase 3 AD trials in the United States.

17.4.2 Participant Engagement, Prescreening, and Trial Screening

Likely determinants for AD trial recruitment are participant/family engagement, primary care physicians (PCPs), and the research team [4]. Unfortunately, 74% of adults in the United States have not discussed medical research with their doctors/healthcare professionals [5]. Thus, recruitment relies heavily on research-center outreach to prompt participation in clinical research. In 2016, GAP launched its innovative GAP GPS program. GPS Liaisons offer their clinical trialist expertise to sites throughout the enrollment period. Through Oct 2020, over 1,200 GPS Liaison/site encounters occurred resulting in the following outcomes in GAP-Net sites with GPS support compared with sites without GPS support (GAP unpublished data):

- 24% faster trial screening rates;
- fewer sites with 0 or 1 randomizations;
- randomization rates up to 20% higher; and
- randomization rates up to 80% higher for academic GAP-Net sites.

GPS Liaison support was also critical during 2020 as the COVID-19 pandemic disrupted typical recruitment efforts. GAP provided trial sponsors with real-time data on site closures and visit restrictions, and rapidly deployed virtual outreach tools to sites to minimize recruitment delays. GPS Liaisons' ongoing efforts are helping sites and sponsors navigate the unique challenges of continuing clinical trials during the pandemic.

17.4.3 Better Characterizing the Funnel – Medicare Advantage

To address a lack of PCP involvement in timely diagnosis of mild cognitive impairment (MCI)/AD and referrals to clinical trials, GAP is leveraging recent changes made to MA insurance plans for >24 million adults in the United States who are 65 years of age or older [6]. In 2019, MA plans were allowed to provide memory fitness benefits and, in 2020, MA plans received increased payments for beneficiaries diagnosed with dementia. For the first time, insurers have a financial incentive to diagnose dementia and improve care. GAP is facilitating MA-organized PCP education, which discusses timely diagnosis and care plans that include clinical trial opportunities. GAP and MA providers are also educating beneficiaries with risk of AD about brain health, with the goal of connecting them with their local AD research centers.

17.4.4 More Representative Trial Participants: Minority Outreach

Black/African Americans and Latinx Americans are under-represented in clinical research even though they are about 2.0 and 1.5 times more likely, respectively, than White Americans to have AD [7]. In two large AD biomarker trials, less than 5% of the population studied were African American [8]. Latinx Americans have a median participation rate of 2% in AD-related dementias (ADRD) clinical trials [9]. These reports are alarming given that Black/

African Americans and Latinx Americans comprise 13.4% and 18.5%, respectively, of the US population [10]. GAP is augmenting community outreach efforts and recruitment programs across GAP-Net, including culturally competent outreach materials, and is facilitating relationships with minority community organizations. These programs will be leveraged on GAP's Bio-Hermes study. A major goal of the Bio-Hermes study is to help understand the specificity and sensitivity of blood-based and digital biomarkers in under-represented minority groups. Recruitment strategies are designed to ensure that 20% of the population contributing outcome data are from minority groups.

17.5 The Role of GAP in Advancing Biomarkers to Assess and Diagnose AD

Digital and blood-based biomarkers have the potential to substantially improve patient cost and burden in treating AD. GAP is developing a program intended to characterize the accuracy of multiple digital and blood-based biomarkers in a diverse population and inform the role of these biomarkers in clinical trials and clinical care.

17.5.1 Recent Advances in Digital and Blood-Based Biomarkers

Biomarkers are characteristics that are objectively measured as an indicator of normal biological processes, pathological processes, or biological responses to therapeutic intervention [11]. In recent years, biomarkers have been developed that enable the diagnosis and assessment of patients with AD based on the presence of amyloid-beta (Aβ) plaques [12] and/or tau deposits in the brain [13]. Both positron emission tomography (PET) scanning and cerebrospinal fluid (CSF) measures have been developed as biomarkers. These biomarkers augment traditional clinical and psychometric assessments and increase the likelihood that participants enrolled in clinical trials have not only the clinical phenotype of AD but the neuropathological hallmarks of the disease [14]. While these biomarkers have greatly improved the diagnostic accuracy of participants entering clinical trials, they are costly, time consuming, and relatively invasive.

Easily administered digital and blood-based assessments of cognition may provide much more cost-effective and generally usable biomarkers for assessment of underlying pathology and cognitive status in patients with AD and in those at risk for AD. As examples, plasma measures of $A\beta_{40}$ and $A\beta_{42}$ have shown strong correlations with the presence of brain amyloid deposits as measured by PET [15]; specific forms of hyperphosphorylated tau (p-tau), particularly $p\text{-}tau_{217}$, have shown strong relationships with both brain amyloid and brain tau levels in selected populations [16]. Blood-based biomarkers thought to reflect neurodegeneration, including neurofilament light chain (NfL) [16] as well as those possibly reflecting brain inflammation [17], are also showing promise.

While several cognitive test batteries have been validated for use in diagnostic assessment and as measures of cognitive effects of drugs [18], these tests require skilled technicians to administer and involve a substantial time commitment from participants. Brief cognitive tests that can be administered remotely on handheld devices [19] as well as passive recording devices, such as those used to analyze speech samples, are under development and may provide digital biomarkers reflecting cognitive and/or functional status without the need for extensive in-person testing. As with the blood-based biomarkers, the appropriate use and interpretation of these biomarkers will depend upon data showing how they should be interpreted in different contexts.

Regulatory guidance describes many of the different ways in which biomarkers can be used and the data needed to support such use [11]. Biomarkers can be diagnostic, prognostic, predictive, or pharmacodynamic, and some biomarkers may be suitable for more than one use.

17.5.2 Need for Validation in Populations Similar to Those Recruited for Trials

Current AD clinical trials are designed for participants with MCI due to AD, preclinical AD, or mild AD [20]. Participant groups are identified through a combination of cognitive tests, clinical evaluation, and, usually, verification of Aβ deposits in the brain by PET scan or CSF measurement. Participants often screen fail during recruitment for trials because they do not have the required cognitive characteristics or are lacking Aβ deposits. Promising blood-based biomarkers and cognitive screening tests have been developed, but few have been validated in clinical trials.

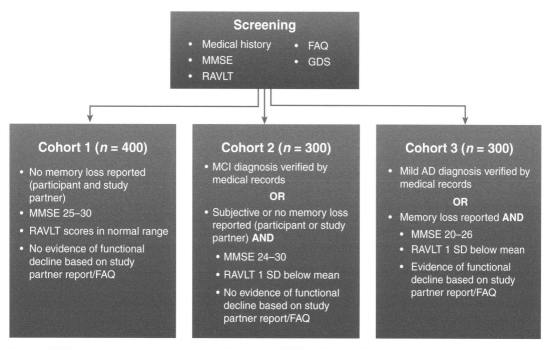

Figure 17.3 Bio-Hermes cohort characterization. Abbreviations: FAQ, Functional Activities Questionnaire; GDS, Geriatric Depression Scale; MMSE, Mini Mental State Examination; RAVLT, Rey Auditory Verbal Learning Test; SD, standard deviation.

GAP's Bio-Hermes study is designed to evaluate several promising digital and blood-based biomarkers that could lower screen fail rates and accelerate enrollment. GAP is recruiting participants that fall into three clinical diagnostic classifications: cognitively normal, MCI, and mild AD (Figure 17.3). Because the rate of amyloid positivity is likely to be lower in cognitively normal participants [21], the cognitively normal cohort is larger to ensure enough amyloid-positive participants. GAP is also recruiting participants who identify as under-represented minority populations (20% of total) to understand the specificity and sensitivity of blood-based biomarkers in minority groups. GAP is obtaining a common set of blood-based and digital biomarkers from each participant and these biomarker results are being compared with centrally read and quantitated Aβ PET scans. Results from this trial will help determine the relative efficiencies of blood-based and digital biomarkers as well as the extent to which different combinations of biomarkers are useful for determining the likelihood of amyloid positivity. Participating GAP-Net sites are uniquely positioned to recruit participants with the required clinical phenotypes as well as the minimum of 20% who identify as Black/African American and/or Latinx so the utility of biomarkers can be assessed in minority groups.

17.6 GAP's Unique Role in Clinical Trials: The Future

New initiatives will enhance how GAP contributes to the speed, quality, and effectiveness of AD clinical trials. GAP is extending its network globally, initially into Europe, and will continue to partner with other site networks to share learnings and, where possible, to implement GAP-enabled trials. GAP has expanded GAP-Net to include GAP-Net PD, a PD trial network that will leverage existing AD programs as well as offer PD-specific programs.

Based on its experiences over the last 5 years, GAP is uniquely positioned to connect clinical trial sites, sponsors, and CROs with patient advocacy groups, academic consortia, government agencies, and trial participants. GAP's efforts to organize site networks, streamline study start-up, enhance trial awareness and recruitment, and foster site efficiency will continue to enhance the speed, efficiency, and quality of clinical trials. Sponsors, investigators, trial participants, and patients all benefit from GAP's efforts.

In response to requests from industry sponsors and sites, GAP established a PD trial network in North America, GAP-Net PD. This network leverages existing site relationships and AD programs including accelerated study start-up and in-person and remote prescreening strategies; it also offers PD-specific programs including recruitment steering committees and outreach committees with community partners. GAP-Net PD is already engaged in several (US) PD studies.

Other new initiatives are being planned that will further enhance how GAP contributes to the speed, quality, and effectiveness of clinical trials. In addition to the Bio-Hermes project described in Section 17.5, GAP is also extending the network globally, initially to Europe, in partnership with approximately 40 sites; many of these sites were formerly part of the European Prevention of Alzheimer's Disease (EPAD) network [22]. The emerging network of European sites subscribe to GAP's mission. The processes developed for GAP-Net have the potential to expand the clinical trial capabilities of the proposed GAP European network, GAP-Net EUR. GAP will also intensify its collaboration with site networks in Japan, Australia, and other countries to share learnings and, where possible, to implement GAP-enabled trials. These efforts will further GAP's aim of achieving a fully global network of sites sharing knowledge to enhance speed, efficiency, and quality of AD and PD clinical trials.

Acknowledgments

In addition to those who contributed to this chapter, GAP thanks several individuals who were instrumental in defining our mission and creating the foundation:

- NYAS leadership including Ellis Rubenstein, BA; Diana van de Hoef, PhD; and Cynthia Duggan, PhD;
- Jeff Cummings, MD, ScD, University of California, Los Angeles – now with University of Nevada and Cleveland Clinic Lou Ruvo Center for Brain Health;
- Drew Holzapfel, MBA, Global CEO Initiative on Alzheimer's Disease (CEOi);
- Janssen Pharmaceuticals leadership including Luc Truyen, MD, PhD; Roy Ervin Twyman, MD, PhD; Michael Ropacki, PhD; and Maike Stenull, MBA;
- Eli Lilly and Company leadership including Phyllis Barkman Ferrell, MBA; Russ Barton, MS; Eric Siemers, MD; and J. Carmel Egan, PhD;
- Randy Bateman, MD, Washington University;
- Paul Aisen, MD, Keck School of Medicine, University of Southern California, San Diego;
- Reisa Sperling, MD, Harvard Medical School, Harvard University;
- Howard Feldman, MD, FRCP, University of British Columbia;
- Andy Satlin, MD, Eisai, Inc.

The work of GAP has been supported by the following industry partners: Biogen, Inc.; Eisai, Inc.; Eli Lilly and Company; Green Valley Pharmaceuticals; Janssen Pharmaceuticals; Lundbeck; Roche; and Takeda, Inc. Philanthropic partners include the Vradenburg Foundation; the Ray and Dagmar Dolby Family Fund; and the Alzheimer's Drug Discovery Foundation. GAP projects have benefited from collaboration and in-kind support from Cogstate, Ltd.; IQVIA, Inc.; the Alzheimer's Therapeutic Research Institute of the University of Southern California; the National Institute on Aging; the European Prevention of Alzheimer's Dementia (EPAD) program; and all of the investigators and staff at GAP-Net sites.

References

1. Vradenburg G. Catalyzing the Landmark G8 Commitment. *HuffPost* 2013; December 23. Available at: www.huffpost.com/entry/catalyzing-the-landmark-g8-commitment_b_4489405 (accessed November 24, 2020).

2. Mathias A, Lamberti MJ, Getz K. 'START' (Start-up Time And Readiness Tracking) study: Working Group final report. Tufts Center for the Study of Drug Development (CSDD). Released June 15, 2012.

3. Amjad H, Roth DL, Sheehan OC, et al. Underdiagnosis of dementia: an observational study of patterns in diagnosis and awareness in US older adults. *J Gen Intern Med* 2018; **33**: 1131–8.

4. Carr SA, Davis R, Spencer D, et al. Comparison of recruitment efforts targeted at primary care physicians versus the community at large for participation in Alzheimer disease clinical trials. *Alzheimer Dis Assoc Disord* 2010; **24**: 165–70.

5. Research!America. Public perception of clinical trials. July 2017. Available at: www.researchamerica.org/sites/default/files/July2017ClinicalResearchSurveyPressReleaseDeck_0.pdf (accessed November 24, 2020).

6. Murphy-Barron C, Pyenson B, Ferro C, Emery M. Comparing the demographics of enrollees in Medicare Advantage and fee for service medicare. Milliman report. October 2020. Available at: www.bettermedicarealliance.org/publication/

comparing-the-demographics-of-enrollees-in-medicare-advantage-and-fee-for-service-medicare/ (accessed November 24, 2020).

7. Alzheimer's Association. 2020 Alzheimer's disease facts and figures. *Alzheimers Dement* 2020; **16**: 391–460.

8. Shin J, Doraiswamy PM. Underrepresentation of African-Americans in Alzheimer's trials: a call for affirmative action. *Front Aging Neurosci* 2016; **8**: 123.

9. National Institutes of Health. NIH RCDC inclusion statistics report. Available at: https://report.nih.gov/RISR/#/ (accessed November 24, 2020).

10. United States Census Bureau. Quick facts United States. 2020. Available at: www.census.gov/quickfacts/fact/table/US/PST045219 (accessed November 24, 2020).

11. US Food and Drug Administration. Qualification process for drug development tools guidance for industry and FDA staff draft guidance. November 2020. Available at: www.fda.gov/media/133511/download (accessed November 24, 2020).

12. Clark CM, Pontecorvo MJ, Beach TB, et al. Cerebral PET with florbetapir compared with neuropathology at autopsy for detection of neuritic amyloid-β plaques: a prospective cohort study. *Lancet Neurol* 2012; **11**: 669–78.

13. Schwarz AJ, Yu P, Miller BB, et al. Regional profiles of the candidate tau PET ligand ^{18}F-AV-1451 recapitulate key features of Braak histopathological stages. *Brain* 2016; **139**: 1539–50.

14. Jack CR, Bennett DA, Blennow K, et al. A/T/N: an unbiased descriptive classification scheme for Alzheimer disease biomarkers. *Neurology* 2016; **87**: 539–47.

15. Nakamura A, Kaneko N, Villemagne VL, et al. High performance plasma amyloid-β biomarkers for Alzheimer's disease. *Nature* 2018; **554**: 249–54.

16. Palmqvist S, Janelidze S, Quiroz YT, et al. Discriminative accuracy of plasma phosphor-tau217 for Alzheimer disease vs other neurodegenerative disorders. *JAMA* 2020; **324**: 772–81.

17. Morgan AR, Touchard S, Leckey C, et al. Inflammatory biomarkers in Alzheimer's disease plasma. *Alzheimers Dement* 2019; **15**: 776–87.

18. Welsh KA, Butters N, Mohs RC, et al. The Consortium to Establish a Registry for Alzheimer's Disease (CERAD). Part V. A normative study of the neuropsychological battery. *Neurology* 1994; **44**: 609–14.

19. Kourtis LC, Regele OB, Wright JM, Jones GB. Digital biomarkers for Alzheimer's disease: the mobile wearable devices opportunity. *NPJ Digit Med* 2019; **2**: 1–9.

20. McKhann GM, Knopman DS, Chertkow H, et al. The diagnosis of dementia due to Alzheimer's disease: recommendations from the National Institute on Aging–Alzheimer's Association workgroups on diagnostic guidelines for Alzheimer's disease. *Alzheimers Dement* 2011; **7**: 263–9.

21. Sperling RA, Donohue MC, Raman R, et al. Association of factors with elevated amyloid burden in clinically normal older individuals. *JAMA Neurol* 2020; **77**: 735–45.

22. Ritchie CW, Molinuevo JL, Truyen L, et al. Development of interventions for the secondary prevention of Alzheimer's dementia: the European Prevention of Alzheimer's Dementia (EPAD) project. *Lancet Psychiatry* 2016; **3**: 179–86.

Chapter 18

Clinical Trial Development in Frontotemporal Lobar Degeneration

Peter A. Ljubenkov and Adam Boxer

18.1 Introduction

Frontotemporal lobar degeneration (FTLD) is a heterogeneous class of neurodegenerative pathological entities which gives rise to a large proportion of early-onset dementia in North America and Europe. While FTLD is comprised of multiple rare individual subtypes, the combined point prevalence of these subtypes is estimated at about 20 per 100,000 for patients [1]. Moreover, this prevalence may be underestimated, as FTLD clinical syndromes tend to be underrecognized and misdiagnosed as psychiatric illness. FTLD-associated syndromes cause a high level of caregiver burden and often impact multiple individuals within the same family, as up to 40% of FTLD is associated with an autosomal-dominant pattern of inheritance [1]. Depending on the pattern of frontal and temporal lobe pathology, FTLD gives rise to a diverse group of clinical phenotypic syndromes, including the spectrum of frontotemporal dementia (FTD) and related motor syndromes, such as FTD with motor neuron disease (FTD-MND) [2], corticobasal syndrome (CBS)[3], and progressive supranuclear palsy (PSP) [4]. Patients with the behavioral variant of FTD (bvFTD) [5] experience debilitating changes in personality and behavior, while progressive loss of language is a key feature of other FTD variants designated as variants of primary progressive aphasia (PPA) [6]. These PPA variants may progressively impair the pronunciation and grammatical formulation of language, as in the non-fluent agrammatic variant of PPA (nfvPPA), or progressively destroy a person's knowledge of the concepts that words represent, as in the semantic variant of PPA (svPPA). Regardless of the resulting initial clinical syndrome, FTLD gives rise to an unrelenting and universally fatal disease course without any approved disease-modifying therapies. There is therefore a crucial need for clinical therapeutic trials targeting the mechanisms of FTLD pathogenesis and progression.

18.2 FTLD Heterogeneity

The pathological heterogeneity of FTLD is a major factor limiting therapeutic development, as each individually rare pathological subtype may reflect unique mechanisms of pathogenesis and modes of disease progression. At autopsy, approximately half of FTLD spectrum disorders are characterized by pathological forms of the microtubule stabilizing protein tau: abnormally misfolded, cleaved, and post-translationally modified (often phosphorylated and acetylated) and in the form of monomers, oligomers, and filamentous aggregates [7]. FTLD-tau pathology can be further subclassified based on the relative preponderance of six tau isoforms, primarily distinguished by alternative splicing of the microtubule-associated protein tau (*MAPT*) gene, which leads to four repeated microtubule binding domains (4R tau) with the inclusion of exon 10, and three binding domains (3R tau) with the exclusion of exon 10 [8]. Moreover, tau conformation and post-translational modifications may differ in further subdivisions of FTLD-tau pathology.

The majority of FTLD without tau pathology falls under another diverse pathological category, FTLD-TDP, with at least four distinct subtypes (A–D) defined by neuronal patterns of intranuclear depletion and cytoplasmic accumulation of a transactive response DNA-binding protein 43 kDa (TDP-43) [9]. Additionally, a minority of patients diagnosed with FTD have alternative pathological features at autopsy, including FTLD with intraneuronal inclusions with FET proteins [2, 10] or Alzheimer's disease (AD) pathology mimicking the phenotypic spectrum of FTLD [2, 3, 11]. Given this diversity of pathology and the possibility of multiple co-pathologies in some cases, it is possible that future disease-modifying therapies may not have broad efficacy, as they may need to be precisely tailored to target the unique mechanism of each individually rare FTLD subtype. Additionally, differences in protein isoforms, post-translational modifications, and conformations may give rise to differences in drug affinity and target engagement in FTLD variants sharing the same pathogenic protein.

18.3 Patient Selection in FTLD Clinical Trials

The pathological heterogeneity of FTLD is also associated with heterogeneity of clinical syndromes, sometimes with limited clinical–pathological correlation. Most FTLD pathological subtypes give rise to multiple clinical phenotypes, and FTD phenotypes may be associated with multiple pathological etiologies. This issue is particularly clear in bvFTD, the most common FTD variant, in which FTLD-TDP only comprises a narrow majority of cases at autopsy [2]. The development of biomarkers to specifically identify FTLD-tau or -TDP pathology during life would transform the ability to conduct trials in bvFTD. Given this context, a majority of recent clinical trials have focused on specific clinical phenotypes and familial cohorts with reliable associations to specific FTLD pathological subtypes on autopsy.

The classic Richardson syndrome of PSP (which involves restricted eye movements, early falls, and atypical parkinsonism) is nearly 100% specific for FTLD-tau [4] with a distinct pattern of 4R tau pathology, and has therefore been the primary focus for multiple, clinical trials, including pivotal previous trials [12] (ClinicalTrials.gov, ID: NCT03413319, NCT03068468). The presence of motor neuron disease with FTD features is also similarly specific for FTLD-TDP (type B) pathology on autopsy [2], though this cohort has so far only been served by clinical trials of therapies rationalized as potential treatments for amyotrophic lateral sclerosis (ALS). Additionally, several clinical phenotypes have received little attention in clinical trials but are associated with sufficient clinical–pathological correlation to enable future trial programs (Table 18.1). Specifically, svPPA and nfvPPA are upwards of 80% specific for FTLD-TDP (typically type C) and FTLD-tau pathology, respectively [11], and CBS is also relatively specific for FTLD-tau, once Alzheimer's pathology has been ruled out [14].

Familial FTLD cohorts, with defined mutations causing autosomal-dominant FTLD, have become a growing point of interest in recent clinical trial development, given their defined candidate mechanisms for therapeutic intervention and firm correlations with specific pathological subtypes.

Defined FTLD risk mutations also firmly predict specific FTLD pathological subtypes on autopsy. Among the major familial causes of FTLD, heterozygous progranulin gene (GRN) mutations have been the focus of several clinical trials [15–17], given their common mechanism of action (progranulin haploinsufficiency) and consistent correlation with FTLD-TDP (type A) [9] pathology after symptom onset. Additionally, the most common mutation to cause FTLD and ALS, hexanucleotide expansion of chromosome 9 open reading frame 72 (C9orf72), is also strongly associated with FTLD-TDP (typically type B) [9] and is currently under investigation in multiple therapeutic programs directed at C9orf72-ALS (NCT03626012) [18]. Patients with pathogenic mutations in the MAPT gene are also firmly associated with FTLD-tau pathology on autopsy (with specific mutations being predictive of the preponderance of 3R or 4R pathology [13]), and have begun to be included in clinical trials targeting tau pathology [19]. Importantly, defined FTLD risk mutations theoretically enable a multitude of future prevention trials, intended to abate the onset (i.e., "phenoconversion") and progression of FTLD pathology in presymptomatic or early symptomatic mutation carriers, though it is unclear how well the results of these trials will generalize to sporadic FTLD. Such trials will require validation of reliable measures of impending phenoconversion and measures of early disease progression (as later discussed in this chapter).

18.4 The Role of Advocacy Groups and Consortia Advancing Clinical Trials in FTLD

A variety of independent advocacy groups, National Institutes of Health (NIH)-funded research consortia, and international research consortia have served crucial roles in supporting patient education, expanding the visibility of FTLD, supporting FTLD research, and coordinating massive multi-center clinical research projects. These organizations also promote the protection of patient rights in clinical research, including familial FTLD cohorts at risk of discrimination based on their genetic status.

The Association for Frontotemporal Degeneration (AFTD; www.theaftd.org), founded in 2002, is the most established patient advocacy group for FTLD and is responsible for significant philanthropic interest in this disease space. AFTD has also

217

Table 18.1 Clinical–pathological correlation in FTLD

Clinical phenotypes associated with FTLD		FTLD-TDP	FTLD-tau	Other FTLD[a]	AD including mixed FTLD and AD
FTD variants	bvFTD [2, 5]	51%	29%	7%	13%
PPA variants	nfvPPA [6, 11]	8%	88%	–	~4% mixed AD + FTLD
	svPPA [6, 11]	86%	14%	–	>1%
	lvPPA [6, 11]	[b]		–	>90%
FTLD-associated motor phenotypes	PSP-RS [4]	>99%	–	–	–
	CBS [3]	52.5% (~81% if AD is excluded)	13.5%	–	35% ~22% primary AD ~7% AD + FTLD
	FTD-MND [2]	>99%	–	<1%	–

Loci for FTLD-associated mutations		FTLD-TDP	FTLD-tau	FTLD-other	AD
Loci for >80% of FTLD mutations	C9orf72 [9]	100%	–	–	–
	GRN [9]	100%	–	–	–
	MAPT [13]	–	100%	–	–
Loci for rare FTLD mutations	TARDBP [9]	100%	–	–	–
	VCP [9]	100%	–	–	–
	TBK1 [9]	100%	–	–	–
	CHMP2B [1]	–	–	100%	–

Note: [a] "Other FTLD" is comprised of FTLD with ubiquitinated inclusions typically containing FET proteins (Fused in liposarcoma [FUS], Ewing Sarcoma [EWS], and TATA binding associated factor 15 [TAF15]). [b] The vast majority of lvPPA represents AD, but some cohorts have described a minority of lvPPA cases with FTLD-TDP.

Abbreviations: bvFTD, behavioral variant frontotemporal dementia; C9orf72, chromosome 9 open reading frame 72; CBS, corticobasal syndrome; CHMP2B, charged multivesicular body protein 2b gene; FTD-MND, frontotemporal dementia with motor neuron disease; GRN, progranulin gene; MAPT, microtubule-associated protein tau; nfvPPA, non-fluent variant primary progressive aphasia; PSP-RS, progressive supranuclear palsy Richardson syndrome; svPPA, semantic variant primary progressive aphasia; TARDBP, transactive response DNA binding protein 43 kDa gene; TBK1, TANK binding kinase 1 gene; VCP, valosin-containing protein gene.

been instrumental in regularly convening meetings of the Frontotemporal Degeneration Study Group (www.theaftd.org/for-researchers/ftsg/) comprised of FTLD experts from academia, government agencies, non-profit foundations, and industry, in order to develop and advance policies in FTLD therapeutic development [20]. The AFTD, in coordination with the Alzheimer's Disease Discovery Fund, is also active in the financial support of multiple early-phase trial programs in FTLD spectrum disease. These opportunities, in conjunction with funding opportunities through the Alzheimer's Association (www.alz.org/partthecloud/research.asp) and the NIH, have formed an important backbone of potential support promoting investigator-initiated trials, often using drugs repurposed for FTLD. Additional independent foundations have provided substantial support

to basic science, translational research, and clinical research that may promote FTLD therapeutic development. The Bluefield Project to Cure FTD (www.bluefieldproject.org) was founded in 2008, largely with an interest in FTLD-TDP (particularly due to GRN haploinsufficiency), and the Tau Consortium (tauconsortium.org) was founded shortly after, in 2009, largely with an interest in FTLD-tau. Both organizations have provided expansive support to a variety of basic scientists and clinical researchers, and have been instrumental in seeing several drugs move into clinical trial. Additionally, several charitable organizations, such as CurePSP (www.psp.org) and CBD Solutions (www.cbdsolutions.se) have emerged to promote patient support and clinical research, particularly in FTLD phenotypes associated with 4R tauopathy (i.e., PSP and CBS). Together, the AFTD and other aforementioned organizations have coordinated with NIH-funded research consortia to found the FTD Disorders Registry (ftdregistry.org), an online registry of patients, family members, and caregivers, intended to promote education, patient support, and participation in clinical research.

Given the rarity of individual FTLD subtypes, multiple NIH-funded, multi-site, research consortia have emerged among academic sites to enroll participants into clinical research over a larger geographic distribution [21]. Similar to efforts in AD (specifically the Alzheimer's Disease Neuroimaging Initiative [ADNI] and the Dominantly Inherited Alzheimer Network [DIAN]) these consortia use harmonized protocols for clinical data collection, imaging data collection, and biospecimen collection, and frequently rely on centralized biospecimen repositories such as the National Centralized Repository for Alzheimer's Disease and Related Dementias (NCRAD). Among the earliest of these consortia, the 4 Repeat Tauopathy Neuroimaging Initiative (4RTNI) is currently in its second cycle and actively recruits patients with 4R-tau-related clinical phenotypes across six sites in North America (NCT02966145). In 2014, a more expansive research effort, the Advancing Research and Treatment of Frontotemporal Lobar Degeneration (ARTFL) Consortium (U54NS092089), initiated a project collecting clinical, imaging, and fluid biomarker data from a variety of FTD syndromes (both sporadic and familial) over 17 clinical sites. In parallel, ARTFL's sister project, the Longitudinal Evaluation of Familial Frontotemporal Dementia Subjects (LEFTTDS) Consortium (U01AG045390), also collected longitudinal data and biospecimens from asymptomatic and symptomatic participants from families carrying the three most common genetic causes of FTLD (mutations in *C9orf72*, *GRN*, and *MAPT* genes). More recently, the ARFTL and LEFFTDS consortia have been renewed as the NIH-funded ARTFL–LEFFTDS Longitudinal Frontotemporal Lobar Degeneration (ALLFTD) project (U19AG063911; www.ALLFTD.org) consortium, which collects longitudinal data in familial and sporadic FTLD cohorts and spans 19 clinical sites in North America.

Outside of the United States, the Genetic Frontotemporal Dementia Initiative (GENFI; www .genfi.org) has formed the largest FTLD research consortium collecting longitudinal clinical, imaging, and fluid biomarker data from familial FTLD cohorts enrolled at 26 sites in the United Kingdom, Europe, and Canada. Together, the ALLFTD and GENFI consortia have greatly advanced efforts to genotype participants in familial cohorts and generally expand the pool of identified trial-ready participants within a variety of FTLD cohorts. Additionally, these consortia have prioritized the discovery and validation of clinical, imaging, and fluid biomarkers for use as measures of therapeutic response in clinical trials, with a particular emphasis on measures that track impending phenoconversion and trend early disease pathology in familial FTLD. Since their inception, FTLD consortia like ALLFTD and GENFI have been committed to the support of biospecimens and data sharing among collaborators (in academia and industry) in an effort to enhance the speed of discovery and validation of disease biomarkers for use in clinical trials. The importance of data sharing also applies to interventional therapeutic trials in rare disease sets, particularly when the number of enrolled participants approaches the magnitude of total participants known to have a specific condition. In order to foster the greater adoption of data-sharing policies worldwide, ALLFTD and GENFI have partnered with the Australian Dominantly Inherited Non-Alzheimer Dementias (DINAD) and Research Dementia Latin America (ReDLat) research consortia to form the Frontotemporal Dementia Initiative (FPI; www .thefpi.org). The FPI will promote the curation of a minimum shared data set across all worldwide genetic FTD studies, including industry-sponsored clinical trials. This collaboration has also spawned several ongoing projects, including greater coordination of efforts to develop predictors of phenoconversion and multimodal disease progression modeling in familial FTLD.

18.5 Clinical Trial Endpoints in FTLD

While patients who meet full clinical criteria for FTD may have clear deficits in executive and language function on formal psychometric testing, a single cognitive measure may not be sensitive to changes in differing phenotypes or subtle symptoms associated with the earliest stages of phenoconversion in familial FTLD. Individualized patient scales present one approach to studying heterogeneous syndromes and allow patients the opportunity to relate the severity or symptoms that are most bothersome or disabling [22]. Potential individualized measures may also include individualized goal attainment scales [23] as well as computerized adaptive testing scales, which adjust to a patient's responses during testing [24]. While individualized assessments remain a potential option for future trials, caregiver interview-based measures of general functional disease impairment, including Clinical Dementia Rating Scale (CDR) derivatives, the Frontotemporal dementia Rating Scale (FRS) [25], and the Functional Activities Questionnaire [26], currently provide the most immediately viable clinical endpoints in FTD trials and allow a method of comparison between patients with differing FTD phenotypes. CDR with National Alzheimer's Coordinating Center FTLD domains (CDR plus NACC FTLD) builds on the traditional CDR (designed for AD clinical studies) with the addition of language and behavioral domains pertinent to FTD [27], but it still remains agnostic to additional clinical features of FTLD, such as parkinsonism, motor neuron disease, and apraxia. The Multidomain Impairment Rating (MIR) builds on the CDR plus NACC FTLD by capturing all aspects of the clinical spectrum of FTLD [28] and is currently under investigation in the ALLFTD consortium. Longitudinal observational studies suggest that, compared to formal psychometric testing, the CDR plus NACC FTLD sum of boxes score (sum of all sub-domains) and similar clinical endpoints may allow for smaller sample sizes in trials enrolling patients with sporadic FTD [29]. CDR plus NACC FTLD and MIR may also provide sensitive consensus methods to score subtle clinical changes with the earliest symptoms of familial FTLD [27].

Several other clinical measures are currently under investigation to expand available clinical endpoints in familial FTLD trials enrolling asymptomatic or mildly symptomatic individuals. Informant-based measures of social and emotional sensitivity, such as the Revised Self-Monitoring Scale (RSMS), may also be sensitive to early symptoms and track rates of early brain atrophy on imaging in familial FTLD [30]. Additionally, The Executive Abilities: Measures and Instruments for Neurobehavioral Evaluation and Research (NIH-EXAMINER), a tablet-based executive function battery utilizing item response theory, may detect, for instance, slopes of cognitive decline in mutation carriers who are otherwise identified to be asymptomatic [31]. This and other tablet-based measures also present the added benefit of facilitating uniformed clinical assessments across a large number

of clinical sites and potentially enabling remote assessment techniques.

Ultimately, future FTLD clinical trials in rare populations may depend on validation of non-clinical surrogate fluid and imaging biomarkers to establish drug efficacy. Ideally, these surrogate fluid and imaging biomarkers may enable prevention trials aimed at abating symptom onset in familial FTD in individuals prior to developing detectable clinical symptoms. The US Food and Drug Administration (FDA) has previously accepted such surrogate biomarkers of efficacy for approval of therapies in a variety of other diseases [32], provided these biomarkers strongly correlate with disease pathology and firmly predict symptom onset or progression. It is possible that familial FTLD prevention trials may not rely on a single primary endpoint but rather a multimodal approach, such as those being pursued by the FPI (including clinical, fluid biomarker, imaging biomarker, and specific genetic information) to provide a more reliable measure of early disease staging or impeding phenoconversion prior to symptom onset.

18.5.1 Fluid Biomarkers in FTLD Clinical Trials

Potential applications for fluid (plasma, serum, and cerebrospinal fluid [CSF]) biomarkers in FTLD trials include the confirmation of pathological diagnosis (aiding design trial inclusion criteria), prognostication, staging of disease severity, and confirmation of pharmacodynamic response. A recent thorough review by Swift et al. [33] identifies a large variety of potential fluid biomarkers, including biomarkers of neurodegeneration, neuroinflammation, lysosomal function, and specific gene products important to familial forms of FTLD. Our discussion in this chapter will primarily focus on current biomarker research with the most immediate impact on upcoming FTLD trials.

Currently, no fluid biomarkers (including blood and CSF measures of TDP-43 and tau species) have been validated to distinguish FTLD-tau from FTLD-TDP with enough specificity to aid enrollment criteria in clinical trials [33]. However, plasma elevations in specific hyperphosphorylated tau (p-tau) species (specifically p-tau$_{217}$ and p-tau$_{181}$) appear to reliably distinguish patients with primary AD pathology from patients with underlying FTLD [34, 35]. Additionally, elevation in CSF total tau to amyloid-beta ratio provides a widely commercially available method to distinguish patients with AD pathology from patients with FTLD pathology [36]. However, the ease of collection of blood-based AD biomarkers may lead to them supplanting CSF biomarkers as the method to exclude patients with AD pathology from future FTLD clinical trials.

Neurofilament light chain (NfL) is an axonal cytoskeletal protein released during neurodegeneration, and has been commonly explored as a candidate measure of FTLD biological response to interventions in recent clinical trials [15, 16, 19]. Elevations in plasma, serum, and CSF NfL clearly distinguish symptomatic FTLD from healthy controls [37–39] (though NfL has less diagnostic value in distinguishing between neurodegenerative diseases and FTLD subtypes). Peripheral and CSF NfL hold potential value as prognostic markers of FTLD aggressiveness and as general measures of disease severity in some forms of FTLD [38, 39]. Additionally, NfL may be of particular value as a candidate biomarker of impeding phenoconversion in familial FTLD [40]. In order to investigate this potential application, The Bluefield Project to Cure Frontotemporal Dementia and the ALLFTD research consortium have partnered with a pre-competitive consortium composed of industry and other non-profit organizations in order to support the Neurofilament Light Surveillance Project (NSP) (NCT04516499). The NSP will collect plasma at 3-month intervals (a total of 13 times per participant) in presymptomatic and early symptomatic carriers of FTLD-associated mutations. This effort will allow a high level of temporal resolution in comparing the dynamics of peripheral NfL and the earliest stages and phenoconversion in FTLD.

In patients with specific mutations associated with FTLD, specific gene products may offer valuable pharmacodynamic measures of therapies tailored to the unique pathogenic mechanism of each mutation. Pathogenic GRN mutations lead to FTLD through the common mechanism of haploinsufficiency [41–44], and may reduce secreted progranulin protein in the plasma [45, 46] and CSF [45] by roughly 50%. Plasma and CSF progranulin have therefore been leveraged as biomarkers of successful target engagement in a variety of clinical trials investigating therapies intended to restore progranulin [15–17]. In patients with

hexanucleotide expansion of the C9orf72 gene, abnormal gene products from the mutant allele may also provide detectable biomarkers, reflecting the toxic gain of function in this cohort. RNA is transcribed from both the sense and antisense strands of the expanded C9orf72 allele, and the guanine- and cytosine-rich regions of RNA expansion are capable of undergoing repeat-associated non-AUG (RAN) translation. This RAN translation gives rise to three distinct dipeptide protein repeats (DPRs) from open reading frames in the sense direction (glycine–arginine, GR; glycine–proline, GP; and glycine–alanine, GA) and the antisense direction (proline–arginine, PR; glycine–proline, GP; and proline–alanine, PA) [47, 48]. Levels of these dipeptides can be measured in the CSF of asymptomatic and symptomatic patients with pathogenic C9orf72 expansion, and these may provide a practical pharmacodynamic biomarker for therapies designed to knock down abnormal gene products for the expanded C9orf72 alleles [49, 50].

18.5.2 Imaging Biomarkers in FTLD Clinical Trials

A variety of imaging-based approaches have been proposed for trials enrolling asymptomatic patients at risk for FTLD or with clear FTD clinical syndromes. Resting-state functional MRI (fMRI) and fluorodeoxyglucose positron emission tomography (FDG PET) appear to be sensitive to early abnormalities in subsets of presymptomatic GRN mutation carriers [51, 52], but their value as longitudinal measures of progression or impending phenoconversion remains unknown. At present, volumetric MRI is the best-studied imaging modality for potential use in clinical trials, and the methodology for harmonization of volumetric imaging information is already well established in multi-site consortia such as ALLFTD and GENFI. A priori MRI volumetric regions of interest (ROIs), such as frontal or temporal lobe composites based on pre-existing brain atlases, likely allow for smaller sample sizes than clinical measures alone in trials enrolling patients with symptomatic FTLD [29]. Additionally, data-driven volumetric ROIs (based on regions most with consistent atrophy progression in longitudinal studies) may allow for even smaller sample sizes than a priori ROIs, particularly in trials enrolling bvFTD cohorts, which contain multiple subtypes of atrophy progression [53].

Heterogeneity in atrophy patterns presents a particular challenge to trials enrolling familial FTLD cohorts, which share the same biological disease mechanism but present with a diversity of atrophy patterns and resulting clinical phenotypes. One solution to adjust for this heterogeneity is to quantify each individual's cumulative burden of atrophy using individual W-scores, which provides a normalized measure of atrophy at each voxel, adjusted for demographic factors. This W-score approach appears to be sensitive to changes in brain atrophy at the earliest stages of familial FTLD and may be useful in predicting impending phenoconversion in presymptomatic mutation carriers [54].

18.6 Recent Clinical Programs in FTLD

18.6.1 Drug Development in Progranulin Deficiency

As previously discussed, patients with heterozygous loss of GRN function experience a high penetrance of FTD due to progranulin haploinsufficiency [45, 46], and several clinical trials have sought to measure the pharmacodynamic effects of therapeutic interventions on progranulin levels in the blood and CSF. The calcium-channel blocker nimodipine was, for instance, shown to raise progranulin levels in a mouse model of disease [17], but failed to raise progranulin levels in participants with GRN haploinsufficiency enrolled in an 8-week, open-label trial. Histone deacetylase (HDAC) inhibitors were also found to substantially increase progranulin transcription in a high-throughput cell screen [55], but the HDAC inhibitor FRM-0334 also failed to raise plasma progranulin levels in participants with GRN haploinsufficiency enrolled in a double-blind placebo controlled trial (NCT02149160) [16]. It is, however, worth noting that FRM-0334 also showed inconsistent oral bioavailability, so it may be difficult to reliably extrapolate the broader impact of consistent HDAC inhibition from this trial. Despite its negative results, the FRM-0334 trial did set a precedence as the first international, multi-site, clinical trial enrolling patients with familial FTLD, and maintained ongoing interest in multi-site trials in GRN deficiency. Subsequent, more encouraging results have been observed in multi-site trials of AL001, a monoclonal antibody against sortilin, a protein central to the degradation of progranulin [56]. So far, AL001 has successfully

normalized progranulin levels in people with GRN haploinsufficiency in open-label Phase 1 and 2 trials [15, 57]. Additionally, early trial data suggest that AL001 may decrease plasma NfL levels in mutation carriers, and may therefore exert a neuroprotective effect [58]. AL001 is now being investigated in the first Phase 3 trial targeting progranulin deficiency, with planned sites in North America, Europe, and Australia (NCT04374136). At least two pharmaceutical companies have announced progranulin gene-therapy programs using intracisterna magna delivery of adeno-associated virus (AAV) vector therapies, including the AAV1-based PBFT02 [59] and the AAV9-based PR006 [60], the latter of which entered its first in-human trial in late 2020 (NCT04408625). Additionally, Denali has recently announced a clinical program centered on DNL593, a peripherally administered recombinant progranulin protein, modified to cross the blood–brain barrier [61]. Interestingly, a small molecule, AZP006, has also reportedly been developed to increase progranulin signaling [62] (though preclinical data have not been published), but this strategy is currently being examined in a Phase 2 trial enrolling patients with PSP due to underlying FTLD-tau (NCT04008355), rather than FTLD-TDP due to progranulin deficiency.

18.6.2 Drug Development in C9orf72 Hexanucleotide Expansion

The pathogenic mechanism of C9orf72 expansion remains unknown, but a variety of mechanisms have been proposed, including toxic inclusions of abnormally expanded RNA, toxic gain of function from dipeptides abnormally transcribed from the expanded RNA, and haploinsufficiency [63]. So far, the leading edge of therapeutic programs targeting C9orf72 expansion have focused on suppression of the abnormally expanded RNA transcript using antisense oligonucleotides (ASOs). ASOs are small, single-stranded, synthetic oligonucleotides designed to hybridize with high specificity to RNA targets (both pre-messenger and mature messenger RNA [mRNA]) and impact gene function via a variety of mechanisms, including suppression expression (via RNAase H-mediated degradation of target mRNA), enhancement expression (by suppressing natural antisense transcripts or binding target promoters), or modulation of alternative splicing of specific exons [64]. ASOs require intrathecal infusion and may be limited in their

Table 18.2 Clinical trial programs pertinent to FTLD-TDP

	Mechanism	Indication	Phase	ClinicalTrials.gov identifier	Status
Potential therapies for GRN haploinsufficiency					
Nimodipine	Calcium-channel blocker	FTLD-GRN	1	NCT01835665	Negative
FRM-0334	HDAC inhibitor	FTLD-GRN	2	NCT02149160	Negative
AL001	Anti-sortilin antibody	FTLD-GRN	3	NCT03987295	Ongoing
PR006	AVV9-based gene therapy	FTLD-GRN	1/2	NCT04408625	Ongoing
PBFT02	AVV1-based gene therapy	FTLD-GRN			Planned
DNL593	Recombinant progranulin	FTLD-GRN			Planned
Potential therapies for c9orf72 expansion					
BIIB078	ASO	ALS-C9orf72	1	NCT03626012	Ongoing
Afinersen	ASO	ALS-C9orf72	Pilot		Ongoing
AL001	Anti-sortilin antibody	FTLD-C9orf72	2	NCT03987295	Ongoing

degree of penetration to some targeted areas of brain parenchyma, but they offer diverse and highly specific mechanisms to target discrete C9orf72 RNA transcripts. There is now a growing precedence for ASOs in the treatment of other rare neurodegenerative disorders, as recent clinical trials have led to FDA approval of eteplirsen [65] for treatment of Duchenne muscular dystrophy and nusinersen [66] for treatment of spinomuscular atrophy. In Phase 1 and 2 trials enrolling patients with ALS due to toxic gain of function mutations in the superoxide dismutase 1 (*SOD1*) gene, the ASO tofersen also successfully suppressed total CSF SOD1 and may have shown preliminary signals of clinical efficacy [67]. Additionally, in bacterial artificial chromosome mouse models of C9orf2 hexanucleotide repeat expansion, ASOs directed against the expanded C9orf72 RNA transcripts suppressed nuclear foci of toxic RNA, suppressed production of atypical dipeptides, and improved cognitive performance [68]. So far, clinical therapeutic trials of intrathecal ASOs designed to target expanded C9orf72 transcripts (including BIIB078 and afinersen) have only occurred in patients with an ALS phenotype, due in part to the relative clarity of clinical measures for drug efficacy in this cohort. BIIB078 is currently being investigated in a Phase 1 trial enrolling patients with ALS (NCT03626012) while afinersen has been investigated in a pilot study enrolling one patient with ALS [18]. While both of these clinical programs have so far excluded patients with cognitive or behavioral features of C9orf72 expansion,

they provide the opportunity to establish important proof-of-concept studies that may lay the foundation for future trials in patients with phenotypes associated with FTLD. Aside from ASO therapies, the anti-sortilin antibody AL001 is also being explored in a Phase 2 trial in symptomatic C9orf72 expansion carriers, in an effort to investigate the impact of increasing progranulin levels in other FTLD-TDP cohorts (NCT03987295) (Table 18.2).

18.6.3 Drug Development in FTLD-Tau

A multitude of potential therapies are currently under consideration for treatment of FTLD-tau, and given the importance of tau pathology in AD, a number of clinical trials in FTLD-tau have sought to repurpose therapies from AD development pipelines. Potential therapeutic mechanisms include enhancement of tau clearance, suppression of the prion-like behavior of toxic tau molecules, mitigation of toxic loss of microtubule function, suppression of tau production, alteration of mRNA splicing, and alteration of tau, post-translational modifications [69] (Table 18.3).

18.6.3.1 Passive and Active Immunization Strategies

Passive immunization, using anti-tau monoclonal antibodies, is a potential modality to improving tau clearance and suppress the prion-like behavior of tau (i.e., the propensity of misfolded tau to propagate

Table 18.3 Clinical trial programs pertinent to FTLD-tau

	Mechanism	Indication	Phase	ClinicalTrials.gov identifier	Status
Passive and active tau immunization strategies					
ABBV-8E12 (C2 N-8E12)	Anti-tau antibody (N-terminus)	PSP	2	NCT03413319	Negative
BIIB092 (BMS-986168)	Anti-tau antibody (N-terminus)	PSP	2	NCT03068468	Negative
		CBS, nfvPPA, TES, MAPT	1	NCT03658135	Negative, terminated
LY3303560	Anti-tau antibody (N-terminus)	AD	2	NCT03518073	Active
JNJ-63733657	Anti-tau antibody (mid domain)	AD	1	NCT03375697	Unavailable
UCB0107	Anti-tau antibody (mid domain)	PSP	1	NCT04185415	On hold
BIIB076	Anti-tau antibody (monomer and filament)	AD	1	NCT03056729	Active
AADvac1	Tau vaccine	nfvPPA	1	NCT03174886	Active
ACI-35	Tau vaccine	AD	1/2	NCT04445831	Active
Microtubule stabilization therapies					
Davunetide	Microtubule stabilizations	PSP	2/3	NCT01110720	Negative
TPI-287	Microtubule stabilizations	AD, PSP, CBS	1	NCT01966666, NCT02133846	Negative
Therapies altering tau expression					
BIIB080	Antisense oligonucleotide	AD	1/2	NCT03186989	Active
NIO752	Antisense oligonucleotide	PSP	1	NCT04539041	Active
Small molecules investigated in FTLD-tau					
TRx0237 (LMTM)	Tau aggregation inhibition	bvFTD	3	NCT03446001	Negative
Tideglusib	Glycogen synthase kinase inhibitor	PSP	2	NCT01049399	Negative
Lithium carbonate	Glycogen synthase kinase inhibitor	PSP/CBS	2	NCT00703677	Negative
Fasudil	ROCK inhibitor	PSP/CBS	2	–	Active
Salsalate	Tau acetylation inhibition	PSP	1	NCT02422485	Negative
ASN001	O-GlcNACase inhibitor	PSP	1	–	Planned
AZP2006	Alteration of progranulin	PSP	2	NCT04008355	Active
Additional therapies investigated in FTLD-tau					
Young plasma transfusions	Altered cell milieu/signaling	PSP	1	NCT02460731	Negative
Autologous mesenchymal stem cells		PSP	1	NCT01824121	Unknown

from neuron to neuron and induce conformation changes in other tau molecules). Unfortunately, it is not clear what epitopes are most important in each of the differing forms of tauopathy, and a multitude of potential therapies may be considered, including antibodies against specific tau fragments (e.g., the N-terminal, proline rich, microtubule binding domain, or C-terminal regions of tau) as well as specific hyperphosphorylated forms of tau, specific conformations of misfolded tau, monomeric tau, and oligomeric tau [7]. Early work in a transgenic mouse model of tauopathy suggested that antibodies against the N-terminal epitopes may alter tau pathology and improve cognition [70]. These encouraging preclinical data led to multiple industry-sponsored trials seeking to target N-terminal tau epitopes in AD, as well as parallel programs investigating the same monoclonal antibodies in patients with PSP. Unfortunately, in two well-powered Phase 2 trials, antibodies directed against *N*-terminal tau epitopes (BIIB092, ABBV-8E12) definitively failed to impact the rate of clinical progression in patients with PSP (NCT03413319, NCT03068468). Moreover, termination of Biogen's BIIB092 program in PSP led to an early termination in the Phase 1 basket trial of BIIB092, enrolling patients with CBS, nfvPPA, *MAPT*-mutations, and traumatic encephalopathy syndrome (TES) (NCT03658135) [19]. The outcomes of the BIIB092 and ABBV-8E12 trials come in the context of recent human studies suggesting that most pathogenic species of tau may be truncated at the *N*-terminus and retain their microtubule binding domains [71]. Several subsequent AD drug-development pipelines now focus on antibodies directed against alternative tau epitopes. LY3303560 binds to *N*-terminal tau but shows preference for tau aggregates. BIIB076 binds to monomeric and fibrillar forms of tau. Additionally, multiple monoclonal antibodies (JNJ-63733657 and UCB0107) bind to mid-domain regions of tau. While it is unclear how well each of these antibodies can engage tau in different forms of tau pathology, they present a theoretical opportunity for additional therapeutic trials in FTLD-tau. So far, a Phase 1 trial of UCB0107 has been planned in patients with PSP (NCT04185415), though the trial's sponsor recently announced a pause in this program in December 2020, with plans to instead focus on UCB0107's AD development pipeline [72].

Active immunization strategies are a less explored pathway for tau therapy, but offer the potential benefits of decreased treatment burden and generation of multiple antibodies against a variety of epitopes. The AADvac1 vaccine (containing tau peptide aa 294–305/4R) has been shown to be safe and well tolerated in an open-label trial enrolling patients with AD [73] and has subsequently been investigated in a Phase 1 trial enrolling patients with nfvPPA (NCT03174886). An additional vaccine containing phosphorylated S396 and S404 tau fragments, ACI-35, is also currently under investigation in a Phase 1 clinical trial enrolling patients with AD [74], and may theoretically be investigated in FTLD-tau cohorts.

18.6.3.2 Microtubule Stabilization

Given tau's role in microtubule stabilization and transport, some therapeutic strategies have sought to mitigate the loss of these functions in FTLD-tau.

Davunetide (AL-108, NAP) is a short, intranasally administered peptide, which was thought to promote microtubule stability. Unfortunately, in 2014 davunetide was not found to be efficacious in an international, Phase 2/3, randomized, placebo-controlled trial enrolling patients with PSP. This trial did, however, provide an important first example of a pivotal trial in PSP [12], and thus provided a template for the design of future trials investigating other therapeutic modalities. TPI-287 (abeotaxane), a repurposed, brain-penetrant, taxane derivative, has also more recently been investigated as a method to stabilize microtubules in tauopathies, including Phase 1 parallel cohort trials enrolling patients with PSP, CBS, and AD (NCT02133846, NCT01966666). Unfortunately, dosing in the AD cohort was discontinued due to multiple anaphylactoid reactions to study drug [75]. Additionally, worsening dementia symptoms and increased falls were noted in the PSP and CBS groups, and TPI-287 was not pursued in follow-up trials in FTLD.

18.6.3.3 Decreasing Tau Expression

Direct alteration of tau expression remains relatively unexplored in FTLD development pipelines, but ASOs offer a diverse range of methods to impact the expression of tau. In non-human primates, intrathecal infusions of an ASO that knocks down tau expression, BIIB080 (IONIS-MAPT$_{Rx}$), were well tolerated and led to a 75% reduction of MAPT mRNA in the cortex [76]. Currently BIIB080 is only being investigated in clinical trials enrolling patients with mild AD (NCT03186989), though it may provide a viable mechanism to suppress tau pathology in FTLD-tau and a mechanistically similar drug, NIO752, is now being investigated in patients with PSP (NCT04539041). Additionally, ASO-mediated splice alteration, impacting the alternative splicing of *MAPT* exon 10, is able to normalize the balance of 4R and 3R tau isoforms [77] and may provide an alternative therapeutic strategy for treatment of FTLD-tau typified by aggregates of 4R tau isoforms (as is found in the majority of patients with PSP, CBS, and nfvPPA).

18.6.3.4 Small-Molecule Therapies in FTLD-Tau

The phenothiazine LMTM (TRx0237) is a proprietary formulation of methylthioninium chloride (MTC, an old treatment for malaria and methemoglobinemia) [78] hypothesized to inhibit tau aggregations, and is the most studied small-molecule therapeutic candidate in patients with FTLD.

Disappointingly, large, Phase 3, therapeutic trials of LMTM in Alzheimer's diease [79] (NCT01689246) and bvFTD (NCT03446001) failed to convincingly establish benefits in primary endpoints. The LMTM trial in bvFTD was, however, an important contribution to the field of FTLD clinical research, as it provided the first example of the feasibility and successful completion of a large, multi-site, international trial in bvFTD, with sufficient power to clearly assess efficacy in primary clinical endpoints.

Among patients with PSP, several other clinical programs provide examples of small-molecule drugs repurposed for potential use in FTLD-tau, many with proposed mechanisms impacting the post-translational modification of tau. Tideglusib (a drug previously investigated in AD) and lithium carbonate (a drug used in the treatment of bipolar disorder) potentially block pathogenic tau phosphorylation via inhibition of glycogen synthase kinases, though tideglusib failed to meet its primary endpoint of efficacy in a Phase 2 trial [80] in PSP. Additionally, in a trial of lithium carbonate in patients with PSP and CBS, a majority of patients discontinued the drug due to poor tolerability (NCT00703677), though this drug is still under investigation for behavioral management in bvFTD, svPPA, and nfvPPA (NCT02862210).

Selective inhibitors of rho-associated protein kinases (ROCK) offer an alternative therapeutic mechanism to inhibit pathogenic tau phosphorylation and may promote tau autophagy via alteration of the mTOR signaling pathway. In preclinical studies, fasudil (a selective ROCK inhibitor already clinically used in Asia to treat cerebral vasospasm) was found to suppress tau phosphorylation in primary cortical neurons from rodents and reduced pathogenic tau in a *Drosophila* model of tauopathy [81]. Given these preclinical data, and the availability of preceding clinical safety and pharmacodynamic data, fasudil will soon be investigated in a Phase 2a trial enrolling patients with PSP and CBS [82].

Other potential therapeutic targets in FTLD-tau include post-pathogenic translational modifications other than phosphorylation, such as acetylation and addition of *O*-Linked β-*N*-acetylglucosamine (*O*-GlcNAc). Salsalate, a repurposed drug long used to treat pain, inhibits pathogenic tau acetylation via p300 acetyltransferase and suppresses tau pathology in a transgenic mouse model of FTLD-tau [83]. Salsalate recently failed to show any preliminary signals of efficacy (compared to historic controls)

in a Phase 1 trial in PSP [84], and is thus unlikely to be investigated in future FTLD-tau trials, but tau acetylation may remain a pathway of interest in trials of other therapies. Additionally, *O*-GlcNAcase inhibitors also suppress tau aggregation in a transgenic mouse model of FTLD-tau [85], and at least one drug in this class, ASN001, will soon be investigated in a trial enrolling patients with PSP [86].

18.6.3.5 Alteration of the Extracellular Milieu in FTLD-Tau

One additional strategy for treatment of FTLD-tau is alteration of the extracellular milieu of cells impacted by tauopathy, including alteration of local neurotrophic factors and local inflammatory signaling pathways. This mechanism forms some of the basis for consideration of autologous mesenchymal stem cells in a previously proposed trial in PSP [87] (NCT01824121). However, the viability and validity of this approach has yet to be established in FTLD cohorts. Studies in aging mice also suggest that plasma-derived factors from young mice may provide another approach to alter the extracellular milieu of neurons, and thereby improve synaptic health, neurogenesis, and cognitive performance [88, 89]. However, pooled whole plasma from young human donors failed to show a therapeutic signal relative to historic controls in a Phase 1 open-label trial enrolling patients with PSP [84]. Therefore, while specific humoral factors may still be examined in future FTLD trials, follow-up trials of whole plasma are unlikely in FTLD-tau.

18.7 Future Directions for Clinical Trial Design in FTLD

To date, the majority of clinical trials in the FTLD disease space have utilized relatively traditional randomized, placebo-controlled formats [90], with a re-occurring emphasis on cross-over designs and open-label extensions, in order to improve recruitments and expand compassionate access to potential FTLD treatments. The heterogeneity of FTD and rarity of each individual FTLD subtype do, however, present unique challenges, which may be better addressed by more novel approaches.

In early-phase trials, chiefly interested in safety, tolerability, pharmacokinetic signatures, and pharmacodynamic effects, the so-called "basket trial" [91] may be an appropriate solution to address the clinical and pathological heterogeneity of FTLD. Basket trials, initially developed for oncology, enroll heterogeneous clinicopathological syndromes with similar molecular markers in order to test a common molecular target for a therapeutic agent. As recently illustrated in the previously discussed Phase 1, placebo-controlled trials of the microtubule stabilizer TPI-287 [75], a basket trial design may be useful in highlighting differences in drug safety and tolerability in distinct diseases sharing common neuropathological features (such as intraneuronal tau pathology). Basket trials may also be helpful in comparing pharmacodynamic measures of target engagement in differing diseases which share the same pathogenic protein, but exhibit different protein conformations and post-translational modifications that may impact drug affinity. For instance, despite early termination, in a recent Phase 1 trial of the anti-tau monoclonal antibody BIIB092 [19], a basket design was helpful in comparing relative levels of anti-tau monoclonal anti body target engagement (i.e., binding of CSF N-terminal tau residues) in four clinical cohorts associated with tau neuropathology (CBS, nfvPPA, symptomatic *MAPT*-mutation carriers, and traumatic encephalopathy).

In later-phase FTLD trials, the rarity of individual clinical syndromes may make it challenging to feasibly enroll large enough samples to allow statistical power and establish efficacy. Moreover, as multiple basic science and preclinical advancements translate into clinical trials, several exciting therapeutic programs may compete for an increasingly small share of the same patient pool. Recently, the DIAN Trials Unit (DIAN-TU) and Healey Center for ALS have adapted a platform trial design [92] for other neurodegenerative diseases with similar constraints as FTD; autosomal-dominant AD (NCT01760005) and ALS (NCT04297683), respectively. Platform trials randomize patients to either a single placebo group or one of multiple therapeutic interventions. This approach allows for efficient enrollment from a precious patient population, and enables response-adaptive randomization rules (typically utilizing Bayesian approaches) to preferentially assign participants to the interventions that perform most favorably during the conduct of the study. Combined with the multi-site infrastructure of large multinational FTLD clinical research consortia (such as ALLFTD, GENFI, and FPI), platform trials may offer the most viable template for more rapid therapeutic development in FTD and related disorders.

References

1. Onyike CU, Diehl-Schmid J. The epidemiology of frontotemporal dementia. *Int Rev Psychiatry* 2013; **25**: 130–7.

2. Perry DC, Brown JA, Possin KL, et al. Clinicopathological correlations in behavioural variant frontotemporal dementia. *Brain* 2017; **140**: 3329–45.

3. Armstrong MJ, Litvan I, Lang AE, et al. Criteria for the diagnosis of corticobasal degeneration. *Neurology* 2013; **80**: 496–503.

4. Höglinger GU, Respondek G, Stamelou M, et al. Clinical diagnosis of progressive supranuclear palsy: the movement disorder society criteria. *Mov Disord* 2017; **32**: 853–64.

5. Rascovsky K, Hodges JR, Knopman D, et al. Sensitivity of revised diagnostic criteria for the behavioural variant of frontotemporal dementia. *Brain* 2011; **134**: 2456–77.

6. Gorno-Tempini M, Hillis A, Weintraub S, et al. Classification of primary progressive aphasia and its variants. *Neurology* 2011; **76**: 1006–14.

7. Jadhav S, Avila J, Schöll M, et al. A walk through tau therapeutic strategies. *Acta Neuropathol Commun* 2019; **7**: 22.

8. Weingarten MD, Lockwood AH, Hwo SY, Kirschner MW. A protein factor essential for microtubule assembly. *Proc Natl Acad Sci USA* 1975; **72**: 1858–62.

9. Mackenzie IRA, Neumann M, Baborie A, et al. A harmonized classification system for FTLD-TDP pathology. *Acta Neuropathol* 2011; **122**: 111–13.

10. Svetoni F, Frisone P, Paronetto MP. Role of FET proteins in neurodegenerative disorders. *RNA Biol* 2016; **13**: 1089–102.

11. Spinelli EG, Mandelli ML, Miller ZA, et al. Typical and atypical pathology in primary progressive aphasia variants. *Ann Neurol* 2017; **81**: 430–43.

12. Boxer AL, Lang AE, Grossman M, et al. Davunetide in patients with progressive supranuclear palsy: a randomised, double-blind, placebo-controlled Phase 2/3 trial. *Lancet Neurol* 2014; **13**: 676–85.

13. Forrest SL, Kril JJ, Stevens CH, et al. Retiring the term FTDP-17 as *MAPT* mutations are genetic forms of sporadic frontotemporal tauopathies. *Brain* 2018; **141**: 521–34.

14. Lee SE, Rabinovici GD, Mayo MC, et al. Clinicopathological correlations in corticobasal degeneration. *Ann Neurol* 2011; **70**: 327–40.

15. Haynes BA, Rhinn H, Yeh FL, et al. AL001 restores CSF PGRN levels and normalizes disease-associated biomarkers in individuals with frontotemporal dementia due to heterozygous

mutations in the progranulin gene. *Alzheimers Dement* 2020; **16**: e046114.

16. Boxer AL, Moebius HJ, Harris B, et al. Phase 2a randomized, double-blind, placebo-controlled trial of the histone deacetylase inhibitor (HDACi), FRM-0334, in asymptomatic carriers of, or patients with frontotemporal lobar degeneration (FTLD) due to progranulin gene mutations. Alzheimer's Association International Conference, Los Angeles, CA, 2019.

17. Sha SJ, Miller ZA, Min S won, et al. An 8-week, open-label, dose-finding study of nimodipine for the treatment of progranulin insufficiency from *GRN* gene mutations. *Alzheimers Dement (N Y)* 2017; **3**: 507–12.

18. The Angel Fund for ALS Research. Research at the day lab. Available at: https://theangelfund.org/research-at-day-lab/ (accessed December 28, 2020).

19. Boxer A, Ljubenkov P, VandeVrede L, et al. A Phase 1b, randomized, double-blind, placebo-controlled, parallel cohort safety, tolerability, pharmacokinetics, pharmacodynamics and preliminary efficacy study of intravenously infused BIIB092 in patients with four different tauopathy syndromes. 13th Clinical Trials on Alzheimer's Disease (CTAD) Congress, November 4–7, 2020.

20. Boxer AL, Gold M, Feldman H, et al. New directions in clinical trials for frontotemporal lobar degeneration: methods and outcome measures. *Alzheimers Dement* 2020; **16**: 131–43.

21. ALLFTD. History. Available at: www.allftd.org/history (accessed December 30, 2020).

22. Richardson E, Burnell J, Adams HR, et al. Developing and implementing performance outcome assessments: evidentiary, methodologic, and operational considerations. *Ther Innov Regul Sci* 2019; **53**: 146–53.

23. Gaasterland CMW, Jansen-Van Der Weide MC, Weinreich SS, Van Der Lee JH. A systematic review to investigate the measurement properties of goal attainment scaling, towards use in drug trials. *BMC Med Res Methodol* 2016; **16**: 99.

24. Guinart D, de Filippis R, Rosson S, et al. Development and validation of a computerized adaptive assessment tool for discrimination and measurement of psychotic symptoms. *Schizophr Bull* 2021; **47**: 644–52.

25. Mioshi E, Hsieh S, Savage S, Hornberger M, Hodges JR. Clinical staging and disease progression in frontotemporal dementia. *Neurology* 2010; **74**: 1591–7.

26. Pfeffer RI, Kurosaki TT, Harrah CH, Chance JM, Filos S. Measurement of functional activities in older adults in the community. *J Gerontol* 1982; **37**: 323–9.

27. Miyagawa T, Brushaber D, Syrjanen J, et al. Use of the CDR® plus NACC FTLD in mild FTLD: data from the ARTFL/LEFFTDS consortium. *Alzheimers Dement* 2020; **16**: 79–90.

28. Boeve B, Rosen H, Boxer A, et al. The Multidomain Impairment Rating (MIR) Scale: initial reliability data on a multidimensional scale for FTLD (P5.1–010). *Neurology* 2019; **92**;https://n.neurology.org/content/92/15_Supplement/P5.1-010.abstract.

29. Staffaroni AM, Ljubenkov PA, Kornak J, et al. Longitudinal multimodal imaging and clinical endpoints for frontotemporal dementia clinical trials. *Brain* 2019; **142**: 443–59.

30. Toller G, Ranasinghe K, Cobigo Y, et al. Revised Self-Monitoring Scale: A potential endpoint for frontotemporal dementia clinical trials. *Neurology* 2020; **94**: e2384–95.

31. Staffaroni AM, Bajorek L, Casaletto KB, et al. Assessment of executive function declines in presymptomatic and mildly symptomatic familial frontotemporal dementia: NIH-EXAMINER as a potential clinical trial endpoint. *Alzheimers Dement* 2020; **16**: 11–21.

32. FDA. Table of surrogate endpoints that were the basis of drug approval or licensure. www.fda.gov/drugs/development-resources/table-surrogate-endpoints-were-basis-drug-approval-or-licensure (accessed December 30, 2020).

33. Swift IJ, Sogorb-Esteve A, Heller C, et al. Fluid biomarkers in frontotemporal dementia: past, present and future. *J Neurol Neurosurg Psychiatry* 2021; **92**: 204–15.

34. Palmqvist S, Janelidze S, Quiroz YT, et al. Discriminative accuracy of plasma phospho-tau217 for Alzheimer disease vs other neurodegenerative disorders. *JAMA* 2020; **324**: 772–81.

35. Thijssen EH, La Joie R, Wolf A, et al. Diagnostic value of plasma phosphorylated tau$_{181}$ in Alzheimer's disease and frontotemporal lobar degeneration. *Nat Med* 2020; **26**: 387–97.

36. Paterson RW, Slattery CF, Poole T, et al. Cerebrospinal fluid in the differential diagnosis of Alzheimer's disease: clinical utility of an extended panel of biomarkers in a specialist cognitive clinic. *Alzheimers Res Ther* 2018; **10**: 32.

37. Meeter LHH, Vijverberg EG, Del Campo M, et al. Clinical value of neurofilament and phospho-tau/tau ratio in the frontotemporal dementia spectrum. *Neurology* 2018; **90**: e1231–9.

38. Rojas JC, Karydas A, Bang J, et al. Plasma neurofilament light chain predicts progression in progressive supranuclear palsy. *Ann Clin Transl Neurol* 2016; **3**: 216–25.

39. Ljubenkov PA, Staffaroni AM, Rojas JC, et al. Cerebrospinal fluid biomarkers predict frontotemporal dementia trajectory. *Ann Clin Transl Neurol* 2018; **5**: 1250–63.

40. Meeter LH, Dopper EG, Jiskoot LC, et al. Neurofilament light chain: a biomarker for genetic frontotemporal dementia. *Ann Clin Transl Neurol* 2016; **3**: 623–36.

41. Gass J, Cannon A, Mackenzie IR, et al. Mutations in progranulin are a major cause of ubiquitin-positive frontotemporal lobar degeneration. *Hum Mol Genet* 2006; **15**: 2988–3001.

42. Baker M, Mackenzie IR, Pickering-Brown SM, et al. Mutations in progranulin cause tau-negative frontotemporal dementia linked to chromosome 17. *Nature* 2006; **442**: 916–19.

43. Shankaran SS, Capell A, Hruscha AT, et al. Missense mutations in the progranulin gene linked to frontotemporal lobar degeneration with ubiquitin-immunoreactive inclusions reduce progranulin production and secretion. *J Biol Chem* 2008; **283**: 1744–53.

44. Kao AW, McKay A, Singh PP, Brunet A, Huang EJ. Progranulin, lysosomal regulation and neurodegenerative disease. *Nat Rev Neurosci* 2017; **18**: 325–33.

45. Meeter LHH, Patzke H, Loewen G, et al. Progranulin levels in plasma and cerebrospinal fluid in granulin mutation carriers. *Dement Geriatr Cogn Dis Extra* 2016; **6**: 330–40.

46. Finch N, Baker M, Crook R, et al. Plasma progranulin levels predict progranulin mutation status in frontotemporal dementia patients and asymptomatic family members. *Brain* 2009; **132**: 583–91.

47. Ash PEA, Bieniek KF, Gendron TF, et al. Unconventional translation of C9orf72 GGGGCC expansion generates insoluble polypeptides specific to c9FTD/ALS. *Neuron* 2013; **77**: 639–46.

48. Mori K, Arzberger T, Grässer FA, et al. Bidirectional transcripts of the expanded C9orf72 hexanucleotide repeat are translated into aggregating dipeptide repeat proteins. *Acta Neuropathol* 2013; **126**: 881–93.

49. Gendron TF, Chew J, Stankowski JN, et al. Poly(GP) proteins are a useful pharmacodynamic marker for C9orf72-associated amyotrophic lateral sclerosis. *Sci Transl Med* 2017; **9**: eaai7866.

50. Cammack AJ, Atassi N, Hyman T, et al. Prospective natural history study of C9orf72 ALS clinical characteristics and biomarkers. *Neurology* 2019; **93**: E1605–17.

51. Lee SE, Sias AC, Kosik EL, et al. Thalamo-cortical network hyperconnectivity in preclinical progranulin mutation carriers. *Neuroimage Clin* 2019; **22**;DOI: https://doi.10.1016/j.nicl.2019 .101751.

52. Jacova C, Hsiung GYR, Tawankanjanachot I, et al. Anterior brain glucose hypometabolism predates dementia in progranulin mutation carriers. *Neurology* 2013; **81**: 1322–31.

53. Binney RJ, Pankov A, Marx G, et al. Data-driven regions of interest for longitudinal change in three variants of frontotemporal lobar degeneration. *Brain Behav* 2017; **7**: e00675.

54. Staffaroni AM, Cobigo Y, Goh S-YM, et al. Individualized atrophy scores predict dementia onset in familial frontotemporal lobar degeneration. *Alzheimers Dement* 2020; **16**: 37–48.

55. Cenik B, Sephton CF, Dewey CM, et al. Suberoylanilide hydroxamic acid (vorinostat) up-regulates progranulin transcription: rational therapeutic approach to frontotemporal dementia. *J Biol Chem* 2011; **286**: 16101–8.

56. Lee WC, Almeida S, Prudencio M, et al. Targeted manipulation of the sortilin–progranulin axis rescues progranulin haploinsufficiency. *Hum Mol Genet* 2014; **23**: 1467–78.

57. Paul R. AL001 Phase 1b/2 update. Alzheimer's Association International Conference, July 26–30, 2020.

58. Alector Inc. Alector showcases progress in immuno-neurology clinical programs and research portfolio at R&D day. Available at: www.globenewswire.com/news-release/2019/12/13/1960338/0/en/Alector-Showcases-Progress-in-Immuno-Neurology-Clinical-Programs-and-Research-Portfolio-at-R-D-Day.html (accessed February 17, 2020).

59. Passage Bio. Pipeline: frontotemporal dementia. Available at: www.passagebio.com/pipeline/frontotemporal-dementia/default.aspx. (accessed June 20, 2020).

60. Prevail Therapeutics. Prevail Therapeutics announces first patient dosed in Phase 1/2 PROCLAIM clinical trial evaluating PR006 for the treatment of frontotemporal dementia patients with *GRN* mutations. Available at: www.globenewswire.com/news-release/2020/12/11/2143673/0/en/Prevail-Therapeutics-Announces-First-Patient-Dosed-in-Phase-1-2-PROCLAIM-Clinical-Trial-Evaluating-PR006-for-the-Treatment-of-Frontotemporal-Dementia-Patients-with-GRN-Mutations.html (accessed December 27, 2020).

61. Denali. Our pipeline. Available at:https://denalitherapeutics.com/pipeline (accessed June 20, 2020).

62. Alzprotect. AZP2006: a mechanism of action with multiple effects, a unique solution for

neurodegeneration. Available at: www.alzprotect
.com/en/pipeline/azp2006?view=article&layout
=alzprotect:hero-article (accessed December 30,
2020).

63. Taylor JP, Brown RH, Cleveland DW. Decoding
ALS: from genes to mechanism. *Nature* 2016; **539**:
197–206.

64. DeVos SL, Miller TM. Antisense oligonucleotides:
treating neurodegeneration at the level of RNA.
Neurotherapeutics 2013; **10**: 486–97.

65. Lim KRQ, Maruyama R, Yokota T. Eteplirsen in the
treatment of Duchenne muscular dystrophy. *Drug
Des Devel Ther* 2017; **11**: 533–45.

66. Hoy SM. Nusinersen: first global approval. *Drugs*
2017; **77**: 473–9.

67. Miller T, Cudkowicz M, Shaw PJ, et al. Phase 1–2
trial of antisense oligonucleotide tofersen for *SOD1*
ALS. *N Engl J Med* 2020; **383**: 109–19.

68. Jiang J, Zhu Q, Gendron TF, et al. Gain of toxicity
from ALS/FTD-linked repeat expansions in
C9orf72 is alleviated by antisense oligonucleotides
targeting GGGGCC-containing RNAs. *Neuron*
2016; **90**: 535–50.

69. Sanders DW, Kaufman SK, DeVos SL, et al. Distinct
tau prion strains propagate in cells and mice and
define different tauopathies. *Neuron* 2014; **82**:
1271–88.

70. Yanamandra K, Kfoury N, Jiang H, et al. Anti-tau
antibodies that block tau aggregate seeding in
vitro markedly decrease pathology and improve
cognition in vivo. *Neuron* 2013; **80**: 402–14.

71. Zhou Y, Shi J, Chu D, et al. Relevance of
phosphorylation and truncation of tau to the
etiopathogenesis of Alzheimer's disease. *Front
Aging Neurosci* 2018; **10**: 27.

72. CurePSP. UCB pauses the development of
bepranemab for progressive supranuclear palsy.
Available at: www.psp.org/ucb-shift-2020/
(accessed December 28, 2020).

73. Novak P, Schmidt R, Kontsekova E, et al.
FUNDAMANT: an interventional 72-week
phase 1 follow-up study of AADvac1, an active
immunotherapy against tau protein pathology
in Alzheimer's disease. *Alzheimers Res Ther* 2018;
10: 108.

74. Hung S-Y, Fu W-M. Drug candidates in clinical
trials for Alzheimer's disease. *J Biomed Sci* 2017;
24: 47.

75. Tsai RM, Miller Z, Koestler M, et al. Reactions
to multiple ascending doses of the microtubule
stabilizer TPI-287 in patients with Alzheimer
disease, progressive supranuclear palsy, and
corticobasal syndrome: a randomized clinical trial.
JAMA Neurol 2020; **77**: 215–24.

76. Mignon L, Kordasiewicz H, Lane R, et al. Design
of the first-in-human study of IONIS-MAPTRx,
a tau-lowering antisense oligonucleotide, in
patients with Alzheimer disease (S2.006).
Neurology 2018; **90**.

77. Rodriguez-Martin T, Anthony K, Garcia-Blanco
MA, Mansfield SG, Anderton BH, Gallo JM.
Correction of tau mis-splicing caused by FTDP-
17 *MAPT* mutations by spliceosome-mediated
RNA trans-splicing. *Hum Mol Genet* 2009; **18**:
3266–73.

78. Wischik CM, Edwards PC, Lai RYK, Roth
M, Harrington CR. Selective inhibition of
Alzheimer disease-like tau aggregation by
phenothiazines. *Proc Natl Acad Sci USA*. 1996; **93**:
11213–18.

79. Gauthier S, Feldman HH, Schneider LS, et al.
Efficacy and safety of tau-aggregation inhibitor
therapy in patients with mild or moderate
Alzheimer's disease: a randomised, controlled,
double-blind, parallel-arm, Phase 3 trial. *Lancet*
2016; **388**: 2873–84.

80. Tolosa E, Litvan I, Höglinger GU, et al. A Phase
2 trial of the GSK-3 inhibitor tideglusib in
progressive supranuclear palsy. *Mov Disord* 2014;
29: 470–8.

81. Gentry EG, Henderson BW, Arrant AE, et al. Rho
kinase inhibition as a therapeutic for progressive
supranuclear palsy and corticobasal degeneration.
J Neurosci 2016; **36**: 1316–23.

82. Woolsey Pharmaceuticals. PSP and CSP patients.
Available at: www.woolseypharma.com/psp-cbs/
(accessed December 28, 2020).

83. Min SW, Chen X, Tracy TE, et al. Critical role of
acetylation in tau-mediated neurodegeneration
and cognitive deficits. *Nat Med* 2015; **21**: 1154–
62.

84. VandeVrede L, Dale ML, Fields S, et al. Open-label
Phase 1 futility studies of salsalate and young
plasma in progressive supranuclear palsy. *Mov
Disord Clin Pract* 2020; **7**: 440–7.

85. Hastings NB, Wang X, Song L, et al. Inhibition of
O-GlcNAcase leads to elevation of O-GlcNAc tau
and reduction of tauopathy and cerebrospinal fluid
tau in rTg4510 mice. *Mol Neurodegener* 2017; **12**:
1–16.

86. Asceneuron. R&D pipeline. Available at: www
.asceneuron.com/pipeline (accessed December 28,
2020).

87. Giordano R, Canesi M, Isalberti M, et al.
Autologous mesenchymal stem cell therapy for

progressive supranuclear palsy: translation into a Phase I controlled, randomized clinical study. *J Transl Med* 2014; **12**: 14.

88. Katsimpardi L, Litterman NK, Schein PA, et al. Vascular and neurogenic rejuvenation of the aging mouse brain by young systemic factors. *Science* 2014; **344**: 630–4.

89. Villeda SA, Plambeck KE, Middeldorp J, et al. Young blood reverses age-related impairments in cognitive function and synaptic plasticity in mice. *Nat Med* 2014; **20**: 659–63.

90. Desmarais P, Rohrer JD, Nguyen QD, et al. Therapeutic trial design for frontotemporal dementia and related disorders. *J Neurol Neurosurg Psychiatry* 2019; **90**: 412–23.

91. Tao JJ, Schram AM, Hyman DM. Basket studies: redefining clinical trials in the era of genome-driven oncology. *Annu Rev Med* 2018; **69**: 319–31.

92. Berry SM, Connor JT, Lewis RJ. The platform trial: an efficient strategy for evaluating multiple treatments. *JAMA* 2015; **313**: 1619–20.

Chapter 19

Statistical Considerations in the Design and Analysis of Alzheimer's Disease Clinical Trials

Suzanne B. Hendrix, Jessie Nicodemus-Johnson, Logan Kowallis, Newman Knowlton, Sean Hennessey, Samuel P. Dickson

19.1 Study Design

A statistician's involvement in clinical trials often begins with the determination of sample size. However, there are many other study design issues that benefit from a statistical perspective, including selection of the study population, study duration, efficacy or biomarker outcomes, interim or adaptive features, randomization ratio, and frequency of assessment. A prudent statistician will take time to review and offer recommendations on these design elements when asked to perform a sample-size calculation, while an effective study team will involve a statistician in the study design process as early as possible and throughout the study. Because of the statisticians' focus on quantifying effect, they often can provide key insights on the specific questions different study designs will address and can help to ensure that, at study completion, the most relevant questions can be answered, and key development program decisions can be made. Proper attention to these variables and others can increase the likelihood of clinical trial success by avoiding the common pitfalls that result in clinical trial failures.

19.1.1 Study Phase

Phase 1 studies include approximately 20–100 participants and are designed to assess safety and tolerability, identify potential side effects, and find the safe dosing range for one or more drug formulations. Phase 2 studies include approximately 50–300 participants and assess drug efficacy, confirm Phase 1 safety findings, and add to the safety database. Additionally, assessment of biomarker or clinical outcome target engagement may be explored. Within Alzheimer's disease (AD) specifically, Phase 1a single ascending dose (SAD) studies are often followed by a combined Phase 1b/2 (proof-of-concept [POC]) study that

includes SAD (Phase 1a) or multiple ascending dose (MAD; Phase 1b) studies for determining the appropriate dosing range for safety and efficacy measures. Phase 3 studies enroll approximately 300–3,000 participants; they assess safety and are designed to confirm Phase 2 efficacy findings.

19.1.2 Study Population

The study population is defined by the inclusion and exclusion criteria. Defining the inclusion and exclusion criteria is a balance between making sure the trial can meet its objectives as efficiently as possible and ensuring that the results can be generalized to all who may benefit from the treatment. Clinical trial populations often exclude patients with co-morbidities that may interfere with achieving or measuring a treatment effect, or that may contribute to safety concerns. In contrast, when the study population is too narrow it can limit the indication approved by regulatory agencies. An AD study population is often defined by the stage of disease, ranging from preclinical to severe AD dementia (Figure 19.1 – top line). As the biological and underlying molecular mechanisms of AD have been deciphered over the years, the definition of AD has changed to incorporate the newfound understanding of the disease and mechanisms. Due to this, the AD research definition has evolved, resulting in studies that may not have the same populations. Specifically, the former AD definition was broader (National Institute of Neurological and Communicative Diseases and Stroke/Alzheimer's Disease and Related Disorders Association [NINCDS–ADRDA] criteria) and more recently the AD definition has been updated, restricting the AD population to only those with amyloid plaques detectable via positron emission tomography standardized uptake value ratio (PET SUVR).

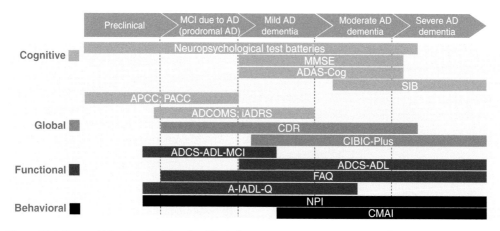

Figure 19.1 Stages of AD and scales. AD scales differ in their sensitivity to progression across disease severity. Scales for measuring cognitive, functional (activities of daily living, ADL), global, and behavioral domains are shown across disease stages.

The updated AD definition works well for treatments that specifically target amyloid, but treatments with a broader mechanism of action may now need to target both AD and dementia without amyloid positivity to include all patients who were included under the original definition. Studies that were conducted under the older definition would benefit from an analysis looking at separate subgroups comprised of the new definition and those included in the old definition and excluded from the new definition. This distinction is more relevant in earlier disease since nearly all moderate or severe AD patients have MRI levels of brain amyloid consistent with the standard cut-offs.

19.1.3 Study Duration, Frequency of Assessment, and Type of Effect

Studies in earlier-stage disease (preclinical or mild cognitive impairment [MCI] stages) generally require a longer study duration than studies in later stages (mild to severe AD) due to the slower progression on clinical disease outcomes in the earlier stages. Measurements are often performed every 3 months but may be less frequent in studies longer than 12 months, in order to reduce the patient burden and attrition. Assessments may be more frequent in studies of shorter duration.

The study duration may also be determined by the anticipated treatment outcome or mode of action. A treatment effect can be expected to be symptomatic, meaning that it directly targets specific symptoms, or disease-modifying, meaning that it targets the entire cascade of AD pathology. Symptomatic effects are generally expected

to be improvements of limited duration, but disease-modifying effects are generally expected to be more subtle, with a slowing of progression over time rather than improvement (Figure 19.2). Treatments targeting amyloid (23% of therapies; Figure 19.3b) are assumed to be disease-modifying since amyloid is a key component of the diagnosis of AD; however, other treatments may also be disease-modifying by indirectly targeting amyloid, such as the plasmapheresis approach [1] or those targeting aging-related mechanisms, such as lifestyle and nutritional approaches [2]. Studies of symptomatic treatments can typically be shorter than studies of disease-modifying treatment because the effects of a symptomatic treatment are expected to present under a shorter timeframe.

A treatment with both symptomatic and disease-modifying effects would be ideal, as it may have both rapid improvement and a long-lasting slowing of the disease process, such as treatments that specifically target cognition. Cognitive treatments may eventually also impact functional and global outcomes through a cognitive mechanism that may be primarily symptomatic or disease-modifying.

One class of symptomatic treatments consists of those treatments that specifically target neuropsychiatric symptoms such as agitation and aggression or AD psychosis (delusions and hallucinations). Unlike cognition and function, which are progressive and affect all patients, psychiatric symptoms differ across patients and are not as progressive. Because these symptoms tend to be episodic, event-based outcomes are more relevant, and studies usually target only patients who experience these specific symptoms. In one well-designed study, only patients who were responders to treatment were randomized to active treatment or placebo, and the outcome was time to relapse [3]. These types of studies are more common in psychiatric illnesses than in neurodegenerative diseases and benefit from a detailed understanding of the patterns of these symptoms in AD patients.

19.1.4   Efficacy Outcomes

Clinical measures for AD include cognitive (Alzheimer's Disease Assessment Scale – cognitive subscale [ADAS-cog] and Severe Impairment Battery [SIB]), functional (Alzheimer's Disease Cooperative Study Activities of Daily Living [ADCS ADL] scale, Functional Activities Questionnaire [FAQ], Amsterdam Instrumental Activities of Daily

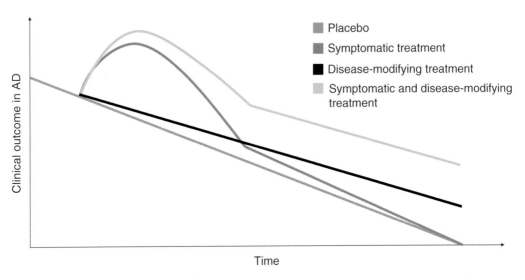

Figure 19.2 Symptomatic and disease-modifying treatment effects. Symptomatic treatment effects occur quickly and improve symptoms, disease-modifying treatment effects slowly accumulate over time, and treatment effects that combine symptomatic and disease-modifying effects have both initial improvement and longer-term separation over time.

Living [aIADL] scale, and Disability Assessment for Dementia [DAD]), behavioral (Neuropsychiatric Inventory [NPI] or targeted behavioral symptom scales), or global (Clinical Dementia Rating – sum of boxes [CDR-sb] and Clinician Interview-Based Impression of Change with Caregiver Input [CIBIC+]) aspects of progression. CDR-sb is often used as a primary outcome in studies targeting effects in MCI or prodromal AD, since it includes both cognitive and functional aspects of disease progression, which are known to change early on. In mild-to-moderate and moderate-to-severe AD, co-primary outcomes are generally required for US Food and Drug Administration (FDA) approval, with a cognitive scale (ADAS-cog or SIB) supported by either a global outcome or functional outcome (CIBIC+, CDR-sb, or ADCS ADL) to establish clinical meaningfulness. The remaining domain, global or functional, is usually designated as a key secondary outcome, and the European Medicines Association (EMA) generally considers all three components in evaluating efficacy.

Global statistical tests (GSTs) have been recently proposed [4, 5] as a way of combining information across cognitive, functional, and global outcomes to assess the overall impact of a treatment on disease progression. This approach is particularly helpful in small studies or as a preliminary analysis intended to support an overall treatment benefit in larger studies. Behavioral assessments are typically only included as secondary assessments.

A composite score measurement may benefit disease stages with subtle progression because a well-constructed composite score can target the most progressive aspects of disease-related change [6, 7]. Ideally, an outcome measure or a composite score should be continuous and aligned with disease progression. The use of highly discrete scales with clinically meaningful separations between categories has been proposed as a method of ensuring clinical meaningfulness at the analysis stage, but in reality the discreteness of the scale handicaps our ability to detect changes and undermines power. This approach is equivalent to using a scale with

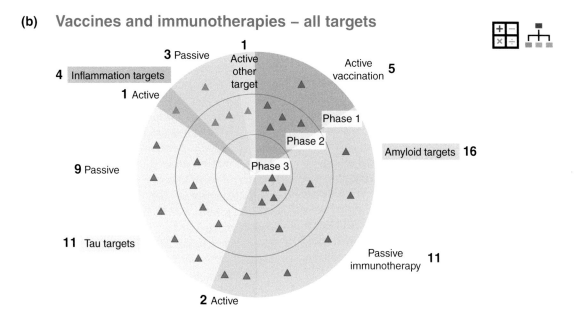

(a) All therapy types except immunotherapies – all targets

4 Procedural intervention 2 DNA/RNA-based

6 Dietary supplement

8 Other

1 Small molecule, other

2 Small molecule, supplementary/dietary

5 Combination, small molecule

88 Small molecule

Phase 1

Phase 2

Phase 3

80 Small molecule only

(b) Vaccines and immunotherapies – all targets

1 Active other target

3 Passive

4 Inflammation targets

1 Active

5 Active vaccination

9 Passive

11 Tau targets

2 Active

Phase 1

Phase 2

Phase 3

Amyloid targets 16

Passive immunotherapy 11

Figure 19.3 Compounds currently in development: (a) non-immunotherapy approaches; (b) immunotherapy approaches. Many compounds are currently in development across phases 1, 2, and 3, with the majority being classified as small molecules.

10-pound increments in a weight-loss study based on the argument that less than a 10-pound weight loss is not meaningful [8]. Cognitive decline is subtle in the preclinical disease stages and composites such as the Alzheimer's Prevention Cognitive Composite (APCC) and the Preclinical Alzheimer's Cognitive Composite (PACC) have been proposed to improve measurement of progression. Functional decline is subtle in the MCI/prodromal stage and the Alzheimer's Disease Composite Score (ADCOMS) [9] and the integrated Alzheimer's Disease Rating Scale (iADRS) [10] have been proposed to combine both functional and cognitive changes in a composite score that is more sensitive to progression over time. Global progression is generally measurable across all clinical disease stages. Some composite measures have been developed by combining items for maximum sensitivity to progression over time

235

using a strictly empirical approach (ADCOMS), combining an empirical and theoretical approach (APCC) [11], or relying solely on a theoretical approach with confirmation of separation of amyloid-positive and -negative groups cross-sectionally (PACC) [12]. Optimal weighting of items can improve performance by increasing the signal-to-noise ratio as implemented for the ADCOMS, which was empirically derived. Overall, the choice of efficacy outcome should be specific to the AD severity included in the study population.

19.1.5 Biomarker Outcomes

Biomarkers are measurable disease markers that may predict or correlate with various aspects of disease progression. AD is a complex disease phenotype that encompasses multiple aspects of an individual's health. To this end, endeavors to understand AD progression and ultimately predict disease occurrences should span multiple areas of disease pathogenesis.

Although clinical measures are vital to identifying onset and characterizing disease progression, plasma and cerebrospinal fluid (CSF) biomarkers have been shown to be altered years before the manifestation of cognitive symptoms. The core AD biomarkers include amyloid beta (Aβ), total tau (t-tau), and hyperphosphorylated tau (p-tau) [13]. Additional biomarkers such as neurogranin (Ng), neurofilament light chain (NfL), and hippocampal volume are also informative. It is important to remember that the type and magnitude of biomarkers will influence the analysis. Both amyloid and tau accumulation are associated with inflammation in the brain at different times during disease progression, with amyloid driving inflammation during early accumulation (MCI cases) and tau appearing after the amyloid load in the brain is near AD levels (prodromal AD) [14]. While $A\beta_{42}$ is reduced in the CSF of AD patients, t-tau and p-tau are increased. NfL [15] and Ng [16] are associated with axonal degeneration and synaptic dysfunction. Although NfL and Ng are broadly associated with common pathways, when paired with Aβ presence, they become more convincingly associated with AD pathogenesis. Finally, hippocampal volume declines over time in individuals with AD at the prodromal stage and later. Hippocampal volume is usually correlated with cognitive and functional changes, making it a useful marker of disease progression.

Singular biomarkers targeting specific aspects of AD are suitable for assessing target engagement along a specific pathway, while downstream biomarkers that are more correlated with clinical progression may provide evidence that is more likely to be confirmed by clinical outcomes. A composite score or global statistical test can be used to combine multiple downstream biomarkers to improve power (the probability of a successful trial given a specified treatment effect size for the chosen outcome) and increase the chance that the biomarker results will be predictive of clinical results in a larger study.

19.1.6 Power/Sample Size

Sample sizes for POC studies (Phase 2) are usually based on 80% or 90% power, a two-sided alpha of 0.05, and an effect size of at least 50% slowing over 12–18 months for a disease-modifying treatment. Symptomatic treatments often expect treatment effects of 100–150% (complete halting of progression, or improvement that is 50% of the placebo worsening over time) over 3–9 months. In small trials, it is often helpful to calculate the effect size that is associated with 50% power, since it corresponds to the observed effect size that would be on the boundary of achieving statistical significance at the end of the study if the rest of the sample size assumptions hold.

Although a mixed model with repeated measures (MMRM) is most used for the primary analysis, most sample-size calculations are based on a simple t-test with the assumption that an MMRM analysis would result in better power. An attrition rate of approximately 15–18% over 6 months, 25–30% over 12 months, and 30–35% over 18–24 months is generally assumed for early through severe AD. Studies in preclinical AD have an expected attrition rate of 30–40% over 3–5 years, since drop-out tends to be higher in more progressed patients.

19.1.7 Interim Analyses or Adaptive Designs

Adaptive clinical trial design allows adjustment or adaptation to aspects of the trial at various stages as the trial progresses. Adjustments are based on predefined rules to avoid undermining the integrity or validity of the clinical trial. Commonly used adaptive designs include group-sequential, sample-size re-estimation, Phase 2/3 seamless designs, and dose-escalation or dose-selection designs. Designs are deployed to reduce the time to market (efficacy) or time spent on ineffective compounds (futility) as well as to reduce trial participant size.

Group-sequential designs (GSDs) allow the premature termination of a trial due to efficacy or futility based on interim analysis results. A multi-arm multistage (MAMS) trial design is a GSD with more than one active arm, with a mechanism that allows active arms to be dropped. This approach allows several agents to be assessed simultaneously against a single placebo arm in a randomized fashion. A pairwise comparison between the placebo and active arms using an appropriate surrogate outcome measure at distinct time points allows assessment of trial outcomes before the trial endpoint. Interim assessment allows the opportunity to discontinue arms that do not show promise (pre-specified effect size, hazard ratio, serious adverse events, cross lower [futility/lack of benefit] boundary, etc.). It also allows an arm to cross the upper (efficacy) bound, and to terminate the trial early due to the detection of significant beneficial associations. If none of the arms cross the efficacy bound, randomization to the placebo arm and active arms that show promise continues. This cycle continues through additional interim analyses or until a single arm crosses the efficacy boundary or the maximum sample size is reached. Futility or efficacy are determined based on various alpha-spending approaches such as O'Brien and Fleming [17], Lan and Demets [18] or the triangular approach of Whitehead and Stratton [19].

Adaptive-randomization designs are becoming more common in clinical trials and utilize real-time data to determine sample-size allocation to arms based on clinical readout while the trial is running. The main purpose is to increase the likelihood of randomizing patients to superior treatment arms and reduce patient exposure to ineffective drugs (less-effective arms). Commonly employed approaches are the "promising-zone" approach and Bayesian adaptive randomization. A promising-zone approach allows an increase in sample size to be made only if the pre-specified interim analysis has a trend toward success but requires more participants to achieve success at the final analysis. If the interim result is clearly weak or negative or if it is very strong, the trial is allowed to accumulate subjects to the originally planned sample size. In contrast to promising zone in which sample-size adjustments are made at specific time points, Bayesian assessments are performed with the addition of each additional participant. Neither adaptive-randomization design is subject to alpha-spending restrictions as required for a GSD; however, Bayesian designs still pay a penalty for frequent looks (formal analyses of efficacy), since the threshold for declaring success is usually adjusted through extensive simulation in the design phase in order to control type I error.

Both GSDs and adaptive-randomization designs are frequently paired with adaptive Phase 2/3 seamless designs in which a Phase 2b dose-finding and Phase 3 confirmatory study are combined into one design. This approach is sometimes termed a "play the winner" design in which the winner of the selection stage (GSD) is carried forward into the confirmation stage (Phase 3). The approach is similar to performing Phase 2 and Phase 3 separately in that new patients are recruited and randomized to receive the best-performing dose, and the final analysis is performed with cumulative data of patients from both stages. The Phase 3 portion frequently begins immediately after Phase 2, as the overall trial design and approval have already been obtained.

19.2 Data Management/Data Formatting

19.2.1 Data Standards

Although not commonly discussed in the context of drug development, the data management process can greatly affect the statistical analysis, because data are the foundation upon which analysis is built. The Clinical Data Interchange Standards Consortium (CDISC) data standards were established for clinical trials in 1997 and have been required for FDA submissions since 2016 [20], are recommended by the EMA (although patient-level data are not required), have been required for the Japanese Pharmaceuticals and Medical Devices Agency (PMDA) submissions since 2016, and have been preferred for the Chinese National Medical Products Agency submissions since 2019. These standards should be applied as early as possible in the data collection process and include standards for the case report form (CRF) design using Clinical Data Acquisition Standards Harmonization (CDASH); raw-data-set structures have also been established, although some owners of proprietary scales have refused to allow official standardization (www.cdisc.org/standards/foundational/qrs). Documentation of the data collection, data-set structures, and conversions are also provided in a standard format. Implementation of data standards later in the study process result in ambiguities in data interpretation, data errors, and delays in timelines.

19.2.2 Level of Detail for Data Collection

For many AD scales, several different levels of data detail can be collected. The least detail would be to collect only the total score. If any subscale is missing, then the total score would also be missing. If more detail is desired, then individual item scores could also be collected. Individual item data allow retrieval of partially missing scores using available data. The most detailed level of data collection would be to keep every word from every word list. This level of detail allows assessment of the probability of remembering each word based on the order it was given, termed primacy and recency. If an analysis of the primacy and recency effect is desired, then this level of detail is required. We recommend collecting detailed data throughout the study, as this allows the opportunity to forge deeper into the data if unexpected results occur.

19.2.3 Risk-Based Data Management

Risk-based monitoring is an industry standard approach that focuses on site performance, data collection, and data cleaning from the clinical monitoring perspective; however, little thought is put into the statistical implications of concerns that arise. For example, each time the data are reformatted from the time of collection through the analysis, there is room for error to be introduced through reformatting. In a worst-case scenario, the original data responses aren't able to be formatted appropriately (i.e., they do not follow CDISC-controlled terminology) for regulatory submission and statisticians are left to alter the clinical responses to match controlled terminology required for FDA submission. Awareness of these standards throughout the CRF design process, site training, query generation, and resolution will result in better-quality data for analysis.

19.2.4 Statistical Perspective in Data Decisions

The data management plan (DMP) should be treated as a living document that is updated and revised throughout the clinical trial process. The data management plan is initially written in the context of a standard data flow, but each study is unique and requires a customized approach. We recommend continuous assessment of the clinical data by both data managers as well as statisticians

with disease-specific knowledge to ensure that all data handling decisions are made in the context of the planned analyses and the type of treatment effect expected. This will ensure that the final statistical analysis can be performed as outlined in the statistical analysis plan (SAP) without concern that data handling decisions may have adversely affected the results by introducing bias or increasing variability in the outcome measures. These practices ensure that high data quality is maintained, and that data are consistent with the assumptions of the planned analysis throughout the performance of the study.

19.3 Simulations and Model Selection

Simulations are critical for selecting outcomes, timing of visits, duration of study, and selection of the analytical model. Any assumptions that are made during the simulation process must be carefully assessed for accuracy since it is easy to make assumptions consistent with the planned analysis, resulting in simulations that are circular and just reconfirm the assumptions that were made. This can be avoided by utilizing several different scenarios for the following conditions:

(1) patient population;
(2) the pattern and size of the treatment effect;
(3) the decline rate and pattern of placebo decline; and
(4) the relationships between outcomes.

19.3.1 Simulations Based on Real Clinical Trial Data

Historical placebo group data from previous clinical trials are essential to form the basis of new clinical trials, as observational data may differ in critical ways from clinical trial data. Differences between the planned study and the historical data, including visit timing, patient population, and the order of the assessments can impact the conclusions in unexpected ways.

19.3.2 Size and Type of Treatment Effect

A treatment effect refers to the point difference between the active and placebo groups. A standardized effect size can be a Cohen's d (the treatment difference divided by a standard deviation) or a percentage slowing (the treatment difference divided by the placebo change from baseline). Because of the progressive nature of AD, we recommend using a percentage slowing from the placebo group as the standardized effect size [21]. Expressing the treatment difference as an extension of the time course may also be helpful, particularly when the placebo group decline is not linear.

A treatment benefit may be a shift effect or a slope effect. A shift effect is associated with a symptomatic benefit that is simply a point difference that is obtained when starting treatment, and then lost when treatment is removed. A slope effect can be assumed to be either vertically proportional or horizontally proportional (i.e., extended). The vertical proportionality is similar to a proportional hazards assumption for a survival analysis, and the horizontal extension is similar to an accelerated failure time survival model. A slope effect for an assumed linear progression can be represented as a proportion slowing or an extension of time, for instance a 50% slowing would be equivalent to a time multiple of 2×, and a 33.3% slowing would mean that the active group progresses by 66.7% of the placebo group, which is equivalent to extending time by 1.5×, since it would take half again as long to progress to the level of the placebo group. The factor by which time is extended can be calculated from the percentage slowing as $1\Big/\left(1-\dfrac{\%\,\text{slowing}}{100}\right)$.

In early disease, the placebo decline is generally not linear, and instead follows a reverse S-curve decline with slow change early on, and then progressively faster decline until a linear phase through moderate AD, and then a slower phase during severe AD (see Figure 19.4a, blue line). With this nonlinearity, a treatment effect that is a proportional slowing, say, 40% (Figure 19.4a, red line), is not the same as a 2.5× extension of time (see Figure 19.4a, green line). A disease-modifying effect would result in slowing of the pathological cascade, which would slow the process over time (horizontally affect the curve, like the green line) or extend the time course by 2.5×. In earlier disease during the downward curvature progression, this results in a larger percentage slowing than 40% but in later disease it is a smaller percentage slowing. Figure 19.4b shows the percentage slowing corresponding to the red and green lines from Figure 19.4a at each time point until the floor effect happens in the placebo group. This specific type of effect – a slowing of time – is also consistent with a disease-modifying effect since it is assumed that disease modification will be stronger in earlier disease than in later disease.

A proportional reduction in the progression curve of 40% implies that the progression is always 60% of what it would have been without treatment, with larger effects during faster-progressing stages and smaller effects in slower-progressing stages. If this model is extended over the course of disease, then this model implies that patients will eventually stabilize 60% through the disease. Because of these inconsistencies of this type of treatment effect, we recommend using a percentage-slowing approach only during disease stages where the assumption of linearity holds.

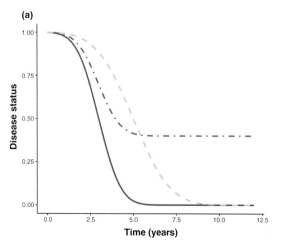
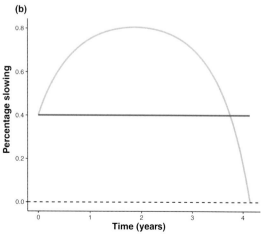

Figure 19.4 (a) Comparison of natural history to proportional and time-delayed treatment effects. (b) Comparison of effect size for proportional and time-delayed treatment effects.

19.3.3 Statistical Models and Assumptions

Several statistical models have been used for analyzing the change from baseline for quantitative outcome scales in AD trials. These include an end-of-study analysis of covariance (ANCOVA), a mixed model with repeated measures (MMRM) analysis with separate means across visits, an MMRM with a linear slope model, and a disease progression model. The ANCOVA model requires imputation of missing data at the end of the study and was used for the cholinesterase inhibitor studies with a last observation carried forward (LOCF) imputation approach. The MMRM approach has been the most commonly used approach for AD clinical trials since the mid 2000s, and the separate-means version of that model requires the fewest assumptions. The assumption of linearity is required for the linear-slope model, but this assumption may be appropriate for some scales across shorter-duration trials. A disease-progression model has recently been proposed, which is similar to the MMRM but has the added assumption of a proportional treatment benefit across the study. This requires a decline in the placebo group, which may not occur if there are learning effects, and the proportionality assumption is a fairly strong assumption.

We have proposed a time-delay model which is more consistent with a treatment effect that corresponds to an extension of time. This type of model would be helpful if a study combines an earlier and later stage of disease, which may result in substantially different decline rates between the two disease stages. Alternatively, the outcome measure could be transformed using a log transformation or something similar to achieve a linear decline rather than the reverse S-curve decline, and then fit a linear or separate-means MMRM model.

19.3.4 Holistic Perspective of Treatment Effect

Simulations should include all primary and key secondary outcomes simultaneously, if possible, to keep the correlations between the scales intact for all decision making. If composite scores and GST approaches are being used, then differences in the correlational assumptions can critically change the conclusions of the simulations.

19.4 Statistical Analysis

All analyses that will be performed for a clinical trial are specified in the SAP. The SAP specifies patient populations for analysis, analysis of subject disposition (which feeds into the CONsolidated Standards Of Reporting Trials [CONSORT] diagram), demographic and baseline characteristics, concomitant medications, efficacy and biomarker outcomes, safety analysis of adverse events, laboratory tests, electrocardiogram results, and vital signs. Since most of these analyses are nearly identical across any disease area, only efficacy and biomarker analyses will be discussed here.

19.4.1 Primary Analysis

The primary analysis model must be specified in the SAP and the same model will generally be fit for all quantitative primary, key secondary, secondary, and exploratory outcomes. Estimated treatment means from the model (least-squares means) at the end-of-study visit and least-squares means of the differences with confidence intervals and p-values are calculated and displayed in tables and figures.

19.4.2 Standardized Effect Sizes

Least-squares differences are also referred to as effect sizes, and standardized effect sizes are often provided: either a Cohen's d (difference divided by either the baseline standard deviation or by the standard deviation of the change score across both groups) or a percentage slowing (difference divided by the placebo standard deviation). If the placebo group shows enough progression over the duration of the study, and if the treatment effect is expected to be disease-modifying rather than improving over baseline, then a percentage slowing is generally preferential. If the study is of short duration, such that the placebo decline is minimal, or the placebo group improves over baseline, then a percentage-slowing calculation may be misleading. The advantage of a percentage-slowing calculation is that it allows us to evaluate the treatment benefit relative to the progression of the disease, and without also factoring in the variability of the scale used to measure it [22]. With a disease-modifying effect, the percentage slowing would be expected to be equivalent across multiple outcome measures, and consistency of the percentage slowing across endpoints provides evidence for a disease-modifying effect.

19.4.3 Interpretation of *p*-Values

Often, *p*-values are relied upon as the most important metric in interpreting the results of a hypothesis test, but this frequently results in misinterpretation. Two-sided *p*-values are the most common and offer incomplete information –an estimate or a difference in means is needed to interpret the *p*-value properly. Two prevalent issues with *p*-value interpretation come from two very human inclinations: (1) an over-emphasis on the magnitude of the *p*-value, and (2) confirmation bias.

First, a *p*-value of 0.96 is often interpreted as "worse" than a *p*-value of 0.20. True, a *p*-value of 0.96 offers no information supporting a positive or negative treatment effect, but a *p*-value of 0.20 can offer some evidence that a treatment had the opposite of the intended effect. In short, a *p*-value of 0.20 in the wrong direction is far more evidence against a positive treatment effect than *p* = 0.96 in either direction. Neutral treatment effects with large two-sided *p*-values can't "cancel out" positive treatment effects (small *p*-value and positive treatment effect) from another outcome or another study of the same underlying hypothesis but will weaken them if the totality of evidence is considered.

Second is people's natural confirmation bias. A *p*-value of 0.11 is often seen as evidence of a "trend" in favor of treatment benefit. Funding, publications, and new studies can be based on a trending *p*-value. But *p*-values "trending" in the opposite direction are often ignored. Confirmation bias can lead to an inaccurate interpretation of *p*-values.

19.4.4 Covariates for Reducing Error

It is commonly known that including covariates in a model can correct for baseline imbalances, and this is illustrated in Figure 19.5a. Baseline imbalances may either exaggerate the treatment effect or underestimate the treatment effect depending on the nature of the baseline imbalance.

Inclusion of covariates in a model is also helpful for reducing error and making treatment differences more detectable. If there is a non-zero correlation between the covariate and the outcome variable, then including the covariate in the primary statistical model will reduce the variability (see Figure 19.5b, top and bottom panels). Inclusion of multiple covariates that are all correlated with the outcome variable may further reduce the variability, even if the covariates are highly correlated with each other (colinear) since any unique contribution will

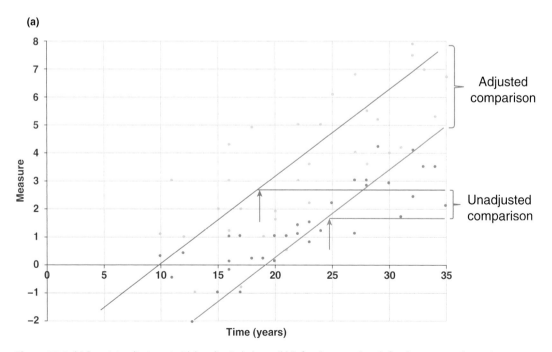

(a)

Figure 19.5 (a) Covariate adjustment with baseline imbalance. (b) Before (top panel) and after (bottom panel) covariate adjustment. The different colors represent different treatment arms or subgroups.

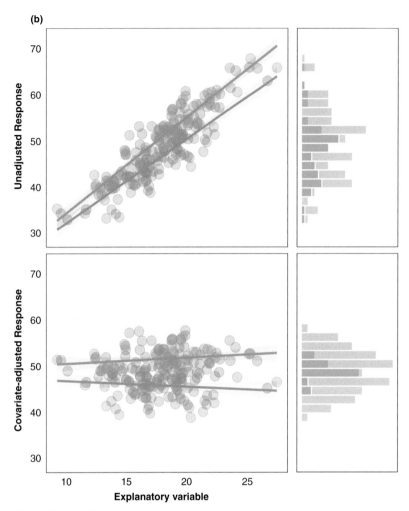

Figure 19.5 (cont.)

be subtracted out of the error estimates and make it easier to detect treatment differences. In AD trials, it is often useful to include baseline ADAS-cog, baseline Mini-Mental State Examination (MMSE), and baseline CDR-sb each as covariates in the primary model when changes from baseline in any of these outcomes are being analyzed.

19.4.5 Subgroups/Covariates: Interaction with Treatment

If covariates or subgroups interact with the treatment group, this means that the treatment effect differs for different values of the covariate, or with different levels of the subgroup variable. Graphically, this is evident with non-parallel lines when plotting the covariate against the outcome variable for a continuous outcome variable,

or different group differences at each level of the subgroup. Ideally, an interaction analysis will be performed first to assess whether the treatment difference statistically differs between groups or across the covariate. If a significant treatment interaction is found, then it is helpful to follow up with subgroup analyses to illustrate the treatment difference separately within the subgroups or for those with higher and lower covariate values for a continuous covariate.

Often, subgroup analyses are used to try to salvage a mostly negative study, but this approach is usually futile since a negative subgroup can often be found that counteracts the positive subgroup that is promoted. Any time one subgroup is presented, the group excluding that subgroup should also be shown, to provide a balanced perspective.

19.4.6 Biomarkers

Quantitative biomarker outcomes are often analyzed with the same statistical model as the primary analysis model. In addition, biomarker outcomes may also be grouped into responder and non-responder categories for analysis, with the proportion responding being compared between active and placebo groups with a proportion test.

19.4.7 Biomarker Relationship with Clinical Outcomes

Assessing the relationship between changes in biomarkers and changes in clinical outcomes is substantially more complicated since the biomarkers and clinical outcomes may not be correlated to begin with. In the "Jack" curves (Figure 19.6), any biomarker that is much earlier than the clinical outcome would not be expected to show a correlation between change in the biomarker and change in the clinical outcome. Figure 19.7 shows that the biomarker and clinical outcome may be totally uncorrelated at both baseline and post baseline (a); uncorrelated at baseline, but correlated at post baseline, if, for instance, the biomarker was on the progressive part of the curve at baseline, but the clinical outcome hadn't started to progress until post baseline (b); correlated at baseline but uncorrelated at post baseline, if, for instance, the clinical outcome

and biomarker were on the progressive part of the curve at baseline, but then the biomarker was on the flat part of the curve by post-baseline (c); or correlated at both visits, if both the biomarker and clinical outcome were on the progressive part of the curve at both visits (d).

Treatment effects on biomarkers and clinical outcomes can occur completely independently of correlations between changes in biomarkers and changes in clinical outcomes (Figure 19.8). One of the best displays for showing the relationship between the change in biomarker and clinical outcome is a scatterplot with an ellipse for the baseline and post-baseline values.

A scatterplot of change from baseline in the biomarker plotted against change from baseline in the clinical outcome may be misleading since equivalent lines in both the placebo and active treatment groups may be consistent with a positive treatment effect on both the biomarker and clinical outcome. Additionally, there is often a correlation between change in biomarker and change in a clinical outcome within the placebo group, and observing a similar correlation in the active group with significant changes in both the biomarker and clinical outcome may be the best result in a clinical study since this suggests a natural relationship between the biomarker and clinical outcome but just an earlier disease stage. In this case, there would be no difference

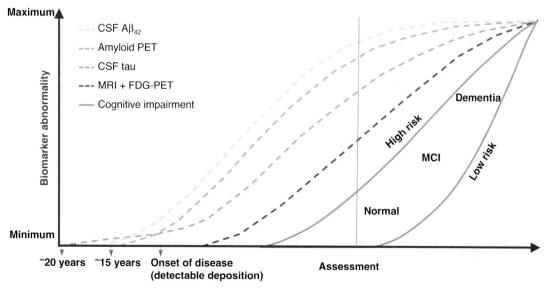

Figure 19.6 Theoretical progression of biomarkers and clinical outcomes. Biomarkers that progress closer in time to clinical outcomes are more likely to correlate with clinical outcomes. Biomarkers that change very early in disease are not likely to correlate with clinical outcomes.

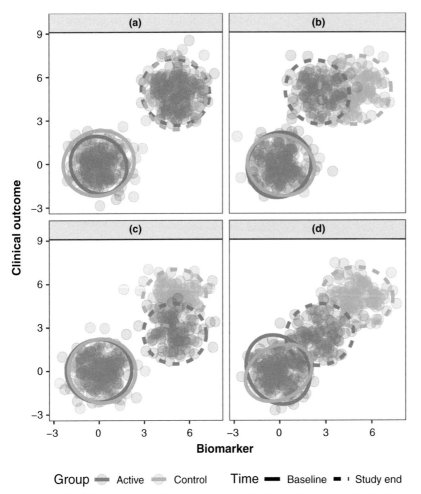

Figure 19.7(a)–(d) Scatterplots for biomarker and clinical outcomes that are correlated and uncorrelated at baseline and post baseline.

in the correlation between the placebo and the active group for the clinical trial since both would have a perfectly natural correlational relationship.

Consider the scenario in Figure 19.7d where there is a correlation at baseline and post baseline, represented by an ellipse for each treatment group. The change-score correlation depends on the path that is taken to get from baseline to post baseline. If the entire distribution of patients at baseline in Figure 19.7d shifted to the right by a fixed amount and shifted up by a fixed amount, to get to the post-baseline position, there would be zero correlation between the change scores for the biomarker and the clinical outcome. There would be a small correlation if the patients were randomly scattered at the post-baseline visit, but this would be due to regression toward the mean. If the ellipse were to flip over the end into the post-baseline position, so that the highest patients at baseline were now the lowest patients at post baseline, then the change scores would have a strong correlation. None of this is directly related to the treatment effect.

Therefore, we recommend using correlations between biomarkers and clinical outcomes only to support a clinical trial interpretation, and not to try to establish a causal relationship between a biomarker and a clinical outcome. Similarly, lack of a correlation between the biomarker and clinical outcome, or between the change from baseline in the biomarker and change from baseline in the clinical outcome cannot rule out a causal relationship when there is otherwise strong evidence for both a biomarker and a clinical treatment benefit.

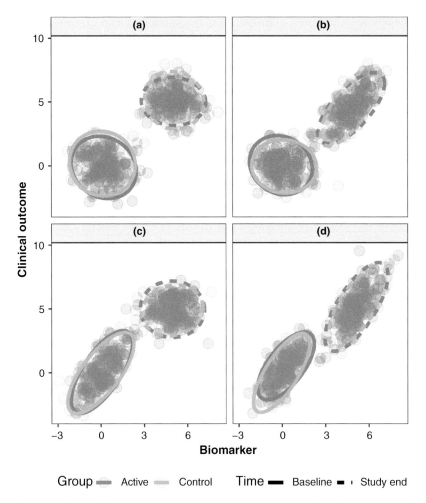

Figure 19.8 (a)–(d) Scatterplots for biomarker and clinical outcomes at baseline and post baseline that have (a) no treatment effect, (b) biomarker effects only, (c) clinical effects only, or (d) both.

19.5 Regulatory Considerations

Regulatory agencies have different statistical perspectives, but all emphasize reducing bias by pre-specification of the alpha-spending approach, primary and secondary outcomes, and the statistical model. It is also important to test model assumptions and robustness of the results using sensitivity analyses. Treatments that are believed to be disease-modifying have more subtle effects than symptomatic treatments, making it more difficult to succeed, but the standards for regulatory approval are generally the same. Regulators are unlikely to give a specific disease-modifying claim despite this additional challenge.

19.5.1 Control of Type I Error

Regulatory agencies are primarily concerned with control of the type I error rate, which is the probability of seeing statistical significance when there is no true treatment effect. The type I error rate is called the alpha level and is typically set at a two-sided 0.05 level, meaning that there is a 5% chance of declaring a treatment significantly better or worse than placebo when there is no true treatment difference.

19.5.2 Control of Type II Error (Protecting Power)

The trial sponsor's primary goal is to protect the power of the study, or the study's probability of achieving statistical significance if the intervention has a true treatment effect. Anything that increases noise in the study will reduce the power: poor rater or site training, frequent data errors, inclusion of the wrong population, using non-equivalent forms for scales, fitting a poor statistical model, and too

245

much data conversion. Since the sample size and alpha level are fixed, any increase in noise will reduce the power of the study.

19.5.3 Consistency of Effect Across Outcomes

Cognitive, functional, and global outcomes are often only weakly correlated ($r \sim 0.30$) with each other, particularly over shorter study durations such as 6 months or less. This often results in differing results across primary and secondary outcomes even with disease-modifying effects that would be expected to affect all aspects of disease similarly.

19.5.4 Disease Modification Designs

Both FDA and EMA guidance observed that randomized-start and randomized-withdrawal trial designs with clinical outcomes can provide evidence of enduring effects consistent with disease modification. The randomized-withdrawal design assesses whether treatment effects are maintained once treatment is withdrawn (Figure 19.9a). The staggered-start design assesses whether a longer and earlier treatment initiation results in a better treatment response, suggesting that the earlier exposure to treatment resulted in a maintained benefit over time (Figure 19.9b).

The FDA has stated that a clinical benefit that is supported by a meaningful effect on a biomarker is consistent with disease modification. In addition, they assert that a treatment should have a lasting effect on the disease course, but that divergence of slope alone is not enough since it might be produced by a pharmacologically reversible effect [23, 24].

The EMA considers a medicinal product to be disease-modifying when it delays the underlying pathological or pathophysiological disease processes. The EMA notes that measurement of the change in rate of decline, as shown by slope analysis and increasing drug–placebo difference, can support a disease-modifying effect.

19.6 Conclusions

AD has a higher clinical trial failure rate than any other common disease due to both drug design issues and study design issues. The complexity of the disease mechanisms and potential targets are well-known challenges in designing drugs, but the complexity of measuring the disease and analyzing the data are similarly challenging and often overlooked. Results that are not clearly positive are often interpreted as clearly negative and the compounds are interpreted as inactive, but AD trials in Phase 2 and Phase 3 are often underpowered, invalidating this conclusion.

Accurately interpreting the results of an AD clinical trial requires an understanding of the progression of and relationships between the outcome measures in the study population, particularly when the results are positive for some outcomes and not positive for others. Subgroup analyses are helpful for understanding whether an observed effect is primarily driven by a specific subpopulation, but they are rarely helpful for salvaging a study that is primarily negative. Phase 2 and some Phase 3 AD clinical trials have unclear results but can be clarified with global test statistics, composite scores, and Bayesian hierarchical meta-analyses, and by basing the interpretation on the totality of evidence across primary and secondary endpoints.

Careful attention to the study design, outcome-measure selection, rater training, data management, and statistical analysis of a clinical trial

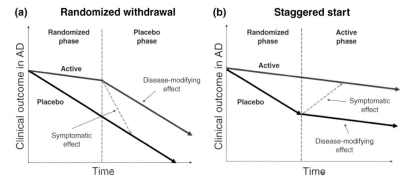

Figure 19.9 (a) Randomized-withdrawal and (b) staggered-start study designs.

improves the chance of success by reducing variability and increasing the power. These decisions vary by patient population, mechanism of action of the drug, study duration, and overall development strategy, and they must be made in that context.

References

1. Boada M, López OL, Olazarán J, et al. A randomized, controlled clinical trial of plasma exchange with albumin replacement for Alzheimer's disease: primary results of the AMBAR study. *Alzheimers Dement* 2020; **16**: 1412–25. https://doi.org/10.1002/alz.12137.

2. Kivipelto M, Mangialasche F, Ngandu T. Lifestyle interventions to prevent cognitive impairment, dementia and Alzheimer disease. *Nat Rev Neurol* 2018; **14**: 653–66. https://doi.org/10.1038/s41582-018-0070-3.

3. Cummings J, Ballard C, Tariot P, et al. Pimavanserin: potential treatment for dementia-related psychosis. *J Prev Alzheimers Dis* 2018; **5**: 253–8. https://doi.org/10.14283/jpad.2018.29.

4. Huang P, Goetz CG, Woolson RF, et al. Using global statistical tests in long-term Parkinson's disease clinical trials. *Mov Disord* 2009; **24**: 1732–9. https://doi.org/10.1002/mds.22645.

5. Dickson SP. Comparison of aducanumab, solanezumab and BAN2401 using a global statistical test for assessing impact on overall strength of evidence. 13th Clinical Trials on Alzheimer's Disease (CTAD) Congress, November 4–7, 2020.

6. Schneider LS, Goldberg TE. Composite cognitive and functional measures for early stage Alzheimer's disease trials. *Alzheimers Dement Diagnosis, Assess Dis Monit* 2020; **12**: 1–9. https://doi.org/10.1002/dad2.12017.

7. Hendrix SB, Dickson SP, Ellison N. Composite endpoints – pro perspective: the key to successful clinical development in Alzheimer's disease. *Alzheimers Dement* 2019; **15**: P1274. https://doi.org/10.1016/j.jalz.2019.06.3660.

8. Hendrix SB, Ellison N. ADCOMS: a sensitive measure of disease progression in early AD supporting better development decisions. *Alzheimers Dement* 2019; **15**: P520. https://doi.org/10.1016/j.jalz.2019.06.4426.

9. Wang J, Logovinsky V, Hendrix SB, et al. ADCOMS: a composite clinical outcome for prodromal Alzheimer's disease trials. *J Neurol Neurosurg Psychiatry* 2016; **87**: 993–9. https://doi.org/10.1136/jnnp-2015-312383.

10. Wessels AM, Siemers ER, Yu P, et al. A combined measure of cognition and function for clinical trials: the Integrated Alzheimer's Disease Rating Scale (iADRS). *J Prev Alzheimers Dis* 2015; **2**: 227–41. https://doi.org/10.14283/jpad.2015.82.

11. Langbaum JB, Ellison NN, Caputo A, et al. The Alzheimer's Prevention Initiative Composite Cognitive test: a practical measure for tracking cognitive decline in preclinical Alzheimer's disease. *Alzheimers Res Ther* 2020; **12**: 1–11. https://doi.org/10.1186/s13195-020-00633-2.

12. Donohue MC, Sperling RA, Salmon DP, et al. The Preclinical Alzheimer Cognitive Composite: measuring amyloid-related decline. *JAMA Neurol* 2014; **71**: 961–70. https://doi.org/10.1001/jamaneurol.2014.803.

13. Blennow K, Zetterberg H. Biomarkers for Alzheimer's disease: current status and prospects for the future. *J Intern Med* 2018; **284**: 643–63. https://doi.org/10.1111/joim.12816.

14. Ismail R, Parbo P, Madsen LS, et al. The relationships between neuroinflammation, beta-amyloid and tau deposition in Alzheimer's disease: a longitudinal PET study. *J Neuroinflammation* 2020; **17**: 151. https://doi.org/10.1186/s12974-020-01820-6.

15. Preische O, Schultz SA, Apel A, et al. Serum neurofilament dynamics predicts neurodegeneration and clinical progression in presymptomatic Alzheimer's disease. *Nat Med* 2019; **25**: 277–83. https://doi.org/10.1038/s41591-018-0304-3.

16. Liu W, Lin H, He X, et al. Neurogranin as a cognitive biomarker in cerebrospinal fluid and blood exosomes for Alzheimer's disease and mild cognitive impairment. *Transl Psychiatry* 2020; **10**: 125. https://doi.org/10.1038/s41398-020-0801-2.

17. O'Brien PC, Fleming TR. A multiple testing procedure for clinical trials. *Biometrics* 1979; **35**: 549–56. https://doi.org/10.2307/2530245.

18. Lan KKG, Demets DL. Discrete sequential boundaries for clinical trials. *Biometrika* 1983; **70**: 659–63. https://doi.org/10.1093/biomet/70.3.659.

19. Whitehead J, Stratton I. Group sequential clinical trials with triangular continuation regions. *Biometrics* 1983; **39**: 227–36. https://doi.org/10.2307/2530822.

20. Hume S, Aerts J, Sarnikar S, Huser V. Current applications and future directions for the CDISC Operational Data Model standard: a methodological review. *J Biomed Inform* 2016; **60**: 352–62. https://doi.org/10.1016/j.jbi.2016.02.016.

21. Hendrix SB, Wilcock GK. What we have learned from the Myriad trials. *J Nutr Health Aging* 2009; **13**: 362–4. https://doi.org/10.1007/s12603-009-0044-7.

22. Hendrix SB. Measuring clinical progression in MCI and pre-MCI populations: enrichment and optimizing clinical outcomes over time. *Alzheimers Res Ther* 2012; **4**: 24. https://doi .org/10.1186/alzrt127.

23. US Department of Health and Human Services, Food and Drug Administration, Center for Drug Evaluation and Research (CDER), and Center for Biologics Evaluation and Research (CBER). Early Alzheimer's disease: developing drugs for treatment. Guidance for industry.

Available at: www.fda.gov/files/drugs/published/ Alzheimer%E2%80%99s-Disease---Developing-Drugs-for-Treatment-Guidance-for-Industy.pdf (accessed January 20, 2021).

24. European Medicines Agency. Clinical investigation of medicines for the treatment of Alzheimer's disease/ CPMP/EWP/553/1995. Available at: www.ema.europa.eu/en/documents/scientific-guideline/guideline-clinical-investigation-medicines-treatment-alzheimers-disease-revision-2_en.pdf (accessed January 20, 2021).

Chapter 20

Alzheimer's Disease Trial Recruitment and Diversifying Trial Populations

Samantha E. John

20.1 Introduction

Alzheimer's disease (AD) drug development and clinical trials testing are of critical importance, given the current public health crisis posed by the disorder. In 2020, as many as 5.8 million Americans were affected by AD, resulting in costs of up to $305 billion in healthcare and long-term care [1]. As cohorts of adults continue to live into advanced age, the public health and economic burden of AD will only continue to increase. Within the AD drug-development ecosystem, researchers and advocacy groups are motivated to discover treatments that alter the course of disease and reduce the global public health burden it imposes. It is in this context that we focus on clinical trial samples and their recruitment.

AD disproportionately affects particular groups, and the field has an incomplete understanding of the underlying causes of this unequal risk and prevalence. Differences in sociodemographic characteristics, such as ethnoracial identity, socioeconomic status, and primary residence, may influence the level of conferred risk [2, 3]. Trial populations must include representative variability across sociodemographic characteristics to capture unequal risk and potentially varied responses to treatment. Diverse participant samples are our best tool for generalizing effects to patient populations. Unfortunately, diverse participant samples are also one of our largest barriers to the timely and complete investigation of new treatments. This chapter explores aspects of AD clinical trial recruitment, the strategies necessary for achieving sufficient and inclusive representation, and the effective models and approaches currently in practice and in need of further research.

20.2 Clinical Trial Recruitment

Clinical trial recruitment is a significant barrier in the development of novel treatments. The recruitment timeline is lengthy, often extends beyond initial trial deadlines, and is subject to complications throughout the process, including differential enrollment, loss to follow-up, and a lack of diversity among potential participants [4]. Knowledge of clinical trial demands can help shape strategies for participant identification and recruitment.

20.2.1 Recruitment Numbers

Enrollment criteria increase and become more specific with each subsequent trial phase. This process produces conflicting demands, where the need for large numbers of diverse participants is in opposition to an ever-narrowing pool of potential enrollees. Comprehensive reviews of trends in clinical trials have shown that up to two-thirds of drug trials will fail to achieve recruitment targets; as many as half of all drug trials will require an extension on recruitment timelines; and up to 85% of trials finish late as a result of low participation [5, 6]. To achieve sufficient sample size for generalizability of results, Phase 3 trials may require thousands of participants, recruited through multiple sites. Sample identification is therefore resource and time intensive; it requires significant time and skill investments to appropriately tailor recruitment approaches to the target population and their motivations [6].

20.2.2 Screening Failures, Competing Trials, and Trial Timelines

Primary- and secondary-prevention trials are increasingly emphasized within the drug-development ecosystem. AD research prioritizes biomarker approaches to diagnosis, which aim to identify patients during the preclinical or asymptomatic phases of disease. Asymptomatic populations may be more difficult to recruit, as they are less likely to seek treatment and less motivated to pursue a trial that may pose risks without providing a clear benefit [7]. Primary- and secondary-prevention trials require thorough screening processes that consist of neuropsychological testing, neuroimaging, and biomarker collection of blood and cerebrospinal fluid samples. Identifying biomarker-positive individuals from an asymptomatic population requires significant time and resources, and results in many screening failures, leading to a recruitment bottleneck that impedes trial progress [8, 9]. For example, the A4 trial required a period of roughly 3 years to recruit a sample of 1,169 older adult participants (aged 65+), who were screened via positron emission tomography scans for evidence of amyloid. The A4 trial recruitment resulted in a screen fail rate of 71% [8]. Within trial timelines, recruitment phases may extend as long as 10 times the duration of actual drug exposure [10]. These figures highlight the connection between potential participants and trial efficacy, where efficiency of recruitment dictates efficiency of discovery.

At any one time, there may be hundreds of clinical trials in progress investigating an AD target. While increased trial numbers will increase the likelihood of successful discovery, they also increase the overall recruitment burden within the AD research ecosystem. As of February 27, 2020, there were 121 agents in 136 trials of AD therapies, consisting of drug targets for cognitive enhancement, neuropsychiatric symptoms, and disease modification [10]. Phase 3 trials represent about one-fourth of registered AD trials, each containing an average of 554 participants at an average trial duration of 240 weeks. These studies are likely vying for many of the same highly restricted and well-characterized samples, further tightening the recruitment bottleneck.

20.2.3   Trial Characteristics

Features of the participant sample may be treated as secondary in importance relative to the study timeline and required sample size. Samples that are easier to identify and characterize have a higher likelihood of being screened and enrolled, reflecting health-disparity trends in access and treatment. Recent approaches to the study of clinical trials have identified the need to prioritize diversity recruitment efforts in the AD drug-development ecosystem [11, 12].

Ethnoracial representation in the country is increasing and clinical trial study samples are failing to match these population trends. Health-disparate populations are often excluded from clinical trials and longitudinal aging research, which limits the generalizability of results to those groups. The majority of AD clinical trial and prospective

research participants are non-Hispanic white [13–15]. According to US Census estimates, however, minority older adults will make up an increasingly large proportion of the population. By 2050, racial and ethnic minorities will make up roughly 42% of the older adult population [16], and by 2060, older adults will make up one in four Americans [17]. In contrast to these numbers, ethnic and racial minorities make up less than 5% of clinical trial samples, with enrollment of roughly 1% Hispanic and roughly 2% African-American participants across projects [18, 19]. Racial and ethnic minorities are also less likely to be retained within longitudinal projects [20]. As a result, we define, monitor, and treat AD according to the non-Hispanic white majority, which both contributes to and maintains disparities in risk and treatment. The development of participant pipelines that account for local and community needs, increase access to disease-specific knowledge, and more efficiently match potential participants to opportunities represents a strategic shift in study planning that promises to reduce trial timelines.

20.3   Diversity in Clinical Trials

Participant samples within clinical trials and longitudinal research projects should reflect the population of interest. The target population for AD clinical trials is therefore wide, varied, and multidimensional. Recruitment of diverse clinical trial participants addresses two primary issues: (1) diverse groups face disproportionate risk for, and prevalence of, AD; and (2) medication safety and efficacy can vary as a function of participant characteristics.

20.3.1   Dimensions of Diversity and Importance of Inclusion

Diversity of clinical trial participants is paramount in AD research, owing to the diverse nature of AD patients and the health disparities associated with diagnosis. Recruitment strategies for obtaining diverse participants must be considered early in trial planning and recurrently throughout implementation. The Food and Drug Administration (FDA) in the United States recommends that sponsors include explicit plans for the inclusion of diverse participants no later than the end of Phase 2 [11]. Conducting analyses by ethnoracial group has shown differential medication responses and population-specific signals in the outcome data

[11]. Therefore, the primary outcomes of interest in clinical trials are dependent upon the ability to recruit, enroll, and retain diverse participants. Diversity characteristics include demographic variables, such as age, sex, race, ethnicity, and location of primary residence (e.g., rural vs. urban). A broader definition of participant diversity includes the individual characteristics that influence disease heterogeneity, including co-morbid conditions, weight or body mass index, disability status, and lifestyle practices such as smoking, diet, exercise, concomitant drug use, and sleep habits.

AD risk and prevalence vary as a function of demographic factors. Because AD is a disorder that manifests in later life, later-phase trials, if not all phases, require recruitment and retention of a group deemed vulnerable by the FDA. Enrollment of participants of advanced age allows for the evaluation of age-dependent physiological changes, disease co-morbidities, and concomitant medication use. The FDA provides guidelines for medication evaluation in the elderly, which must include strict evaluation of dose and drug response as well as assessment of drug–drug interactions [11]. Females have nearly double the lifetime risk of AD at ages 45 and 65 when compared to males [21]. Roughly two-thirds of current dementia patients are female [22] and females will make up the majority of diagnosed patients throughout older adulthood [23]. Hispanics and African/Black Americans face disproportionate risk for AD, with Hispanics at a roughly 1.5-fold risk and African Americans at a roughly 2-fold risk, relative to non-Hispanic whites [24]. Rural Americans also possess greater risk for cognitive impairment and dementia [25]. Rural-dwelling older adults tend to experience worse overall health as well as worse health outcomes, relative to their urban-dwelling counterparts [26]. This is true for both risk of disease as well as increased rates of mortality as a result of AD [27].

Groups facing disproportionate risk also have unique risk factors and characteristics that influence how we measure disease progression and treatment effects. For females specifically, several causative factors have been associated with increased rates of AD, including greater life expectancy, decreased educational attainment and cognitive reserve within older female cohorts, increased genetic risk, and/or the influence of estrogen on genetic risk [1]. For ethnoracial minorities, rates of co-morbid conditions, language barriers, quality of education, and cultural lifestyle factors, such

as diet and exercise trends, have been implicated. For those living in rural areas, access to healthcare, limited knowledge about brain health, economic distress, and low levels of education are associated with AD risk [28–30]. Individual characteristics likely also influence the safety and effectiveness of medication, particularly if they modify pharmacokinetics, pharmacodynamics, and, ultimately, therapeutic dose. Ignoring these individual features during the early phase of a drug trial all but guarantees that the resulting influence of these factors will be realized only in later trial phases, increasing the likelihood of negative side effects and unintended adverse events.

20.3.2   Barriers to Trial Diversity

Only limited research has examined barriers to diverse recruitment among AD participants. Of the existing research, the majority of studies have emphasized or solely evaluated AD trial recruitment within African/Black American samples. In recent years, the AD ecosystem has begun to broaden its recruitment and retention efforts to include a focus on Hispanic/LatinX communities and, to a lesser extent, Asian Americans and indigenous communities [11]. Preliminary evidence from these limited studies suggests that examination and elimination of community-specific barriers can be effective for increasing diversity of study participants, but more research is needed [12, 31].

For AD research and clinical trials in particular, biomarker collection and brain-donation requirements have a significant influence on ethnic-minority participation [3, 32]. Within a targeted self-study of one AD center, African-American enrollment in research projects declined by more than 50% in the 2 years following implementation of required lumbar puncture [33]. Among potential participants who responded to an initial study advertisement, of those who provided a reason for declining participation, African Americans, more so than their non-Hispanic white counterparts, stated that concerns about the lumbar puncture were the deciding factor in their decision; roughly 46% of African-American potentials who declined study participation named lumbar puncture as the reason for declining versus only 25% of non-Hispanic white participants [34]. Brain donation is also a common requirement of longitudinal AD research. Postmortem autopsy and pathology evaluations provide necessary and important details about the severity and spread of disease relative

251

to clinical presentations, especially among those decedents without a clinical diagnosis [32]. Given the recognition that biomarker and tissue-donation requirements create barriers to participation, requirements are sometimes waived for minority participants to increase enrollment [35].

20.3.3 Trial Biases Limit Diversity

There are also systematic biases in clinical trial processes that contribute to the lack of diverse participants. Populations needing accommodations are less likely to be represented within trials, despite the fact that these accommodations may not pertain to the disease process specifically. Trial participation is an outcome influenced by access, education, and primary language [4].

Existing patient streams are often the first source for potential participants. Participating clinical trial sites, including academic and urban medical institutions, can enroll existing patients. Existing patients may already be well characterized and they may be able to roll study visits into already scheduled clinical visits [31]. Though efficient for recruitment and enrollment, this practice privileges certain kinds of AD patients, typically those in urban areas with higher education and higher socioeconomic status.

Factors such as time of day and availability of trial participation time slots can also influence study access. Potential participants with full-time jobs and other employment limitations or those with caregiver responsibilities during the day may be prevented from attending required in-person sessions. Other potential participants will be excluded from participation as a result of transportation barriers to and from the trial site. Education requirements may be necessary for certain aspects of study participation, including independent consent and neuropsychological testing. Consent and neuropsychological testing also typically require familiarity and comfort with the English language. Unfortunately, studies may not be equipped to provide translators or to support bilingual patient participation [11].

20.4 Trial Recruitment Approaches and Strategies to Increase Diversity

The most effective recruitment approaches create long-term, stable infrastructures that support and engage potential participants, reduce barriers to entry, and anticipate causes of attrition.

Actions taken locally through community-based participatory approaches can increase engagement at particular sites. These efforts fuel the enrollment into, and use of larger, national initiatives aimed at matching potential participants to specific trials.

Academic institutions and centers with relevant patient populations are the most common sites for study recruitment. For AD specifically, there are networks of federally funded aging-focused research centers that serve to engage and study AD patients. In addition to local research sites, clinical trials may be advertized nationally through earned media coverage, paid advertisements, social media, and other online methods. Participant registries and matching services represent promise for creating and sustaining contact with potential participants. The online environment allows for efficient digital enrollment and ongoing communication with potential participants, providing a high-touch engagement method that can be iteratively updated to target evolving project goals [6, 36].

20.4.1 Trial Registries

To support recruitment efforts, several initiatives have created online registries and platforms for recruiting, characterizing, tracking, and matching potential participants to clinical trials in need of recruits. These websites increase the transparency and accessibility of trials across the nation and aim to decrease or remove the recruitment bottlenecks delaying results and discovery.

Alzheimer's Association TrialMatch: The TrialMatch is a service that connects individuals living with AD, caregivers, and healthy volunteers to current research studies. The service consists of an updated database of AD clinical studies, both non-pharmacological and pharmacological. The service encourages any adult to register and be matched to studies in active recruitment. Study matches are based on personal characteristics, diagnostic status, and treatment history.

ClinicalTrials.gov: ClinicalTrials.gov is a web-based resource that provides patients, their family members, healthcare professionals, researchers, and the public with easy access to information on publicly and privately supported clinical studies on a wide range of diseases and conditions. The website is maintained by the National Library of Medicine at the National Institutes of Health (NIH). Principal investigators and study sponsors submit information to the website and are responsible for registering studies and reporting updates and details. The site serves as a study registry and a database of results.

Trial-Ready Cohort for Preclinical and Prodromal Alzheimer's Disease (TRC-PAD): The TRC-PAD is a launching pad to advance prevention trials in AD research, by matching potential participants to trials. This initiative grew out of the online-only Alzheimer's Prevention Trials web study, which characterizes online volunteers according to self-reported cognitive functioning, brief medical history, and a quarterly unsupervized cognitive assessment. If study criteria are met, participants join the Trial-Ready Cohort, a group of potential volunteers that receive routine assessment for AD indicators. The cohort is a participant stream for multiple trials and allows for ongoing tracking of potential participants [8, 37].

Healthy Brains Initiative: The Healthy Brains Initiative (healthybrains.org) is an online resource center with a quantitative assessment tool, the Healthy Brains Index, which characterizes brain health through the domains of nutrition, sleep, physical activity, social connection, and medical and cognitive health. The website includes scientific news, customized questionnaires, and recommendations, and it encourages yearly assessments. Potential participants can endorse an interest in research and provide their contact information for recruitment into relevant projects.

20.4.2 Strategies to Increase Diversity and Inclusion

Increasing the diversity of clinical trial participants requires a concerted approach that addresses the historical and logistical barriers to participation and systematically installs a sustained infrastructure. Among the stakeholders motivated to achieve equity and efficiency in clinical trials, the NIH's National Institute on Aging and the FDA have both convened reports outlining best practices for recruitment planning and achieving diversity among participants [11, 31]. Several common goals underlie all of the strategies discussed: increased accessibility, reduction of participant and caregiver burden, and allowance for greater variability among participants.

One of the most effective ways to increase accessibility to clinical trials is to broaden eligibility criteria, which can widen the recruitment bottleneck by increasing the number of potential participants. Eligibility criteria can be broadened through the use of specific measurable exclusion parameters. Exclusion criteria can more specifically define the subsets of individuals at greatest study risk, and only these individuals should be excluded rather than all individuals carrying a particular concomitant diagnosis [11]. Modifications can also be made to the overall trial design and methodology. Use of adaptive trial design and sample enrichment can shorten study timelines and achieve generalizable results. In an adaptive trial design, pre-specified changes to study design can be implemented during the trial in response to interim analyses. These changes might allow for broadened eligibility criteria, mid trial. Sample enrichment strategies, both prognostic and predictive, can be effective for reducing overall sample-size requirements, though they often require a greater upfront burden through participant screening [38]. In prognostic enrichment, participants are enrolled based on the increased likelihood of reaching study endpoints or demonstrating drug effectiveness. In predictive enrichment, participants are enrolled based on characteristic responsiveness to treatment. Reducing the study burden for both participants and participant informants is also a priority, and this can be achieved through reducing the frequency of study visits, allowing for remote data collection, and providing reimbursement for travel and time [11].

20.5 Retention

Exposure periods for clinical trials commonly span a year or longer, with multiple observations. Time- and resource-intensive monitoring places a burden on participants and their study partners, often resulting in loss to follow-up. Study attrition can extend trial timelines and lead to incomplete trials. Non-random attrition in trials can produce underpowered, biased, and potentially invalid analytic results [39]. Few studies have examined retention in longitudinal projects and clinical trials in a systematic way. Fewer still have emphasized ethnoracial minorities in studies of retention. Available study evidence suggests that clinical trials should plan retention strategies prior to trial initiation and utilize inclusive, tailored, and multidimensional approaches to improve retention rates.

Evaluation of longitudinal retention within prospective observational studies of AD can provide some insights. Utilizing data from the National Alzheimer's Coordinating Center, Burke and colleagues [40] found that increasing age, greater neuropsychiatric symptoms, and more severe cognitive impairment are all associated with greater levels of attrition. Pathological signs of disease severity may also be associated with greater attrition in longitudinal AD research, including reduced hippocampal volume, greater levels of white-matter lesion volume, and greater declines in hippocampal volume between study visits [41].

Grill and colleagues evaluated retention strategies utilized by the Alzheimer's Disease Research Centers and found that a variety of techniques have been employed, usually in combination, to retain non-trial participants for annual visits. Common retention strategies across centers include financial incentives, reimbursements for travel and meals, non-financial incentives, and specialized tracking methods (e.g., participant phone-trees for contact, following on social media, attending clinical visits) [20]. A meta-analysis of five clinical trials implementing retention strategies revealed minimal impact from intervention approaches. When individual studies within the meta-analysis were evaluated, only one intervention showed a significant benefit to retention. The use of community health advisors produced an almost two-fold improvement to retention [42]. Of the available research evaluating retention among minority populations, most studies have focused on African-American/Black participants. African Americans have 24% lower odds of being retained relative to non-Hispanic whites within longitudinal, prospective observational studies. Other characteristics, including lower education, younger age, and more co-morbidities, also predict decreased retention [20]. More research is needed in this area.

20.6 Recruitment and Diversity in the AD Drug-Development Ecosystem

In conducting clinical trials, we evaluate the most promising findings from translational research, gain perspective about mechanisms of action, and strive to identify treatments that are both effective and safe for a wide range of AD patients. To assess the effectiveness of any clinical trial drug, we must first identify, screen, and follow representative participants through multiple trial phases, a year-long duration between discovery and efficacy. Sufficient sample sizes at each phase are necessary for detecting meaningful clinical differences in symptoms [12]. To reflect the complexity and heterogeneity of AD presentations, clinical trials depend upon large, diverse, and well-characterized participant samples [31].

Recruitment and retention receive some of the blame for the long, protracted timeline of clinical trials. Finding solutions for recruitment challenges will therefore improve the overall efficiency of study trials and the speed of drug discovery. With respect to diversity and inclusion, steps taken at the beginning of study planning benefit not only the trials process but also the broader healthcare system responsible for access and delivery of treatment. The AD drug-development ecosystem is therefore well positioned to innovate and deliver a model of research that is effective, adaptive, and inclusive.

References

1. Alzheimer's Association. 2020 Alzheimer's disease facts and figures. *Alzheimers Dement* 2020; **16**: 391–460.

2. Babulal GM, Quiroz YT, Albensi BC, et al. Perspectives on ethnic and racial disparities in Alzheimer's disease and related dementias: update and areas of immediate need. *Alzheimers Dement* 2019; **15**: 292–312.

3. Wong R, Amano T, Lin S-Y, Zhou Y, Morrow-Howell N. Strategies for the recruitment and retention of racial/ethnic minorities in Alzheimer disease and dementia clinical research. *Curr Alzheimer Res* 2019; **16**: 458–71.

4. Ashford MT, Eichenbaum J, Williams T, et al. Effects of sex, race, ethnicity, and education on online aging research participation. *Alzheimers Dement (N Y)* 2020; **6**: 1–9.

5. McDonald A, Knight R, Cambell M, et al. What influences recruitment to randomized controlled trials? A review of trials funded by two UK funding agencies. *Trials* 2006; **7**: 1–8.

6. Dowling NM, Olson N, Mish T, Kaprakattu P, Gleason C. A model for the design and implementation of a participant recruitment registry for clinical studies of older adults. *Clin Trials* 2012; **9**: 204–14.

7. Hsu D, Marshall GA. Primary and secondary prevention trials in Alzheimer disease: looking back, moving forward. *Curr Alzheimer Res* 2016; **14**: 426–40.

8. Aisen PS, Sperling RA, Cummings J, et al. The Trial-Ready Cohort for Preclinical/Prodromal

Alzheimer's Disease (TRC-PAD) project: an overview. *J Prev Alzheimers Dis* 2020; 7: 208–12.

9. Rafii MS, Aisen PS. Alzheimer's disease clinical trials: moving toward successful prevention. *CNS Drugs* 2019; 33: 99–106. https://doi.org/10.1007/s40263-018-0598-1.

10. Cummings J, Lee G, Ritter A, Sabbagh M, Zhong K. Alzheimer's disease drug-development pipeline: 2020. *Alzheimers Dement (N Y)* 2020; 6: e12050.

11. US Food and Drug Administration. Enhancing the diversity of clinical trial populations: eligibility criteria, enrollment practices, and trial designs guidance for industry. November 2020. www.fda.gov/regulatory-information/search-fda-guidance-documents/enhancing-diversity-clinical-trial-populations-eligibility-criteria-enrollment-practices-and-trial. Available at: https://www.fda.gov/media/127712/download (accessed November 17, 2020).

12. National Institute on Aging. Alzheimer's disease and related dementias: clinical studies recruitment planning guide. Available at: www.nia.nih.gov/sites/default/files/2019-05/ADEAR-recruitment-guide-508.pdf (accessed June 17, 2020).

13. Heredia NI, Strong LL, Hatten V. Community perceptions of biobanking participation: a qualitative study among Mexican-Americans in three Texas cities. *Public Health Genom* 2017; 20: 46–57.

14. Nuño MM, Gillen DL, Dosanjh KK, et al. Attitudes toward clinical trials across the Alzheimer's disease spectrum. *Alzheimers Res Ther* 2017; 9: 81–90.

15. Zhou Y, Elashoff D, Kremen S, et al. African Americans are less likely to enroll in preclinical Alzheimer's disease clinical trials. *Alzheimers Dement (N Y)* 2017; 3: 57–64.

16. Barnes LL, Bennett DA. Alzheimer's disease in African Americans: risk factors and challenges for the future. *Health Aff* 2014; 33: 580–6.

17. Matthews KA, Xu W, Gaglioti AH, et al. Racial and ethnic estimates of Alzheimer's disease and related dementias in the United States (2015–2060) in adults aged ≥65 years. *Alzheimers Dement* 2019; 15: 17–24.

18. Faison WE, Schultz SK, Aerssens J, et al. Potential ethnic modifiers in the assessment and treatment of Alzheimer's disease: challenges for the future. *Int Psychogeriatr* 2007; 19: 539–58.

19. Olin JT, Dagerman KS, Fox LS, Bowers B, Schneider SL. Increasing ethnic minority participation in Alzheimer's disease research. *Alzheimer Dis Assoc Disord* 2002; 16: S82–5.

20. Grill JD, Kwon J, Teylan MA, et al. Retention of Alzheimer disease research participants. *Alzheimer Dis Assoc Disord* 2019; 33: 299–306.

21. Chêne G, Beiser A, Au R, et al. Gender and incidence of dementia in the Framingham Heart Study from mid-adult life. *Alzheimers Dement* 2015; 11: 310–20.

22. Hebert L, Weuve J, Scherr PA, Evans D. Alzheimer's disease in the United States (2010–2050) estimated using the 2010 Census. *Neurology* 2013; 80: 1778–83.

23. Plassman BL, Langa KM, Fisher GG, et al. Prevalence of dementia in the United States: the aging, demographics, and memory study. *Neuroepidemiology* 2007; 29: 125–32.

24. Mehta K, Yeo G. Systematic review of dementia prevalence and incidence in US racial/ethnic populations. *Alzheimers Dement* 2017; 13: 72–83.

25. Weden MM. Secular trends in dementia and cognitive impairment of U.S. rural and urban older adults. *Am J Prev Med* 2018; 54: 164–72.

26. Jaffe S. Aging in rural America. *Health Aff* 2015; 34: 7–10.

27. Singh GK, Siahpush M. Widening rural–urban disparities in all-cause mortality and mortality from major causes of death in the USA, 1969–2009. *J Urban Health* 2014; 91: 272–92.

28. Borak J, Salipante-Zaidel C, Slade M, Fields C. Mortality disparities in Appalachia: reassessment of major risk factors. *J Occup Environ Med* 2012; 54: 146–56.

29. Galvin J, Fu Q, Nguyen J, Glasheen C, Scharff D. Psychosocial determinants of intention to screen for Alzheimer's disease. *Alzheimers Dement* 2009; 4: 353–60.

30. Wiese LK, Williams CL, Tappen RM. Analysis of barriers to cognitive screening in rural populations in the United States. *Adv Nurs Sci* 2014; 37: 327–39.

31. National Institute on Aging. Together we make the difference: national strategy for recruitment and participation in Alzheimer's and related dementias clinical research. Available at: www.nia.nih.gov/research/recruitment-strategy (accessed October 22, 2020).

32. Marquez DX, Glover CM, Lamar M, et al. Representation of older Latinxs in cohort studies at the Rush Alzheimer's Disease Center. *Neuroepidemiology* 2020; 54: 404–18.

33. Williams MM, Meisel MM, Williams J, Morris JC. An interdisciplinary outreach model of African American recruitment for Alzheimer's disease research. *Gerontologist* 2011; 51: 134–41.

34. Howell JC, Parker MW, Watts KD, et al. Research lumbar punctures among African Americans and Caucasians: perception predicts experience. *Front Aging Neurosci* 2016; 8: 1–7.

35. Boise L, Hinton L, Rosen HJ, Ruhl M. Will my soul go to heaven if they take my brain? Beliefs and

worries about brain donation among four ethnic groups. *Gerontologist* 2017; **57**: 719–34.

36. Walter S, Clanton TB, Langford OG, et al. Recruitment into the Alzheimer Prevention Trials (APT) Webstudy for a Trial-Ready Cohort for Preclinical and Prodromal Alzheimer's Disease (TRC–PAD). *J Prev Alzheimers Dis* 2020; **7**: 219–25.

37. Jimenez-Maggiora GA, Bruschi S, Raman R, et al. TRC-PAD: accelerating recruitment of AD clinical trials through innovative information technology. *J Prev Alzheimers Dis* 2020; **7**: 226–33.

38. Grill JD, Monsell SE. Choosing Alzheimer's disease prevention clinical trial populations. *Neurobiol Aging* 2014; **35**: 1–16.

39. Weuve J, Sagiv SK, Fox MP. Quantitative bias analysis for collaborative science. *Epidemiology* 2018; **29**: 627–30.

40. Burke SL, Hu T, Naseh M, et al. Factors influencing attrition in 35 Alzheimer's disease centers across the USA: a longitudinal examination of the National Alzheimer's Coordinating Center's Uniform Data Set. *Aging Clin Exp Res* 2019; **31**: 1283–97.

41. Glymour MM, Chěne G, Tzourio C, Dufouil C. Brain MRI markers and dropout in a longitudinal study of cognitive aging: the three-city Dijon study. *Neurology* 2012; **79**: 1340–8.

42. Crocker JC, Ricci-Cabello I, Parker A, et al. Impact of patient and public involvement on enrolment and retention in clinical trials: systematic review and meta-analysis. *BMJ* 2018; **363**: 1–17.

Chapter 21

The Role of Online Registries in Accelerating Alzheimer's Disease Drug Development

Sarah Walter, Jessica Langbaum, and Rachel Nosheny

21.1   Introduction

21.1.1   Alzheimer's Disease Therapeutics

Alzheimer's disease (AD) is the most prevalent fatal neurological condition, impacting an estimated 5.8 million people in the United States [1]. The challenges facing AD clinical trials are significant [2, 3]. There is limited participation in research, driven by the burden of the disease, complexity of trials, under-diagnosis of dementia, and for those that are diagnosed, the stigma of dementia. Clinical trials enroll very few people from African-American and Latinx communities, despite research showing an elevated risk [4]. However, recent advances in AD research are generating opportunities; the most impactful being the ability to measure in vivo the key proteinopathies of AD (amyloid plaques and tau tangles) using positron emission tomography imaging. This has led to an increased understanding of the disease progression prior to the development of cognitive symptoms [5]. Population studies have revealed the key risks for AD, including hypertension and high cholesterol, which if managed could result in reduced incidence of AD [6]. A long-awaited blood test to confirm diagnosis and potentially predict AD is on the horizon [7, 8]. These advances emerged during the same decade when multiple large Phase 3 studies in symptomatic AD have failed, posited in part as due to intervening too late in the disease progression. Each of these above-mentioned factors have pushed the field towards developing interventions to delay or prevent symptoms of AD in individuals with an elevated risk.

21.1.2   The Role of the Registries in the AD Drug-Development Ecosystem (Overview)

In the ecosystem of AD drug development, registries play an important role of identifying large groups of individuals – referred to in this chapter as participants – who may be eligible for clinical trials [9]. Major advantages include scalability, the ability to reach many individuals with few resources, and the ability to connect with individuals who may not otherwise engage in research. Major challenges include generalizability, data integrity, data validity, and study drop-out.

21.2   Registries in AD Drug Development

21.2.1   Medical Registries

A medical registry in its simplest form is a list of individuals that includes health, demographic, or biological information. A common use of registries is to identify participants potentially eligible for research studies. When recruited through population-based methods, a registry is typically much more reflective of the population as a whole and can be used to understand the applicability of a clinical trial to the general population [10].

21.2.2   AD Registries

A registry for AD will typically include measures of cognition, as well as factors that contribute to an elevated risk (e.g., family history of AD or dementia, heart disease, blood pressure, and high cholesterol). When a registry aims to refer participants to clinical trials, common inclusion criteria will also be collected, in particular the availability of a friend or relative that can serve as a study partner. Outside the United States, three key registries are pioneering the endeavor to connect research participants to clinical trials: Step up for Dementia Research in Australia (www.stepupfordementia research.org.au), Join Dementia Research in the UK (www.joindementiaresearch.nihr.ac.uk), and the Dutch Brain Research Registry in the Netherlands (https://hersenonderzoek.nl). In this chapter we provide an overview of the approach and status of the four largest online registries in the United States: the Brain Health Registry (BHR), Alzheimer's Prevention Registry (APR) and Genematch, Healthy Brains, and TrialMatch (Table 21.1).

Each takes a different approach to (1) utilize online assessments to study and characterize their cohorts, (2) engage and inform participants through providing updates on current research, and (3) refer participants into clinical trials. We then describe the Trial-Ready Cohort for Preclinical and Prodromal Alzheimer's Disease (TRC-PAD) program, which leverages online registries to establish a biomarker-confirmed cohort to accelerate clinical trial recruitment. We still have much to learn about the best registry design and methods for recruitment and retention, and ongoing collaboration will be key [11, 12].

21.2.3   The Brain Health Registry

21.2.3.1 Overview

The BHR (brainhealthregistry.org) is an online registry developed to recruit, screen, assess, and longitudinally monitor participants for clinical research [13]. BHR collects longitudinal demographic, cognitive, functional, health, lifestyle, genetic, and plasma biomarker data using online self- and study-partner-report questionnaires, online cognitive tests, and remote biofluids collection. BHR was launched in 2014 and currently has over 80,000 participants. BHR is led by Michael Weiner MD, Scott Mackin PhD, and Rachel Nosheny PhD, with funding from the National Institutes of Health (NIH) and a number of private foundations and individual donors. Published papers describe the overall structure [14], construct

Table 21.1 AD registries in the United States (November 2020)

Registry	Engage and Inform	Remote study	Refer to clinical trials	Enrolled	Target age	Follow-up	Women	Under-represented groups
BrainHealth REGISTRY	✓	✓	✓	>80,000	18+	6 months	73.9%	19%
ALZHEIMER'S **PREVENTION** REGISTRY	✓		✓	352,453	18+	NA	75%	24%
trialmatch alzheimer's association CenterWatch iConnect	✓		✓	370,000	18+	NA	64.91%	26%
Cleveland Clinic **Healthy Brains**	✓	✓	✓	28,255	18+	12 months	69%	22%
apt webstudy Trial-ready cohort for preclinical/prodromal AD (TRC-PAD)	✓	✓	✓	34,696	50+	3 months	73.0%	7.5%

validity of unsupervised cognitive tests [15] and study-partner assessments [16, 17], prediction of brain amyloid levels using BHR data [18], associations between sociodemographic factors and registry behaviors [19], remote collection of blood for apolipoprotein-E (*APOE*) genotyping [19], and the relationship between cognitive measures and various medical conditions [8]. BHR facilitates clinical AD research by: (1) referral of BHR participants to collaborator studies, (2) co-enrollment of collaborator participants into BHR, with data linkage between in-clinic and online data, (3) sharing of de-identified BHR data with qualified investigators, and (4) software-as-a-service, in which collaborators conduct studies using the BHR platform. The BHR Caregiver and Study Partner Portal is a novel, scalable, web-based tool for obtaining study-partner data remotely, currently with data from >7,000 BHR participant–study-partner dyads [16]. This tool is a portal within the BHR that allows current participants to nominate a potential study partner, who is automatically contacted, invited to consent and to answer questions about the participant.

21.2.3.2 Recruitment Strategies and Demographics

BHR participants are recruited from a variety of sources, including owned, paid, earned media and digital advertising. A number of current initiatives are aimed at the recruitment of under-represented populations using community-engaged research techniques and culturally tailored materials. Of these, 27.7% are under the age of 50, 25.5% are in their 50s, and 30.3% are in their 60s (Figure 21.1) [13]. The majority of participants are female (74%), have 16 years of education or more (63%), and identify as White (81%); 5.3% identify as Hispanic/Latinx, 4.5% as Black/African American, 3.2% as Asian, 0.4% as Native American, 3.6% as mixed race, and 7.3% as either another race or declined to report [9, 13]. Forty-nine percent report a subjective memory concern and ~6% report a diagnosed memory disorder.

21.2.3.3 Engagement Strategies and Retention

BHR participants receive emails after enrollment and are emailed reminders to complete tasks and return every 6 months to BHR for longitudinal follow-up. Approximately 48% of participants return to complete at least one follow-up visit. Participant engagement includes: (1) e-newsletters that describe BHR news, results, and brain health education resources, sent every 2–3 months; and

(2) new features, including new questionnaires and/or new neuropsychological tests.

21.2.3.4 Referral to Clinical Trials

Over 86,500 current BHR participants have been referred to other studies, and approximately 4,100 have been enrolled in a total of 25 different aging and AD-related dementia observational studies and treatment trials [14].

21.2.4 The Alzheimer's Prevention Registry

21.2.4.1 Overview

The APR (www.endalznow.org) is an internet-based participant recruitment registry (ClinicalTrials.gov, ID: NCT02022943) for adults ages 18 and older developed by Banner Alzheimer's Institute (BAI) researchers, leaders of the Alzheimer's Prevention Initiative (API) program [20, 21]. The APR was launched in 2012 with the goal of efficiently and effectively raising awareness about AD-focused studies, engaging members, and connecting potentially eligible volunteers to studies. Members initially provide their name, email address, zip/postal code, and year of birth. After enrollment, members can provide additional information (sex, race/ethnicity, family history of AD or other dementia, self-reported cognitive status, and whether they are a caregiver). The APR served as a foundation for GeneMatch, a novel, trial-independent program launched in 2015 to refer cognitively healthy adults (age 50–90) to AD prevention studies based in part on their *APOE* test results (NCT02564692) [22].

21.2.4.2 Recruitment Strategies and Demographics

As of November 2020, 352,453 people had joined the APR, with 91,377 also enrolled in GeneMatch, and 62,928 with *APOE* genotype results. Approximately 80,000 (22%) are considered "actively engaged," meaning they have opened a registry email during the past 6 months. Of these, 9.1% are under the age of 50, 13.7% are in their 50s, and 57.9% are in their 60s and 70s (Figure 21.1), with a mean age of 63.3 years (standard deviation [SD] 11.7). APR members are predominately women (75%) and self-report being cognitively unimpaired (94%); half (50%) report a family history of AD/dementia (12% are unsure, 18% prefer not to answer). Fifteen percent of APR members do not report their race/ethnicity, but of those that do, 76% are non-Hispanic white. The APR and GeneMatch have used community talks, brochures, paid social media advertisements (e.g., Facebook advertisements), and earned media coverage (e.g., newspaper articles) to raise awareness of the programs and enroll participants, targeting adults aged 50 and older where feasible. Paid social media has been the most successful recruitment strategy (leading to 39% of total APR members), followed closely by people visiting the website directly (e.g., learning about the APR in a news article, being referred by a friend, attending a community talk) (32%).

21.2.4.3 Engagement Strategies and Retention

Immediately after enrollment into the APR, members receive a series of emails over 1 week welcoming and orienting them to the APR. This is followed by monthly newsletters, announcements about local events, and study opportunities via email for engagement and retention purposes. The APR developed a four-part re-engagement campaign for members who fall below an established engagement threshold. If a member does not open the re-engagement email, they are removed from the email distribution list. During the past 12 months, the APR monthly newsletter had an average open rate of 39.8% (non-profit healthcare industry average is 16%), and click rate (percentage who clicked on the emailed link in relation to emails opened) of 19.9% (industry average is 1.6%).

21.2.4.4 Referral to Clinical Trials

The APR assists a range of AD-focused studies to meet their recruitment goals, including prevention trials, observational studies, online studies, studies for caregivers, and clinical trials for individuals with cognitive impairment. In 2014, the APR began notifying members when new study opportunities were available. The APR team works directly with the study team to design email campaigns to meet their recruitment objectives. These campaigns have ranged from small, targeted emails to APR members based on information provided at sign-up (e.g., age, zip code) to large, "spread the word" campaigns that encourage APR members to tell friends and family about a study. Initially, these emails provided members with instructions for next steps if interested (often requiring them to contact a study coordinator). Beginning in 2019, study announcements transitioned to allowing members to share their contact information directly and securely to the study via the APR website, with the added benefit of better referral tracking. As of November 2020, APR has 37 active study recruitment campaigns out of a total of 98; GeneMatch has helped 8 studies with their recruitment goals. The "contact form" strategy was launched in late 2019, during a time when many studies were impacted by COVID-19. Despite this, 525 APR members shared their information for a total of 19 studies, 208 participants have been contacted for screening, and 121 have enrolled.

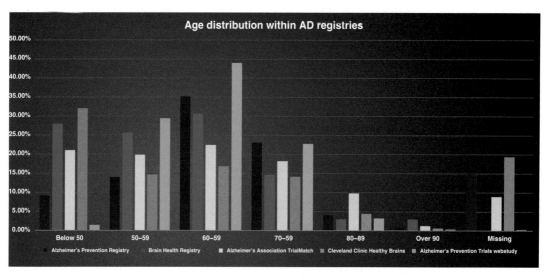

Figure 21.1 Age distribution of US registries for AD (November 2020). This graph illustrates distribution by age for the four largest US registries for AD clinical trials, and the APT Webstudy, the remote webstudy that refers participants into the TRC-PAD. A majority of participants are over 50, with more younger participants engaging with the registries focusing on brain health.

21.2.5 Cleveland Clinic Healthy Brains Registry

21.2.5.1 Overview

The **Cleveland Clinic Healthy Brains Registry (healthybrains.org)** is a longitudinal online registry that includes symptomatic and lifestyle assessments. Healthy Brains aims to (1) reduce the risk of late-life cognitive decline through education about a brain healthy lifestyle, (2) collect preliminary lifestyle and demographic information about participants, and (3) engage potential participants to join a registry aimed at recruiting into clinical trials [23]. Healthy Brains is led by Marwan Sabbagh MD, Jeffrey Cummings MD, ScD, and Aaron Ritter MD, and is coordinated by the Cleveland Clinic Lou Ruvo Center for Brain Health. Funding is provided by Caesar's Foundation.

Healthy Brains is organized around the six pillars of brain health: physical exercise, food and nutrition, medical health, sleep and relaxation, mental fitness, and social interaction. Participants can learn about brain healthy strategies and clinical trials without registering, but can also sign up for email updates, newsletters, and a copy of "Cleveland Clinic's: A Brain Health Guide." Participants are invited to complete the brain health questionnaires, resulting in a brain health index (BHI), a score between 0 and 100. The average assessment time is 15 minutes, with repeat visits requested every 12 months. Cognitive testing includes the cognitive function index (CFI) [24]. Healthy Brains is available in both English and Spanish, and can be accessed either through an internet browser or through the mobile application (iOS application launched in 2015 and Android in 2020).

21.2.5.2 Recruitment Strategies and Demographics

Recruitment strategies for Healthy Brains include efforts based in the community, clinic, and online. The Healthy Brains website began recruiting to their registry in May 2015 through a collaboration with Caesars Entertainment and their employees on a day deemed by Las Vegas Mayor, Carolyn Goodman, as Healthy Brains Day, recognized annually by Caesars Corporation. Recruitment strategies include earned media, clinic recruitment and education programs, community-based health fairs and education events at local senior community centers, YMCAs, retirement communities, and at faith-based sites. In-person engagement includes the use of electronic tablets for data collection and availability of printed education materials both in English and Spanish. Community engagement and education has focused on under-represented populations, both urban and rural groups. The effort to effectively reach these populations includes local brain-health radio shows and paid advertising through the Spanish-language Univision television network plus the formation of a community advisory board, providing gatekeeper support and guidance.

As of mid September 2020, 1.2 million users visited the Healthy Brains website, with 88% new users and 12% returning users. A total of 9,022 users have viewed the Spanish language version of the website. Nearly 21,000 individuals have signed up for newsletter subscriptions and 28,255 registered for a BHI assessment. Of these, 57% completed the BHI, with 30% of those going on to complete the CFI. A majority (69%) of Healthy Brains participants are women, and the mean age of participants is 55. Many participants have more than a high school education (70%), with 78% identifying as White, 8% as Asian, 6% as African American, 1% as Native American/Native Alaskan, 1% as Hawaiian/Pacific Islander, and 6% identify as another race. Nearly 80% indicate a family history of AD or memory loss.

21.2.5.3 Engagement Strategies and Retention

Retention tools include the BHI, a personalized brain health report and interactive dashboard, newsletter engagement, and community education events. The interactive dashboard displays scores for: physical exercise, food and nutrition, medical health, sleep and relaxation, mental fitness, and social interaction plus memory test scores (CFI) and body mass index. Users are able to retake tests and learn brain health tips for each pillar from the dashboard.

21.2.5.4 Referral to Clinical Trials

Referral to clinical trials is a primary aim of the Healthy Brains registry, and 60% of participants express interest in learning more about clinical research opportunities. Participants can opt to be contacted about a clinical trial and receive an email when a study is available near them. Those located in Cleveland, OH, and in Las Vegas, NV, can be pre-screened for studies directly from the clinical trials webpage. As of November 2020, 1,169 Healthy Brains participants have been referred to clinical research studies and 405 have enrolled.

21.2.6 TrialMatch

21.2.6.1 Overview

The Alzheimer's Association TrialMatch™ (trialmatch.alz.org) is a free, online clinical studies matching service that connects individuals living with AD, caregivers, and healthy volunteers with more than 700 active studies in AD and other dementias. Users can access TrialMatch independently in one of three ways; through a web-based widget, over the phone by contacting a dedicated TrialMatch representative, or by mailing their information to the Alzheimer's Association. The information they provide is then used to generate a custom report of clinical trials for which they may be a good fit. Users can elect to be guided through the search process by answering a few simple questions, search through the study database on their own, and register to be notified about future trials. TrialMatch was initiated in 2010 and underwent significant revisions in the summer of 2020 to improve user experience and expand the studies listed. Funding is provided through donations made to the Alzheimer's Association, and is led by Maria Carrillo PhD, Chief Science Officer, Medical and Scientific Relations. As of spring 2020, TrialMatch has more than 370,000 users [25].

21.2.6.2 Recruitment Strategies and Demographics

Demographic information is only collected for the users that create an account through the website (134,148 participants). Just over half indicate they are a healthy volunteer (52.8%), a third of users are caregivers looking for clinical trials for someone else such as a family member with AD (31.7%). Thirteen percent are individuals living with a diagnosis of AD or another dementia. A small percent (2.2%) of users are entered into TrialMatch by a physician or researcher. Individuals under 50 comprise 35% of the healthy volunteers and 20% of all TrialMatch participants (Figure 21.1). Sixty-nine percent are over the age of 50. Participants are 73.4% White, 4.5% Hispanic/Latinx, 3.2% Black/African American, and 65% are women. Twenty-two percent of TrialMatch users either care for someone with a diagnosis of AD or have a diagnosis of AD.

21.2.6.3 Referral to Clinical Trials

Individuals can find clinical trials by independently locating a study and a site, or through longitudinal engagement emails. In terms of independent searches, an average of 550 users search each month, with nearly half choosing to contact a study, by phone or email, directly within the TrialMatch platform. Seventy-five percent of TrialMatch users provide their information and permission to be contacted by TrialMatch, either by phone or by email. TrialMatch users are engaged longitudinally through alerts when new studies matching their profiles become available as well as tailored email campaigns for individual studies. This direct-contact approach has been utilized by TrialMatch for more than 400 studies, with an email open rate of 35%.

21.3 Trial-Ready Cohort for Preclinical and Prodromal Alzheimer's Disease

21.3.1 Overview

The TRC-PAD program shares the aim of accelerating clinical trial enrollment, by recruiting a cohort of 2,000 individuals that have been confirmed to be eligible for clinical trials through biomarker and cognitive phenotyping. The program was born out of the urgent need to accelerate enrollment for clinical trials, particularly those evaluating presymptomatic interventions [26]. The first stage was to develop and recruit to the Alzheimer Prevention Trials (APT) Webstudy (aptwebstudy.org) [25]. Participants are followed with quarterly assessments, and through an algorithm are identified as potentially at high risk, then referred to clinical sites [27, 28]. Referral from APT to the clinical site is tracked through a site referral system, where staff at sites review the list of participants, conduct pre-screening, and refer them for in-person screening. TRC eligibility involves cognitive testing, *APOE* genotyping and, where appropriate, amyloid biomarker testing. TRC participants are followed every 6 months until a clinical trial becomes available, and the participant elects to join. Both for efficiency and to minimize participant burden, the TRC utilizes a US Food and Drug Administration (FDA) CFR part 11 compliant data system and the consent includes permission to share data with a downstream clinical trial. The TRC-PAD program is the result of extensive collaboration between multiple principal investigators, partnering registries, the coordinating center, and the network of clinical trial sites. TRC-PAD is led by Paul Aisen MD, Reisa Sperling MD, and Jeff Cummings MD ScD, and is coordinated by the Alzheimer's

Therapeutic Research Institute at the University of Southern California. TRC-PAD is affiliated with the Alzheimer's Clinical Trials Consortium (ACTC) with scientific guidance provided by the ACTC steering committee, and is funded by a grant from the National Institute on Aging, NIH.

21.3.2 Recruitment Strategies and Demographics

Registries are the primary source of APT Webstudy participants, with 69.69% consenting after being referred by a registry. Other forms of outreach include central media efforts like Facebook advertisements and earned media. In the initial 2 years of the program, APR referred the most participants into the APT Webstudy with 15.9% of the APR participants that were contacted consenting to APT, followed by TrialMatch with 9.8% [25]. Most participants in the APT Webstudy have normal cognition [29], with a majority in their 50s (28.9%) and 60s (44.1%) (Figure 21.1). Most participants identify as women (73.0%), White (92.5%), have more than high-school level education (85.0%), with a family history of AD (62.6%). Of the total APT Webstudy participants, 2.3% self-describe as Hispanic/Latinx. The APT Webstudy has a broad geographic distribution, with participants residing in 60% of US counties.

21.3.3 Engagement Strategies and Retention

A key tool of the APT Webstudy is the ability to track scores on the clinical and cognitive assessments. The participant is encouraged to print out memory scores to share with their primary care provider. This ability to see one's scores over time and the potential to be referred to a clinical trial are both expected to motivate return visits. Other strategies include a quarterly newsletter of AD research updates, emailed to participants, with an average open rate of 50%. Retention is a challenge in the APT Webstudy, with 38.9% returning for a second CFI assessment [29]. Once participants do return for a quarterly assessment, they are more likely to return again, and a loyal band of 792 participants have completed 10 visits. A study to test different retention interventions is under development.

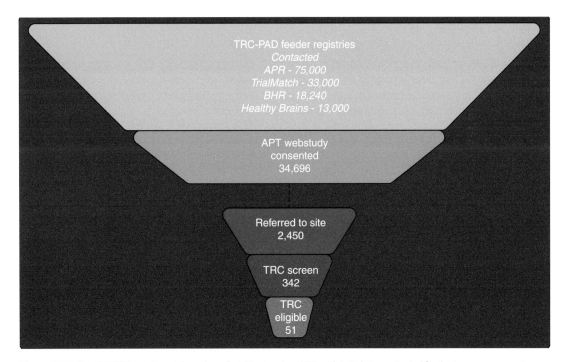

Figure 21.2 The TRC-PAD enrollment funnel, as of mid September 2020, with initial sites activated for the in-person screening assessments. Recruitment is ongoing and will include referrals to clinical trials beginning in late 2020. The rate of referrals from the APT Webstudy to clinical sites is determined by site capacity, significantly impacted by spread of COVID-19 in the United States.

21.3.4 Referral to Clinical Trials

Currently, 50% of the APT Webstudy participants live within 50 miles of a clinical trial site and are eligible to be referred. As of fall 2020, the process of referring and evaluating participants for TRC-PAD is underway, but has been impacted by a pause on in-person research due to the spread of COVID-19 (Figure 21.2). In order to minimize participant burden and streamline screening, TRC-PAD is exploring the potential of blood-based biomarkers (plasma amyloid beta 42/40 ratios and plasma hyperphosphorylated tau 217) to predict amyloid eligibility.

21.4 Lessons Learned from Registries for AD Drug Development

It is clear from this summary that a registry must be large in order to identify enough eligible participants interested in clinical trials. The rapid recruitment to each of these registries illustrates the high level of enthusiasm for information across all ages (Figure 21.2). Furthermore, recruitment to the APT Webstudy demonstrates that registries can be used to recruit a large number of participants remotely (Figure 21.2) [25]. The limited number of research sites reduces the pool of potential participants by 50%. A move to remote and decentralized trials with no in-person component could facilitate a much larger, and more representative, group of participants to be recruited to clinical trials. We will soon learn whether incorporating blood-based biomarkers can reduce the screening burden for participants and reduce costs for researchers. Retention has been a significant challenge, with between 20% and 50% of participants remaining engaged. Further study is needed to evaluate interventions that best retain participants.

Across each of these registries, we can see that women are more readily engaged than men, and a significant proportion (50–80%) have a family history of AD or dementia. The two registries with a focus on brain health have recruited younger participants than those focused on AD or clinical trials. A registry or online study must be compatible with smartphones or risk disproportionate exclusion of under-represented communities, since lower-income Americans, those with less than college education, and Black and Hispanic populations, are more likely to use a cell phone to access the internet [30]. It is critical to study different recruitment and communication strategies in these under-represented groups. Researchers should obtain direct feedback from the individuals in these registries; in particular, participants who sign up for clinical trials. Why did they sign up for the registry, and did the experience meet their expectations or fall short? What are the pain points from their perspective? What information was clearly presented, and what was missing? Ultimately, we must design clinical trials that are accessible to all, where participants reflect the US population; registries are an important tool to achieve this goal.

Acknowledgments

Our thanks to APR, BHR, Healthy Brains, TrialMatch, the APT Webstudy and TRC-PAD participants and their families. Many thanks to Cleveland Clinic Healthy Brains' Katurah Hartley, and to the Alzheimer's Association's Stephen Hall, Carl Hill, Heather Snyder, and Maria Carrillo.

References

1. Alzheimer's Association. 2020 Alzheimer's disease facts and figures. *Alzheimers Dement* 2020; **16**: 391–460.

2. Fargo KN, Carrillo MC, Weiner MW, Potter WZ, Khachaturian Z. The crisis in recruitment for clinical trials in Alzheimer's and dementia: an action plan for solutions. *Alzheimers Dement* 2016; **12**: 1113–15.

3. Grill JD, Karlawish J. Addressing the challenges to successful recruitment and retention in Alzheimer's disease clinical trials. *Alzheimers Res Ther* 2010; **2**: 34.

4. Tang M-X, Cross P, Andrews H, et al. Incidence of AD in African-Americans, Caribbean Hispanics, and Caucasians in northern Manhattan. *Neurology* 2001; **56**: 49–56.

5. Sperling RA, Aisen PS, Beckett LA, et al. Toward defining the preclinical stages of Alzheimer's disease: recommendations from the National Institute on Aging–Alzheimer's Association workgroups on diagnostic guidelines for Alzheimer's disease. *Alzheimers Dement* 2011; **7**: 280–92.

6. Norton S, Matthews FE, Barnes DE, Yaffe K, Brayne C. Potential for primary prevention of Alzheimer's disease: an analysis of population-based data. *Lancet Neurol* 2014; **13**: 788–94.

7. Ovod V, Ramsey KN, Mawuenyega KG, et al. Amyloid beta concentrations and stable isotope labeling kinetics of human plasma specific to central nervous system amyloidosis. *Alzheimers Dement* 2017; **13**: 841–9.

8. Mattsson-Carlgren N, Janelidze S, Palmqvist S, et al. Longitudinal plasma p-tau217 is increased in early stages of Alzheimer's disease. *Brain* 2020; **143**: 3234–41.

9. Aisen P, Touchon J, Andrieu S, et al. Registries and cohorts to accelerate early phase Alzheimer's trials. A report from the E.U./U.S. Clinical Trials in Alzheimer's Disease Task Force. *J Prev Alzheimers Dis* 2016; **3**: 68–4.

10. Kluding PM, Denton J, Jamison TR, et al. Frontiers: integration of a research participant registry with medical clinic registration and electronic health records. *Clin Transl Sci* 2015; **8**: 405–11.

11. Grill JD. Recruiting to preclinical Alzheimer's disease clinical trials through registries. *Alzheimers Dement (N Y)* 2017; **3**: 205–12.

12. Jeon YH, Fargo K, Smith A, et al. Comparison of digital platforms for participant recruitment in dementia research: lessons and future directions from a global collaborative: epidemiology/innovative methods in epidemiology (i.e., assessment methods, design, recruitment strategies, statistical methods, etc.). *Alzheimers Dement* 2020; **16**: e046401.

13. Weiner MW, Nosheny R, Camacho M, et al. The Brain Health Registry: an internet-based platform for recruitment, assessment, and longitudinal monitoring of participants for neuroscience studies. *Alzheimers Dement* 2018; **14**: 1063–76.

14. Mackin RS, Insel PS, Truran D, et al. Unsupervised online neuropsychological test performance for individuals with mild cognitive impairment and dementia: results from the Brain Health Registry. *Alzheimers Dement (Amst)* 2018 **10**: 573–82.

15. Nosheny RL, Camacho MR, Insel PS, et al. Online study partner-reported cognitive decline in the Brain Health Registry. *Alzheimers Dement* 2018; **4**: 565–74.

16. Nosheny RL, Camacho MR, Jin C, et al. Validation of online functional measures in cognitively impaired older adults. *Alzheimers Dement* 2020; **16**: 1426–37.

17. Ashford MT, Neuhaus J, Jin C, et al. Predicting amyloid status using self-report information from an online research and recruitment registry: the Brain Health Registry. *Alzheimers Dement (Amst)* 2020; **12**: e12102.

18. Ashford MT, Eichenbaum J, Williams T, et al. Effects of sex, race, ethnicity, and education on online aging research participation. *Alzheimers Dement (N Y)* 2020; **6**: e12028.

19. Fockler JK, Ashford MT, Flenniken D, et al. Brain Health Registry GenePool study: a novel approach to online genetics research. *Alzheimers Dement (N Y)* 2021; **7**: e12118.

20. Langbaum JB, High N, Nichols J, et al. The Alzheimer's Prevention Registry: a large internet-based participant recruitment registry to accelerate referrals to Alzheimer's-focused studies. *J Prev Alzheimers Dis* 2020; **7**: 242–50.

21. Reiman EM, Langbaum JB, Tariot PN. Alzheimer's Prevention Initiative: a proposal to evaluate presymptomatic treatments as quickly as possible. *Biomark Med* 2010; **4**: 3–14.

22. Langbaum JB, Karlawish J, Roberts JS, et al. GeneMatch: a novel recruitment registry using at-home *APoE* genotyping to enhance referrals to Alzheimer's prevention studies. *Alzheimers Dement* 2019; **15**: 515–24.

23. Zhong K, Cummings J. Healthybrains.org: from registry to randomization. *J Prev Alzheimers Dis* 2016; **3**: 123–6.

24. Amariglio RE, Donohue MC, Marshall GA, et al. Tracking early decline in cognitive function in older individuals at risk for Alzheimer disease dementia. *JAMA Neurol* 2015; **72**: 446.

25. Walter S, Clanton TB, Langford OG, et al. Recruitment into the Alzheimer Prevention Trials (APT) Webstudy for a Trial-Ready Cohort for Preclinical and Prodromal Alzheimer's Disease (TRC–PAD). *J Prev Alzheimers Dis* 2020; **7**: 219–25.

26. Sperling RA, Donohue MC, Raman R, et al. Association of factors with elevated amyloid burden in clinically normal older individuals. *JAMA Neurol* 2020; **77**: 735.

27. Aisen PS, Sperling RA, Cummings J, et al. The Trial-Ready Cohort for Preclinical/Prodromal Alzheimer's Disease (TRC-PAD) project: an overview. *J Prev Alzheimers Dis* 2020; **7**: 208–12.

28. Langford O, Raman R, Sperling RA, et al. Predicting amyloid burden to accelerate recruitment of secondary prevention clinical trials. *J Prev Alzheimers Dis* 2020; **7**: 213–18.

29. Walter S, Langford OG, Clanton TB, et al. The Trial-Ready Cohort for Preclinical and Prodromal Alzheimer's Disease (TRC-PAD): experience from the first 3 years. *J Prev Alzheimers Dis* 2020; **4**: 234–41.

30. Perrin A, Turner E. Smartphones help blacks, Hispanics bridge some – but not all – digital gaps with whites. Available at: www.pewresearch.org/fact-tank/2019/08/20/smartphones-help-blacks-hispanics-bridge-some-but-not-all-digital-gaps-with-whites/ (accessed April 2020).

Chapter 22

Data Safety Monitoring Boards in Alzheimer's Disease Trials

Emily D. Clark and Anton P. Porsteinsson

22.1 Introduction

The data safety monitoring board (DSMB), also known as the data monitoring committee (DMC), is a multidisciplinary team of scientific experts that serve an advisory role within the operation of clinical trials. The principle responsibility of a DSMB is to monitor the conduct of trials for concerns related to participant safety and data quality through the review of interim data analyses, and then to advise trial leadership whether a study is appropriate to continue, needs to modify procedures, or should be terminated. An emphasis is placed on the responsibility of the DSMB to safeguard the rights and well-being of study participants, so it is common to see the incorporation of a DSMB into a study protocol when a trial explores an intervention with high participant risk, a trial is working with a large number of participants, or when a study is working with a particularly vulnerable population, like Alzheimer's disease (AD) patients.

22.2 History of DSMBs

DSMBs have played a role in the regulation of federally funded research since the 1960s, initially starting in the setting of large multi-center clinical trials with the primary objectives of improving survival or reducing the risk of major morbidity. One of the earliest mentions of an external monitoring body is found in the Greenberg Report, an advisory report from the Heart Special Project Committee to the National Heart Advisory Council released in 1967. Amongst the guidelines provided by the Heart Special Project Committee in improving conduct, organization, and operation of large, multi-site clinical trials was the recommendation to include a "policy board or advisory committee" made up of senior scientists who were considered experts in the field of study. This committee's role would be to assist in reviewing the study's overall plan, protocol, and operating procedures, and provide advice

as needed with the goal of improving the quality of data collection while minimizing bias by removing those directly involved in data collection from the interim data interpretation. Advice that could be rendered by this committee included guidance on early trial termination if "accumulated data answer the original question sooner than anticipated; if it is apparent that the study will not or cannot achieve its stated aims; or if scientific advances since initiation render continuation superfluous" [1]. The first trial to incorporate the recommendations from the Greenberg Report and utilize interim data review by an independent advisory committee was the Coronary Drug Project in 1975, which helped to lay the groundwork for DSMBs becoming more commonplace in large, federally funded, multi-institutional trials [2].

Becoming more aware of improvements needed in monitoring of data and safety in clinical research, the National Institutes of Health (NIH) updated the policy on clinical trial conduct in 1979, specifying "every clinical trial should have a provision for data and safety monitoring" [3]. The policy would go on to note "large or multi-center trials, and trials in which the protocol requires blinding of the investigators, should have a data and safety monitoring unit" but did not make any specifications as to whether this unit should be independent from the trial sponsor or not. No formal or direct mandates for the inclusion of an independent DSMB existed within any federal agencies until 1996 when the United States Code of Federal Regulations (CFR) specified that an independent DMC should be established for the protection of the rights and welfare of subjects participating in clinical research in emergency situations in which informed consent cannot be obtained (21 CFR 50.24). The settings in which these guidelines served were mostly limited to emergency settings involving trauma or cardiac arrest but, nonetheless, highlighted the general need for a higher level of protection for vulnerable individuals/populations.

As DSMB use continued to grow, another NIH policy update followed in 1998, announcing a formal requirement for the use of an independent DSMB in all Phase 3 clinical trials involving potential participant risk [4]. The International Conference on Harmonization also addressed a role for DMCs and statistical monitoring issues for DSMBs within their 1998 release of E6 guidelines on good clinical practice and E9 guidelines on statistical principles [5, 6]. The most substantive guidance on the use of formal data and safety monitoring boards came in 2006 from the US Food and Drug Administration (FDA) in their "Guidance for clinical trials sponsors on the establishment and operation of clinical trial data monitoring committees." This guidance was directed at study sponsors of trials utilizing drugs, biologics, and medical devices and addressed matters of DSMB benefits and limitations, organization, and operation of a DSMB, and communications between the DSMBs and study sponsors or sponsor representatives [7].

Since 2006, no formal federal recommendations have been released that focus on the use of DSMBs in clinical research. Several editorials, case reports, and meeting summaries have been published and a few consortia have convened, including the Clinical Trials Transformation Initiative (CTTI) and the Clinical and Translational Science Awards (CTSA) Collaborative DSMB Workgroup, to address best-practice guidelines for DSMBs. Nonetheless, a great deal of variety continues to be seen in the roles and responsibilities of DSMBs especially as randomized controlled trials report an expanded use of DSMBs in comparison to what was seen just 20 years ago [8].

22.3 Roles and Responsibilities of DSMBs

Most agree that the primary responsibility of the DSMB is to protect research participants [9]. A DSMB addresses this responsibility by serving as an independent, multidisciplinary, advisory committee composed of scientific experts who perform regular risk–benefit assessments on interim safety and efficacy data as a study is being conducted. From these risk–benefit assessments, a DSMB will formulate recommendations for a study sponsor or steering committee specifying if a trial can continue, continue but with modification, or needs early termination (either due to overwhelming benefit, safety hazards, or futility). As opposed

to the safety monitoring role served by the institutional review board, the DSMB is in a unique position of having access to blinded data while a study is still being conducted, and observing early trends in adverse effects or efficacy by treatment group, to make their determination. It is critical that confidentiality within the DSMB is maintained because of the risk of introducing bias when this information is shared with individuals funding or conducting the study. As a unified definition of the roles and responsibilities of DSMBs does not exist, different sponsors may seek additional oversight and guidance from the DSMB to enhance trial integrity through review of study protocol adherence and study deviations, monitoring the completeness and quality of data, tracking individual site performance when multiple sites are involved, and observing recruitment population trends [10]. For those serving on a DSMB, clarification on the specific roles and responsibilities you will be expected to serve for a particular study will be outlined by the study sponsor or study steering committee in the DSMB charter – a topic that will be covered later in this chapter.

22.4 When to use a DSMB

All clinical studies require a level of safety monitoring, but not all studies require a DSMB. The decision to incorporate a DSMB into a data monitoring plan is guided to a limited degree by federal agencies but is largely at the discretion of the study sponsor and/or the study steering committee when no formal guidance exists. In these circumstances, the decision is determined by the anticipated risk posed to the study population and the need for additional monitoring. As discussed previously, there are few federal mandates guiding the use of a DSMB, and much variability is present in the use of DSMBs by industry sponsors. This variability and absence of comprehensive federal guidance has resulted in a general lack of consensus as to when a DSMB should be used. The use of a DSMB will often be seen in Phase 3 multi-site clinical trials involving any degree of risk to participants, regardless whether the study is privately or publicly funded. The use of DSMBs in smaller or early trials is more equivocal and is more likely to be determined by factors such as the trial complexity, the number of sites involved, blinded data collection, the degree of intervention risk, and the vulnerability of the study population (children, pregnant women, elderly, or cognitively impaired) [10]. More specific guidance in determining the need for a DSMB has been published by various governing bodies, including the FDA, NIH, the Department of Veterans Affairs (VA), and independent consortia like the CTTI and the CTSA Collaborative DSMB Workgroup and is reviewed below.

22.4.1 Food and Drug Administration

The only FDA mandate on the use of a DSMB in clinical trials is established under 21 CFR 50.24, in which it specifies that trials conducted in emergency settings, where an informed consent cannot be obtained, must have an independent monitoring committee observing data accumulation to protect participant rights. The decision to utilize a DSMB in other settings is at the discretion of the study sponsor. The FDA advises study sponsors to consider the use of a DSMB based on three areas of consideration: What is the risk to the participant? Is a DSMB practical for the study? Will a DSMB assure scientific validity of a trial? [7] Studies comparing mortality or major morbidity, of any size, are encouraged to use a DSMB. The FDA suggests that a DSMB may not be practical in circumstances where the risk is minimal, or the study duration is short. The cost of hiring experts to serve on a DSMB and the added level of administrative complexity must also be considered in the decision to use a DSMB in studies where the need is not as apparent. Lastly, trial leadership may consider the use of a DSMB to help assure scientific validity of the study through minimization of bias, which can occur when changes made to trial design are shaped by the trial organizer's knowledge of unblinded data.

22.4.2 National Institutes of Health

Currently, the only held requirement regarding DSMBs in NIH-funded clinical research is that Phase 3 clinical trials must have an independent DSMB. While Phase 1 and 2 studies are exempt from this mandate, a policy update released in June 2000 announced that Phase 1 and 2 studies still have to submit a general description of some form of a data and safety monitoring plan for approval [11]. This permits a large degree of flexibility for trial sponsors, steering committees, or primary/principal investigators (PIs) to determine the most appropriate level of monitoring for a specific study. Similar to other agencies, the NIH emphasizes that the decision to use a DSMB should be commensurate with the size, complexity, potential risks, and nature of the anticipated trial [11]. They note that in situations where the potential risk is high, or when vulnerable populations are involved, additional monitoring safeguards should be considered, but they do not specify that this requires a DSMB.

22.4.3 Department of Veterans Affairs

The VA Office of Research and Development and the Director of Clinical Science Research and Development (CSRD) released updated DMC guidance in June 2020 [12]. In this document, the VA and the CSRD specify that the decision to incorporate a DSMB into the operations of a study funded by the CSRD will be determined by the Director of the CSRD, with input as deemed necessary by program staff. Factors cited by the VA that would lean more in favor of utilizing a DSMB include: multi-site trials, medication trials, and trials considered to have greater than minimal risk to the study population. The VA has also released its own standardized DSMB charter for use by studies conducted under the CSRD.

22.4.4 Clinical Trials Transformation Initiative

The CTTI, a public–private partnership cofounded by Duke University and the FDA, is among a few agencies that have released their own recommendations on the operation and utilization of DSMBs in clinical research [13]. In 2014, the CTTI conducted online surveys and focus groups consisting of DSMB organizers, DSMB members, and statistical data analysis center (SDAC) representatives (a third-party data analysis center that receives trial data and prepares reports for DSMBs) to assess the current use and conduct of DSMBs. Based on data collected directly from those involved in DSMBs, the CTTI found that no clear consensus existed on criteria for when a DSMB should be utilized [9]. Additionally, respondents in the CTTI focus groups expressed a belief that DSMBs may be over-utilized in some settings where a comprehensive monitoring plan could suffice. Taking these perspectives into account, the CTTI's DMC Project developed a guiding principle that suggests utilizing a DSMB when a need exists in a study to periodically review accumulating, unmasked, safety and efficacy data by treatment group, and to provide guidance to trial sponsors to continue, modify, or terminate a trial on the basis of informed benefit–risk assessments [14].

22.4.5   CTSA Collaborative DSMB Workgroup

The CTSA Collaborative DSMB Workgroup is a committee consisting of faculty and staff from nine CTSA-awarded institutions with a common goal of providing guidance, training, and resources for DSMB practice in investigator-led trials [15]. This workgroup has published a DSMB training manual and released a number of training videos to further the education and development of future DSMB members. Amongst the recommendations for best practice of DSMBs, the CTSA Collaborative DSMB Workgroup has recommended the consideration of a DSMB in trials deemed "high risk." Studies considered "high risk" include those that involve a risk of permanent physical or mental harm, hospitalization, or death. Other trial situations that may be considered high risk include interventions in which the likelihood or severity of adverse effects is unknown, study procedures that involve more than a minimal amount of risk, studies that involve a large number of participants, complex study designs with multiple sites, or studies that involve outcomes that would alter current standard-of-care practices [15]. All Phase 3 clinical trials are considered high risk, as well as blinded Phase 1 and 2 trials. Trials that are considered low or moderate risk are encouraged to consider data and safety monitoring directly by the investigator or through the use of a safety officer, respectively.

22.5   DSMB Composition

The study sponsor and/or the study steering committee is responsible for establishing a DSMB and recruiting DSMB members. An average DSMB is made up of three to seven members and is composed of at least one to two clinicians with expertise in the disease being studied and a biostatistician with expertise in clinical research. Individuals with other areas of expertise may be needed depending on the complexity of the research and study intervention and the degree of risk posed to the study population. These individuals may include professionals such as ethicists, pharmacists, patient advocates, or other clinical sub-specialists. It is generally suggested that all members of the DSMB have some experience with clinical research, but this is not always the case. An odd number of members is favored for voting purposes and a smaller committee is preferred when possible to limit the degree of administrative complexity.

The DSMB chair and the biostatistician are two of the few clearly defined roles in the composition of a DSMB. The DSMB chair is responsible for many aspects of the DSMB operation, including input and approval on committee members, leading meeting deliberations, signing off on official meeting minutes, and serving as the point person for communication with the sponsor. As the main facilitator for the activities of the DSMB, it is highly advised that the chair has experience sitting on previous DSMBs. The DSMB biostatistician is also highly advised to have some previous experience working in clinical trials and with DSMBs, particularly if there is only one biostatistician on the board.

22.6   Conflicts of Interest

It is important that conflicts of interest are discussed prior to selection of committee members and that no member have significant financial, personal, or administrative conflicts of interest. As the pool for finding scientific experts in clinical research and the field of study can be small, it is not uncommon for there to be already established relationships between a DSMB member and a sponsor, or amongst the DSMB members themselves. Finding committee members completely free of conflicts of interest may not be feasible in all situations, but it is encouraged, and when not possible, the conflicts should be known to all parties. It is imperative for DSMB members to carefully review any new relationships with the sponsor or related parties to avoid conflicts of interest or even the appearance thereof. The opportunity to disclose any new or change in conflict of interest usually occurs at the beginning of each DSMB meeting. If a conflict of interest is felt to be serious, a committee member may be asked to resign to avoid the introduction of bias or undue influence.

22.7   DSMB Charter

The DSMB charter is a formal document that articulates the roles, responsibilities, and standard operating procedures for the DSMB. A charter should outline key aspects of the DSMB's operations, such as meeting frequency and format, data reporting to the DSMB, communication between the board and trial sponsor, confidentiality measures, statistical monitoring guidelines, and DSMB membership and conflicts of interest. While a charter will outline key aspects of the operation, it is not expected to outline every action of the DSMB and should be seen as a general guidance for the DSMB, not a legal contract or instruction manual. The charter's first draft is developed by either the study sponsor or the DSMB, depending on whether the sponsor already utilizes a preferred charter template. Before the initiation of the study, both parties should be given the opportunity to review, make amendments to, and formally sign the charter. No universal template exists for DSMB charters but, as mentioned earlier, there are a number of federal and academic institutions that produce their own charter outlines. A standard charter should generally include an introduction, a delineation of DSMB responsibilities, a list of DSMB members and conflicts of interest, a general meeting schedule and format, specifics on communication between the DSMB and the study sponsor, confidentiality measures, statistical monitoring guidelines, and report templates.

It is highly important that the communication pathway between the DSMB and study leadership is explicit in the charter to allow for a timely report of recommendations from the DSMB, particularly in the instance of recommended study termination or modification. It is also important that the charter is not too rigid when it comes to the decision-making process as the decision to terminate, modify, or continue a study should come from a group evaluation and consideration of multiple factors, not purely be based on statistical guidelines. As a study proceeds, DSMB meetings should provide an opportunity for regular review of the DSMB charter with the sponsor or study steering committee and allow for the proposal of amendments as necessary.

22.8 DSMB Meetings

The anticipated schedule and format for DSMB meetings will be outlined in the charter. The average meeting frequency occurs anywhere between every 6–12 months [16]; however, meetings may take place at a higher frequency given the particular degree of participant risk in a study. Some sponsors or DSMBs may choose to schedule meetings around a pre-specified percentage of data gathered instead of calendar dates; for example, the percentage of subjects enrolled or percentage of subjects entering treatment. Overall, the minimum frequency required for a DSMB to meet is usually on an annual basis and this is more often seen in circumstances with longer trial durations and lower

risk profiles. Ad hoc meetings can be requested in circumstances where a DSMB chair or a sponsor wants to gather sooner than the schedule calls, to address any urgent issues that may arise. Some ad hoc meetings may exclude the open session invitation to study sponsors and/or PIs in an effort to preserve data blinding and reduce bias when new issues arise.

The initial meeting of the DSMB takes place prior to patient recruitment and should be conducted in person if possible. This meeting allows for DSMB members to familiarize themselves with one another and with their roles, to review important trial-related documentation, and report any modifications that may need to take place prior to trial initiation. Documents to be reviewed during this time include the DSMB charter, the study protocol, the data collection protocol, and data analysis plans. DSMB members should particularly look to establish clarification on the main safety and efficacy outcome measures, prior knowledge of treatment-related adverse effects, the manner in which adverse effects are being monitored, safety monitoring on drop-out participants, and early termination guidelines that are clear and reasonable for different termination rationale (e.g., overwhelming benefit, safety concerns, or futility) [17]. Once the initial DSMB meeting has concluded and all parties have reached an agreement on the aforementioned topics, a trial can begin enrollment and routine DSMB meetings will commence. As opposed to the initial meeting, at which in-person attendance is usually preferred, routine DSMB meetings are generally held via webinar or teleconference.

All DSMB meetings are composed of open and closed sessions. The open meeting session can include trial sponsors, steering committee members, ad hoc specialists, and other trial representatives in addition to the DSMB members. Closed meeting sessions are limited strictly to the DSMB members, independent biostatistician, and ad hoc specialists if requested to help the committee develop well-informed recommendations. Ad hoc specialists can be invited to either session to provide expert insights to the DSMB as needed. The content covered in open meeting sessions includes an update from the PI or study sponsor on the study and pertinent recent literature, a review of blinded data and generalized safety events, a review of enrollment, discussions from ad hoc specialists invited to the meeting, and an opportunity for

DSMB members to ask the study leadership other pertinent questions to help inform their recommendations. Closed meeting sessions allow for the DSMB and the independent biostatistician to discuss and review blinded data, formulate input or additional questions for the PI or sponsor, and vote on their recommendation to continue, modify, or terminate the study.

The data reviewed during these meetings are usually sent to DSMB members about 7–14 days prior to the meeting to allow for individual review. During DSMB meetings, a member will be tasked with keeping meeting minutes on both open and closed sessions. Following the completion of each DSMB meeting, a formal meeting report and recommendation for the study sponsor or PI will be documented and signed off by the DSMB chair. Even if the recommendations are to continue the trial without modification, it is important that these reports are sent in a timely manner to the trial leadership to avoid unnecessary delays in study procedures.

22.9   Interim Data Analyses

The statistical approach to analyzing interim data will be designated by the sponsor or steering committee and should be documented in the DSMB charter for the committee to review for agreement. A DSMB may request a completely independent, external entity to perform interim data analyses and DSMB reports, such as a SDAC; or a sponsor may assign biostatisticians employed under the sponsor but not directly involved in the study being analyzed to perform these tasks. Routine statistical approaches to analyzing interim data in clinical trials include methodologies such as group-sequential design, stochastic curtailment, or Bayesian methods [18]. We will not delve into recommendations or a breakdown of the advantages or disadvantages of these different statistical approaches; instead, we note these analytical approaches to highlight that a DSMB needs to be mindful of what approach is being used in data analyses, and how this can impact the manner in which data are to be interpreted. A particular concern that should be kept in mind is the potential for inflated type I error when group differences are subject to repeated analyses and what adjustments are being made to account for it in the data plan [19].

The manner in which the reports are presented to the DSMB is determined between the independent biostatistician or SDAC and the DSMB. Prior to receiving the first interim report, the DSMB will have an opportunity to view a template of the data report outline and propose modifications if desired. A typical interim report will contain both aggregate and individual data. Data tables include information such as screened and enrolled patients, time in study, protocol deviations, inclusion/exclusion criteria, abnormal laboratory findings, adverse events by grade, serious adverse events, and participants removed early from the study [8]. Data should be grouped based upon cohorts and labeled in a generic manner (e.g., "group a," "group b") with the opportunity for the DSMB to request unblinding of the groups when necessary. The use of figures and graphs to aid in interpreting data analyses performed by the biostatistician/SDAC is highly encouraged.

22.9.1   Safety and Efficacy Monitoring

Prior to trial start-up, a consensus should exist on monitoring parameters and the criteria for early trial termination on the bases of safety, efficacy, and futility. The criteria should be explained as guidelines for the DSMB and not absolute stopping rules as the determination to terminate a trial should consider a broad picture of the risk–benefit assessment and evolving trial factors.

Safety analyses will focus on interim and cumulative occurrences of adverse and serious adverse events, assessing for significant harm associated with the study treatment (as opposed to incidental events or events related to the disease course). As a DSMB's primary role is to protect participant safety, the parameters for study termination due to safety concern will be less conservative than termination for benefit. A recent example of a DSMB recommending trial termination due to safety in AD clinical research occurred in the Phase 3 trial of the gamma-secretase inhibitor semagacestat [20]. The double-blinded, randomized, placebo-controlled trial for semagacestat in patients with mild-to-moderate AD was intended to assess two different doses of semagacestat over a 21-month period. Early interim analyses were performed as a response to emerging differences in the treatment groups as observed by the DSMB in predetermined p-value cut-off for between-group differences. Interim analyses revealed a dose-related clinical worsening in multiple primary and secondary outcome measures and an increase in adverse effects in both treatment arms vs. placebo. Early trial termination was recommended by the DSMB and the study was halted at week 79 [20].

22.9.2 Monitoring for Efficacy

Interim analyses for efficacy or futility will consist of a variation of the end-of-study efficacy analyses to identify early trends that may support early termination. Trial termination for overwhelming benefit is not common but can be seen in fields where there is an urgent need for intervention or few pre-existing treatment options are available. An example of this was seen recently in the HARMONY trial, a Phase 3, double-blinded, randomized, placebo-controlled study of pimavanserin in dementia-related psychosis. The HARMONY trial was terminated early due to overwhelming benefit when pre-planned interim analyses by the DSMB revealed pimavanserin had met its primary endpoint by significantly reducing the time to relapse of psychosis by 2.8-fold compared to placebo [21]. While terminating early for benefit is considered a positive development in a study's trajectory, a DSMB must consider the criticisms a study may face and the quality of the data at the point of termination. Even after communicating the recommendation to terminate early for benefit, considerable discussions should be had between the DSMB and the sponsor/steering committee to discuss whether the shortened trial will lead to acceptance of the results in the scientific community and/or practicing clinicians [22, 23].

22.9.3 Monitoring for Futility

Interim analyses for futility are a particularly important task of the DSMB, especially in long-term studies where standards of care for a particular disease may change during the course of a trial. When data reveal no significant difference between the intervention and control groups, the DSMB has an important decision to make about the operation of a trial. Maintaining participants in a study that is showing signs of futility can lead to indirect harm by preventing them from enrolling in other trials with a potential for benefit, especially in environments where standards of care have changed. Alternatively, terminating a trial due to futility without a well-informed data review and consideration of influencing factors may result in hindering further scientific development or discovery with a particular intervention, as it will be harder to justify the development of additional studies. A recent example of DSMB interim futility analyses leading to early trial termination

was seen in the ENGAGE and EMERGE trials sponsored by Biogen and Eisai. ENGAGE and EMERGE were both Phase 3, double-blinded, randomized, placebo-controlled trials investigating the efficacy of aducanumab in participants with either mild cognitive impairment due to AD or mild AD. When interim futility analyses were examined by the DSMB, it was found that neither trial was anticipated to meet primary endpoints and trial termination was advised. Halting these trials also resulted in Biogen terminating the Phase 2 EVOLVE trial and dropping plans for the long-term extension of the PRIME study (both studies involving aducanumab) [24]. Months later, Biogen announced that futility analyses were inaccurate and additional analyses on the complete trial data revealed that the EMERGE trial had, in fact, met primary endpoints of reducing decline on the Clinical Dementia Rating – sum of boxes scale. Despite the positive findings in the EMERGE trial, damage was done as Biogen found limited support from the FDA advisory committee in November 2020 to bring the drug to market due to the sustained findings of futility in the ENGAGE trial [25]. On June 7, 2021, the FDA moved to approve aducanumab under the accelerated approval program, using the reduction of amyloid beta as a surrogate endpoint. While this allows for the initial market release of aducanumab, Biogen is still required to perform a post-approval trial confirming clinical efficacy in order to maintain aducanumab's approval status. While this is a ground-breaking development in the field of AD treatment options, the initial DSMB findings of futility in the ENGAGE and EMERGE trials, and the absence of a completed Phase 3 trial, has left an indelible mark on the name of aducanumab and hesitancy in the minds of providers faced with the decision to prescribe aducanumab or not [26].

Ultimately, the decision to recommend trial termination for safety, efficacy, or futility is a complicated matter and must be balanced with the anticipated outcome this decision will have on future research development. Regardless of the nature of the decision, it is preferred that all DSMB recommendations are made by consensus vote (and preferably that this is unanimous). If a committee is facing a particularly difficult decision, or having difficulty reaching a consensus, access to additional data should be made available to the committee to help guide a well-informed decision.

22.10 DSMB Reporting of Recommendations

Once recommendations have been agreed upon, a DSMB will draft a formal report to the study sponsor or steering committee reporting their advice. Communications are preferred to be in writing, and a documentation of recommendations can be as brief as a few sentences if the recommendation is to continue a study without modification. This report will be much more extensive if modification or termination is being recommended. In the event that study modification or termination is recommended, communicating these recommendations must be done in a timely manner and through the communication pathways outlined in the charter. As an advisory board, and not an executive one, a DSMB is only responsible for communicating their recommendations, and it is up to the sponsor or steering committee to make a determination. It is not often the case that a study sponsor or steering committee disagrees with DSMB recommendations. In fact, 97% of respondents in the CTTI's survey of DSMB members in 2014 indicated that their recommendations were accepted by study sponsors always or most of the time [9]. If there is a disagreement, the charter should outline what the next steps should be in this situation, such as a third-party assessment.

22.11 Training DSMB Members

A topic discussed in multiple publications is the lack of formal DSMB training opportunities. As it currently stands, there is no system of training or certification accepted globally by regulatory, academic, and industry sponsors, and many currently serving DSMB members have never received formal training themselves [9]. Proposed ideas to address this problem include a formal training curriculum, which would include didactic learning, case-review discussions, and mentorship. A central database of DSMB members has also been proposed to expand the pool of applicants that a sponsor or steering committee has from which to choose. Some institutions and independent authors have developed didactics and case-review series for DSMB education, but we found little in our search for current mentoring programs.

22.12 DSMBs in AD Research

As illustrated earlier in this chapter, DSMBs have already had an active role in monitoring and regulating AD research. The use of DSMBs in Phase 3 clinical trials in AD have followed the common practice of other Phase 3 clinical trials. The need for DSMBs in Phase 1 and 2 AD trials is less clear, however, and worth consideration given the vulnerable state of our study population. Shorter, lower-risk AD trials examining preclinical, prodromal, and even mild AD populations may not require monitoring as meticulous as a DSMB, as these patients will have the cognitive capacity to provide consent and are not likely to see much progression of disease in studies spanning weeks to a few months. Trials lasting several months or years, or trials including moderate-to-severe AD populations, should strongly consider the use of a DSMB due to an increased level of vulnerability in these particular circumstances. While the addition of a study partner/legally authorized representative is generally included in these studies to protect a patient's interests and safety, this does not account for all risk. A particular concern is in the loss of capacity to provide informed consent as the disease progresses, something that can take place within a longer study timeframe. Thus, in research that targets participants with or at risk of cognitive impairment, a comprehensive data and safety monitoring plan is an imperative part of the study design and execution.

References

1. Heart Special Project Committee. Organization, review, and administration of cooperative studies (Greenberg Report): a report from the Heart Special Project Committee to the National Advisory Heart Council, May 1967. *Control Clin Trials* 1988; **9**: 137–48.

2. DeMets DL, Ellenberg SS. Data monitoring committees expect the unexpected. *N Engl J Med* 2016; **375**: 1365–71.

3. National Institutes of Health. NIH guide for grants and contracts. 1979. Available at: https://grants.nih.gov/grants/guide/historical/1979_06_05_Vol_08_No_08.pdf (accessed November 14, 2020).

4. National Institutes of Health. NIH policy for data and safety monitoring. 1998. Available at: https://grants.nih.gov/grants/guide/notice-files/not98-084.html (accessed November 14, 2020).

5. International Conference on Harmonisation of Technical Requirements for Pharmaceuticals for Human Use. Integrated addendum to ICH E6(R1): guideline for good clinical practice. 2016. Available at: https://ichgcp.net/ (accessed November 14, 2020).

6. International Conference on Harmonisation of Technical Requirements for Pharmaceuticals

for Human Use. Statistical principles for clinical trials. 1998. Available at: https://database.ich.org/sites/default/files/E9_Guideline.pdf (accessed November 14, 2020).

7. Food and Drug Administration. Guidance for clinical trial sponsors: establishment and operation of clinical trial data monitoring committees. March 2006. Available at: www.fda.gov/regulatory-information/search-fda-guidance-documents/establishment-and-operation-clinical-trial-data-monitoring-committees (accessed November 18, 2020).

8. Gewandter JS, Kitt RA, Hunsinger MR, et al. Reporting of data monitoring boards in publications of randomized clinical trials is often deficient: ACTTION systematic review. *J Clin Epidemiol* 2017; **83**: 101–7.

9. Calis KA, Archdeacon P, Bain RP, et al. Understanding the functions and operations of data monitoring committees: survey and focus group findings. *Clin Trials* 2017; **14**: 59–66.

10. Sartor O, Halabi S. Independent data monitoring committees: an update and overview. *Urol Oncol* 2015; **33**: 143–8.

11. National Institutes of Health (NIH). Further guidance on data and safety monitoring for Phase I and Phase II trials. 2000. Available at: https://grants.nih.gov/grants/guide/notice-files/not-od-00-038.html (accessed November 18, 2020).

12. US Department of Veterans Affairs. Clinical Science Research & Development (CSRD), data monitoring committee guidance. 2015. Available at: www.research.va.gov/services/csrd/data-monitoring.cfm (accessed December 3, 2020).

13. Calis KA, Archdeacon P, Bain R, et al. Recommendations for data monitoring committees from the Clinical Trials Transformation Initiative. *Clin Trials* 2017; **14**: 342–8.

14. DMC Project. CTTI recommendations: data monitoring committees. 2016. Available at: www.ctti-clinicaltrials.org/files/recommendations/dmc-recommendations.pdf (accessed November 18, 2020).

15. CTSA Collaborative DSMB Workgroup. DSMB training manual. 2018. Available at: https://tuftsctsi.wpengine.com/research-services/regulatory/data-and-safety-monitoring-board-training-manual-for-investigator-initiated-studies (accessed December 3, 2020).

16. Grant AM, Altman DG, Babiker AG, et al. A proposed charter for clinical trial data monitoring committees: helping them to do their job well. *Lancet* 2005; **365**: 711–22.

17. Neaton JD, Grund B, Wentworth D. How to construct an optimal interim report: what the data monitoring committee does and doesn't need to know. *Clin Trials* 2018; **15**: 359–65.

18. Ellenberg SS, Fleming TR, DeMets DL. *Data Monitoring Committees in Clinical Trials: A Practical Perspective*. Newark, NJ: John Wiley & Sons Inc.; 2019.

19. Kim K. Sequential designs for clinical trials. In *Designs for Clinical Trials: Perspectives on Current Issues*, Harrington D (ed.). New York, NY: Springer; 2012: 57–80.

20. Doody RS, Raman R, Farlow M, et al. A Phase 3 trial of semagacestat for treatment of Alzheimer's disease. *N Engl J Med* 2013; **369**: 341–50.

21. Yunusa I, El Helou ML, Alsahali S. Pimavanserin: a novel antipsychotic with potentials to address an unmet need of older adults with dementia-related psychosis. *Front Pharmacol* 2020; **11**: 1–5.

22. Wilhelmsen L. Role of the data and safety monitoring committee (DSMC). *Stat Med* 2002; **21**: 2823–9.

23. Acadia Pharmaceuticals. ACADIA pharmaceuticals presents positive top-line results from pivotal Phase 3 harmony trial of pimavanserin in patients with dementia-related psychosis. 12th Clinical Trials on Alzheimer's Disease (CTAD) Meeting, December 4-7, 2019. Available at: https://ir.acadia-pharm.com/news-releases/news-release-details/acadia-pharmaceuticals-presents-positive-top-line-results?field_nir_news_date_value (accessed December 3, 2020).

24. Alzforum.org. Biogen/Eisai halt Phase 3 aducanumab trials. Available at: www.alzforum.org/news/research-news/biogeneisai-halt-phase-3-aducanumab-trials (accessed December 10, 2020).

25. Alzforum.org. Aducanumab still needs to prove itself, researchers say. Available at: www.alzforum.org/news/research-news/aducanumab-still-needs-prove-itself-researchers-say (accessed December 10, 2020).

26. Karlawish J. If the FDA approved Biogen's Alzheimer's treatment, I won't prescribe it. Available at: www.statnews.com/2021/05/30/if-the-fda-approves-biogens-alzheimers-treatment-i-wont-prescribe-it/ (accessed July 8, 2021).

Chapter 23

Globalization of Alzheimer's Disease Clinical Trials

Huali Wang, Tao Wang, Shifu Xiao, and Xin Yu

23.1 Introduction

Alzheimer's disease (AD) has become a significant challenge in the medical and social care system as a progressing neurodegenerative condition in aging societies. The enormous burden due to caring for people with AD impacts our society both financially and emotionally [1]. Investment in early treatment and intervention will slow down the progression and save costs eventually [2]. Therefore, advancing drug discovery to delay the onset, slow the progression, and improve the symptoms of AD is urgently needed.

Around two-thirds of people with dementia live in low- and middle-income countries, with a tremendous burden on Asia, Africa, and Latin America [3]. As the disease is a worldwide epidemic, there is a substantial need to conduct clinical trials in the developing world. Globalization is a process whereby countries, companies, and relevant stakeholders integrate and interact globally by sharing information and resources. It is only through globalization that people with dementia will get access to novel therapeutics in a coordinated and efficient manner [4].

23.2 Drivers of Globalization in Drug Development

The number of clinical trials on AD has been proliferating [5]. The growth of the world's AD population, particularly soaring in low- and middle-income countries, is driving the increasing trend toward globalization of clinical trials [6]. Globalization may aid the process of drug development as it takes advantage of cost-saving and speeding up patient recruitment [7].

23.2.1 Growth of the World's Population of AD

With the growth of the aging population worldwide, the number of people with dementia is predicted to rise rapidly in the next decade. AD accounts for 60–70% of all-cause dementia. According to Alzheimer's Disease International, over 50 million people were living with dementia in 2020 [8]. Sixty percent of people with dementia live in low- and middle-income countries, but by 2050 this will rise to 71%. A recent survey in China estimated that about 9.83 million people aged 60 years or older had AD, and 38.77 million had mild cognitive impairment (MCI) [9]. Furthermore, because of extended lifespans and the improved diagnostic criteria accuracy, the age-specific prevalence of AD is predicted to increase dramatically [10].

23.2.2 Need for Larger Samples in Trials

Non-publication was common for large randomized clinical trials registered with ClinicalTrials.gov, with unsatisfactory enrollment status possibly partially contributing to results not being published [11]. The recruitment and retention of patients, particularly in the asymptomatic and early stage, account for the failure in trials for AD drugs [12]. Collaboration between industry and the academic and clinical fields in conducting trials in the United States and the European countries might accelerate drug innovations from the research pipeline to patients [13]. However, low- and middle-income countries may make additional contributions to global trials. First, recruitment of participants from diverse background could be increased. For example, in China, the memory clinic in a single site receives more than 200 patients with dementia per month. The case registry in the memory clinic constitutes a large patient pool [14, 15]. Second, a large portion of treatment-naïve patients in low- and middle-income countries may be helpful in assessing the actual efficacy of a drug rather than an additive effect on top of previous medications. Therefore, randomized AD clinical trials are increasingly recruiting patients globally in order to provide reliable, conclusive overall findings on treatment efficacy and safety.

23.2.3 Ethnography and Ethnobiology

Patients from international sites differ ethnically and in biological (e.g., genetics) and social aspects from the United States and European countries. The genetic differences may influence AD pathophysiology and progression or response to treatment. For instance, apolipoprotein-E ε4 (ApoE-4) may mediate AD risk through several pathways: (1) impacting amyloid pathology, (2) modulating tau pathology and tau-related neurodegeneration, (3) modulating immune and microglial response, (4) directly affecting neurons and neuronal networks, and (5) modulating blood–brain barrier integrity [16]. The frequency of the *APOE-4* allele is higher in Caucasians than that in Chinese [17]. Thus, the potential ApoE-4-dependent drug response may influence the findings of a clinical trial in different countries.

The sociocultural context and healthcare system in different countries may also influence the interpretation of cognitive and neuropsychiatric symptoms and functional levels. For example, apathy, one of the strongest predictors of conversion from MCI to AD dementia, varies across different ethnic populations [18]. Testing new therapies in diverse cultures provides insight into the variation in drug response from the ethnographic perspective. Global recruitment provides the opportunity to explore potential ethnobiological variations in treatment effect, and it may enhance the generalizability of a trial's findings to a diverse population of patients.

23.3 Difference between Global Sites

23.3.1 Differences in the Trial Operations

Site-related factors have a significant effect on the quality of data generated in a trial. With more sites involved, global trials will have more variability than the trials conducted in a single country or region.

The variation in making a diagnosis of AD or MCI is one of the primary reasons for such differences between sites. Petersen et al. examined the variability in performance in randomized controlled trials for MCI. They found that the implementation of criteria varied a great deal across the study sites despite similar criteria being adopted by the studies [19]. The same MCI criteria were used in all seven trials for amnestic MCI participants, but most studies included participants with multidomain amnestic MCI, and the degree of impairment of non-memory domains varied. There may also have been differences between academic and commercial sites. Health workers with less specialized training assessed and diagnosed dementia based on history and physical examination alone, which might lead to more screening failure for clinical trials. A central review of diagnostic approaches may help reduce the variability associated with differences between sites.

People with dementia get access to diagnosis and care through different pathways across sites. For example, in the United States, volunteers register to participate in clinical trials through the Alzheimer's Disease Research Center funded by the National Institute on Aging (NIA). Such a long-term funding mechanism increases the accessibility of support for those in high-risk or early AD stages. In contrast, seeking a medical diagnosis of AD was delayed for an average of 2 years in China [20]. People with asymptomatic or very early-stage AD are not likely to visit memory clinics promptly. Community outreach and supporting community-based memory clinics offer one means to promote subject recruitment and screening [15]. However, the equipment in the community is not sufficient for confirming the diagnosis. Liaison between specialists and community doctors is indispensable for the successful implementation of an AD trial protocol.

Familiarity in administering cognitive assessment varies across international sites. The instruments commonly used in global trials, e.g., the Clinical Dementia Rating (CDR) scale, Alzheimer's Disease Assessment Scale – cognitive subscale (ADAS-cog), the Neuropsychiatric Inventory (NPI), and the Alzheimer's Disease Cooperative Study Activities of Daily Living scale (ADCS ADL), are not routinely used in European and Asian centers [21, 22]. However, the CDR, NPI, and ADCS ADL are included in the assessment package in Alzheimer's Disease Research Center in the United States. The use of a centralized assessment workstation increases the inter-rater reliability and reduces the variability. Rater surveillance and an endpoint reliability enrichment program might ensure quality data collection.

Besides this, investigators in different countries may interpret the criteria defining patient outcomes, such as reported adverse events, differently.

For instance, hospitalization (due to the deterioration of a disease) as a severe adverse event could have different thresholds for its occurrence, depending on the healthcare system and local practice in different countries.

23.3.2   Differences in the Trial Participants

International recruitment provides the opportunity to explore potential geographic variations in treatment effect. There may be several types of geographic variations [23–25]: patient selection, medical practice, and outcomes evaluation. Data pooled from three 24-week, randomized, double-blinded, placebo-controlled studies in mild-to-moderate AD found that there was regional heterogeneity, in terms of study conduct, patient characteristics, and outcomes [26].

Ethnic (e.g., genetic, as noted above) or environmental differences that result in varying disease incidence and severity could influence how a treatment affects disease progression in different regions. It could also affect the risk–benefit ratio. The difference in healthcare systems and other practicalities of how patients present, and how clinical teams select whom to include in a trial may generate real between-country differences in patient characteristics. Patient management, such as ancillary patient care, and including other drug and interventional treatments, may be markedly different across countries. For instance, herbal medicine is commonly prescribed in Asian countries, but it remains unclear whether the concomitant use of such medicines benefits people with AD.

Subjects in international trials differ by sociodemographic statuses, such as age, gender, and educational level [27]. Brain and cognitive-reserve levels, interacting with modifiable risks of dementia, may have a meaningful impact on the clinical outcomes in AD trials [28, 29]. Subjects with a higher cognitive reserve may have a better cognitive performance at the asymptomatic stage but have rapid progression due to the severely compromised brain network than patients with lower reserve.

In a pooled analysis of four similarly designed randomized controlled trials with mild or moderate AD, Henley et al. found that disease severity measured by CDR and ADAS-cog was numerically worse for Eastern Europe/Russia than other regions, including Japan, Asia, and South America/Mexico [30].

Ethnic factors may affect pharmacokinetic and pharmacodynamic profiles in global trials. For instance, ethnic differences in the distribution of polymorphism affecting the cytochrome P450 enzyme system may affect drug metabolism levels. The variation in this regard should be noted in the interpretation of the response to the investigational drug.

As noted above, an accurate diagnosis of AD remains a significant challenge for clinical settings in most countries. A standardized diagnostic work-up flow substantially improves the clinical diagnostic accuracy. In several ongoing AD clinical trials, the use of biomarker-supportive AD diagnosis ensures that the trial participants have the underlying neuropathology relevant to the investigational product's mechanism of action [31, 32]. Such a strategy is essential, especially for trials that aim to modify the disease progression from the asymptomatic stage.

23.4   Global Regulatory Agencies

Regulatory policies differ across countries and are not completely harmonized. With the evolution of the scientific understanding of AD, sponsors of global trials started to incorporate biomarkers in the protocol, particularly for the trials targeting the earlier stages of the disease and individuals without detectable functional impairment.

23.4.1   FDA Guidance

The US Food and Drug Administration (FDA) considered that these efforts are critical because of the opportunity to intervene very early in the disease process, given the development of characteristic pathophysiological changes that greatly precede clinically evident findings and the slowly progressive AD course. According to AD pathophysiology, the FDA issued guidance to assist sponsors in the clinical development of drugs to treat the early stages of sporadic AD.

23.4.2   EMA Guidance

In the European Medicines Agency (EMA) guidance, from a regulatory perspective, both the International Working Group and the NIA–Alzheimer's Association sets of criteria are accepted for diagnosis of AD for research purposes and trial enrichment. The EMA acknowledges that it is challenging to prove a disease-modifying effect without validated biomarkers. A slower or delayed clinical decline demonstrated by innovative trial designs may be acceptable as an alternative development goal.

23.4.3   Chinese NMPA: Actions and Policies

In the "Technical guidelines for clinical trials of drugs for the treatment of Alzheimer's disease (draft 2007)" of the Chinese National Medical Products Agency (NMPA), there are three primary purposes of drug intervention for AD: improving symptoms, controlling disease progression, and primary prevention. The NMPA considers that significant differences exist in the response and prognosis between mild and moderate patients and severe patients. The neuropsychological tests and clinical evaluation scales used to judge the curative effect are also different. Therefore, when preparing for clinical trials, a drug must have a defined target: for example, to improve symptoms or control disease progression or prevention; to use for mild-to-moderate patients, or for severe patients. Accordingly, the study protocol should be designed to meet the requirement of the NMPA guidance.

In terms of the clinical trials for preventing and controlling disease progression, meeting the general requirements for clinical trials of symptomatic therapeutic drugs is mandatory. Due to the trial's different objectives, special issues should be considered, such as the target population, the duration of treatment, and endpoint measures. In addition to cognitive tests, neuroimaging examination should be deployed as the therapeutic index. For example, regular evaluation of brain structure or functional imaging can provide direct evidence for brain tissue-structure and functional changes. Still in the exploratory stage is judging the curative effect by examining biological markers in cerebrospinal fluid or blood.

23.5   Global Innovation

23.5.1   New Therapies

Cholinesterase inhibitors and N-methyl-D-aspartate receptor antagonists are the main approaches of AD treatment targeting the clinical features of AD. In the last two decades, many new drugs focusing on AD's pathogenesis have been tested or are being tested, such as amyloid-beta monoclonal antibodies, gamma-secretase inhibitors, and compounds inhibiting the formation of neurofibrillary tangles or tau-related antibodies.

There are also some potential candidates such as plant-derived medicines that might have a different mechanism of action.

Sodium oligomannate (GV-971) is a marine-derived oligosaccharide. It is a mixture of linear, acidic oligosaccharides with a degree of polymerization ranging from dimers to decamers. GV-971 might reconstitute the dysbiosis of gut microbiota, reduce metabolite-driven peripheral infiltration of immune cells into the brain, and inhibit neuroinflammation [33]. A recently completed 36-week multi-center, randomized, double-blinded, and placebo parallel-controlled Phase 3 clinical trial observed a significant statistical difference in the change of the primary endpoint measured by the total score ADAS-cog12 between the 900-mg group and the placebo control group [34]. The pivotal trial supported the NMPA to issue conditional approval for GV-971 as a novel AD drug.

23.5.2   New Trial Technologies

A concern in the globalization of trials is the reliability and quality of data collection. Stimulated by the advance of information technology, electronic data capture systems, including e-tool assessment workstations, have been commonly used in global clinical trials.

During the unprecedented times of COVID-19, research participants were unable to keep their appointments within protocol-specified windows [35]. It stimulated the development of remote assessment of cognitive performance and patient-reported outcome measurement. As the resource for biomarker testing is limited, it remains a challenge to recruit new subjects during this socially distanced period.

23.6   How Globalization Contributes to the AD Drug-Development Ecosystem

The results of these drugs' clinical trials have made us more aware of the complexity of the pathogenesis of AD. Although the amyloid and tau protein hypotheses are the mainstream to explain the onset of AD, it is possibly only the tip of the iceberg in the whole pathogenesis of AD. With an increased number of emerging new therapies, globalization will play a more critical role, with reciprocal benefits among participating sites, academia, and industry. For example, introducing new biomarkers or diagnostic criteria to developing countries may facilitate more timely diagnosis for the local population. Regular monitoring of site performance may increase dialogue with experts and improve the competence of the local clinician. Testing in the lesser-developed countries may expedite the marketing process once the regulatory agencies approve the new therapies.

23.7 Lessons Learned for AD Drug Development from a Globalization Perspective

As noted above, ensuring the quality of data collection remains a priority in global trials. To improve the quality of international multi-center clinical trials, we would like to make the following recommendations:

(1) **improved site performance** by adequate training of clinicians and site personnel involved in trials, enriched training of outcome measuring and rater surveillance, increasing use of biomarkers, and performing regular monitoring;

(2) **enhanced infrastructure development** by adopting an e-tool platform and creating an educational platform for the investigators and clinicians;

(3) **reinforced information sharing among investigators** by encouraging best practice of subject recruitment and retention, reaching consensus on culturally insensitive cognitive tests, and facilitating communication between investigators; and

(4) **promotion of a universal regulatory mechanism** by encouraging harmonization of international drug-development guidelines from regulatory agencies, ensuring a standard institutional review board review process, and encouraging uniform protection procedures.

There is a tidal increase in the globalization of AD clinical trials. Developing a constructive mechanism will minimize the geographic variation and help develop novel therapies for people with AD.

References

1. Wimo A. The worldwide costs of dementia 2015 and comparisons with 2010. *Alzheimers Dement* 2017; **13**: 1–7.

2. Gustavsson A, Green C, Jones RW, et al. Current issues and future research priorities for health economic modelling across the full continuum of Alzheimer's disease. *Alzheimers Dement* 2017; **13**: 312–21.

3. Prince M, Ali G, Guerchet M, et al. Recent global trends in the prevalence and incidence of dementia, and survival with dementia. *Alzheimers Res Ther* 2016; **8**: 23.

4. Thiers FA, Sinskey AJ, Berndt ER. Trends in the globalization of clinical trials. *Nat Rev Drug Discov* 2008; **7**: 13–14.

5. Cummings J, Lee G, Ritter A, Sabbagh M, Zhong K. Alzheimer's disease drug-development pipeline: 2020. *Alzheimers Dement (N Y)* 2020; **6**: e12050.

6. Nichols E, Szoeke CEI, Vollset SE, et al. Global, regional, and national burden of Alzheimer's disease and other dementias, 1990–2016: a systematic analysis for the Global Burden of Disease Study 2016. *Lancet Neurol* 2019; **18**: 88–106.

7. Qiao Y, Alexander GC, Moore TJ. Globalization of clinical trials: variation in estimated regional costs of pivotal trials, 2015–2016. *Clin Trials* 2019; **16**: 329–33.

8. Alzheimer's Disease International. Dementia statistics. Available at: www.alzint.org/about/dementia-facts-figures/dementia-statistics/ (accessed June 29, 2021).

9. Jia L, Du Y, Chu L, et al. Prevalence, risk factors, and management of dementia and mild cognitive impairment in adults aged 60 years or older in China: a cross-sectional study. *Lancet Public Health* 2020; **5**: e661–71.

10. Jia L, Quan M, Fu Y, et al. Dementia in China: epidemiology, clinical management, and research advances. *Lancet Neurol* 2019; **4422**: 1–12.

11. Jones CW, Handler L, Crowell KE, et al. Non-publication of large randomized clinical trials: cross sectional analysis. *BMJ* 2013; **347**: 1–9.

12. Gauthier S, Albert M, Fox N, et al. Why has therapy development for dementia failed in the last two decades? *Alzheimers Dement* 2016; **12**: 60–4.

13. Goldman DP, Fillit H, Neumann P. Accelerating Alzheimer's disease drug innovations from the research pipeline to patients. *Alzheimers Dement* 2018; **14**: 833–6.

14. Jia J, Zuo X, Jia XF, et al. Diagnosis and treatment of dementia in neurology outpatient departments of general hospitals in China. *Alzheimers Dement* 2016; **12**: 446–53.

15. Wang H, Xie H, Qu Q, et al. The continuum of care for dementia: needs, resources and practice in China. *J Glob Health* 2019; **9**: 020321.

16. Long JM, Holtzman DM. Alzheimer disease: an update on pathobiology and treatment strategies. *Cell* 2019; **179**: 312–39.

17. Wang X, Wang H, Li H, Li T, Yu X. Frequency of the apolipoprotein E ε4 allele in a memory clinic cohort in Beijing: a naturalistic descriptive study. *PLoS One* 2014; **9**: e99130.

18. Zhang M, Wang H, Li T, Yu X. Prevalence of neuropsychiatric symptoms across the declining memory continuum: an observational study in a memory clinic setting. *Dement Geriatr Cogn Dis Extra* 2012; **2**: 200–8.

19. Petersen RC, Thomas RG, Aisen PS, et al. Randomized controlled trials in mild cognitive impairment: sources of variability. *Neurology* 2017; **88**: 1751–8.

20. Zhao M, Lv X, Tuerxun M, et al. Delayed help seeking behavior in dementia care: preliminary findings from the Clinical Pathway for Alzheimer's Disease in China (CPAD) study. *Int Psychogeriatr* 2016; **28**: 211–19.

21. Paulino Ramirez Diaz S, Gil Gregório P, Manuel Ribera Casado J, et al. The need for a consensus in the use of assessment tools for Alzheimer's disease: the Feasibility Study (assessment tools for dementia in Alzheimer centres across Europe), a European Alzheimer's Disease Consortium's (EADC) survey. *Int J Geriatr Psychiatry* 2005; **20**: 744–8.

22. Shen JHQ, Shen Q, Yu H, et al. Validation of an Alzheimer's disease assessment battery in Asian participants with mild to moderate Alzheimer's disease. *Am J Neurodegener Dis* 2014; **3**: 158–69.

23. Pocock S, Calvo G, Marrugat J, et al. International differences in treatment effect: do they really exist and why? *Eur Heart J* 2013; **34**: 1846–52.

24. Mentz RJ, Kaski J-C, Dan G-A, et al. Implications of geographical variation on clinical outcomes of cardiovascular trials. *Am Heart J* 2012; **164**: 303–12.

25. Kristensen SL, Martinez F, Jhund PS, et al. Geographic variations in the PARADIGM-HF heart failure trial. *Eur Heart J* 2016; **37**: 3167–74.

26. Cummings JL, Atri A, Ballard C, et al. Insights into globalization: comparison of patient characteristics and disease progression among geographic regions in a multinational Alzheimer's disease clinical program. *Alzheimers Res Ther* 2018; **10**: 116.

27. Cummings J, Reynders R, Zhong K. Globalization of Alzheimer's disease clinical trials. *Alzheimers Res Ther* 2011; **3**: 24.

28. Wang H. Nexus between cognitive reserve and modifiable risk factors of dementia. *Int Psychogeriatr* 2020; **32**: 559–62.

29. Wang J, Gu Y, Dong W, et al. Lower small-worldness of intrinsic brain networks facilitates the cognitive protection of intellectual engagement in elderly people without dementia: a near-infrared spectroscopy study. *Am J Geriatr Psychiatry* 2020; **28**: 722–31.

30. Henley DB, Dowsett SA, Chen YF, et al. Alzheimer's disease progression by geographical region in a clinical trial setting. *Alzheimers Res Ther* 2015; **7**: 43.

31. Jack CR, Bennett DA, Blennow K, et al. NIA–AA Research Framework: toward a biological definition of Alzheimer's disease. *Alzheimers Dement* 2018; **14**: 535–62.

32. Hampel H, Vergallo A, Flores Aguilar L, et al. Precision pharmacology for Alzheimer's disease for the Alzheimer Precision Medicine Initiative (APMI). *Pharmacol Res* 2018; **130**: 331–65.

33. Wang X, Sun G, Feng T, et al. Sodium oligomannate therapeutically remodels gut microbiota and suppresses gut bacterial amino acids shaped neuroinflammation to inhibit Alzheimer's disease progression. *Cell Res* 2019; **29**: 787–803.

34. Xiao S, Chan P, Wang T, et al. A 36-week multicenter, randomized, double-blind, placebo-controlled, parallel-group, Phase 3 clinical trial of sodium oligomannate for mild-to-moderate Alzheimer's dementia. *Alzheimers Res Ther* 2021; **13**: 62.

35. Editorial. Alzheimer's disease research enterprise in the era of COVID-19/SARS-CoV-2. *Alzheimers Dement* 2020; **16**: 587–8.

Chapter 24

The Use and Development of Clinical Measures of Alzheimer's Disease Trials

John Harrison

24.1 Importance of Cognitive and Functional Measures in AD Clinical Drug Trials

Many disorders of the central nervous system (CNS) can cause a decline in cognitive function. The type and magnitude of the observed deficits is understood to be a function of the physiological systems that subserve specific cognitive skills. In the case of Alzheimer's disease (AD) there is good evidence to show that amongst the structures most susceptible to early pathological damage are those subserving an individual's ability to encode and recall new information. These episodic memory deficits are often the presenting sign for individuals who have developed AD. It is perhaps therefore unsurprising that the traditional measures of cognitive function used in AD are heavily weighted toward memory assessment. This is particularly true of instruments commonly employed in clinical drug trials of putative new therapies such as the Alzheimer's Disease Assessment Scale – cognitive subscale (ADAS-cog) and the Mini Mental State Examination (MMSE) [1, 2]. In these two scales more than half of the possible score tally is derived from measures of episodic memory, with the remaining subtests providing indices of language and praxis function. However, AD research in the past decade has repeatedly highlighted that cognitive functions either not well or not at all indexed by the ADAS-cog and MMSE can also be impaired early in the disease process. There is now good evidence of early impairments of attention, executive function, and working memory, deficits often manifested in individuals living with AD, as well as deficits of concentration, problem-solving, and navigation. This variable presentation of early AD is well understood by specialist centers, expert groups, and third-party stakeholders, such as advocacy groups and drug-approval regulators.

The cognitive assessment of individuals with AD has a role in a number of therapeutic and research contexts. AD is a prima facie disorder of cognition, and a key role of assessment has been in the detection and identification of individuals who exhibit deficits consistent with the presentation of AD. However, it is important to note that cognitive tests are not diagnostic of AD. Other pathological processes, such as Lewy body dementias, stroke, and traumatic brain injury, can also cause cognitive deficits if neurophysiological structures that subserve episodic memory, attention, etc. are damaged. Nevertheless, as a cheap, safe, and non-invasive method of screening at-risk individuals, cognitive assessment has a useful role to play.

An extension of the screening role is the use of cognitive measures in helping to understand the presentation and evolution of cognitive change in at-risk cohorts. In this context, researchers employ cognitive testing primarily as a means of characterizing the endophenotype of AD. However, these endeavors are as much concerned with monitoring changes in cognition as the identification of deficits.

24.2 A Critical Review of Current Clinical Trial Measures

The MMSE, originally designed as a bedside measure of general cognition, is comprised of brief tests of memory, attention, praxis, and language. It has been commonly employed as an inclusion measure and as a means of stratifying clinical trial cohorts. The earliest trials of AD therapies were designed to assess treatment effects in patients labeled as having "mild-to-moderate" disease severity, typically a range of 14–26 on the MMSE. The MMSE is ranged from 0 to 30, with higher scores indicating superior performance. An informal scheme has evolved by which patients with scores in the 0–13 range are classified as "severe," 14–20 as "moderate," and 21–26 as "mild."

The ADAS-cog has for the past 20 years near-universally been employed as the primary cognitive efficacy measure in AD trials [3, 4]. Like the MMSE, it is also comprised of memory, language, and praxis subtests. A major limitation of the ADAS-cog is the omission of working memory, attention, and executive function tests, a deficiency highlighted by Mohs et al. [5]. These domains are known to be compromised early in the disease process and have repeatedly been specified for evaluation by expert groups [6, 7].

In an attempt to remedy these deficiencies, Mohs et al. recommended the inclusion of the Maze and Number Cancellation subtests, as well as a Delayed Recall component of the Word Recall subtest [5]. These additional measures are referred to as ADAS-cog+ tests and have on occasion been augmented by the Concentration/Distractibility element of the ADAS-noncog. These additional measures have been variously added to the original 11 ADAS-cog subtests to create new configurations, the most common of which is the ADAS-cog13. The components and standard running order of the ADAS-cog13 are shown in Table 24.1 (for a review of ADAS-cog variants see Podhorna et al., 2016 [8]).

24.2.1   ADAS-cog Content

Memory assessment accounts for 45 out of 70 of the available points in the original 11-item ADAS-cog. Word Recall and Word Recognition, tests of episodic verbal memory, account for 22 possible points. Remembering Test Instructions relates to the need for reminders whilst completing Word Recognition, though was originally for reminders needed across the whole scale. A significant element of the Commands subtest is the ability to recall the instructions. The Orientation subtest requires the patient to recall elements of orientation to time, place, and self. The worst possible score for the orientation test is 8, with 7 points for episodic memory items (What is the date?, day?, month?, etc.) and just one related to semantic memory ("What is your name?"). Semantic memory is also assessed in the context of the Object and Finger Naming and Word-Finding Difficulty subtests. The addition of Delayed Word Recall adds a further 10 points of episodic memory

measurement. When employed, this test is typically inserted after the Object and Finger Naming and Commands subtests, which yields a delay of approximately 5 minutes between the immediate and delayed recall tasks.

Language skills are assessed subjectively, largely through an opening conversation with the patient, but also during the administration of other ADAS-cog subtests. On the basis of these interactions, the patient is rated on a 0–5 scale for their spoken language ability and language comprehension skills. Word Finding Difficulty is classed as a language measure, though is perhaps better considered as a measure of semantic memory. A 0–5 severity rating is also a feature of the Concentration/Distractibility subtest.

24.2.2   Criticisms of the ADAS-cog

A substantial literature exists with regard to the challenges, quirks, and inadequacies of the ADAS-cog in its different versions. A key challenge with the Word Recall subtest is when the word list is unchanged across study visits. Best practice requires that equivalent parallel word lists be used when word recall tasks are repeated. However, crucially, the different versions of the test must be demonstrably equivalent. Recent data suggest that the standard variants employed in AD drug trials may not have this attribute. Data from Expedition 1, 2, and 3 have clearly illustrated the problem. Word list 4 typically yields higher scores than the others employed [9]. Also, the frequent use of the ADAS-cog in mild, and even prodromal patients, can lead to learning effects, and it is evident that the invariant content of several subtests can lead to artificially sustained levels of performance [10].

A further issue with the continued use of the ADAS-cog is the insensitivity of many subtests across the full range of disease severity. Performance on the ADAS-cog subtests of praxis, language, and those of semantic memory, attention, and executive function, is at ceiling in more than three-quarters of mild-stage patients [11]. This gives the false impression that these cognitive skills are unimpaired in prodromal and even mild-stage patients. Working memory is not indexed by the ADAS-cog in any of its variants [12]. When cognitive domains are measured by items that are at ceiling for most study

Table 24.1 Cognitive coverage of tests commonly employed in AD clinical trials

Domain/skill	ADAS-cog subtest	NTB	RBANS	Digital test examples
Episodic verbal memory	Immediate Word Recall	RAVLT	List learning	ISLT
Episodic verbal memory	Delayed Word Recall (+)	Visual Paired Associates	Story memory	Paired associative learning
Episodic verbal memory	Word Recognition	Verbal Paired Associates	List recognition	Word recognition
Episodic memory	Remembering Test Instruction	–	Figure recall	Picture recognition
Episodic memory	Orientation	–	–	–
Semantic memory	Orientation	–	–	–
Semantic memory	Word-Finding Difficulty	–	–	–
Confrontation naming	Naming Fingers and Objects	–	Picture naming	–
Comprehension/praxis	Commands	–	–	–
Constructional praxis	Constructional Praxis	–	Figure copy	–
Ideational praxis	Ideational Praxis	–	–	–
Language production	Spoken Language Ability	–	–	–
Language comprehension	Language Comprehension	–	–	–
Attention	Number Cancellation (+)	Digit span forwards	Digit span/ coding	Identification/detection/rapid visual information/simple reaction time/choice reaction time
Executive function	Maze (+)	COWAT and CFT	Semantic fluency	GMLT/spatial working memory/ SOC
Working memory	–	Digit span backwards	Semantic fluency	Numeric working memory
Spatial working memory	–	–	–	Spatial working memory
Visuospatial function	–	–	Figure copy	Spatial working memory

Abbreviations: CFT, Category Fluency Test; COWAT, Controlled Oral Word Association Test (aka "phonological fluency"); GMLT, Groton Maze Learning Test; ISLT, International Shopping List Test; NTB, Neuropsychological Test Battery; RBANS, Repeatable Battery for the Assessment of Neuropsychological Status; RAVLT, Rey Auditory Verbal Learning Test; SOC, Stockings of Cambridge; + denotes a later addition to the ADAS-cog.

participants, there is a risk that changes seen on these scales may reflect more noise than true signal. In mild disease, using eight items from the ADAS-cog has been shown to be more sensitive to AD progression over time than the full 1-item ADAS-cog score [13].

As well as issues with content and administration, ADAS-cog scoring conventions have also received criticism. For example, performance on the three administrations of the 10-item Word Recall subtest is averaged across the three trials to yield a score of 0–10, where 10 represents the worst possible performance. This requirement reduces the dynamic range of the test from 0–30 to 0–10. As the Word Recognition subtest has near universally

been reduced to a single trial, averaging performance is not a requirement for scoring this subtest. With respect to the Remembering Test Instructions subtest, in spite of the potential for 22 reminders per Word Recognition trial, the ADAS-cog scoring scheme specifies a worst possible scaled score of 5, which occurs when seven reminders have been given. The reduction of raw score values to scaled scores is also a characteristic of the Object and Finger Naming test. In this subtest, the patient's ability to name the five fingers and twelve objects has the potential to yield a score with a 0–17 range. However, the ADAS-cog scoring scheme requires that this be compressed to a 0–5 range, again resulting in further loss of information.

24.3 Neuropsychological Test Battery

The development of the first anti-amyloid active immunotherapy, AN1792, provided an opportunity to augment the use of the ADAS-cog with a cognitive assessment focused not just on episodic memory, but also on working memory and executive function. The author, while employed at CeNeS Pharmaceuticals, had discussed with the study sponsors the possibility of employing digital tests of episodic memory, working memory, and attention from the Cambridge Neuropsychological Test Automated Battery (CANTAB) system. It was proposed that the CANTAB Choice Reaction Time, Paired Associative Learning, and Spatial Working Memory tasks be augmented with paper-and-pencil measures of executive function to include tests of both semantic and phonological fluency. For logistical reasons, it did not prove possible to employ this test combination. Instead, well-known "paper-and-pencil" measures of episodic memory and executive function were employed. The emergence of serious adverse events led to the trial being halted. However, by this time, a significant cohort had been dosed with AN1792, and these individuals and those in the placebo arm continued to be assessed using the Neuropsychological Test Battery (NTB). These data indicated a positive treatment effect on AN1792, with preservation of cognition as a function of antibody titer levels [14]. No positive treatment effects were observed on the ADAS-cog.

Since the use of the NTB in the AN1792 trial, a number of studies have employed the original "classic" version of the assessment. Additionally, a number of assessments with a strong "family resemblance" to the original have been employed with varying degrees of success with respect to the detection of treatment efficacy. Notable successes have been the FINGER study and more recently the proof-of-concept (POC) study of neflamapimod [15]. Test combinations titled "cognitive composites," with task content similar to variants of the NTB, have also been a recent feature of the AD literature, as well as in other indications, such as Parkinson's disease and major depressive disorder.

Use of the NTB in studies of AN1792 helped to open the door to the use of measures other than the ADAS-cog. However, due to the length of the assessment and the inclusion of lengthy and cumbersome measures drawn from clinical psychology

insensitive to disease progression, we would not advocate use of the classic NTB. Evidence suggests that the Controlled Oral Word Association Test (COWAT), Category Fluency Test (CFT), and Rey Auditory Verbal Learning Test (RAVLT) Immediate Recall elements are usefully sensitive to disease progression and exhibit assay sensitivity [16].

24.4 Stage Specificity of Measures: Test Selection and Disease Severity

Earlier in this chapter the issue of range restrictions was discussed in the context of both the floor and ceiling effects frequently observed on ADAS-cog subtests. It has been noted that the "sweet spot" with regard to the MMSE score for detecting impairments on the ADAS-cog is a score of around 15 and that individuals living with AD in the severest stage appear to have significant difficulties comprehending the instructions for ADAS-cog subtests and other cognitive measures. Conventionally we have marked the transition between moderate- and severe-stage performance at MMSE scores of less than 14 and clinical trials of individuals in this severe-impairment category have typically employed the Severe Impairment Battery to assess cognition.

It is evident from the foregoing and earlier discussion of these issues that there is a precedent within AD clinical trials for selecting severity-appropriate measures. Nevertheless, until very recently, the inclination of most sponsors has been to specify the inclusion of "mild-to-moderate" patients, equivalent to an MMSE range of 14–26, for clinical trials of putative symptomatic-relieving compounds. This runs the risk of yielding floor effects on the ADAS-cog Word Recall and Word Recognition tests in the moderate-stage patients and ceiling effects on a large proportion of the Praxis and Language subtests. As outlined previously, this is regrettable for a number of reasons.

While less prone to floor effects on memory measures, the use of the ADAS-cog in mild and prodromal individuals yields a high proportion of ceiling performance in a number of individuals, often in excess of 70% of a study cohort, and in the case of the Mazes subtest, greater than 90% [11]. The lack of parallel forms of these tests compounds the issue of ceiling effects, as any progressive decline can be masked by improvement due to practice and task familiarity. We would therefore strongly recommend the use of the assessments free of these restrictions.

24.5   Regulatory Perspectives

Further stakeholders in the approval process are regulators, such as the US Food and Drug Administration (FDA) and the European Medicines Agency (EMA). Both agencies have opined on the selection of cognitive outcome measures for use in dementia drug trials. The most recent EMA guidance offers the following advice to organizations seeking marketing approval [17]:

> Applicants may need to use several instruments to assess efficacy of putative drugs for treatment of dementing conditions because there is no ideal measurement instrument at the present time. Whilst a large number of methods for evaluation of cognitive and functional changes have been suggested, none has convincingly emerged as the reference technique, satisfying the above set of requirements. Hence the choice of assessment tools should remain open, provided that the rationale for their use is presented and justified.

The inclination of study sponsors has been to employ the instruments critically reviewed earlier in this chapter, such as the ADAS-cog. It is notable that the guidance does not specify use of the ADAS-cog, though the authors pointedly note that:

> Currently used cognitive scales have demonstrated a ceiling effect which makes them not sensitive enough to detect small changes in cognition and complex neuropsychological batteries may be difficult to implement in large clinical trials.

The guidance does not specify which cognitive domains the agency requires assessment of, but word recall, word recognition, and executive functions are listed as being "sensitive to detect disease progression in earlier stages of AD (e.g. world [sic] recall, world [sic] recognition, executive functions)." Reference is also made to "complex attention, executive function, learning and memory, language, perceptual motor, or social cognition" in the guidance references.

In 2018, the FDA produced a new guidance document [18]. Earlier guidance from the FDA and its representatives has specifically listed specific cognitive measures for use. For example, in 1991, Leber referenced use of the ADAS-cog

[19]. Later FDA guidance included references to both the ADAS-cog and NTB as scales, as well as other popularly used scales including the Clinical Dementia Rating – sum of boxes (CDR-sb) scale [20]. The 2018 FDA guidance represents a marked departure from this position. The agency has instead placed an emphasis on "sensitive neuropsychological measures," which are repeatedly called for throughout the guidance. The guidance establishes a taxonomy of severity based on a system of staging:

- Stage 1 patients are in part defined as having no "detectable abnormalities on sensitive neuropsychological measures."
- Stage 2 patients are defined as those who exhibit "detectable abnormalities on sensitive neuropsychological measures" but in whom "there is no evidence of functional impairment."
- Stage 3 patients are in part defined as exhibiting "subtle or more apparent detectable abnormalities on sensitive neuropsychological measures, and mild but detectable functional impairment."

The authors of the 2018 guidance suggest in the context of Stage 2 patients that the "FDA will consider strongly justified arguments that a persuasive effect on sensitive measures of neuropsychological performance may provide adequate support for a marketing approval." So, what would the FDA find sufficiently persuasive to grant marketing approval for Stage 2 patient treatment? This is not specified, though the guidance authors suggest that this requires "a pattern of putatively beneficial effects demonstrated across multiple individual tests" and that: "a large magnitude of effect on sensitive measures of neuropsychological performance may also increase their persuasiveness." The guidance authors do not provide an indication of how substantive a treatment would have to be. Some speculation on this topic is engaged later in this chapter in the context of our recent comments regarding the use of effect size as a common vocabulary for discussing treatment impact [21].

A further key theme of the guidance is the implied dichotomous relationship between cognition and function, about which the guidance authors state: "FDA rejects this dichotomy and finds such usage inappropriate, because it implies that an effect on cognition itself, regardless of the nature of the observed effect and the manner in

285

which it is assessed, cannot be clinically meaningful. This is certainly not the case." I concur with this view. For me, it is axiomatic that cognition is the substrate of function and that the rescue and/or preservation of function is necessarily accompanied by rescue and/or preservation of cognition. I hold to the view that the relatively modest correlations between traditionally employed measures of cognition and function are a further legacy of the poor cognitive-domain coverage. Support for this view is that elsewhere in the psychological literature robust correlations between cognition and function are observed. For example, performance on the Trail Making Test is a useful proxy measure of various driving behaviors [22]. This is in contrast to the poor correlations typically observed between the ADAS-cog and activities of daily living (ADL) scales (typically correlations of less than 0.4) [23]. Modest levels of correlation are also observed between ADAS-cog scores and performance on clinical global impression of change scales such as the Alzheimer's Disease Cooperative Study (ADCS)–Clinical Global Impression of Change (CGIC). The same explanations of incomplete coverage likely account for this lack of correlation, but here this might extend to coverage of the cognitive domain absent from the ADAS-cog. CGIC scales are free from restrictions with regard to content focus. Consequently, it is expected that CGIC raters will index attention, working memory, problem solving, various aspects of executive function, and spatial skills, none of which are indexed by the ADAS-cog. Small wonder, therefore, at the lack of correlation with CGIC scales.

24.6 A Regulatory Path? Validating New Test Combinations

Recent evidence from successful POC studies has supported the notion that brief assessments that exhibit good reliability, and which index the key cognitive domains at risk in early AD, represent our best chance of capturing efficacy. A further characteristic of these reliable and valid measures is their sensitivity. Latency measures such as reaction-time tests yield scores reckoned in thousandths of a second. Similarly, the dynamic range of number of correct measures such as the COWAT when used in patients with mild-to-moderate AD typically yields a substantially variable range (around 50 words). The use of these POC tools also

provides validation of that most critical test characteristic, assay sensitivity, a topic to which we will return shortly.

So, what is the FDA's stance on the selection of cognitive measures for use in clinical trials? As stated, the most recent guidance described above placed a heavy emphasis on the use of sensitive neuropsychological measures. While agency representatives have been reluctant to specify particular tests, they have previously publicly stated that measures other than the ADAS-cog are acceptable. For example, Dr. Russell Katz, in a 2008 presentation, stated in reply to the question "Besides the ADAS-cog, to what extent are alternative measures now accepted as are primary cognitive endpoints?": "The NTB has been accepted. Alternative measures have always been accepted, though rarely used. Formal validation is increasingly becoming more common" [24]. This was a clear and unequivocal statement of the agency's position, which, to the best of the author's understanding has remained unchanged. The "rarely used" observation is just as true now as it was in 2018. Less clear is what might constitute validation in the eyes of the agency. Here, Dr. Katz's statement confirming the acceptability of the NTB offers clarification on the issue of validation. In the year prior to the 2008 roundtable at which Dr. Katz spoke, Harrison et al. published a validation of the NTB that had been successfully employed in the clinical trial of AN1792 [25]. In this study the authors calculated and reported rudimentary psychometrics of the NTB (see Section 24.3). In spite of the limitations of the published study, the NTB was included in agency guidance in advance of formal publication of the manuscript.

24.7 Establishing a Method: POC, Exploratory, and Confirmatory Trials

So, with earlier comments in mind, how best might we embark on the process of nurturing a new molecule into and through clinical development? Decision making must be driven by available evidence. Mechanism of action and preclinical cognitive data are two principles that can be employed to inform cognitive test selection [26]. In Phase 1 trials there is value in showing that the compound is cognitively safe. To do so requires the incorporation of a broad assessment that maps the basic cognitive domains listed in Table 24.1. These same tests have the capacity to show positive effects of treatment. As an example, nicotinic compounds have a rich history of capturing pro-cognitive effects in typical controls. Similarly, it seems likely that compounds which induce long-term potentiation may well exhibit pro-mnemonic effects comparable to the behavioral induction of this same phenomenon [27]. Data from these studies can inform test selection for POC in studies of the target indication. Preclinical evidence and typical volunteer results can suggest a specific cognitive test or domain as a clear efficacy target for a Phase 2a study. An alternative approach is to conduct an exploratory study with a cognitive assessment that maps all the key domains.

A major challenge for POC studies has been how best to interpret study data. Some compounds appear to have general non-specific positive effects on cognition. This was our experience in studies of vortioxetine conducted in people living with major depressive disorder [28, 29]. However, it might be that cognitive effects are specific to one or more cognitive domain, or even that the cognitive profile is of benefit to one or more cognitive domain but deficits in others. Analyzing a single cognitive composite can be a fruitful approach in circumstances such as those seen in the aforementioned vortioxetine studies, but less helpful in the other scenarios described (interested readers are directed to a recent discussion of the pros and cons of composite score use [30, 31]). A further major challenge when interpreting Phase 2a data is the risk of reporting type I errors. This is an issue when multiple tests are used and reported individually, with the probability of making type I errors a function of the number of tests and outcome measures employed. In response to this challenge, we recommend analyzing and reporting cognitive data by domain. Such an approach avoids the issue of oversimplification, whilst mitigating the risk of false-positive findings. This process involves grouping test outcome measures according to primary domain and then combining scores from tests of this domain. Test scores often have different scalar properties and correcting for this is an important step in ensuring that no one test dominates the domain score. Our preferred methodology for achieving this has been to calculate each study participant's score as a change from baseline z-score using mean and standard deviation data for the selected measures (see Harrison and Hendrix for a more detailed discussion of these issues [32]). A

further opportunity exists to support test groupings through the use of statistical techniques such as factor analysis.

Results from POC studies of the kind described in the last section provide a principled means of selecting a primary cognitive outcome measure for confirmatory Phase 2b and 3 studies. This follows the premise of being guided by empirical findings. However, such an approach is very much at odds with the typical approach of selecting traditional measures such as the ADAS-cog and leaves the issue of seeking evidence of functional benefit unresolved. One approach to this is to propose the use of a composite of functional and cognitive measures similar to the Alzheimer's Disease Composite Score methodology and, more recently, development of the Cognitive Functional Composite [33–35]. In the case of the latter the authors employed episodic memory ADAS-cog elements combined with the NTB and other cognitive measures of attention, working memory, and executive function. To this was added performance on the Amsterdam Instrumental Activities of Daily Living scale to yield a cognitive and functional composite score.

How best to proceed with the selection of cognitive outcome measures? The selection of measures with robust psychometric characteristics has been the clear recommendation of expert groups dating back to at least 1997 [36]. Cognitive domain coverage has also been the focus of consideration of expert groups, which have consistently advocated the assessment of episodic memory, working memory, and executive function. I would endorse this view and, like Ritchie et al., would mandate the inclusion of attentional tests [7]. However, the fundamental principle for test selection must be the use of measures capable of successfully testing hypotheses developed from (i) preclinical findings, (ii) a compound's mode of action, and (iii) the results of exploratory studies. This approach has been rarely employed beyond the general hypothesis that the new chemical entity will preserve and/or rescue cognition. Due to its inadequate cognitive-domain coverage the ADAS-cog is not fit for purpose as a primary measure of this hypothesis. It seems unlikely that the extraordinary failure rate of putative AD drugs is entirely due to poor outcome-measure selection. However, the consistent failure to measure executive function, attention, and working memory in clinical trials

287

means that we simply cannot know whether failed compounds may have had undetected, positive effects on these domains. There is good evidence to suggest that the assessment of these domains of function are impacted by pharmacological interventions, as discussed in the following section.

In spite of the lack of late-stage AD trial success, a number of exploratory studies have yielded positive cognitive results. These results are summarized in Table 24.2.

An interesting characteristic of a number of the studies reported in Table 24.2 is the tendency of authors to express treatment versus placebo differences in effect size. Grove et al. for example focus on the positive treatment impact of 0.35 at week 16 on episodic memory. This tendency is also a characteristic of the Nathan et al. study in which treatment-effect sizes are reported by dose level and by test, together with 95% confidence intervals for each effect-size value. I find this to be a very useful method of reporting observed effects and would strongly encourage the use of this reporting methodology as the basis of a common vocabulary for comparing treatment effects across different tests and different studies. To return briefly to the earlier theme of what can be regarded as evidence of treatment efficacy, currently marketed drugs for AD tend to yield positive cognitive effect sizes of about 0.3 [43]. However, we are mindful of the fact that in the eyes of many this represents a very modest treatment benefit. Furthermore, it is more than 15 years since

marketing approval was given for a new symptom-relieving AD drug and regulators may now require a more robust effect to grant marketing approval. In a recent commentary on the 2018 FDA guidance, I speculated that a stand-alone cognitive effect of a symptomatic-relieving treatment might require positive effect sizes of at least 0.3 across a number of domains, with a 0.5 positive effect on a key domain, such as episodic or working memory [21]. A full discussion of the utility of effect size is beyond the scope of this chapter, but interested readers are directed to a detailed consideration of this issue [44].

Evident also from Table 24.2 is that tests of executive function, working memory, and attention have yielded evidence of positive treatment effects in a number of studies. As we acknowledged earlier, these cognitive domains have only rarely been assessed. This is to be regretted, as evidence suggests that executive function can be improved by already marketed drugs. Rockwood et al. inquired of healthcare practitioners their experience of anticholinergic therapy in patients with AD. Those responding stated that the most conspicuous change was on the patients' ability to organize their thoughts, synonymous with executive skills, which, as the authors comment, have not been systematically assessed in clinical drug trials [45]. A final comment on Table 24.2 is that the tests listed appear to be capable of detecting treatment effects or "assay sensitivity." We have discussed elsewhere the importance of this test characteristic [46].

Table 24.2 Putative AD treatments POC studies showing assay sensitivity of non-ADAS-cog measures

Study	Year	Compound	Measure(s)	Domain
Gilman et al. [14]	2005	AN1792	NTB	Episodic memory; executive function
Lannfelt et al. [37]	2008	PBT2	NTB	Executive function
Hilt et al. [38]	2009	EVP-6124	COWAT	Executive function
Scheltens et al. [39]	2012	Souvenaid	RAVLT and verbal paired associates	Episodic memory
Nathan et al. [40]	2013	GSK239512	Detection	Attention
Nathan et al. [40]	2013	GSK239512	Identification	Attention
Nathan et al. [40]	2013	GSK239512	One-Back Task	Working memory
Nathan et al. [40]	2013	GSK239512	ISLT Immediate Recall	Episodic memory
Grove et al. [41]	2014	GSK239512	ISLT and CPAL	Episodic memory
Scheltens et al. [42]	2018	PQ912	Identification	Attention
Scheltens et al. [42]	2018	PQ912	One-Card Learning	Working memory

Abbreviations: CPAL; Continuous Paired Associate Learning. For other abbreviations, see Table 24.1.

Final Comments – Personal Perspectives from 20 Years of Consulting

Over the past 25 years I have worked on a good number of CNS clinical drug trials, the vast majority of which have been studies of putative AD treatments. In this time, I have worked with some of the most able, educated, and driven individuals I have ever encountered. At an individual and group level these people have been driven by sound scientific principles and clinical evidence. However, an early lesson for me was that cognitive test selection for clinical drug trials is driven by overly conservative interpretations of regulatory guidance, inaccurate perceptions of third-party stakeholder perceptions, and, not unusually, an odd blend of folklore and superstition.

Cognitive tests are simply measurement instruments, no different in kind from thermometers, sphygmomanometers, and electrocardiograms. The same principles of reliability, validity, and sensitivity ought to be applied to their selection; and yet cognitive tests are employed with limitations that would be unthinkable in other areas of medicine. If we were seeking to test an antipyretic, we would never countenance the use of a thermometer that had a maximum value of 37 °C, and yet the use of cognitive tests with range restrictions has been commonplace in AD trials and conveniently obscured by the use of composite scores. Similarly, whilst clinical trials in non-CNS indications are often focused on specific signs or symptoms, other disease-relevant dimensions are also routinely evaluated. It is curious then that in clinical trials of putative therapies for AD, prima facie a cognitive disorder, we omit entirely measures of key cognitive skills known to be impaired early in the disease process and for which there is good reason to suppose a possible positive response to treatment.

Ultimately our enterprise is a simple one – we have the hypothesis that our treatment will either preserve or rescue cognition. All that good science requires is that we proceed to test that hypothesis with the use of measurement instruments that meet basic standards of reliability, validity, and sensitivity.

References

1. Rosen WG, Mohs RC, Davis KL. A new rating scale for Alzheimer's disease. *Am J Psychiatry* 1984; **141**: 1356–64.

2. Folstein MF, Folstein SE, McHugh PR. "Mini-mental state": a practical method for grading the cognitive state of patients for the clinician. *J Psychiatr Res* 1975; **12**: 189–98.

3. Wesnes KA, Harrison JE. The evaluation of cognitive function in the dementias: methodological and regulatory considerations. *Dialog Clin Neurosci* 2003; **5**: 77–88.

4. Hobart J, Cano S, Posner H, et al. Putting the Alzheimer's cognitive test to the test I: traditional psychometric methods. *Alzheimers Dement* 2013; **9**: S4–9.

5. Mohs RC, Knopman D, Petersen RC, et al. Development of cognitive instruments for use in clinical trials of antidementia drugs: additions to the Alzheimer's Disease Assessment Scale that broaden its scope. The Alzheimer's Disease Cooperative Study. *Alzheimer Dis Assoc Disord* 1997; **11**: 13–21.

6. Vellas B, Andrieu S, Sampaio C, et al. Endpoints for trials in Alzheimer's disease: a European task force consensus. *Lancet Neurol* 2008; **7**: 436–50.

7. Ritchie K, Ropacki M, Albala B, et al. Recommended cognitive outcomes in pre-clinical Alzheimer's disease: consensus statement from the European Prevention of Alzheimer's Dementia (EPAD) project. *Alzheimers Dement* 2017; **13**: 186–95.

8. Podhorna J, Krahnke T, Shear T, et al. Alzheimer's Disease Assessment Scale – cognitive subscale variants in mild cognitive impairment and mild Alzheimer's disease: change over time and the effects of enrichment strategies. *Alzheimers Res Ther* 2016; **8**: 1–13.

9. Hendrix S, Ellison N. Are Alzheimer's treatment failures due to inactive compounds or are we doing something wrong? *Alzheimers Dement* 2017; **13**: P617.

10. Sevigny JJ, Peng Y, Liu L, et al. Item analysis of ADAS-cog: effect of baseline cognitive impairment in a clinical AD trial. *Am J Alzheimers Dis Other Demen* 2010; **25**: 119–24.

11. Winblad B, Gauthier S, Scinto L, et al. Safety and efficacy of galantamine in subjects with mild cognitive impairment. *Neurology* 2008; **70**: 2024–35.

12. Hort J, Andel R, Mokrisova I, et al. Effect of donepezil in Alzheimer disease can be measured by a computerized human analog of the Morris water maze. *Neurodegener Dis* 2014; **13**: 192–6.

13. Hendrix SB, Wells BM, and the Alzheimer's Disease Neuroimaging Initiative (ADNI). Time course of cognitive decline in subjects with mild Alzheimer's disease based on ADAS-cog subscales and neuropsychological tests measured in ADNI. *Alzheimers Dement* 2010; **6**: e50.

14. Gilman S, Koller M, Black RS, et al. Clinical effects of Abeta immunisation (AN1792) in patients with AD in an interrupted trial. *Neurology* 2005; **64**: 1553–62.

15. Rosenberg A, Ngandu T, Rusanen M, et al. Multidomain lifestyle intervention benefits a large elderly population at risk for cognitive decline and dementia regardless of baseline characteristics: the FINGER trial. *Alzheimers Dement* 2018; **14**: 263–70.

16. Harrison JE, Rentz D, Brashear HR, et al. Psychometric evaluation of the Neuropsychological Test Battery in individuals with normal cognition, mild cognitive impairment, or mild to moderate Alzheimer's disease: results from a longitudinal study. *J Prev Alzheimers Dis* 2018; **5**: 236–44.

17. European Medicines Agency. Guideline on the clinical investigation of medicines for the treatment of Alzheimer's disease. CPMP/EWP/553/95 Rev.2 2018. Avaailable at: www.ema.europa.eu/en/documents/scientific-guideline/guideline-clinical-investigation-medicines-treatment-alzheimers-disease-revision-2_en.pdf (accessed December 31, 2020).

18. Food and Drug Administration. *Early Alzheimer's Disease: Developing Drugs for Treatment. Guidance for Industry*. US Department of Health and Human Services Food and Drug Administration Center for Drug Evaluation and Research (CDER) Center for Biologics Evaluation and Research (CBER); 2018.

19. Leber P. What is the evidence that a dementia treatment works? Criteria used by drug regulatory authorities. In *Evidence-Based Dementia Practice*, Qizilbash N, Schneider LS, Chui H, et al. (eds.). Oxford: Blackwells; 2003: 376–87.

20. Food and Drug Administration. *Guidance for Industry Alzheimer's Disease: Developing Drugs for the Treatment of Early Stage Disease* (FDA-2013-D-0077) Draft; 2013.

21. Harrison JE. Cognition comes of age: comments on the new FDA draft guidance for early Alzheimer's disease. *Alzheimers Res Ther* 2018; **10**: 61.

22. Szlyk JP, Myers L, Zhang YX, et al. Development and assessment of a neuropsychological battery to aid in predicting driving performance. *J Rehabil Res Dev* 2002; **39**: 483–96.

23. Liu-Seifert H, Siemers E, Selzler K, et al. Correlation between cognition and function across the spectrum of Alzheimer's disease. *J Prev Alzheimers Dis* 2016; **3**: 138–44.

24. Katz R. Presentation to the Alzheimer's Association Research Roundtable Scales for Alzheimer's Disease Meeting. April 2008, Washington, reported in R. Black, B. Greenberg, J.M. Ryan et al. Perspectives scales as outcome measures for Alzheimer's disease. *Alzheimers Dement* 2009; **5**: 324–39.

25. Harrison J, Minassian S, Jenkins L, et al. A neuropsychological test battery for use in Alzheimer disease clinical trials. *Arch Neurol* 2007; **64**: 1323–9.

26. Wessels AM, Edgar CJ, Nathan PJ, et al. Cognitive go/no-go decision-making criteria in Alzheimer's disease drug development. *Drug Discov Today* 2021; **26**: 1330–6.

27. Harrison JE, Bradford E, Edgar C, et al. Testing compounds which facilitate learning: a new proof of principle paradigm from CDR. XXV CINP Congress, Chicago, July 9–13, 2006.

28. McIntyre RS, Harrison JE, Loft H, et al. The effects of vortioxetine on cognitive function in patients with major depressive disorder (MDD): a meta-analysis of three randomized controlled trials. *Int J Neuropsychopharmacol* 2016; **19**: pyw055.

29. Harrison JE, Lophaven S, Olsen CK. Which cognitive domains are improved by treatment with vortioxetine? *Int J Neuropsychopharmacol* 2016; **9**: pyw054.

30. Schneider L, Goldberg TE. Composite cognitive and functional measures for early stage Alzheimer's disease trials. *Alzheimers Dement* 2020; **12**: e12017.

31. Harrison JE. Commentary: composite cognitive and functional measures for early-stage Alzheimer's disease trials. *Alzheimers Dement: Cogn Behav Assess* 2020; **12**: 1–3.

32. Harrison JE, Hendrix SB. The assessment of cognition in translational medicine: A contrast between the approaches used in Alzheimer's disease and major depressive disorder. In *Translational Medicine in CNS Drug Development. Handbook of Behavioral Neuroscience, Volume 25*, Nomikos G (ed.). Amsterdam: Elsevier; 2019: 297–308.

33. Wang J, Logovinsky V, Hendrix SB, et al. ADCOMS: a composite clinical outcome for prodromal Alzheimer's disease trials. *J Neurol Neurosurg Psychiatry* 2016; **87**: 993–9.

34. Jutten RJ, Harrison JE, Brunner AJ, et al. The Cognitive–Functional Composite is sensitive to clinical progression in early dementia: longitudinal findings from the Catch–Cog study cohort. *Alzheimers Dement (N Y)* 2020; **6**: e12020.

35. Jutten RS, Harrison JE, Lee Meeuw Kjoeet PR, et al. Assessing cognition and daily function in early dementia using the Cognitive–Functional Composite: findings from the Catch–Cog study cohort. *Alzheimers Res Ther* 2019; **11**: 45.

36. Ferris SH, Lucca U, Mohs R, et al. Objective psychometric tests in clinical trials of dementia drugs. Position paper from the International

Working Group on Harmonization of Dementia Drug Guidelines. *Alzheimers Dis Assoc Disord* 1997; **11**: 34–8.

37. Lannfelt L, Blennow K, Zetterberg H, et al. Targeting Aβ as a modifying therapy of Alzheimer's disease: safety, efficacy and biomarker findings of a Phase IIa randomised, double-blind placebo-controlled trial of PBT2. *Lancet Neurol* 2008; **7**: 779–86.

38. Hilt D, Gawryl M, Koenig G, et al. EVP-6124: safety, tolerability and cognitive effects of a novel A7 nicotinic receptor agonist in Alzheimer's disease patients on stable donepezil or rivastigmine therapy. *Alzheimers Dement* 2009; **5**: P4-348.

39. Scheltens P, Twisk JWR, Blesa R, et al. Efficacy of souvenaid in mild Alzheimer's disease: results from a randomized, controlled trial. *J Alzheimers Dis* 2012; **31**: 225–36.

40. Nathan PJ, Boardley R, Scott N, et al. The safety, tolerability, pharmacokinetics and cognitive effects of GSK239512, a selective histamine H_3 receptor antagonist in patients with mild to moderate Alzheimer's disease: a preliminary investigation. *Curr Alzheimer Res* 2013; **10**: 240–51.

41. Grove RA, Harrington CM, Mahler A, et al. A randomized, double-blind, placebo-controlled, 16-week study of the H_3 receptor antagonist, GSK239512 as a monotherapy in subjects with mild-to-moderate Alzheimer's disease. *Curr Alzheimer Res* 2014; **11**: 47–58.

42. Scheltens P, Hallikainen M, Grimmer T, et al. Safety, tolerability and efficacy of the glutaminyl-cyclase inhibitor PQ912 in Alzheimer's disease: results of a randomized, double-blind, placebo-controlled Phase 2a study. *Alzheimers Res Ther* 2018; **10**: 107.

43. Rockwood K. Size of the treatment on cognition of cholinesterase inhibitors for Alzheimer's disease. *J Neurol Neurosurg Psychiatry* 2004; **75**: 677–85.

44. Cummings J, Scheltens P, McKeith I, et al. Effect size analyses of souvenaid in patients with Alzheimer's disease. *J Alzheimers Dis* 2016; **55**: 1131–9.

45. Rockwood K, Black SE, Robillard A, et al. Potential treatment effects of donepezil not detected in Alzheimer's disease clinical trials: a physician survey. *Int J Geriatr Psychiatry* 2004; **19**: 854–60.

46. Harrison JE, Lam R, Baune BT, et al. Selection of cognitive tests for trials of therapeutic agents. *Lancet Psychiatry* 2016; **8**: 1–13.

Chapter 25

Tele-Trials, Remote Monitoring, and Trial Technology for Alzheimer's Disease Clinical Trials

Rhoda Au, Honghuang Lin, and Vijaya B. Kolachalama

25.1 Introduction

While still in a relatively nascent stage, technology use in healthcare is already widespread. Consumer-level electronics are allowing monitoring of disease-related symptoms outside the doctor's office. Recognizing the transformative possibilities, the US Food and Drug Administration (FDA) has implemented the Digital Health Innovation Action Plan [1] to promote the development and use of digital health technologies because of their ability to reduce inefficiencies, improve access, reduce costs, increase quality, and create individualized treatment plans [2, 3].

Mobile and wearable devices contain within them high-fidelity microphones, accelerometers, high-definition lenses, global positioning systems (GPS) locators, and gyroscopes, which can potentially capture an endless stream of medically relevant information. Recent reviews summarize how they are being used to assess cognition [4, 5], detect and monitor preclinical symptoms in the home [6, 7], and derive novel digital biomarkers from multi-sensor data [8, 9]. Highlighted below is work being done in each of these three arenas because of their implications for clinical trials at the point of recruitment and screening, as primary and secondary outcomes, and as methods for detecting drug side effects. Emphasis is placed on the role of digital biomarkers and their potentially explosive impact on compressing trial timelines, increasing accuracy of determining drug treatment efficacy, and accelerating the path to precision medicine. FDA regulatory considerations are also addressed, without which the promise of digital technology may not be realized. This chapter also addresses the importance of data science and artificial intelligence (AI) in the process of deriving, validating, and integrating digital metrics into meaningful tools for clinical trials from beginning to end.

25.2 Current Alzheimer's Disease Assessment Methods Using Existing Technologies

The pragmatic reality of doing clinical trials today has led to the use of technologies predominantly as an alternative method to collecting FDA-approved data points through an in-person visit. The most commonly used approaches include (1) integrating digital data collection instruments into the existing test protocols and (2) conducting remote monitoring outside of the clinic. Table 25.1 provides some exemplars of these methods, which are also summarized as follows.

Examples of using technologies to enhance current protocols include using a digital pen in place of a regular ballpoint pen and a digital voice recorder to capture spoken responses to traditional tests that elicit written or spoken responses, respectively [10, 11]. Additional examples include using devices and wearables that measure functional behavior such as gait/walking speed [12], balance [12], posture [13], fall risk [14], tremors [15], and eye movement/tracking using digital retinal scanning [16]. Risk factors for Alzheimer's disease (AD), such as cardiovascular, can also be collected digitally in the clinic, such as sleep [17], blood pressure [18], body composition/weight [19], medications [20], blood glucose levels [21], and medical history [22]. While these technologies provide "gold standard" metrics, they also provide novel metrics such as the time to complete each test item/movement and the length of pauses in between each action, which allows construction of multidimensional performance profiles that capture inter-subject variability as well as highly precise intra-subject profiles.

Remote monitoring largely has centered on converting in-clinic assessment methods into those that can be conducted over the phone or via video conference, administering self-reported questionnaires and cognitive assessments using

Table 25.1 Examples of collecting AD-related data via remote testing methods

Metric	Type of remote testing method									
	Mailing	Telephone	Videoconference	On-line	Home computer	Tablet	Smartphone	Wearable	Sensor	Other device
Self-reported questionnaire	✓	✓	✓	✓	✓	✓	✓			
Cognition: neuropsychological tests	✓	✓	✓	✓	✓	✓	✓			
Cognition: keyboard behavior				✓	✓	✓	✓			
Cognition: derived digital profile					✓	✓	✓	✓	✓	✓
Functional behavior: physical activity							✓	✓	✓	
Functional behavior: gait variables							✓	✓	✓	
AD risk factor: sleep							✓	✓	✓	
AD risk factor: blood pressure								✓	✓	
AD risk factor: blood glucose								✓		✓

computers (e.g., online websites, downloaded software), tablets, and/or smartphones [23, 24]. The key advantage of using digital technologies for remote assessment includes opportunities to collect longitudinal data in real time that is not possible in the clinic [23, 25–27]. For example, sleep clinics can only measure a few nights of sleep at a time, while digital sleep devices used in the home can better capture variability in sleep patterns and the factors associated with them over a period of weeks, if not months and even years. Smartphone-based assessments also provide a means for reducing AD clinical trial disparities given their deep penetration, not just in the general elderly population but also within the communities that are typically under-represented (e.g., low-income, rural, racial/ethnic minorities). While each of these methods reduce the subject burden of travel to a clinic and can also lead to better adherence to study protocol through fewer missed appointments, the likely advances they will lead to will be modest. Using technology to do what is already being done represents incremental change rather than a revolutionary one. Given the current regulatory stipulations for drug treatment approval, however, these methods represent the best near-term options without jeopardizing drug trials already in the pipeline.

The distinguishing innovations of digital technology in clinical trial use will be to (1) reduce reliance on user-initiated engagement technologies that typically capture a limited range of data streams, by introducing more practical, scalable, and sustainable monitoring systems that collect clinically interpretable data through use of ambient technologies; and (2) develop technology platforms that are feasible to do across historically under-represented groups, regardless of age, education, income, place of residence, and/or language/culture. Such transformative approaches can lead to a broader clinical impact.

Passive monitoring of clinically relevant behavior can be done via smartphones, wearable devices, or smart-home anchored sensors. The key advantage to passive assessment is that it does not depend on a participant's ongoing active engagement to input information. The primary types of passive data collected are those associated with activities of daily living. Since all human behavior is mediated through the brain, using digital technologies to track movement as a person moves through his/her natural environment provides a means to collect digital data that can be interpreted into

clinically meaningful endpoints (e.g., digital biomarkers). Surprisingly, despite the relative ubiquity of smartphones, little has been done to date to capitalize on the multiple sensors in the phone for passive behavioral monitoring. The primary use of smartphones has been through use of active engagement applications that produce discrete measures [28].

Wearables have been primarily used to measure various types of physical activity through collection of accelerometer, gyroscope, and GPS location data, and interpreting them into measures of mobility [29], walking speed/gait [30], including in those who are cognitively impaired [31]. The other popular metric of behavior is sleep, which can easily be measured through a wrist-worn actigraph and in those with impaired cognitive function [27]. The efficacy of using wearables in clinical trials, however, is still unclear. Only one study has reported use of a wearable in a large-scale study, with longitudinal follow-up [29].

The majority of contemporary digital biomarker studies rely on sensors embedded in the home environment. The most common methods include using infrared and motion sensors that are installed at various locations throughout the home [26, 32, 33]. Of significance is when these sensors are paired with other digital data collection methods including wearables [15, 25, 32] and computer-interaction behavior [15, 32]. These combined technologies provide a more robust profile of functional/cognitive status through multidimensional high-frequency measurement rather than reliance on a single-source digital stream. Given the passive input of digital data involving minimal to no additional subject burden, longitudinal follow-up was feasible for up to 4 years [33, 34]. Of note, most of these studies were done with relatively small sample sizes (e.g., $n < 50$), reflecting the still largely exploratory nature of these methods. But Dodge et al. observed results from a larger sample size ($n = 100–200$) to be like those observed on smaller numbers ($n < 30$) because high-frequency measurement provided sufficient power to detect clinically meaningful changes necessary for clinical trials [34].

While sensors are providing novel digital outcomes that are relevant to clinical trials, their efficacy has not been fully determined. The FDA, while enthusiastic about their potential, has not provided a clear regulatory path for inclusion of these passive acquired metrics as primary or secondary outcomes. Thus, the current state of the digital health platform will need to be comprised of both active and passive engagement technologies. Active engagement as described earlier provides discrete measures that mimic those typically attained in traditional clinic-based trials. These digital measures are much more readily acceptable clinical endpoints because they can be tied to a large body of research that supports their clinical utility. The few clinical trial studies that have used digital technology [24, 30] have all used them as a remote method for collecting similar behavioral and/or functional measures; these measures are similar to the ones collected during in-person studies.

A key barrier to bold, paradigmatic shifting acceptance of passive engagement technologies into clinical trials is the lack of certainty, given that none of these methods have received the FDA stamp of approval.

25.3   Regulatory Perspective: Current State

Although the FDA realizes the potential impact digital technologies have on healthcare in general and brain health in particular, most digital technologies are still under development. For digital technologies to really penetrate the clinical trial arena it is important and necessary for the FDA to provide clear guidance on the approval pathway, thereby providing both technology developers and clinical trialists a roadmap for what standards must be met. As an important step toward achieving this goal, the FDA's Center for Devices and Radiological Health laid out their vision for fostering digital health innovation in the Digital Health Innovation Action Plan [1]. A key component of this plan includes launching an innovative pilot pre-certification program to work with technology manufacturers (or customers) to develop a new approach to digital health technology oversight (FDA Software Precertification [Pre-Cert] Pilot Program). More recently, the agency also formed the Digital Health Center of Excellence (DHCoE) to align and coordinate digital health work across the FDA [35]. The DHCoE provides services in several functional areas for digital health including digital health policy, medical device cybersecurity, AI and machine learning, regulatory science advancement, review support and coordination, advanced manufacturing, clinical studies,

and strategic partnerships. Currently, the FDA encourages device and technology manufacturers to contact them during any phase (preferably early) of product development. For example, companies such as Apple, Fitbit, Johnson & Johnson, Pear Therapeutics, Phosphorus, Roche, Samsung, Tidepool, and Verily were selected to participate in the development of the FDA Pre-Cert pilot program. With these exciting advancements, it is encouraging to know that the FDA is setting a precedent and proactively participating in the evolution of digital transformation of technologies for healthcare.

25.3.1   Regulatory Needs for Anticipated Outcomes

To seek regulatory approval, digital health technology manufacturers need to provide several forms of evidence that demonstrate data quality, security, measurement effectiveness, and integration with other parties within the ecosystem. To achieve these goals, a key barrier they need to overcome is mitigating risk with timely coordination across different parties. The FDA's DHCoE can precisely help in this scenario as it can serve as a catalyst to facilitate coordination with different parties and enable efficient, transparent, and predictable product review. This will ensure that cutting-edge technologies can be rapidly developed and reviewed. At the same time, by acting as an independent body for oversight, the FDA will protect the population's interests and create trust and awareness across all the parties. These initiatives are expected to incentivize the technology companies to seek FDA guidance early on in their product life cycle and continue to communicate with various parties to bring their products to the market in the least burdensome timeline. An anticipated outcome of these efforts is an accelerated shift toward creating value-based healthcare systems and digital health technologies that can play an important role in this transition.

25.3.2   Regulatory Barriers to Innovation

While clinical trials using digital technologies have the same objective, to evaluate whether the potential medical treatment offers benefit to patients, replication of clinical trial outcomes cannot be the only end goal. For example, opportunities now include using video or hand-motion data that can be paired with a smart pill box to track adherence to medication use; capturing patient-reported outcomes that are inherently biased by self-reporting, with the use of objective metrics such as side effects of mood and depression, by monitoring physical activity and digital voice features; and the identification of digital biomarkers as surrogate markers to expensive and invasive imaging and fluid ones. The FDA is grappling with how to develop the regulatory path that will likely lead to new gold standards for validating and approving digitally acquired outcomes, which are unlike those currently being used.

25.4 Current Methods for Validating Digital Technology

In the past decade, a variety of digital technologies have been developed to collect both structured-derived measures and unstructured digital data streams for cognitive and functional assessments. The effectiveness of many devices, however, has not been rigorously validated. The validation is typically performed through two steps. First, the effectiveness and accuracy of the device is tested in a controlled environment, for example in a research laboratory. The results are more interpretable and replicable in such an environment, and the device could be recalibrated with gold-standard measurements. Second, and more importantly, the real-time effectiveness of digital devices can be validated by different users in the clinical setting.

In addition to effectiveness, it is also important to validate the power consumption under different use cases for portable devices. The power usage is typically done through the measure of the current (in microamperes) and the voltage (in microvolts). The update period for both measurements varies by devices and is usually in the order of a few hundred milliseconds. Monitoring 24/7 will lead to excessive power consumption as well as too much uninformative data; thus "continuous monitoring" really requires determining the frequency of measurement based on the device capacity and the user's activities.

25.4.1 Data Analytics Is the Future for Digital Technology Validation

No one technology will likely be sufficient to generate valid and reliable outcomes at the level of precision that will make the investment of a shift to digital clinical trials timely and cost effective. The

digital platforms comprised of multiple technologies are expected to generate massive amounts of multimodal data. Thus, it is important to develop data analytic frameworks that can systematically tackle the complexities and nuances related to inter- and intra-individual variability and derive assessments on their cognitive/functional status. To build such frameworks, one needs to first appreciate the various forms of data that could be collected, such as from remote applications, wearable devices, and via in-clinic assessments. Data from these sources can be collected via active or passive engagement. While active data collection relies on the "end-user" to engage with the technology, it also poses an inherent limitation on the amount of data that can be accumulated over time. On the other hand, passive data collection might not necessarily rely on the user expertise per se but would demand more hardware and software resources. Despite the engagement modality, the goal for drug treatment monitoring needs to capture behavioral features that, in combination, can serve as surrogate measures of cognition/function and better detect subtle treatment effects than traditional sporadic test methods. The strengths and bounds of these data resources, and their ability to capture and process data from ambient data streams, need to be appreciated and, importantly, data analytic frameworks need to be developed to efficiently process all the forms and modalities of data.

The recent surge of interest in using advanced analytic tools such as machine learning is allowing researchers to develop cutting-edge algorithms to analyze complex data sets. Machine-learning approaches can decompose the complexities of observed data sets into learnable patterns and interactions. Once these interactions are learned, refined, and formalized by exposure to a training data set, fully trained models leverage their "experience" of prior data to make predictions about new cases or outcomes. Thus, these approaches offer powerful decision-making potential due to their ability to rapidly identify low-level signatures of disease from large data sets, and quickly apply them at scale. This capacity enables fusion of various features generated from ambient data streams, whose sheer volume or complexity would previously have made analyzing them unimaginable. Such technologies can provide detailed, accurate, data-driven insights in an efficient fashion. These methods can potentially streamline data analysis and have a potential of reducing inter-sample/

inter-subject/inter-expert variability. Depending on the type of data that are being collected, it is possible to select a machine-learning framework for analysis. While there is no strict protocol for selecting the right analytic methodology for a data set, the expertise of the user and the availability of the computational resources often drive these choices. For example, if active engagement leads to data collection that can be formatted in a row–column structure (rows designate observations and columns describing properties about the observations), then users can employ traditional machine-learning algorithms such as support vector machines or decision-tree-based approaches. On the other hand, if passive-engagement-based data collection leads to a more continuous (or raw) form of data, then the so-called deep-learning frameworks can be employed [36]. While certain traditional machine-learning approaches can be developed using standard computing workstations or central-processing-unit computing servers, hardware infrastructure involving graphics processing units are desirable to implement deep-learning approaches. Also, recently, federated machine-learning approaches are being explored to create a decentralized computing framework, thus addressing critical issues such as data security and privacy, and access to data sets from multiple heterogeneous resources.

25.4.2 Lessons Learned from New Technologies for AD Drug Development

Despite current advances, there are several challenges to fully recognize the potential of digital technologies.

- **Data security**. A risk to any system that captures mobile health is the inadvertent release of medical data. A top priority of any digital trial plan is to ensure data are always encrypted in real time, so losing a device or having an application hacked will not expose the collected digital data. Potential security risks should be constantly investigated as new devices and operating systems with new sensory capabilities and application programming interfaces emerge.
- **Use of raw data**. As digital technology is evolving rapidly, best-of-class today may be obsolete tomorrow. Thus, collection of raw digital files in addition to derived measures will allow re-analysis of digital data using

improved computational algorithms and ensure longitudinal measures are always meeting contemporary standards. In this way, data collected from a later model of the device can be aligned with data obtained from an earlier version.
- **Device/application agnostic**. Rapid obsolescence and emergent technologies necessitate needing continuous evaluation of different combinations of technologies. In designing any digital platform, it is important to be device/application-agnostic to allow swapping in and out to maximize the trial effectiveness and efficiency.
- **Focus on passive technologies**. The transition from active engagement technologies to low-to-no engagement technologies requires investment in collecting and validating ambient data collection approaches, as was described earlier.
- **More inclusive of participants from diverse ancestries and socioeconomic backgrounds**. Most of the existing studies are based on participants of European ancestry. It is important to expand the income/racial/ethnic mix of participants for future technology development to reduce longstanding health disparities in clinical trial studies. Additional testing is needed to assess the robustness of technologies for use in these subpopulations and identify technological solutions that are better suited to them. The inherent intrusiveness of digital technology, however, could also potentially exacerbate issues of trust. But technology also could provide customized messaging that is relevant and responsive to the concerns of the participant to build the trust needed prior to clinical trial engagement.

25.5 Role of New Technologies in the Drug-Development Ecosystem

The opportunities that digital technologies can provide across the entire clinical trial operations (e.g., recruitment, monitoring, drug efficacy outcomes, etc.) has been previously well described [37–39]. Existing precedent, however, is limited to using technology within individual components of the drug trial ecosystem rather than its entirety. Figure 25.1 depicts an end-to-end digital clinical trial solution that relies on the trialist selecting a suite of

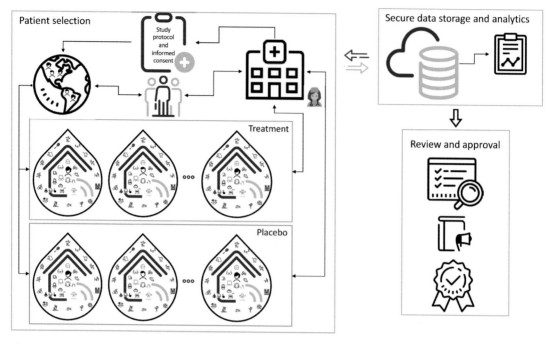

Figure 25.1 Depiction of a future remote AD clinical trial.

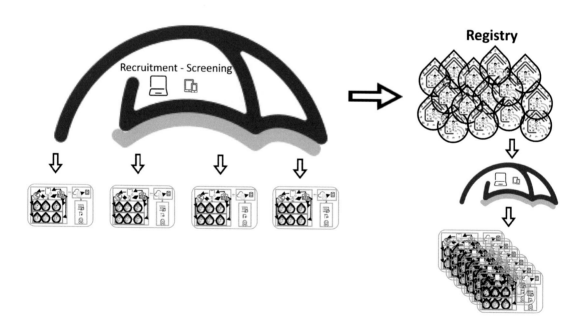

Figure 25.2 Future vision of rapid, concurrent, remote clinical trials.

commercially available technologies, each of which addresses one specific function. Some redundancy is built in to protect against any momentary technology glitch from any one device/application and to allow easier transition to newer, emerging technologies without affecting the foundational clinical trial infrastructure. The trialist is able to track participant adherence and treatment/placebo impact through various digital data streams over the length of the trial, in real time, which could lead to a significant compression of time to detect clinically meaningful primary and secondary endpoints. Figure 25.2

illustrates the significant opportunity to mobilize multiple trials simultaneously using the same technology platform, which would lead to a cost-effective multiple-shots-on-target approach that would accelerate the pace of both positive discovery and faster failures. This operational efficiency will also significantly reduce the overall price tag for the average trial, the savings of which could also translate into less expensive treatment to the patient.

Figures 25.1 and 25.2 do not reflect a pipe dream. The technologies exist, the multidisciplinary expertise is available, and AD healthcare expenditures are increasing exponentially. The time is now for a major sea change to dramatically shift the course of current practices today.

References

1. Food and Drug Administration. Digital Health Innovation Action Plan. Available at: www.fda.gov/media/106331/download (accessed 2018).

2. Food and Drug Administration. Software as a medical device (SAMD): clinical evaluation. Available at: www.fda.gov/regulatory-information/search-fda-guidance-documents/software-medical-device-samd-clinical-evaluation (accessed 2017).

3. FDA–NIH Biomarker Working Group. *BEST (Biomarkers, Endpoints, and Other Tools) Resource.* Silver Spring, MD and Bethesda, MD: Food and Drug Administration and National Institutes of Health; 2016.

4. Chinner A, Blane J, Lancaster C, Hinds C, Koychev I. Digital technologies for the assessment of cognition: a clinical review. *Evid-Based Ment Health* 2018; **21**: 67–71.

5. Koo BM, Vizer LM. Mobile technology for cognitive assessment of older adults: a scoping review. *Innov Aging* 2018; **3**: igy038.

6. Lussier M, Lavoie M, Giroux S, et al. Early detection of mild cognitive impairment with in-home monitoring sensor technologies using functional measures: a systematic review. *IEEE J Biomed Health Inform* 2019; **23**: 838–47.

7. Thabtah F, Mampusti E, Peebles D, Herradura R, Varghese J. A mobile-based screening system for data analyses of early dementia traits detection. *J Med Syst* 2019; **44**: 24.

8. Piau A, Wild K, Mattek N, Kaye J. Current state of digital biomarker technologies for real-life, home-based monitoring of cognitive function for mild cognitive impairment to mild Alzheimer disease and implications for clinical care: systematic review. *J Med Internet Res* 2019, **21**: e12785.

9. Kourtis LC, Regele OB, Wright JM, Jones GB. Digital biomarkers for Alzheimer's disease: the mobile/wearable devices opportunity. *NPJ Digit Med* 2019; **2**: 9.

10. Piers RJ, Devlin KN, Ning B, et al. Age and graphomotor decision making assessed with the digital clock drawing test: the Framingham Heart Study. *J Alzheimers Dis* 2017; **60**: 1611–20.

11. Thomas JA, Burkhardt HA, Chaudhry S, et al. Assessing the utility of language and voice biomarkers to predict cognitive impairment in the Framingham Heart Study cognitive aging cohort data. *J Alzheimers Dis* 2020; **76**: 905–22.

12. Moon S, Song HJ, Sharma VD, et al. Classification of Parkinson's disease and essential tremor based on balance and gait characteristics from wearable motion sensors via machine learning techniques: a data-driven approach. *J Neuroeng Rehabil* 2020; **17**: 125.

13. Leach JM, Mancini M, Kaye JA, Hayes TL, Horak FB. Day-to-day variability of postural sway and its association with cognitive function in older adults: a pilot study. *Front Aging Neurosci* 2018; **10**: 126.

14. Tulipani LJ, Meyer B, Larie D, Solomon AJ, McGinnis RS. Metrics extracted from a single wearable sensor during sit–stand transitions relate to mobility impairment and fall risk in people with multiple sclerosis. *Gait Post* 2020; **80**: 361–6.

15. Dorsey ER, Omberg L, Waddell E. Deep phenotyping of Parkinson's disease. *J Parkinsons Dis* 2020; **10**: 855–73.

16. Hunfalvay M, Roberts CM, Murray NP. Vertical smooth pursuit as a diagnostic marker of traumatic brain injury. *Concussion* 2020; **5**: CNC69.

17. Regalia G, Gerboni G, Migliorini M, et al. Sleep assessment by means of a wrist actigraphy-based algorithm: agreement with polysomnography in an ambulatory study on older adults. *Chronobiol Int* 2021; **38**: 400–14.

18. Kuwabara M, Harada K, Hishiki Y, Kario K. Validation of two watch-type wearable blood pressure monitors according to the ANSI/AAMI/ISO81060-2:2013 guidelines: Omron HEM-6410 T-ZM and HEM-6410 T-ZL. *J Clin Hypertens (Greenwich)* 2019; **21**: 853–8.

19. Collier SR, McCraw C, Campany M, et al. Withings body cardio versus gold standards of pulse-wave velocity and body composition. *J Pers Med* 2020; **10**: 17.

20. Mosnaim GS, Stempel DA, Gonzalez C, et al. The impact of patient self-monitoring via electronic medication monitor and mobile app plus remote clinician feedback on adherence to inhaled corticosteroids: a randomized controlled trial. *J Allergy Clin Immunol Pract* 2021; **9**: 1586–94.

21. Jafri RZ, Balliro CA, El-Khatib F, A three-way accuracy comparison of the Dexcom G5, Abbott Freestyle Libre Pro, and Senseonics Eversense continuous glucose monitoring devices in a home-use study of subjects with type 1 diabetes. *Diabetes Technol Therapeut* 2020; **22**: 846–52.

22. Vandenberk T, Storms V, Lanssens D, et al. A vendor-independent mobile health monitoring platform for digital health studies: development and usability study. *JMIR mHealth uHealth* 2019; **7**: e12586.

23. Seelye A, Mattek N, Sharma N. Weekly observations of online survey metadata obtained through home computer use allow for detection of changes in everyday cognition before transition to mild cognitive impairment. *Alzheimers Dement* 2018; **14**: 187–94.

24. Sano M, Zhu CW, Kaye J, et al. A randomized clinical trial to evaluate home-based assessment of people over 75 years old. *Alzheimers Dement* 2019; **15**: 615–24.

25. Thomas N, Beattie Z, Marcoe J, et al. An ecologically valid, longitudinal, and unbiased assessment of treatment efficacy in Alzheimer disease (the EVALUATE-AD trial): proof-of-concept study. *JMIR Res Protoc* 2020; **9**: e17603.

26. Ahamed F, Shahrestani S, Cheung H. Internet of things and machine learning for healthy ageing: identifying the early signs of dementia. *Sensors (Basel)* 2020; **20**: E6031.

27. Cavuoto MG, Kinsella GJ, Ong B, Pike KE, Nicholas CL. Naturalistic measurement of sleep in older adults with amnestic mild cognitive impairment: anxiety symptoms do not explain sleep disturbance. *Curr Alzheimer Res* 2019; **16**: 233–42.

28. Øksnebjerg L, Woods B, Ruth K, et al. A tablet app supporting self-management for people with dementia: explorative study of adoption and use patterns. *JMIR mHealth uHealth* 2020; **8**: e14694.

29. Buchman AS, Dawe RJ, Leurgans SE. Different combinations of mobility metrics derived from a wearable sensor are associated with distinct health outcomes in older adults. *J Gerontol A Biol Sci Med Sci* 2020; **75**: 1176–83.

30. Mueller A, Hoefling HA, Muaremi A, et al. Continuous digital monitoring of walking speed in frail elderly patients: noninterventional validation study and longitudinal clinical trial. *JMIR mHealth uHealth* 2019; **7**: e15191.

31. De Vito AN, Sawyer RJ 2nd, LaRoche A, et al. Acceptability and feasibility of a multicomponent telehealth care management program in older adults with advanced dementia in a residential memory care unit. *Gerontol Geriatr Med* 2020; **6**: 2333721420924988.

32. Seelye A, Leese MI, Dorociak K, et al. Feasibility of in-home sensor monitoring to detect mild cognitive impairment in aging military veterans: prospective observational study. *JMIR Form Res* 2020; **4**: e16371.

33. Lyons BE, Austin D, Seelye A, et al. Pervasive computing technologies to continuously assess Alzheimer's disease progression and intervention efficacy. *Front Aging Neurosci* 2015; **7**: 102.

34. Dodge HH, Zhu J, Mattek NC, et al. Use of high-frequency in-home monitoring data may reduce sample sizes needed in clinical trials. *PloS One* 2015; **10**: e0138095.

35. Food and Drug Administration. Digital Health Center of Excellence. Available at: www.fda.gov/medical-devices/digital-health-center-excellence (accessed November 2020).

36. Xue C, Karjadi C, Paschalidis IC, Au R, Kolachalama VB. Detection of dementia on voice recordings using deep learning: a Framingham Heart Study. *Alzheimers Res Ther* 2021; **13**: 146.

37. Inan OT, Tenaerts P, Prindiville SA, et al. Digitizing clinical trials. *NPJ Digit Med* 2020; **3**: 1–7.

38. Steinhubl SR, Wolff-Hughes DL, Nilsen W, Iturriaga E, Califf RM. Digital clinical trials: creating a vision for the future. *NPJ Digit Med* 2019; **2**: 1–3.

39. National Academies of Sciences, Engineering, and Medicine. *The Role of Digital Health Technologies in Drug Development: Proceedings of a Workshop*. Washington, DC: The National Academies Press; 2020.

Chapter 26

Expanded Access and Compassionate Use in Alzheimer's Disease Drug Development

Diana Kerwin

26.1 Introduction

In the United States, Alzheimer's disease (AD) is highly prevalent, affecting more than 5.8 million individuals who are currently living with AD or some form of dementia. This statistic is expected to reach 14 million Americans by 2050. AD is the sixth leading cause of death and is quickly overwhelming our aging population, their caregivers and families, and our healthcare systems [1].

The recent approval of aducanumab is the first potentially disease-modifying treatment (DMT) and is the first new treatment for AD on the global market since 2003. The drug-development process in the United States is lengthy for a single new medicine, easily spanning 16–20 years and an average cost to research and develop each successful drug is estimated to be $800 million to $1 billion. This number includes the cost of the thousands of failed trials: for every 5,000–10,000 compounds that enter the research and development pipeline, only one receives approval. These barriers add significant time and costs to the overall clinical trial process, which hinders the overall goal of AD drug development. Drug development in AD has proven to be a slow process. The enrollment in AD clinical trials has been seen as a rate-limiting factor, with extensive screening criteria to properly identify the appropriate subjects often limiting access to participation as well as posing financial challenges for both large pharmaceutical and small biotech companies for the prolonged time needed for clinical development. Five-year projections estimate that more than 54,000 participants will be needed for AD drug testing of the current drug pipeline [2]. The drug-development process may take several more years to provide the likely cocktail of target therapies needed to halt the progression or prevent the onset of cognitive impairment for persons with AD pathology present. For this reason, alternative pathways to access potential treatments and early data collection may help to facilitate the drug-development process in AD, much as it has in the past for oncology and infectious diseases. This chapter focuses on the use of expanded-access and compassionate-use pathways for patients to access potentially beneficial, investigative drugs and the use of these pathways in early-stage drug development.

26.2 Role of Expanded Access in Drug Development

The US Food and Drug Administration (FDA) oversees the premarket assessment of the safety and efficacy of investigational new drugs and biologics. Randomized, clinical trials remain the gold standard for the protection of participants and collection of data that provides the supporting evidence for the approval of investigational drugs for clinical indications. However, in some areas of drug development, enrollment in clinical trials may not be possible for reasons related to the disease (rare diseases, rapidly progressive) or due to patient factors such as eligibility for ongoing trials or lack of access to trials due to geographic limitations. Expanded access is the use of an investigational new drug (IND) outside of a clinical trial in patients for the diagnosis, monitoring, or treatment of a serious disease or condition. The expanded-access pathway was highlighted most recently in 2020 during the COVID-19 pandemic and was used to facilitate access and treatment development for severely ill patients. The expanded-access pathway has historically been associated with facilitating drug development in oncology and access to unapproved cancer treatments for patients with life-threatening cancer. The FDA expanded-access programs demonstrate the commitment of the FDA to facilitate access, and openly look for mechanisms to facilitate access. In 2019, the US FDA Oncology Center of Excellence announced Project Facilitate, a new program to assist healthcare providers on how to request access to unapproved therapies for patients with cancer diagnoses [3].

The FDA formalized the process for its expanded-access programs in 1987 for drugs and biologics. An expanded-access program for devices was formalized in 1996 and the expanded-access programs were made law by the Food and Drug Administration Modernization Act (FDMA) of 1997. Outside of the United States, several countries have developed regulations for access to unapproved drugs, and use the term "compassionate use," including Canada, Australia, Brazil, and many European Union countries (France, Italy, Germany, Spain) under the European Medicines Agency's (EMA's) Guideline on Compassionate Use of Medicinal Products. The FDA no longer uses the term "compassionate use"; however, this term is still used to generally describe any pathway to access of investigational drugs outside of clinical trials, and now includes the US Right-To-Try (RTT) laws; many drug makers and patient advocacy groups use the term, as well as access programs outside of the United States.

The use of expanded access in neurology remains limited, with most expanded-access studies in AD designed to provide access to investigational drugs at the conclusion of a clinical trial (ClinicalTrials.gov). This chapter focuses on the expanded-access programs for drugs and biologics and identifies the role of stakeholders and the impact of expanded access on the stakeholders as well as the potential effect on the AD research and the drug-development ecosystem.

26.3   Definition and History of Expanded Access in the United States

The term expanded access, access, and treatment use are used interchangeably by the FDA to refer to the use of an investigational drug when the primary purpose is to diagnose, monitor, or treat a patient's disease or condition. The term compassionate use is used by regulatory agencies outside of the United States and has been used informally by industry and patient advocacy organizations when indicating access programs in general. The expanded-access term was formalized by the FDA Code of Federal Regulations (CFR) and updated most recently in October 2009 to the guidance

in place currently. The FDA's history of facilitating access to investigational therapies outside of clinical trials reaches back to the 1970s; however, regulations did not specifically describe a pathway for access to unapproved drugs until 1987[4]. The 1987 IND regulations were criticized for lacking clear criteria and submission requirements, which resulted in inconsistent policies, inequitable access, and preferential access for certain categories of patients. In response to this criticism, Congress included in the Food and Drug Administration Modernization Act of 1997 (FDAMA) (Public Law 105–115), which amended the Federal Food, Drug, and Cosmetic Act, specific provisions concerning expanded access to investigational drugs for treatment use [5]. This codified expanded access into law.

The current FDA expanded-access regulations provide guidance for the key stakeholders: industry (pharmaceutical companies, biotech, drug manufacturers), researchers, physicians, institutional review boards (IRBs), and patients, for the process and documentation requirements for the program. The expanded-access program provides a process for patients and their treating physician, to obtain authorization to use an investigational drug for treatment under an expanded-access IND when certain criteria have been met as defined by the FDA. In the United States, an expanded-access IND must also include approval and oversight by an IRB; this requirement is not uniformly required in compassionate-use programs outside of the United States.

The FDA guidance states that expanded access may be appropriate when all the following circumstances apply:

- the patient has a serious disease or condition, or their life is immediately threatened by their disease or condition;
- there is no comparable or satisfactory alternative therapy to diagnose, monitor, or treat the disease or condition;
- the patient enrollment in a clinical trial is not possible;
- the potential patient benefit justifies the potential risks of treatment; and/or
- if the investigational medical product will not interfere with investigational trials that could support a medical product's development or marketing approval for the treatment indication.

Expanded-access programs emerged in the 1970s and 1980s in the early drug development stages of oncology and HIV, and for infectious disease outbreaks such as the Ebola, H1N1, and COVID-19 pandemics. The evolution of the expanded-access program in the FDA has often been driven by patient advocacy movements, and this has resulted in legislation and governmental initiatives to expand and improve access:

1970s: Cancer patients advocate for access to INDs. The FDA introduced the Group C Cancer Investigational New Drug Program in 1976. This program was established for oncologists to use IND cancer drugs to treat patients outside of clinical trials.

1980s: AIDS played a significant role in the development of expanded access. Patient advocacy placed pressure on the FDA, and as a result, the FDA made major strides to make experimental drugs for life-threatening diseases more available to severely ill patients.

1990s: The FDMA of 1997 codified the FDA expanded-access regulations and practice to increase patient access to experimental drugs and medical devices, and the law provided an expanded clinical trial database to include results of expanded-access studies [6].

2000s: Congress created the Reagan-Udall Foundation (https://navigator.reaganudall.org), an independent not-for-profit organization for the FDA to promote collaboration. In 2017, the expanded-access navigator created an online resource for patients, caregivers, physicians, advocacy groups, and industry with live and updated guidance of the expanded-access process.

The FDA most recently revised CFR, Part 312, in October 2009, with the addition of new expanded-access regulations to include broad and equitable patient access to INDs for treatment. This addition established the criteria currently used today for expanded access, as well as offering safeguards and submission requirements.

There are currently four categories of expanded access:

- a single-patient IND, for treatment of individual patients for emergency situations;
- a single-patient IND, for treatment of individual patients for non-emergency situations;

- an intermediate-sized-patient-population IND, for treatment of more than one patient, yet smaller than a treatment IND or protocol; or
- a treatment IND or protocol for treatment of a large patient population.

26.4 FDA's Expanded Access Program Guidance

The FDA regularly updates guidance for stakeholders of the expanded-access programs based upon external reviews of the programs and gap analysis. Most recently, the FDA commissioned an external panel to complete and publish the 2018 expanded-access program report. Based upon feedback from stakeholders, several initiatives to broaden or facilitate access have been implemented such as the Reagan-Udall Foundation Expanded Access Navigator and the US FDA Oncology Center of Excellence Project Facilitate. In the most recent FDA expanded-access program report in 2018 [7], the FDA identified the stakeholders of expanded access and developed guidance based upon the regulations and feedback for stakeholders that is available online and updated regularly. The FDA has identified eight stakeholders in the expanded-access process:

- patients;
- patient's advocates and caregivers;
- treating physician (most often is the sponsor for the single-patient IND);
- industry (pharmaceutical, biotech, drug manufacturers);
- payers;
- health systems;
- IRBs; and
- FDA staff.

Based upon the expanded-access program report, the FDA streamlined requirements for supporting documentation for expanded-access requests, lessening the administrative burden for sponsors (typically physicians) to reduce time to complete the application and simplified IRB review requirements.

26.4.1 Obtaining Access

Expanded access is authorized through the submission of a new protocol to either an existing or new IND application. This can be for a single patient, an intermediate-sized patient population, or a larger treatment population.

1. **Patient**: Diagnosed with a serious or life-threatening condition. Consults with a licensed physician to explore and decide about alternative options.
2. **Licensed physician**: Agrees to oversee the patient's treatment and works with industry (e.g., medical product developer), files paperwork with FDA and IRB (for many expanded-access request types), and is responsible for patient care and reporting.
3. **Industry**: Willing to provide the investigational medical product and either sponsors the expanded access, allows the FDA to cross-reference to their industry IND (for drugs and biologics) or investigational device exemption (IDE) on behalf of the expanded-access sponsor-investigator through the use of a letter of authorization, or provides the necessary investigational medical product information for the sponsor-investigator to submit to support an expanded-access request.
4. **IRB**: Reviews the expanded-access protocol and consent to ensure that the patient is informed about the nature of the treatment.
5. **FDA**: Reviews the expanded-access request and determines if the treatment may proceed.

Due to the multiple stakeholders involved in the expanded-access process, the FDA has developed guidance for stakeholders on the requirements of each in the process.

26.4.2 Role of the Treating Physicians

The primary criteria for expanded access are to provide a pathway for a patient with a serious or life-threatening disease access to an unapproved drug, outside of a clinical trial and when all other treatment options have been exhausted. The determination of whether a disease is serious is a matter of clinical judgment and the determination that all treatment options have been exhausted falls to the treating physician. The expanded-access approval process rests on the treating physician's shoulders, and based upon the 2018 Program Report, the FDA streamlined the administrative burden for physician/sponsors (see Box 26.1). Prior to the changes, a typical expanded-access IND application took an average of 8 hours; with the creation of online portals, the submission time was reduced to 45 minutes [8].

26.4.3 Role of Industry

For single-patient expanded-access IND applications, the drug manufacturer is responsible for reporting updates to their safety and clinical data resulting from the expanded-access study, in the form of the investigator's brochure filed with the FDA. The most important aspect of industry is to provide a letter of authorization for the expanded-access IND application. The letter of authorization

---

Box 26.1 Expanded-access approval process (physician guidance)

1. Identify the patient with limited treatment options and a desire to participate in clinical trial.
2. Determine that the patient is not eligible for any currently enrolling studies in a reasonable geographic area (ClinicalTrials.gov).
3. Request access to the drug from the sponsor or drug maker.
4. Develop a protocol with the drug maker and request a letter of authorization to submit an application to the FDA.
5. Request a pre-assigned IND, register for an account with the Center for Drug Evaluation and Research (CDER) NextGen Portal, navigate to https://edm.fda.gov.
6. Open an FDA IND application for expanded access (form 1571).
7. Describe the patient in the protocol and rationale for the expanded-access application (form 3926).
8. Submit through the eCTD platform (directly or via a third-party vendor).
9. Once the application is received by the FDA, there is a 30-day review period; if no clinical hold is placed, the study can proceed at the end of the 30 days, once IRB approval is obtained.
10. An annual report to the FDA is required by the sponsor to report any changes to protocol, safety data, and benefit data to justify continuation of the study, with a risk–benefit analysis.

permits the FDA to refer to the drug manufacturer's submitted information, including safety/toxicity data, dosing information, and totality of the data to determine if the risk–benefit for the patient is favorable to allow the study to proceed. A review of expanded-access applications in the fiscal years 2010–2015 shows that the FDA authorized 99% of single-patient expanded-access applications. Although the expanded-access program is regulated by the FDA, the decision to allow access to the IND remains the responsibility of the company.

The 21st Century Cures Act [9], passed in December 2016, brought sweeping reforms to expedite the discovery, development, and delivery of new treatments and cures. That law included new requirements that industry publicly make available their policies and procedures for processing requests by patients and physicians, for expanded access.

While companies are not required to offer expanded access, they are required to provide the following information:

- contact information for the developer, manufacturer, or distributor;
- procedures for making the expanded-access request;
- the anticipated time it will take to acknowledge receipt of a request;
- general criteria used to evaluate the request; and
- a hyperlink or reference to the clinical trial record in ClinicalTrials.gov, containing information about expanded access for their drugs that may be available through the expanded-access request process.

It is important to reiterate that the posting of policies does not serve as a guarantee of access to any specific investigational treatment. Expanded access can only occur if a drug company agrees to provide the IND. The FDA cannot require a manufacturer to provide its drug, and there are valid reasons why a manufacturer may not do so, such as an ongoing clinical trial the patient can join and limited drug supply. The fear that adverse events that occur during expanded access will lead to clinical holds and have an unfavorable impact upon the overall drug-development program is a concern sometimes raised. A review of almost 11,000 expanded-access requests over a 10-year period, however, demonstrated that only two drug-development programs were placed on clinical

hold due to adverse events observed in patients receiving expanded access, and even these were temporary. Updated guidance on the use of data for the expanded access released in October 2017 [10] stated that "FDA will evaluate any adverse event data obtained from an expanded-access submission within that context." Published literature shows that there have been no instances in which expanded access has led to a negative regulatory decision regarding a drug application [11]. Therefore, it is very rare for an adverse event occurring during expanded access to adversely affect drug development. Nevertheless, this has been cited by manufacturers as the top consideration to deny access. If a company does provide drug for an expanded-access study, the company may decide to cover the cost of the IND or may charge for the drug; the costs must be justified and limited to those necessary to recover costs of manufacture, research, development, and handling.

26.4.4　Role of Institutional Review Boards and Ethics Committees

Independent review of biomedical research is a generally accepted practice for ethical and safety protections of research participants, and all major international ethical and legal guidelines contain this principle, including those of the World Medical Association, Council of Europe, and International Council for Harmonisation Good Clinical Practice (ICH GCP) [12]. All FDA authorized expanded-access trials require IRB/ethics committee (EC) approval and oversight; however, IRB/EC review is mandatory in only a few countries outside of the United States. As with randomized clinical trials, expanded-access studies also require the patient to sign an informed consent form and all the usual regulatory documentation is required. Based upon the 2018 expanded-access program report, the FDA simplified the IRB review requirements as outlined in 21 CFR 312.310, for single-patient expanded-access IND studies to be reviewed by a single member, such as the IRB chair, rather than requiring full board approval. The licensed physician submitting a non-emergency individual-patient expanded-access IND may request a waiver from full IRB review. The waiver also applies to any changes/amendment review of the original treatment plan or for a continuing review of the expanded-access IND. This promoted consistency between emergency-use expanded-access

IND and all expanded-access programs. Due to the public health crisis of the COVID-19 pandemic and a significant increase in single-patient INDs for emergency use, the FDA provided updated guidance focused on the IRB review of the risks and benefits of treatment with the IND for the particular patient [13].

26.5 Relationship to Compassionate Use

Compassionate use, like expanded access, has a general meaning of a program or pathway in which the primary purpose is to provide patients with access to potentially beneficial but unapproved treatment. In the United States, compassionate use applies to the FDA's Expanded Access Program for Investigational Drugs and RTT laws; outside of the United States, regulatory agencies, such as the EMA, use the term compassionate use for their access programs. The EMA, under Article 83 of Regulation (EC) No. 726/2004, defines compassionate use as a treatment option that allows the use of an unauthorized medicine; under strict conditions, products in development can be made available to groups of patients who have a disease with no satisfactory authorized therapies and who cannot enter clinical trials. The EMA provides recommendations through the Committee for Medicinal Products for Human Use, but these do not create a legal framework. Compassionate-use programs are coordinated and implemented by the member states, which set their own rules and procedures. Drug makers with clinical development programs often use expanded access and compassionate use interchangeably when posting their access policies, which is now mandated by the 21st Century Cures Act of 2016 [9].

26.6 Right-to-Try Laws

The first RTT law was drafted and introduced in 2017–2018 session of Congress by Trickett Wendler, Frank Mongiello, Jordan McLinn, and Matthew Bellina. The RTT Act was introduced and signed into law on May 30, 2018. The RTT was developed by the Goldwater Institute and designed to persuade states and Congress to pass laws giving patients with life-threatening illnesses access to unapproved INDs. The RTT law provided a second pathway for compassionate use in the United States. By 2018, 40 states had passed forms of RTT legislation, with Alaska becoming the 41st, passing the RTT law 2 months after the federal law was signed. By January 2019, there were two examples of the use of RTT requests. The RTT pathway is similar in many ways to expanded access; however, the RTT differs from current expanded-access programs in that review and approval by the FDA and an IRB are not required [14], and there is no requirement for reporting adverse events, or safety/efficacy data to the FDA. The RTT pathway is similar to compassionate-use programs outside of the United States, in that it is viewed as a way to provide access to unapproved drugs for the treatment of patients with serious or life-threatening diseases, and not used for data collection due to the lack of reporting requirements. The responsibility for oversight lies with the treating physician to certify that the patient must have:

- been diagnosed with a life-threatening disease or condition; and
- exhausted approved treatment options and is unable to participate in a clinical trial involving the eligible investigational drug (this must be certified by a physician who is in good standing with their licensing organization or board and who will not be compensated directly by the manufacturer for certifying).

In some states (Arizona, Florida, Ohio, Oregon, and Virginia), RTT laws require a second physician to confirm the diagnosis and/or prognosis of the patient, but these laws do not require that the second physician agrees with the decision to use the IND.

It is entirely up to the company developing the investigational product as to whether they will participate in an expanded-access or RTT request. The RTT law removes any liability on the part of the manufacturer for providing access or choosing not to provide access via this pathway. The key elements of both the RTT and expanded-access pathways are outlined in Table 26.1.

26.7 Relationship to Research

Enrollment in clinical trials is preferred whenever possible for patients to gain access to INDs. Single-patient (n-of-1) trials are particularly useful for situations where randomized clinical trial participation is not feasible or appropriate, such as for patients with rare diseases, co-morbid conditions that exclude eligibility, or for life-threatening diseases without DMT options available [15]. The CDER currently receives over 1,000 applications

Table 26.1 Key differences between single-patient expanded-access and RTT pathways

	Expanded access	RTT
Patient eligibility	Immediately life-threatening or serious disease or condition	Life-threatening disease or condition
	No other treatment or research options (including eligibility for clinical trials)	No treatment options; not eligible for clinical trial of the investigational drug or biologic of interest
Required support	Treating physician	Treating physician
	Manufacturer or sponsor	Manufacturer or sponsor
	FDA	
	IRB	
Drug or biological eligibility	No restrictions	Completed a Phase 1 trial and in current clinical development
Charging regulations	This pathway allows charging only for direct costs; documentation must be submitted to the FDA	This pathway allows charging only for direct costs; however, the requirements for documentation are unclear
Informed consent	Requirements in the CFR must be met	Written consent is required, but specific requirements are unclear

From Chapman et al. [14]. Permission granted for use.

for expanded access each year. The majority are for single patients, non-emergency use, and the vast majority, 99.7%, are allowed to proceed [16]. In a review of the FDA expanded-access data from 2010–2014, 5,394 unique patient expanded-access IND applications were submitted, and 408 were requests for access to unique drugs or drug combinations [17]. The expanded-access pathway, although designed for access, can impact drug development and approval. Over the past 5 years, the three centers that oversee pre-market development in the FDA, the CDER, Center for Biologics Evaluation and Research, and the Center for Devices and Radiological Health, have authorized approximately 9,000 applications through the expanded-access programs with 98% of requests of all expanded-access application types authorized to proceed [7]. A study of the CDER from the fiscal years 2010–2014 showed that 20% of INDs used in expanded-access applications received marketing approval within 1 year from the initial submission, and 33% were approved by 5 years from the initial submission [17].

26.8 Role of Expanded Access in the AD Drug-Development Ecosystem

The top 10 review divisions that received expanded-access INDs account for 95% of all expanded-access INDs. A review of expanded-access IND filings since 2010 show the top five review divisions were for antiviral, anti-infective, hematology, oncology, and gastroenterology, with neurology products accounting for 2% of expanded-access INDs [17]. A review of ClinicalTrials.gov for registered expanded-access studies in AD shows one single-patient expanded-access study, three intermediate-sized studies for subjects that completed the clinical trial, and one cancelled study. Although neurology products have not been a common expanded-access filing, the similarities between AD and oncology make expanded access a potential pathway for a patients with AD to access an IND and facilitate early drug development.

The parallels between cancer and AD include:

(1) incurable disease;
(2) limited treatments available; and
(3) often, the disease is diagnosed at a late stage and patients are not eligible for the current early-stage focus.

The challenges of AD clinical trials, both in enrollment and in costs, have resulted in a slow drug-development process for DMTs. With more than 121 therapies currently in the drug-development pipeline, the urgency to gather early biomarker, proof-of-concept, and safety data makes the expanded-access pathway for AD drug development a potential mechanism to facilitate the drug-development process. Expanded-access studies offer unique opportunities to gather clinically meaningful, patient-centered data, including patient-reported outcomes such as patient satisfaction, piloting of new technology that can measure quality of life and patient burden factors. Expanded-access studies are significantly less costly than randomized clinical trials, and may benefit smaller biotech and drug manufacturers that are financially limited in development programs and without data to support further development and investments. The expanded-access process is uniquely dependent upon multiple stakeholders and provides a collaborative approach between patients, physicians, and industry. Expanded-access in AD drug development may provide a fast-track for drug development as well as an increased sense of hope and advancement of the drug-development process.

References

1. Alzheimer's Association. 2020 Alzheimer's disease facts and figures. *Alzheimers Dement* 2020; **16**: 391–460.

2. Cummings J, Lee G, Ritter A, Sabbagh M, Zhong K. Alzheimer's disease drug development pipeline: 2019. *Alzheimers Dement (N Y)* 2019; **5**: 272–93.

3. Food and Drug Administration. Project Facilitate: assisting healthcare providers with expanded access requests for investigational oncology products. Available at: www.fda.gov/about-fda/oncology-center-excellence/project-facilitate (accessed October 31, 2020).

4. Jarlow JP, Moscicki R. Impact of expanded access on FDA regulatory action and product labeling. *Ther Innov Regul Sci* 2017; **51**: 1–2.

5. Food and Drug Administration. Expanded access to investigational drugs for treatment use: final rule. *Fed Regist* 2009; **74**: 40900–45.

6. Food and Drug Administration. FDA backgrounder on FDAMA. Available at: www.fda.gov/regulatory-information/food-and-drug-administration-modernization-act-fdama-1997/fda-backgrounder-fdama (accessed October 31, 2020).

7. Food and Drug Administration. Expanded Access Program Report. 2018. Available at: www.fda.gov/

8. Center for Drug Evaluation and Research. CDER NextGen Portal. Available at: https://edm.fda.gov/ (accessed October 31, 2020).

9. Food and Drug Administration. 21st Century Cures Act. Available at: www.fda.gov/regulatory-information/selected-amendments-fdc-act/21st-century-cures-act (accessed October 31, 2020).

10. Center for Drug Evaluation and Research. *Guidance for Industry: Expanded Access to Investigational Drugs for Treatment Use-Questions and Answers*, Maryland: FDA; 2017.

11. Jarow JP, Lurie P, Crowley Ikenberry S, Lemery S. Overview of FDA's expanded access program for investigational drugs. *Ther Innov Regul Sci* 2017; **51**: 177–9.

12. Borysowski J, Ehni H-J, Górski A. Ethics review in compassionate use. *BMC Med* 2017; **15**: 136–42.

13. Food and Drug Administration. IRB review of individual patient expanded access requests for investigational drugs and biological products during the COVID-19 public health emergency. June 2020. Available at: www.fda.gov/regulatory-information/search-fda-guidance-documents/institutional-review-board-irb-review-individual-patient-expanded-access-requests-investigational (accessed October 31, 2020).

14. Chapman CR, Eckman J, Bateman-House AS. Oversight of right-to-try and expanded access requests for off-trial access to investigational drugs. *Ethics Hum Res* 2020; **42**: 2–13.

15. Porcino A, Shamseer L, Chan A-W, et al. SPIRIT extension and elaboration for *n*-of-1 trials: SPENT 2019 checklist. *BMJ* 2020; **368**: m122.

16. Jarow JP, Lemery S, Bugin K, Khozin S, Moscicki R. Expanded access of investigational drugs: the experience of the center of drug evaluation and research over a 10-year period. *Ther Innov Regul Sci* 2016; **50**: 705–9.

17. McKee AE, Markon AO, Chan-Tack KM, Lurie P. How often are drugs made available under the Food and Drug Administration's expanded access process approved? *J Clin Pharmacol* 2017; **57**: S136–42.

media/119971/download (accessed October 31, 2020).

The Role of the Contract Research Organization in Alzheimer's Disease: The Vital Link in the Clinical Drug-Development Program

John J. Sramek, Henry Riordan, Michael F. Murphy, and
Neal R. Cutler

27.1 Introduction

Neurodegeneration resulting in Alzheimer's disease (AD) is the main type of dementia encountered and is a crisis not only for the patient and family but also for society [1]. Currently approved therapies provide only modest symptomatic improvement but fail to halt the unrelenting progression of the disease [2]. Research into the mechanisms underlying AD has been painfully slow. Although research has revealed a complex pathogenesis, it has nonetheless consistently pointed to abnormalities in amyloid and tau processing, giving hope that disease-modifying agents (DMAs) that affect these proteins may be on the horizon, which can halt the progression of neurodegeneration. To date, clinical trials with DMAs have failed to show consistent results but have also spurred the refinement of new agents and a critical examination of study processes, with a focus on early AD subtypes which may show better therapeutic response to DMA interventions. While it is a Herculean task to develop new therapies, it is also now clear that attention to patient selection and study design are also critical to demonstrating their potential.

This chapter reviews the critical role that a contract research organization (CRO) plays in optimizing the promise of new therapeutics. Late-phase AD clinical trials are lengthy (typically 6–18 months), expensive, and require extensive expertise on all fronts, from protocol design to selection of psychometric assessments, multiple choices of imaging technologies, relevant biomarkers, patient recruitment and retention, and relationships with established investigators and regulatory bodies, often on a global basis. Certainly, many small to medium biotechnology companies will be lacking in such expertise, but even large pharmaceutical companies may not have all the tools available at their disposal. A scientifically and medically oriented CRO having both extensive hands-on AD experience as well as applicable expertise can work seamlessly with any size of pharmaceutical company (hereafter termed the sponsor) to execute a nuanced and complex protocol and effectively fulfill the promise of novel AD therapeutics by placing the drug in the experimental milieu that optimizes the chances of success. A good CRO will speed efficiency in trial conduct, such as speed of enrollment, without sacrificing quality, and it will measurably enhance signal detection by careful adherence to well-thought-out study methodology, conduct, and oversight, particularly in regard to valuable neuropsychological outcome measures.

27.2 Definition of the Contract Research Organization

As outlined in Table 27.1, pharmaceutical companies can outsource any number of clinical drug-development infrastructure components, in part or whole, to a CRO, ranging from preclinical to post-marketing services. There are CROs that specialize in providing only one or several services, and those which can virtually span the entire development life cycle. Decades ago, large pharmaceutical companies would routinely undertake the majority of the clinical drug-development components, with typical exception of centralized clinical laboratories, but this became increasingly untenable due to rapidly changing drug pipelines, with a consequent need for specialized staff in new therapeutic areas. Large CROs, with highly trained staff in specialized therapeutic areas, often provide unified services more cost efficiently and

Table 27.1 Overview of CRO clinical drug-development services

	Phase 1	Phase 2	Phase 3	Phase 4
Protocol development	X	X	X	X
Assistance with regulatory bodies	X	X	X	X
Clinical supplies, importation for global studies	X	X	X	X
Healthy volunteers and specialized patient populations	X			
Pharmacy good manufacturing	X			
Investigator sites and established therapeutic experts		X	X	
Site management and budgets	X	X	X	
Site initiation meeting and staff training	X	X	X	
Clinical monitoring	X	X	X	
Data collection; case report forms or electronic monitoring	X	X	X	
Medical monitoring	X	X	X	
Medical writing (protocols, study reports)	X	X	X	
Assistance with patient recruitment and retention		X	X	
Quality assurance		X	X	
Rater training		X	X	
Biostatistics		X	X	
Bioanalytical laboratory tests: method development and validation analysis of clinical and pharmacokinetic samples pharmacokinetic analysis and reports biomarkers	X	X	X	
Post approval services				X
Drug safety and pharmacovigilance				X
Registries and observational studies				X

meet ever-demanding study timelines. Private and academic consortiums are not able to manage and enroll the required number of patients, particularly for protocols having ever-increasing complexity, which is now the norm in AD programs for DMAs. There are currently over 130 compounds in AD clinical trials, of which nearly 100 involve DMAs [3]. This chapter will highlight a number of the specialized services a CRO provides and include examples relevant to AD trials.

27.3 CRO Role in Protocol Design and Development

Clinical development begins with a well-thought-out protocol, but the protocol is merely the template and a number of moving parts must be deftly coordinated in order for the desired outcomes to be realized. A CRO, whose key people have worked in pharmaceutical companies and as investigators, can bring a vast experience based on prior

AD compounds, methodology, outcome, and patient selection criteria. Confirmation of target engagement early in the clinical program, and careful selection of early AD patients – including amnestic mild cognitive impairment and prodromal AD – offer the possibility of enhanced signal detection over later AD stages. Biomarkers, including structural MRI, amyloid and tau imaging, and cerebrospinal fluid (CSF) amyloid-beta 42 ($A\beta_{42}$) and tau determinations, can offer greater precision in defining the study population than cognitive testing alone, although the latter is crucial as well for regulatory approval. The CRO with a solid history of AD expertise can help guide sponsors on optimal biomarker selection and the employment of cognitive measures that are sensitive to change, as well as carefully thought-out inclusion/exclusion criteria which are compatible with both research and clinical care, helping to foster both patient recruitment and retention. Novel study designs, introducing biomarkers early in the clinical program, and integrating study phases can also be contemplated. For example, Cummings et al. have advocated for early studies that integrate the objectives of both Phase 1 (tolerability) and Phase 2 (initial efficacy). Likewise, adaptive designs, using ongoing data to feed back into protocol design and guide modifications, such as the elimination of a study treatment arm or modifying the length of the study, can result in greater overall efficiency toward achieving study objectives [4, 5]. A protocol must address the primary, secondary, and exploratory objectives with precision, but it is only a template for a comprehensive systems approach that entails many nuances and adjustments which invariably must be made along its execution. The right CRO works as a partner with the sponsor to help guide all the processes that will unfold before and during study conduct. This also includes advice on regulatory investigational new drug submissions and regulatory meetings which often focus on safety monitoring.

An innovative, flexible, and responsive CRO can also structure the protocol to facilitate transitions within phases, which saves valuable time. For example, a good CRO can facilitate a smooth transition between single- and multiple-dose cohorts of AD patients in a late Phase 1 multi-center study with demanding entrance criteria, by creating a virtual waiting room of eligible patients who could be enrolled simultaneously into a single cohort across the sites, while continuing to recruit for the next cohort. Proprietary interactive response programming technology ensures that desired cohort metrics, such as AD severity and gender, are uniformly distributed across all cohorts [6]. An advantage of this methodology is that sites do not have to be shut down and started back up, and the time between cohorts is minimized.

27.4 Site Selection

Prior to selecting sites, the CRO will typically undertake a blinded feasibility assessment of the protocol with potential study sites. This primarily assesses how the protocol assessments and procedures will impact patient recruitment and study execution; findings will be discussed with the sponsor to determine whether any aspects of the protocol can be potentially modified to improve these parameters, long before study launch, and may reduce the need for time-consuming protocol amendments. Of particular interest is prior

experience in AD trials that the site has conducted, in specific AD subtypes similar to those sought in the upcoming study. Site capabilities, access to quality scale raters, neuroimaging, enrollment metrics, and potential institutional review board (IRB) issues will also be reviewed. After a site is vetted on a preliminary basis, the CRO may execute a confidentiality agreement with the site for more detailed discussions, budget approval, and IRB review; these last two issues, if not handled properly, can cause significant delays in getting a site ready to begin recruiting patients [7]. A CRO that has wide experience in AD trials will have many established investigator relationships, but even these need to be reviewed systematically to ensure that the site has access to the AD phenotype required for the trial, as well as no competing interests that would hamper patient enrollment. Of note, studies compete with each other in terms of enrollment of appropriate patients but also compete in terms of securing access to the best site staff, and the CRO is uniquely qualified to assess the true number of competitive studies and workload at a given site. The CRO may also seek advice on the protocol from opinion leaders, who will be valuable to the sponsor for their scientific input as well as for future endorsements and recognition in the medical and neurological community, such as through scientific publications and presentations.

27.5 Study Planning and Site Initiation

Once the protocol has been solidified and potential sites selected, the CRO works to put a large number of logistics in place for study execution, including expert medical monitors, project managers, capable and experienced clinical research associates (CRAs), development of case report forms, IRB approvals, clinical and laboratory study supplies, drug depots for storage, and biostatistical plans. The protocol schedule of study events will be carefully reviewed and tested for smooth progression and to minimize – for example, with psychometric testing – patient fatigue by careful construction of the types and order of psychometric measures. Optimally, the sponsor will also oversee this background work, which will drill down to the smallest detail.

For a large-scale multi-center study, an initiation meeting will occur so that sites are crystal clear on the often-complex protocol procedures, inherent timelines for study visits, and the need for good documentation. With the demanding inclusion and exclusion criteria increasingly common in AD studies of DMAs with accompanying high screen fail rates, sites will often face many recruitment challenges, which an AD-focused CRO can navigate to avoid dismal screen failure rates. The elderly AD population will also have a number of medical co-morbidities and be receiving multiple prescription and over-the-counter medications. Protocols which allow or even mandate the prior use of acetylcholinesterase inhibitors and memantine can positively affect recruitment rate. A detailed patient history – particularly for patients new to a site – will consume much time and effort. A successful strategy, however, can be employed to "prescreen" potential subjects prior to their first visit, so that the most common reasons for study exclusion can be quickly identified [8]. A hierarchical approach to patient eligibility can be employed so that less costly procedures are performed first. As an example, one can also conduct brief memory assessments by telephone (for example, episodic memory), which can be supplemented by home-based computer testing prior to the visit. Such an approach can decrease the screen failure rate in a complex prodromal AD study from the expected 80% to less than 50%. In recent years, late-phase AD global trials investigating changes in cognition have seen significant increases in cognitive screen failure rates. Involving cognitive and therapeutic experts, as part of a cognitive task force, leads to substantial mitigation of these increases in screen failures. Prior studies utilizing this methodology have shown an average 24% reduction in screen failure rates, significantly reducing recruitment timelines, overall study cost, and patient burdens.

The CRO can also assist with recruitment strategies, including community outreach, social media, and forums, in order to promote study awareness and boost referrals [9]. Ongoing discussions will assist sites to retain enrolled patients in the study, streamline procedural events to avoid patient fatigue, deal with behavioral problems that can arise in this population, and engage caregivers effectively throughout the often-lengthy study duration [10]. If a specific AD subtype is sought, it will be important that sites do not enroll patients who could dilute the effect of a highly targeted therapeutic approach, and the sponsor may consider having the CRO implement a centralized

recruitment program wherein third-party experts give the final sign-off on a potential candidate prior to randomization. Our group implemented such an approach in a large double-blinded controlled trial in mild AD, preventing 11% of subjects cleared by the sites for randomization from entering the study and potentially negatively impacting the reliability of the data [11].

Above all, the site initiation meeting begins the process of communication between the site and CRO personnel, so that ongoing issues can be resolved efficiently and effectively. The CRO develops a clear plan for the escalation and resolution of issues to be referred to the CRO experts best able to deal with such issues in a most expeditious manner so that no momentum is lost on the part of the site. The site initiation also – even if quite familiar to established investigators – reviews the basics of good clinical practice (GCP), including ethical conduct and benefit–risk assessment [12]. Patient confidentiality will also be paramount in AD studies, in as much as a number of outcome measures such as imaging and biomarkers will be done by outside vendors, and the CRO must ensure confidentiality in the coding of transmitted data.

Beyond a review of study procedures during the site initiation visit, the CRO must ensure that site staff are trained to carry out the full range of study procedures, from dispensing study medications, to packaging and shipping biological samples, to delicate and complex tasks such as drawing a CSF sample for biomarkers. A CSF procedure would normally be conducted by an experienced neurologist, and the CRO can assist to ensure that it is done in a controlled and safe environment. As an example, our CRO is very experienced with this procedure, whether single or serial CSF sampling, and has an informative video that the site reviews to reinforce the proper technique, puncture site, needle size, types of collection vials, and management of potential (although rare) complications.

27.6 Site Monitoring

Site monitoring is carried out on a regular basis by the CRO's capable and experienced CRAs. Monitoring will normally be more intensive as the first patients are screened and enrolled but, in any case, the project manager will adjust the schedule depending upon feedback from the CRA as well as from ongoing data entry and management. Adhering to GCP, CRAs assess the quality and completeness of written documentation, and have ongoing discussions with the principal investigator and other staff regarding inclusion and exclusion criteria as it pertains to individual subjects. The CRA reviews all data, including completeness of the informed consent and prior medical and drug history, ensures there are no conflicts internally within the documentation, and that confidentiality has been preserved. A proactive approach should be employed throughout, so that protocol deviations and, most importantly, protocol violations can assiduously be avoided. Rapid communication between study staff and the CRO is essential to prevent any deviations and can best be accomplished by establishing rapid communication escalation schemes so that the site receives timely and precise feedback from experts within the CRO and, if necessary, the sponsor.

The US Food and Drug Administration (FDA) has strongly advocated that such a proactive monitoring approach is necessary for ensuring patient safety throughout conduct of the study [13], combining on-site monitoring with centralized CRO and sponsor activities which can flexibly adjust to changes in risks that are identified as the study progresses. This could involve special attention to potential risks that were identified in preclinical and early human testing, as well as those that occur either by extension or unexpectedly as the study progresses. A well-conceived plan can then adjust monitoring activities across sites to better define and detect such risks as new information is available. The CRO must have definitive data management technologies in place and possess strong AD therapeutic experience to continually assess and adjust to any new development in risk. In the best sense, the CRO's approach to monitoring is simultaneously a systems-wide and a reductive approach: while monitoring ensures that all the boxes are checked, it also continually loops feedback from the site to the CRO and sponsor and back again, and disseminates findings that are important to other sites in the study.

Risk-based monitoring (RBM) is a technique that has emerged in recent years in central nervous system clinical trials and has particular application in AD trials. RBM differentiates from the traditional approach of frequent on-site visits and 100% source-data verification (SDV). It implements a blended monitoring model assuming reduced SDV and a continuous risk assessment based on findings from on-site and remote data reviews. This approach allows for proper oversight, ongoing

data surveillance, and a flexible site-visit schedule, tailored to enable extra time for high enrolling sites or sites that require more attention due to a higher rate of data queries or compliance issues. A central monitoring group consisting of several functional groups, such as a project manager, a clinical statistician, a medical monitor, and site management, establishes a central monitoring group committee, which serves as the central risk-detection and mitigation team. The central monitoring group collects and reviews metrics and data trends generated and drives mitigation actions including the on-site monitoring-visit schedule and frequency.

The RBM approach assures adequate and cost-effective oversight and execution of the trial; the reduction in study costs are realized by the decreased number of site visits and related travel pass-through costs. Sites also welcome the RBM approach as it decreases the burden on them from time-consuming monitoring visits. Regulatory authorities including the FDA are also recognizing the value of RBM to improve the conduct of clinical studies. As many AD studies include multiple rating scales as part of the clinical assessments, those rating scales are often performed/completed on electronic tablets. Most clinical assessment technology vendors collaborate with data management to develop and implement specific data flags. Those data flags together with RBM and a centralized data collection have been found very successful in recent trials as they have enabled the identification of signals which indicate potential challenges with the data quality and integrity.

Virtual patient site visits have increased of late, owing to the COVID-19 global pandemic, and are also applicable, especially for patients with advanced dementia who are not flexible for travel times to a site, or who live in remote areas. Trial activities taking place at home for dementia patients can include a complete safety assessment, the tracking of concomitant medication, vital signs, routine physical examinations and electrocardiogram (ECG), blood and urine sampling, conduct of clinical assessments, and investigational product administration including home infusions, as well as many other study-related assessments. Technology systems such as electronic clinical outcome assessments and/or electronic patient-reported outcomes to support simplified site workflows facilitate real-data availability for CROs and sponsors. Digital health technologies that can support virtual patient site visits can assist the remote monitoring visit and ensure real-time clinical data and data integrity while safeguarding patient safety by continuous tracking of safety data and adverse events.

Yet virtualized clinical trials also come with challenges. As more patient data are available electronically, patient privacy can be at risk and the CRO should ensure that no patient identifiers reach the sponsor. One should also not under-estimate the importance of face-to-face contact between the doctor and the patient and therefore a videoconference or video call, if permitted by the local regulations, should be the preferred method for performing the patient tele-visit. Where local regulations and patient consent permits, video calls can be recorded so that a participant's body language and facial expressions can be captured along with their responses to questions. It is impor-tant that sponsors partner with a CRO to carefully design the virtual model that will be used for the specific needs of their study. The ability to be flex-ible and innovative is a key.

27.7　Rater Training

The CRO must ensure that site raters are experi-enced, capable (Master's degree or higher), and skilled to evaluate potential patients with the neu-ropsychiatric measures that will be employed in a given study. These measures serve two main func-tions: to assess disease severity and as outcome measures of efficacy.

A good CRO should be facile in a variety of rater training methods, depending upon the situ-ation, including: training at the investigator meet-ing; self-paced web portal training, which entails raters reviewing didactic presentations and videos, and then taking subsequent quizzes on a special project website; on-site face-to-face training pro-vided by an expert rater; group web-based confer-ence training where a number of sites attend a live presentation simultaneously; and individualized web-based conference training, which entails an individual rater or site attending a live presentation given by an expert rater [14]. In order to determine the relative superiority of five selective training methods on data accuracy operationalized in a blinded review of deviation, violation, and query rates, various rater training methodologies were evaluated across two early-phase double-blinded, randomized, placebo-controlled clinical trials, which were designed to assess the effects of a novel drug on AD. Rater errors were examined by clini-cians' review of the data as well as electronic data

capture (EDC) database queries. From a total num-ber of 36 sites, data from 143 raters across 5 coun-tries were evaluated and included in the analyses. Sites whose raters were trained during an on-site visit by the expert rater yielded minimal EDC data queries regarding the clinical assessments, with no deviations or violations identified by the clini-cian review of the assessment data. On-site rater training provided by an expert rater appears to be the most effective method of ensuring data are captured correctly in a timely fashion, using query rates and severity as the dependent measure.

Regardless of the type of training it is important for the CRO staff to not only oversee initial train-ing, such that the raters fully understand the rating concepts and techniques, but also provide ongo-ing sessions to prevent rating drift internally and between study sites [15]. Subtle differences in scor-ing on crucial ratings can lead to high screen failure rates, which can greatly increase the cost of a multi-center trial. For example, our CRO was called in on an ongoing multi-center study because the screen failure rate was very high, and few patients had been randomized during the first months of the study. Our neuropsychologist and team found that sites were wrongly interpreting scoring on free and cued recall measures, which primarily led to the high screen failure rate. After 5 weeks of meetings and teleconferences with site raters, the randomi-zation rate increased over four-fold compared to the same pre-training period. Thus, it is important that initial training also be followed up throughout the study by expert psychologists, using site visits and also cost-effective supplementary measures such as teleconferences and web-based seminars.

27.8　Challenges in Global AD Studies

When a CRO facilitates a large global trial – often a necessity for enrolling large study numbers and for future regulatory considerations – the accompany-ing challenges escalate exponentially compared to a single-country trial. Of course, the CRO must already have experienced personnel on the ground and regional offices globally, established relation-ships with known investigators and regulatory agencies, and be aware of differences in standard of care and cultural practices across the various countries and continents. Nonetheless, even with known investigators, the CRO should ensure that processes are in place that facilitate smooth study

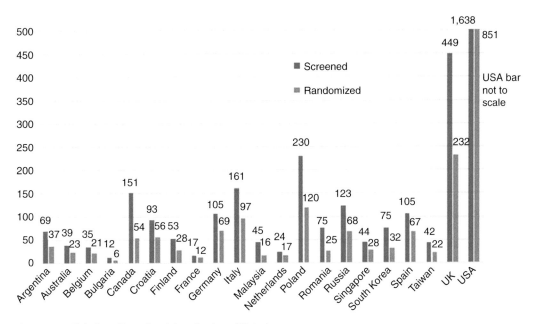

Figure 27.1 Global enrollment breakdown in a large AD study.

conduct in the event key staff leave a site in the middle of the trial. However large the CRO is, it must also rely on established outside expertise to provide quality laboratory and imaging services, or language-translation services. Specialty analytical laboratories will often be initiated by the sponsor early in development of an AD compound, and the CRO will often need to incorporate such vendors into the global program. We have found that a governance model with preferred providers works well to drive compliance, timelines, and quality of the service. Service-level agreements are put in place which hold external providers accountable for deliverables. As an example of the extent with which an AD study is conducted on a global basis, see Figure 27.1, which summarizes enrollment in a large AD study (over 1,300 patients randomized) conducted by our CRO across the United States, UK, Canada, Europe, South America, Australia, and various Asian countries.

The extensive planning for a global trial requires, first, that the CRO ensures its various internal project teams are well structured and managed, and that information processes are in place for timely updates to all teams and sites. Second, the CRO must have all external vendors in place for laboratory, drug supply depots, imaging, translations, regulatory, advertising, and other needs. For study drug needs, vendors who can perform packaging, labeling, distribution, and storage needs on a global basis are used, pending

verification that they also have robust processes in place to navigate import and export processes, and have a network to facilitate distribution. There are many nuances in this process, as these vendors may hold different licenses in different geographical regions depending upon the classification (i.e., schedule) of the study drug. AD trials often require engaging specialty vendors for imaging services, including those who specialize in the morphometric quantification of various brain structures and the presence of amyloid-related imaging abnormalities (ARIA) through standard MRI protocols, as well as other more novel imaging techniques such as magnetization transfer imaging, and magnetic resonance spectroscopy. All vendor services need to be constantly monitored for quality and all activities synchronized such that data transfer to the CRO occurs in a timely fashion to ensure that any remaining monitoring queries at the conclusion of the study can be resolved prior to database lock.

27.9 Overcoming Operational Complications: The Impact of the COVID-19 Crisis on a Large Global Multi-center AD Trial

The COVID-19 pandemic created enormous disruptions in most economic areas, including the delivery of medical care, especially to elderly and

315

frail populations. Our CRO was in the midst of conducting a placebo-controlled study of a novel DMA with the goal of randomizing over 1,500 patients across 14 countries and 250 investigator sites when the pandemic occurred. This is a challenging study with strict neuropsychiatric entry requirements in patients with mild cognitive impairment or mild AD confirmed by positron emission tomography (PET) or CSF amyloid assessment and stratified by current AD medications and apolipoprotein-E ε4 status, with safety MRI scans at predefined time points. Patients receive study medication by intravenous infusion regularly for the 18-month trial period, with the option for further open-label extension. Aside from travel restrictions and lockdowns in most countries, such as Italy, there was initially great difficulty obtaining personal protective equipment and intravenous supplies needed by the investigator sites.

Our CRO quickly devised action plans, in conjunction with the sponsor, and drafted protocol amendments for IRB approval, which extended the screening period, allowed for home infusions and remote clinical assessments in places where site visits were not an option, and provided guidance on visual or phone visits and in-home clinical assessments, with raters often assisted by the in-home infusion nurse. A priority was given to safety checks, vital signs, and sample collections. Third-party vendors were contracted in only several weeks to accomplish these measures, which also provided for deployment of MRI scanners and central ECG, as well as travel arrangements for patient visits and shipment of tracers for the PET studies.

Tremendous efforts were expended to put these plans into action, aided by adaptability of the CRO to increase enrollment efforts in countries that were less affected by the pandemic. The results were very successful given the circumstances: while study screens were down about 50% during the worst period (mid-March to mid-May 2020) compared to the earlier period, they had rebounded to about 75% of pre-pandemic levels by mid-June; study randomizations had decreased by about 10% during this worst period, but were back to 100% of pre-pandemic levels by mid-June. This success was a direct result of the excellent communication streams between the CRO, sponsor, and sites, and could only have been realized by a CRO staff with unwavering dedication to their work.

27.10 Study Flow and Communication

The CRO will undertake extensive planning, in conjuncture with the sponsor, well prior to initiating any study conduct. Key CRO personnel will know what issues need advance attention, for example, which potential sites are not close to imaging centers and will need transportation assistance for patients in order to maintain study timelines. If PET imaging studies are involved, plans for transporting key ligands to sites at the correct time must be put in place well in advance. Ideally, the CRO builds a close working partnership with the sponsor. This requires purposeful and frequent communication, often daily, particularly before and during the early start-up phase of the study when metrics reviewed by the CRO manager and sponsor typically concern site selection, budgets, and contracts. As the study moves forward, the communication metrics shift toward enrollment and enrollment projections, protocol deviations, and recruitment and retention. Patient caregivers are often key to retention, and plans must be formulated in advance to accommodate their needs, especially in light of long study visits (sometimes up to 6 hours) and study duration (6–18 months). The CRO must also develop close ties with the sites, in order to quickly identify sites that are not screening or enrolling within predetermined timelines and offer assistance, although some sites may need to be closed down if they cannot improve within a given timeframe.

CRAs who visit the site frequently to monitor study data also work closely with the investigator and site staff to assure timely data entry and query resolution; CRAs constantly work to remind staff, without being a nuisance. Especially at a time of global pandemic, there may be missed or partial visits which the CRAs need to quickly identify; teleconferencing can be used so that key assessments can be secured. Additionally, the CRO will often suggest that a key sponsor executive – such as the vice president of clinical development – also participates with sites from time to time in order to keep scientific momentum and motivation high. When it comes to finally terminating the study, the CRO ensures that all data are complete prior to data lock. In one study of over 1,000 AD patients, our CRO was able to accomplish this within 10 days after the last completed patient; statistics on key study outcomes (such as the Clinical Dementia Rating scale and Clinician Interview-Based Impression of Change) were then available only 3 days later. CRO medical writers also need to plan in advance by aligning to sponsor standard operating procedures for study reports and communicating with appropriate sponsor personnel so that these reports can be completed without delay.

27.11   CROs in the AD Development Ecosystem

It is well understood that those who labor in research have an obligation to advance science in their field, and the work of a CRO is no exception. With wide-ranging experience across multiple study drugs and methodologies, a CRO working in the AD spectrum should seek to constantly improve study design and conduct to enhance signal detection. Even if results are not always published, past lessons can be put to advantage in future trials as the true advantage of a CRO comes in its vast experience and facility in clinical trial methodology. A CRO's website should include a listing of scientific publications and presentations that reflect its innovative and creative contributions to AD research. CROs should also look to the larger picture, bridging the gap between research and clinical practice. Randomized clinical trials are constructed to optimize signal detection, but results may not transfer to the broader AD population who may be excluded from participation based on co-morbid illnesses, excluded medications, or behavior. We have advocated to bridge this gap by creating real-world evidence studies which link the fragmented research data sets to model a virtual study population or create protocols which extend certain key observations on those who fail screening or drop out early [16]. We have also advocated using emerging digital technologies to create a master global AD data repository in an effort to increase the generalizability of AD data [17].

27.12   Conclusion

We have endeavored in this brief chapter to emphasize the important role a CRO can play in AD drug development as a trusted agent of the sponsor. While we have highlighted various CRO functions performed before and during a trial, it is likely evident that there is a great deal of overlap among the various activities, which are linked by planning, communication, and ongoing evaluation of methodology. For a successful study, all the elements of

science, medicine, operations, logistics, and communication must be firmly in place, and constantly monitored from a medical and scientific perspective infused with a strong desire and drive to combat the tragedy of this dreadful disease.

Acknowledgment

The authors thank Irene Chalofti, Natalia Drosopoulou, Andrew Kuhlman, Stephen Coates, and Tom Doherty for their assistance. Correspondence should be sent to Neal R. Cutler, MD, Worldwide Clinical Trials, 401 N. Maple Dr., Beverly Hills, CA 90210, neal.cutler@worldwide .com.

References

1. Oxford AE, Stewart ES, Rohn TT. Clinical trials in Alzheimer's disease: a hurdle in the path of remedy. *Int J Alzheimers Dis* 2020; **2020**: 5380346.

2. Murphy MF, Sramek JJ, Kurtz NM, et al. *Alzheimer's Disease: Optimizing the Development of the Next Generation of Therapeutic Compounds.* Oxford: Oxford University Press; 1998.

3. Cummings J, Lee G, Ritter A, et al. AD drug development pipeline: 2019. *Alzheimers Dement (NY)* 2019; **5**: 272–93.

4. Cummings J, Aisen P, DuBois B, et al. Drug development in AD: the path to 2015. *Alzheimers Res Ther* 2016; **8**: 39.

5. Satlin A, Wang J, Logovinsky V, et al. Design of a Bayesian adaptive Phase 2 proof-of-concept trial for BAN2401, a putative disease-modifying monoclonal antibody for the treatment of Alzheimer's disease. *Alzheimers Dement (N Y)* 2016; **2**: 1–12.

6. House A, Drosopoulou NE, Riordan HJ. Technology-assisted cohort optimization of early phase multi-centre patient studies. *Int Pharmaceut Ind* 2017; **9**: 46–9.

7. Krafcik BM, Doros G, Malikova MA. A single center analysis of factors influencing study start-up timeline in clinical trials. *Future Sci OA* 2017; **3**: FS0223.

8. Babic T, Riordan HJ. Improving screen failure and recruitment rates in AD clinical trials. *J Clin Stud* 2016; **8**: 38–40.

9. Watson JL, Ryan L, Silverberg N, et al. Obstacles and opportunities in Alzheimer's clinical trial recruitment. *Health Aff* 2014; **33**: 574–9.

10. Zupancic B. Driving patient engagement in alzheimer disease clinical research to achieve trial success. *World Pharma Today* 2017. Available at: www.worldpharmatoday.com/Articles/ driving-patient-engagement-in-alzheimer-s-

disease-clinical-research-to-achieve-trial-success/ (accessed December 9, 2020).

11. Carbo MA, Rock C, Doyle K, et al. An evaluation of independent subject eligibility review to ensure enrollment of high-quality appropriate subjects in mild Alzheimer's disease. Alzheimer's Association International Conference, Chicago, IL, July 2018.

12. World Health Organization. Handbook for good clinical research practice. Available at: https:// apps.who.int/iris/handle/10665/43392 (accessed December 9, 2020).

13. Food and Drug Administration. Guidance for industry. Oversight of clinical investigations: a risk-based approach to monitoring. August 2013. Available at: www.fda.gov/regulatory-information/ search-fda-guidance-documents/oversight-clinical-investigations-risk-based-approach-monitoring (accessed December 9, 2020).

14. Kornsey E, Friedmann B, Bartolic E, et al. An examination into the effects of five rater training modalities on the project conduct in international AD trials. International Society for CNS Clinical Trials and Methodology Meeting, Marina Del Ray, CA, Oct 1–3, 2012.

15. Avrumson R, Carbo MA, Riordan HJ, et al. Effectiveness of rater training and data surveillance in Alzheimer disease clinical trials. Clinical Trials in Alzheimer's Disease (CTAD) Congress, Boston, MA, November 2017.

16. Riordan HJ, Perakslis E, Roosz S, et al. Utilizing large data sets and extended trial observation to close the AD evidence gap. *J Clin Stud* 2019; **11**: 46–50.

17. Perakslis E, Riordan H, Friedhoff L, et al. A call for a global 'bigger' data approach to Alzheimer disease. *Nat Rev Drug Discov* 2019; **18**: 319–20.

Chapter 28

The Role of Regulatory Agencies in Alzheimer's Disease Drug Development

Cristina Sampaio and Swati Sathe

28.1 Introduction

Alzheimer's disease (AD) is a neurodegenerative disease of high prevalence and incidence, particularly in populations older than 65, which is the fastest-growing population subset in Western countries as discussed elsewhere in this book. AD is humanly and financially devastating at personal, family, and societal level. AD consequences can only be mitigated by preventing or delaying the pathogenic process (secondary prevention) and treating the symptoms. Public health measures aiming at primary prevention and physio or cognitive therapies do not need approval from a regulatory agency. Still, all other means of interventions, here generically designated as "drugs" (small molecules, antibodies, gene therapy, and medical devices) do.

The regulatory requirements of a future license tailor the drug development, defined as the process of bringing a new drug to the market once a lead compound has been identified through the process of drug discovery. The hope for curtailing AD consequences hangs on successful drug developments, which are dependent on the existence of validated targets, drugs being able to action those targets and elicit a clinically relevant effect, and sponsors willing to invest time and money into their developments.

Until Biogen's controversial submission to the US Food and Drug Administration (FDA) of aducanumab for the treatment of mild AD in 2020 [1], and its subsequent accelerated approval, there had been no other submissions since 2002 when memantine was approved to treat mild-to-moderate AD in 2006 by the European Medicines Agency (EMA) [2]. In 2019, the Chinese National Medical Products Agency (NMPA) conditionally approved the Green Valley Pharmaceuticals drug, Oligomannate, but the supporting efficacy data are limited [3]. This time lag of 18 years means that all regulatory interactions in the field of AD in almost two decades happened outside the formal review processes that lead to acceptance or rejection of marketing authorization. Such a long period without a single submission for marketing authorization is relevant because regulatory requirements are usually standardized based on success cases. In AD drug development, the success cases consisted of modest benefit in treating the disease symptoms. This paradigm does not translate well when the goal is to demonstrate a delay in the progression of a pathogenic process. Standardized regulatory requirements provide reassurance to the sponsors but frequently clash with what can be done in practice given current clinical and scientific circumstances. These tensions have a positive side because they act as a catalyst for developing new regulatory paradigms. The FDA [4], EMA [5], and the Japanese Pharmaceuticals and Medical Devices Agency (PMDA) [6] showed they have a good understanding of the AD field evolution by issuing the recent guidance documents (2016, 2018) for drug development in early AD disease before the dementia stage, embracing the amyloid, tau, and neurodegeneration (A/T/N) classification [7] and dropping the efficacy requirement of two co-primary endpoints for trials in early disease phases. These changes are critical forward steps in resolving roadblocks in AD drug development that are linked to difficulties in showing drug effects in clinically relevant measures when the disease process has not advanced to the point of determining more than subtle clinical manifestations.

In this chapter, we review the existing regulatory guidance documents that inform clinical development for AD. We characterize the mechanisms of interaction with the regulatory agencies outside the formal review of a license dossier. We also describe the structure, function, and scope of the large and well-recognized regulatory agencies – the FDA, EMA, PMDA – as well as the emergent NMPA (former "FDA-CHINA"). We choose these agencies, all of which are members of the International Conference of Harmonization (ICH; www.ich.org), because of the substantial contributions they have made for regulatory science and their impact in significant markets. However, we should recognize that the world is now globalized, and there are many critical initiatives for international cooperation in regulatory matters. In addition to the work coordinated by the World Health Organization (WHO), the ICH, the Pharmaceutical Inspection Co-operation Scheme (PIC/S), the International Pharmaceutical Regulators Forum (IPRF), and the International Coalition of Medicines Regulatory Authorities (ICMRA) are examples of this growing number of international regulatory initiatives. "Connecting the dots" is an EMA-led project that maps international cooperative projects in four nuclear regulatory areas of interest: supply-chain integrity, crises management, pharmacovigilance, and information technology systems. There is an apparent global effort toward harmonization and cooperation [8].

A fundamental process associated with drug development is reimbursement, which determines the true accessibility to a licensed treatment. Reimbursement mechanisms vary substantively across countries and regions. In the European Union, reimbursement is decided at a national level. In general, the regulatory agencies that supervise the licensing are not involved in reimbursement decisions. The analysis of the reimbursement mechanisms is out of the scope of this chapter.

28.2 The Scope of Regulatory Supervision on Drug Development

Regulatory agencies are legal entities empowered to supervise drug development and use to protect public health. As such, the processes by which the supervision is executed are formal and follow well-established rules. Historically, the regulatory formalism and the enormous financial consequences of the regulatory decisions lead to unyielding relationships between regulators and applicants/sponsors. Those interactions used to be enveloped by a courtroom-like atmosphere. During the last decade, a very systematic effort has been made to change that type of interaction between regulators and applicants/sponsors toward a collaborative activity that should, ideally, start very early in the drug-development process and be nurtured along the way toward licensing and beyond. There were essential modifications in the regulatory ecosystem to support the regulatory changes in attitude

and strategy. In the United States, a crucial piece of legislation was the 21st Century Cures Act (Cures Act) [9], signed into law on December 13, 2016, which is designed to help accelerate medical product development and bring innovations and advances to patients who need them, faster and more efficiently.

The Cures Act builds on the FDA's ongoing work to incorporate patients' perspectives into the decision-making process. It enhances the ability to modernize clinical trial designs, including real-world evidence, and clinical outcome assessments, which will speed the development and review of novel medical products. Similarly, in 2015, the European Union (EU) adopted a regulatory science strategy for 2020 [10], which led to the launch of the PRIME (Priority Medicines) scheme to enhance support for the development of medicines that target an unmet medical need. PRIME is a voluntary scheme based on enhanced interaction and early dialog with developers of promising medicines, to optimize development plans and speed up evaluation, to reach patients earlier. In March 2020, the EMA issued an updated regulatory strategy to 2025, to build a more adaptive regulatory system that will encourage innovation in human and veterinary medicine [11].

In Asia, in 2018, the NMPA in China was rebranded from the former CHINA-FDA, and a revision of the drug administration law was enforced in 2019 [12]. These efforts approximate some of the FDA and EMA changes toward greater interactivity with stakeholders and patients. However, the main concern is still focused on drug safety and the fight against counterfeited medicines.

The PMDA (www.pmda.go.jp/english) was established in Japan in 2004, following a national reorganization of public services (corporations). It is a recent organization, but it has already had a critical impact on Japan's regulatory environment. Many improvements have been seen at the PMDA, resulting from the various types of consultations available to pharmaceutical sponsors throughout the drug-development process, similar to the evolution described for the FDA and EMA. The PMDA had vastly increased the number of reviewers over the past years, compared to the 1990s when the Japanese agency (then known as "KIKO") was understaffed and much more conservative when it came to optimizing Japanese timelines. The situation today is much improved for pharmaceutical manufacturers operating in Japan [13].

In general, regardless of where they are geographically, regulatory agencies are in charge of (1) licensing new medicines and (2) correlated activities associated with the licensing and maintenance of medicines in the market.

1. **Licensing new medicines**. The primary objectives of the regulatory review are to evaluate a drug's quality, safety, and effectiveness and determine whether its benefits outweigh its risks, in which case the new drug receives a "market authorization." The data that allow the evaluation are submitted by the applicant/sponsor. The regulator will not only approve the drug but will also take great care to ensure that the accompanying information reflects the evidence that has been presented. This document is known as the summary of product characteristics (SPC), which is a "label" that provides detailed information about indications, dosage, adverse effects, warnings, monitoring, etc.
2. **Correlated activities**. These can happen before the evaluation of the marketing authorization (scientific advice, rolling reviews, FDA formal

meetings); after the marketing authorization is granted (pharmacovigilance); or are ongoing throughout the conduct of studies (regulating clinical trials; inspecting and maintaining standards of drug development and manufacture).

28.3 Regulatory Processes That Precede Marketing Authorization Submissions

Regulatory agencies are focused on collaborating and being a partner in drug development rather than being just the examiner at the end of the process. There are different mechanisms in place to allow for the interactions along the way. These are summarized in Table 28.1. Table 28.2 describes the various procedures and programs the four agencies have regarding the terms and programs in use.

Unfortunately, the field of AD drug development has not registered many successes, not even early wins that could trigger the expedited programs listed in Table 28.1. The scarcity of designated products can be due to a lack of candidates that meet the designation criteria. Still, it is also possible that this is due to the lack of ability by

Table 28.1 Comparison of regulatory interactions before submission of marketing authorization request interactions

	FDA (USA)	EMA (EU)	PMDA (Japan)	NMPA (China)
Pre-IND application	Yes	No	Yes	No[f]
IND application	Yes	No	Yes	No[f]
CT application	No	Yes	No?	Yes
EOP1/EOP2	Yes	No	Yes	No[f]
Scientific advice (or protocol assistance)	No[a]	Yes[d]	Yes[e]	No[f]
SPA	Yes	No	No	No[f]
Opportunities for expedited review programs				
Adaptive	No[b]	Yes	No	No
Breakthrough designation	Yes[c]	No	No	Yes
Fast Track designation	Yes	No	No	Yes
Priority review	No[c]	Yes[c]	No	No
Rollover	Yes	No	No	No
Sakigake designation	No[c]	No	Yes[c]	No

[a] EMA scientific advice can be similar to EOP1/EOP2. [b] Adaptive assessment at EMA is similar to rollover at FDA. [c] Breakthrough at FDA, PRIME at EMA, and Sakigake at PMDA have similar goals. [d] Scientific advice in Europe can be national or centralized. [e] PMDA pharmaceutical affairs consultation on research and development strategy. [f] From the available documentation it seems the effort is centered in the CT application process. Abbreviations: IND, investigational new drug; CT, clinical trial; EOP1, end of Phase 1 meeting; EOP2, end of Phase 2 meeting; SPA, special protocol assessment.

Table 28.2 Categories and eligibility requirements of regulatory interactions before submission of marketing authorization request

Agency	Regulatory Programs/ Processes	Definition	Criteria	Ref
FDA	Pre-IND/IND	An IND application is for drugs (or biological products) not previously authorized for marketing in the United States that are intended to be used for the purposes of clinical investigation or, in certain cases, for the purposes of clinical treatment when no approved therapies are available. Pre-IND advice may be requested for issues related to data needed to support the rationale for testing a drug in humans; the design of non-clinical pharmacology, toxicology, and drug-activity studies; data requirements for an IND application; initial drug-development plans, and regulatory requirements for demonstrating safety and efficacy.		[14]
	EOP1/ EOP2	EOP1 meetings review several topics: pharmacokinetics and pharmacodynamics, proposed Phase 2 protocol, identification of populations for Phase 3 trials, pediatric studies. EOP2 meeting should be held before Phase 3 trials begin, and topics include: determination of the safety of proceeding to Phase 3, evaluation of the Phase 3 plan and protocols for adequacy and to assess pediatric safety and effectiveness, identification of information necessary to support a marketing application.		[15]
	SPA	SPA is a process to reach agreement on the design and size of certain clinical trials, clinical studies, or animal studies. An SPA agreement indicates concurrence by the FDA with the adequacy and acceptability of specific critical elements of overall protocol design (e.g., entry criteria, dose selection, endpoints, and planned analyses) for a study intended to support a future marketing application.	Types of eligible protocols: • animal carcinogenicity protocols • drug substance and drug product stability protocols • animal efficacy protocols, protocols for trials intended to form the primary basis of an efficacy claim • protocols for any necessary clinical study or studies to prove biosimilarity and/or interchangeability.	[16]
	Breakthrough designation	Breakthrough therapy designation is intended to expedite the development and review of drugs for serious or life-threatening conditions.	A drug that is intended to treat a serious condition AND preliminary clinical evidence indicates that the drug may demonstrate substantial improvement on a clinically significant endpoint(s) over available therapies.	[17]
	Fast Track designation	Fast Track designation is intended to expedite the development and review of drugs for serious or life-threatening conditions.	A drug that is intended to treat a serious condition AND non-clinical or clinical data demonstrate the potential to address unmet medical need.	
	Priority review	Any drug, including those that have received a Fast Track designation, breakthrough therapy designation, or those being evaluated for accelerated approval, can be granted priority review. Priority review does not change the review process, it shortens the review time.	A drug that treats a serious condition AND, if approved, would provide a significant improvement in safety or effectiveness.	
	Accelerated approval	It is used for speeding the development and approval of promising therapies that treat a serious or life-threatening condition and provide meaningful therapeutic benefit over available therapies. Accelerated approval allows approval of a drug that demonstrates an effect on a "surrogate endpoint" that is reasonably likely to predict clinical benefit, or on a clinical endpoint that can be measured earlier than an effect on irreversible morbidity or mortality that is reasonably likely to predict an effect on irreversible morbidity or mortality, or other clinical benefit.	A drug that treats a serious condition AND generally provides a meaningful advantage over available therapies AND demonstrates an effect on a surrogate endpoint that is reasonably likely to predict clinical benefit or on a clinical endpoint that can be measured earlier than irreversible morbidity or mortality that is reasonably likely to predict an effect on irreversible morbidity or mortality, or other clinical benefit (i.e., an intermediate clinical endpoint).	

Table 28.2 (cont.)

Agency	Regulatory Programs/ Processes	Definition	Criteria	Ref
EMA	CT application	Clinical trials in the EU must get authorization from the member states where they will be conducted, and these countries have the responsibility to supervise those clinical trials. The clinical trial regulation of 2014 harmonizes the processes related with clinical trials and introduces specific requirements. The EMA is in charge of application of several requirements imposed by the regulation.		[18]
	Scientific advice	For human medicines, scientific advice and protocol assistance are given by the Committee for Medicinal Products for human use on the recommendation of the Scientific Advice Working Party. At any stage of a medicine's development, a developer can ask guidance and direction from the EMA on the best methods and study designs to generate robust information on how well a medicine works and how safe it is, regardless of whether the medicine is eligible for the centralized authorization procedure or not. Scientific advice helps to ensure that developers perform the appropriate tests and studies, so that no major objections regarding the design of the tests are likely to be raised during the evaluation of the marketing authorization application. Scientific advice is prospective in nature. The EMA does not pre-evaluate the results of the studies and in no way concludes on whether the benefits of the medicine outweigh the risks.		[19]
	Adaptive pathways	Adaptive pathways can be defined as a prospectively planned, iterative approach to bringing medicines to market. The approach is based on three principles: 1. Iterative development – this is either (a) staggered approval from an initial restricted patient population in which the benefit outweighs the risk, to increasingly wider populations (expansion of the indication); or (b) confirmation of the benefit–risk balance of a product authorized under conditional marketing authorization with early or surrogate endpoints. 2. Gathering of evidence through real-world data to supplement clinical trial data. 3. Involvement of patients and health technology assessment bodies in the discussion of the product development program.		[20]
	Priority review (PRIME)	PRIME is a scheme to enhance support for the development of medicines that target an unmet medical need. The EMA offers early and proactive support to medicine developers to optimize the generation of robust data on a medicine's benefits and risks and enable accelerated assessment of medicines applications.	Medicines that may offer a major therapeutic advantage over existing treatments, or benefit patients without treatment options.	[21]
	Conditional approval	Conditional marketing authorizations are valid for 1 year and can be renewed annually. Once a conditional marketing authorization has been granted, the marketing authorization holder must fulfill specific obligations within defined timelines.	The benefit–risk balance of the medicine is positive. It is likely that the applicant will be able to provide comprehensive data post-authorization. The medicine fulfills an unmet medical need. The benefit of the medicine's immediate availability to patients is greater than the risk inherent in the fact that additional data are still required.	[22]
	Exceptional circumstances	A type of marketing authorization granted to medicines where the applicant is unable to provide comprehensive data on the efficacy and safety under normal conditions of use, because the condition to be treated is rare or because collection of full information is not possible or is unethical. The authorization under exceptional circumstances is granted subject to a requirement for the applicant to introduce specific procedures, in particular concerning the safety of the medicinal product, notification to the competent authorities of any incident relating to its use, and action to be taken.		[23]

Table 28.2 (cont.)

Agency	Regulatory Programs/ Processes	Definition and Criteria		Ref
PMDA	CT application	It is necessary to submit clinical trial protocol notifications to PMDA in the following instances: (1) drugs with new active ingredients (2) drugs with new administration routes (excluding bioequivalence studies) (3) new combination drugs, drugs with new indications or new dosage and administration (excluding bioequivalence studies) (4) drugs containing the same active ingredients with the drugs with new active ingredients, for which the re-examination period has not been completed yet (excluding bioequivalence studies) (5) drugs considered to be biological products – excluding (1) to (4) (excluding bioequivalence studies) (6) drugs manufactured using gene recombinant technology – excluding (1) to (5) (excluding bioequivalence studies).		
	Clinical studies consultation system	There is a large array of possible consultations, which include equivalents to INDs at FDA, i.e., before starting Phase 1, and equivalents to EOP1 and EOP2, i.e., before starting Phase 2, and before starting Phase 3.		
	Scientific advice	There is a consultation system for many other topics besides clinical trials including on (1) preliminary assessment of new drugs; (2) eligibility for priority review or conditional approval; (3) applicability of pharmacogenomic markers or biomarkers; and (4) epidemiological surveys.		
	Sakigake designation	It aims to advance early practical applications for innovative new medicines and other products. In principle, the designated product must have the potential for novel treatment effectiveness or reduction in symptoms based on a different mechanism of action from already approved products. Designated products are eligible for prioritized consultation services and reviews for regulatory authorizations.	Medical products for diseases in urgent need of innovative therapy, which may satisfy the following two conditions: having firstly been developed in Japan and with a planned application for approval (desireable to have a PMDA consultation from the beginning of research and development); and prominent effectiveness (i.e., radical improvement compared to existing therapy) can be expected based on the data of mechanism of action, nonclinical study, and the early phase of clinical trials (Phase 1–2).	[24–26]
	Priority review	Applies to accelerate the review time based on the seriousness of indicated disease: diseases with important effects on patient's survival (fatal diseases); progressive and irreversible diseases with marked effects on daily life; other; AND overall assessment of therapeutic usefulness: there is no existing method of treatment, prophylaxis, or diagnosis. Therapeutic usefulness with respect to existing treatment from (a) a standpoint of efficacy; (b) a standpoint of safety; or (c) a standpoint of physical and mental burden on the patient.		
	Conditional approval	For the drugs for treating serious diseases which occur in a small number of patients and for which effective treatment methods are limited.	The drug is indicated for serious diseases. The medical usefulness is high. Confirmatory clinical trials are difficult to conduct. The results of clinical trials, etc., other than confirmatory clinical trials, suggest some efficacy and safety.	
NMPA	CT application	Clinical trials are considered studies to support registration applications for marketing; this appears to exclude investigator-initiated trials. After receiving the initial clinical trial approval, the applicant does not need to apply to the NMPA for additional clinical trial approval for subsequent phases of trials. The sponsor of the clinical trial only needs to obtain approval from the ethics committee and file the relevant protocol and supporting documents with the Center for Drug Evaluation.		[27–29]
	Breakthrough designation (must be applied at the stage of clinical trials)	Applies to innovative drugs or improved new drugs that are used for the prevention and treatment of diseases that seriously endanger life or seriously affect the quality of life, for which there is no effective measure of prevention and treatment or, compared with existing measures of treatment, there is sufficient evidence proving the obvious clinical advantages.		

Table 28.2 (cont.)

Priority review	Applies to (1) urgently needed drugs in short supply, and innovative drugs and improved new drugs for the prevention and treatment of serious infectious and orphan diseases; (2) new varieties of pediatric drugs, dosage forms, and specifications that meet the physiological characteristics of children; (3) urgently needed and innovative vaccines; and (4) drugs approved under the Breakthrough or conditional approval programs.
Conditional approval (must be applied at the stage of clinical trials)	Applies to (1) drugs that treat life-threatening injuries with no effective treatment, and early trial data indicate efficacy and potential clinical value; (2) urgently needed drugs for the public health with clinical trial data that indicate efficacy and potential clinical value; or (3) urgently needed vaccines for major public health emergencies, or that are deemed by the National Health Commission as urgently needed, for which the benefits outweigh the risks. The NMPA will place post-marketing conditions on drugs under this program and a timeline for completion.

small companies to pursue a global regulatory development strategy and to keep up with many regulatory authorities' interactions. Another unlikely possibility is that a designation might have been granted, but it is not in the public domain. The EMA and PMDA post lists of the medicinal products that received PRIME or Sakigake designation, but the FDA only posts the Breakthrough designated products that went on and received market approval. Companies almost always publicize the designations in press-release format, which makes identifying all instances unwieldy. As far as we could ascertain, Biogen's aducanumab is the only product that got the three designations: Breakthrough (FDA), PRIME (EMA), and Sakigake (PMDA); aducanumab had also received special protocol assessment (SPA) from the FDA. There are no other AD-related designations by PRIME or Sakigake. There are few other examples of Breakthrough designation from the FDA, namely for the N-methyl-D-aspartate receptor antagonist from Axsome Therapeutics, intended to treat AD-related agitation, and for pimavanserin from Acadia Pharmaceuticals for the treatment of dementia-related psychosis. The more recent breakthrough device designation program has scored several AD-related products: for example, digital therapies like the Dthera/ALZ device for reminiscence therapy of agitation and depression or MemorEM, a wearable head device from NeuroEM Therapeutics, Inc., so far the only product with direct therapeutic intent on AD; diagnostic tests for screening in the blood (C_2N Diagnostics) and for diagnosis in the cerebrospinal fluid (CSF) (Roche-Elecsys); software systems like Cortical Disarray Measurement (CDM) software device from Oxford Brain Diagnostics Ltd; and Optina Diagnostics' retinal imaging platform uses artificial intelligence to detect biomarkers of AD.

28.3.1 Regulatory Processes That Expedite the Marketing Authorization Evaluation

Table 28.3 summarizes the processes for expedited review for marketing authorizations in the four agencies and the median review times. We separated the discussion of processes that apply before submitting a request of marketing authorization (Table 28.1) from the ones that may be deployed

Table 28.3 Types of approvals and expedite review modalities

	FDA (USA)	EMA (EU)	PMDA (Japan)	NMPA (China)
Standard approval	Yes	Yes	Yes	Yes
Median approval time 2019 (days)[a]	243	423	304	510[b]
Expedited approvals	Yes	Yes	Yes	Yes
Priority review	Yes	No	Yes	Yes
Accelerated assessment	No	Yes	No	No
Conditional approval	No	Yes	Yes	Yes
Exceptional circumstances	No	Yes	No	No
Median expedited approval time 2019 (days)[a]	238	270	256	510[b]

[a] Source: Centre for Innovation in Regulatory Science Briefing 77, 2020) [30]. Median approval time counted from date of submission to the date of approval (includes agency and company time). For the EMA, approval time includes European Commission time. [b] Source: globalforum.diaglobal.org [31].

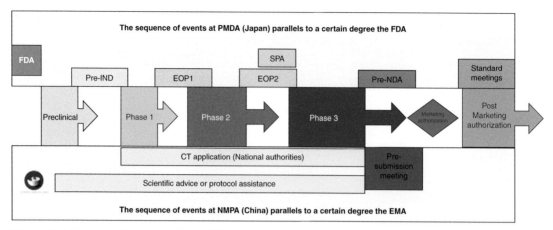

The sequence of events at PMDA (Japan) parallels to a certain degree the FDA

FDA

Pre-IND · EOP1 · SPA · EOP2 · Pre-NDA · Standard meetings

Preclinical · Phase 1 · Phase 2 · Phase 3 · Marketing authorization · Post Marketing authorization

CT application (National authorities)

Pre-submission meeting

Scientific advice or protocol assistance

The sequence of events at NMPA (China) parallels to a certain degree the EMA

Figure 28.1 Alignment of processes within the FDA, EMA, PDMA, and NMPA.

for after the submission (Table 28.3). There is, however, a degree of overlap among processes. The criteria for the different designations and accelerated or exceptional types of reviews and approvals are quite similar, favoring treatments that target life-threatening diseases, and the existence of preliminary evidence is of significant benefit. Almost every single process/designation or program may apply to AD-intended drugs. We excluded from these analyses the emergency-use processes that exist in the four agencies and are designed to cover for severe risks to public health like the COVID-19 pandemic.

Figure 28.1 illustrates how the different processes align in time for the FDA and EMA.

28.4 Qualification and Letters of Support for Drug-Development Tools: Biomarkers, Rating Scales, and Other Outcomes

A drug-development program's success depends on the ability to provide a robust evidentiary base to support a positive benefit–risk relationship for the treatment. The pathway from target validation to the nomination of a lead candidate through all preclinical development is arduous and prone to failure. Suppose a candidate drug makes it to the clinical phase. In that case, there are critical steps to overcome: (1) demonstration that there is target engagement; for AD this implies proving that the drug crosses the blood–brain barrier and has a desireable action on the intended target; (2) demonstration that there is an effect on a correlate of clinical efficacy (early efficacy) and; (3)

demonstration of a dose–response relationship; (4) ability to design an informative pivotal trial, which implies the selection and enrichment of the study population and a definition of endpoints.

These activities are so fundamental to success that regulatory agencies have created mechanisms to support developing the tools (drug-development tools [DDTs]) that are instrumental in achieving the stated goals. DDTs include fit-for-purpose biomarkers, rating scales, and digital endpoints, among others. The regulatory mechanisms to facilitate the development of DDTs include the qualification programs that both the FDA [32] and EMA [33] have in place, a letter of support, and other consultation opportunities in the context of specific drug development. Additionally, the FDA and the European Commission created institutions, the Critical Path Institute (C-Path; https://c-path.org) and the Innovative Medicines Initiative (IMI; www.imi.europa.eu), respectively, dedicated to advancing the pre-competitive research on tools to support drug development. Both C-Path and IMI have several extensive, well-supported projects dedicated to AD.

Several of these research efforts culminated in the qualification of biomarkers to enrich trials populations and a simulator for trial design. Table 28.4 summarizes the Drug-Development Tools for Alzheimer Disease programs that got a letter of support or were qualified by the FDA or EMA [34, 35].

The qualification process leads to regulatory acceptance across diverse development programs, but it is complex to develop and requires a level of evidentiary basis that takes a long time to obtain. The FDA and EMA established an intermediary

Table 28.4 List of qualified biomarkers and letters of support

DDT	Intended use	Agency	Date
Low hippocampal volume (atrophy) by MRI	Enrichment in clinical trials for regulatory purpose – in pre-dementia stage of AD	EMA (Q), FDA (LOS)	2011, 2015
CSF-related biomarkers for drugs affecting amyloid burden	For enrichment in clinical trials for regulatory purpose – in pre-dementia stage of AD	EMA (Q), FDA (LOS)	2011, 2015
Amyloid PET imaging (positive/negative).	Biomarker for enrichment, for use in regulatory clinical trials in pre-dementia AD	EMA (Q)	2012
CSF amyloid beta 42 and total tau and/or PET amyloid imaging (positive/negative)	Biomarkers for enrichment, for use in regulatory clinical trials in mild and moderate AD	EMA (Q)	2012
Data-driven model of disease progression and trial evaluation	Use in drug development as a longitudinal model for describing changes in cognition in patients with mild and moderate AD, and for use in assisting in trial designs in mild and moderate AD	EMA (Q), FDA (endorsement)	2013, 2013

Abbreviations: Q, qualification; LOS, letter of support; endorsement is a non-standardized FDA mechanism that implies the tool was reviewed and the context of use is deemed acceptable.

approach through the issuance of "letters of support," a letter issued to a requester that briefly describes the agency's thoughts on the potential value of a biomarker and encourages further evaluation. This letter of support does not imply a biomarker qualification and does not endorse a specific biomarker test or device. It is meant to enhance the biomarker's visibility, encourage data sharing, and stimulate additional studies.

The different agencies' qualification programs have been described and compared multiple times [36–38]. They are an essential mechanism to avoid duplicative efforts and to achieve comprehensive data sharing among stakeholders.

28.5 The Marketing Authorization Processes

The regulatory evaluation of a marketing authorization request has very well-established processes that can be easily consulted on each agency's website, and comparative analyses are available [39].

The essence of the evaluation of the marketing authorization is to establish if the drug: (1) has quality, which refers to the pharmaceutical formulation(s) characteristics and the manufacturing processes; (2) is efficacious, meaning that it produces a clinically relevant benefit; and (3) is safe in the defined conditions of use. Safe does not mean that there are no established risks, but that the benefits outweigh the known and potential risks. The evaluation of the benefit–risk relationship is one of the most challenging judgments that regulators must make. Frequently, the

benefit–risk assessment differs at the individual and societal level because individuals' values vary. The benefit–risk evaluation is always a matter of fallible human judgment. To reduce the fallibility, regulatory agencies created mechanisms to help standardize the benefit–risk assessment process. These mechanisms include formal, structured benefit–risk analyses [40–42] and committees' use in the decision/making process. Committees' decisions tend for consensus, and to eliminate extreme perspectives. The FDA frequently uses advisory boards of experts; the meetings and decisions are public, which is an excellent contribution to the transparency of the process. The EMA Committee for Human Medicines Products (CHMP) occasionally assembles ad-hoc groups of experts – scientific advisory groups – to contribute to the evaluation. The deliberations of these groups are confidential.

28.6 Regulatory Guidance Documents on AD Drug Development

The EMA, FDA, and PMDA issued guidance documents [4–6] to inform the drug development in AD. Guidance documents are vital to the field even if in draft versions because they synthesize the agencies' understanding regarding the matters discussed. Guidance documents are usually "not-binding" in the sense that science evolves, and new approaches may become acceptable. That is why all the four agencies entertain consultation approaches specific to each drug development, which can be used when there are any doubts or alternatives to the guideline's recommendations. Nevertheless, the guidance documents are revelatory, and particularly useful when they show a convergence of solutions across regions. These guidance documents were recently reviewed comparatively [43]. The main convergence areas are the recognition of (1) the AD continuum, including the pre-dementia phases that are considered appropriate as a target for drug development; (2) the role of biomarkers in the definition of the target populations and, potentially, as endpoints, although none of the documents yet accepts a biomarker in the situation of the primary endpoint; and (3) the need for alternatives for trials in the pre-dementia phases, to the two co-primary clinical primary endpoints, the accepted paradigm for trials in the dementia phase. There are still many areas related to regulatory science that are evolving. For example, FDA guidance settles on a simplified, numeric staging system distilled from the National Institute on Aging–Alzheimer's Association (NIA–AA) one, suggesting that the FDA expects populations in registration trials to be mapped to this staging system. Simultaneously, the EMA recognizes the utility of both NIA–AA and International Working Group systems but advocates that the populations defined on one and other might not be equivalent.

28.7 Regulatory Agencies That Supervise the Large Market Regions: USA, Europe, Japan, China

The majority of the regulatory agencies in the world, including the FDA, PMDA, and NMPA, have a hierarchical organization where the top of the pyramid has the ultimate power and responsibility for the regulatory decisions that are issued. At the FDA, that person is the commissioner by delegation, while the PMDA and NMPA have the tutelage of a governmental ministry. The EMA is a unique organization that has a network structure as a consequence of the political nature of the EU, which avoids structures that may compromise the power of member states. The central body at the EMA has an executive director, but the CHMP is responsible for signing the opinions rendered that are related to marketing authorizations for human medicines. These opinions regarding the direction of the decision should be conveyed to the European Commission that issues the legally binding decisions. The commission may challenge the CHMP opinions, and occasionally they are what triggers a revision of the process that led to the opinion, reaffirming or revising it. A vast European regulatory network supports all activities of the EMA committees. Importantly, each EU member state holds a national regulatory agency that operates in areas that are out of the remit of EMA; decentralized marketing authorizations are still possible in several medical indications but not in AD because all novel therapies for neurodegenerative disease are entirely under the remit of the EMA. From January 1, 2021, the Medicines and Healthcare products Regulatory Agency became the standalone medicines and medical devices regulator of the UK because the EMA/EU lost the UK's regulatory authority after "Brexit."

Table 28.5 compares and contrasts the four regulatory agencies' main organizational characteristics under discussion in this chapter.

Table 28.5 Comparison of the main organizational features among the four regulatory agencies: FDA, EMA, PMDA, and NMPA

	FDA	EMA	PMDA	NMPA
History	1906 – Food and Drugs Act – focused adulteration 1930 – The designation FDA was established 1949 – First guidance for industry 1962 – Kefauver–Harris drug amendment requiring proof of drug efficacy and safety 1988 – FDA Act 2012 – FDA Safety and Innovation Act	1995 – Foundation – to harmonize the work of existing national medicine regulatory bodies 2000 – Expansion of the EMA's remit to medicines for rare disease 2004 – Expansion for herbal medicines 2006 – Expansion for medicines for children 2007 – expansion for advanced-therapy medicines 2012 – PRAC creation	2004 – Establishment of the PMDA There were several organizations working in drug regulation prior to 2004 1979 – The Fund for relief of adverse drug reactions suffering 1994 – Organization for Pharmaceutical Safety and Research 1997 – The Pharmaceuticals and Medical Devices Evaluation Center	2013 – Establishment of the NMPA, after a reorganization of the former China-FDA

Table 28.5 (cont)

	FDA	EMA	PMDA	NMPA
Scope	Food Drugs Biologics Medical devices Radiation-emitting products Veterinary products Tobacco products	Centralized procedure is mandatory for novel human medicines to treat HIV, cancer, diabetes, neurodegenerative diseases, auto-immune and other immune dysfunctions, viral diseases Medicines derived from biotechnology processes Advanced therapy medicines Orphan medicines Veterinary medicines for use as growth or yield enhancers Centralized procedure is optional for all novel substances targeting other indications	Drugs Medical devices Cellular and tissue-based products	Food Drugs (includes biologics and traditional Chinese medicines) Cosmetics Medical devices
Structure (relevant divisions)	Center for Biologics Evaluation and Research Center for Devices and Radiological Health Center for Drug Evaluation and Research (includes Office of New Drugs, which includes the Office of Neuroscience and, within it, the Division of Neurology I that oversees AD drugs)	CHMP PRAC CVMP COMP HMPC CAT PDCO Working parties, and other groups	Center for Product Evaluation Center for Regulatory Science	Department of Drug Registration, Department of Drug Regulation, Department of Medical Device Registration, Department of Medical Device Regulation
Decision holding power	The FDA is an agency within the Department of Health and Human Services	The EMA, through the committees, produces opinions that are made in decisions by the European Commission	The PMDA is an agency of the Ministry of Health, Labor and Welfare	The NMPA has ministerial-level decision-making power
Core procedures related with drug development	Pre-IND, IND, EOP1/EOP2, SPA, Breakthrough designation, Fast Track designation, rollover, NDA	CT application, scientific advice, PRIME, marketing authorization	IND, EOP1/EOP2, scientific advice, Sakigake designation, NDA	CT application, Breakthrough designation, Fast Track designation, NDA
Approved drugs for mild-to-moderate AD	Donepezil Rivastigmine Galantamine Memantine Aducanumab (2021)	Donepezil Rivastigmine Galantamine Memantine	Donepezil Rivastigmine Galantamine Memantine	Donepezil Rivastigmine Galantamine Memantine Oligomannate (2019)

Abbreviations: CAT, Committee for Advanced Therapies; CHMP, Committee for Human Medicines Products; COMP, Committee for Orphan Medicinal Products; CT, clinical trial; CVMP, Committee for Medicinal Products for Veterinary Use; EOP1, end of Phase 1 meeting; EOP2, end of Phase 2 meeting; HMPC, Committee on Herbal Medicinal Products; IND, investigational new drug; NDA, new drug application; PDCO, Pediatric Committee; PRAC, Pharmacovigilance Risk Assessment Committee; PRIME, Priority Medicines; SPA, special protocol assessment.

28.8 Conclusions

The AD pipeline of therapeutic interventions [44] remains reasonably strong despite decades of clinical-stage failures. Interactions among sponsors/applicants and regulatory agencies had multiplied since the early days when most of the interfacing almost only happened when a dossier was submitted with the intent of obtaining a marketing authorization. Several DDTs were qualified or received "letters of support." From 2002 to 2020 there were no approvals of novel AD drugs by FDA, EMA, or PMDA. In 2021, aducanumab was approved for the treatment of AD to be initiated in the mild cognitive impairment or mild dementia phase of the illness. The NMPA reviewed and conditionally approved Oligomannate in 2019. Despite the drought regarding new applications, all agencies have expedited programs to facilitate drug development for serious and life-threatening diseases, including AD. Furthermore, the FDA, EMA, and PMDA have published either finalized or draft guidance documents on drug development for AD, emphasizing the need to target the early phases of the disease before the dementia stage. There have been multiple instances of formal scientific advice to AD drug programs.

Overall, the regulatory environment is now much more interactive and attuned to sponsors/applicants' needs, than when acetylcholinesterase inhibitors and memantine were developed.

References

1. Food and Drug Administration. Peripheral and Central Nervous System Drugs Advisory Committee meeting. Available at: www.fda.gov/advisory-committees/human-drug-advisory-committees/peripheral-and-central-nervous-system-drugs-advisory-committee (accessed January 2021).

2. European Medicines Agency. Ebixa (memantine). Available at: www.ema.europa.eu/en/medicines/human/EPAR/ebixa (accessed January 2021).

3. Chinese National Medical Products Agency. Treatment for Alzheimer's available by end of 2019. Available at: http://english.nmpa.gov.cn/2019-11/04/c_422037.htm (accessed January 2021).

4. Food and Drug Administration. Alzheimer's disease: developing drugs for treatment. Guidance for industry. 2018. Available at: www.fda.gov/regulatory-information/search-fda-guidance-documents/alzheimers-disease-developing-drugs-treatment-guidance-industy (accessed January 2021).

5. European Medicines Agency. Guideline on the clinical investigation of medicines to treat Alzheimer's disease, 2018. Available at: www.ema.europa.eu/en/documents/scientific-guideline/guideline-clinical-investigation-medicines-treatment-alzheimers-disease-revision-2_en.pdf (accessed January 2021).

6. The University of Tokyo Hospital. Project to promote the development of innovative pharmaceuticals, medical devices, and regenerative medical products (Ministry of Health, Labour, and Welfare) regulatory science research for the establishment of criteria for clinical evaluation of drugs for Alzheimer's disease, issues to consider in the clinical evaluation and development of drugs for Alzheimer's disease. Available at: www.pmda.go.jp/files/000221585.pdf (accessed January 2021).

7. Jack CR, Bennett DA, Blennow K, et al. NIA–AA Research Framework: toward a biological definition of Alzheimer's disease. *Alzheimers Dement* 2018; **14**: 535–62.

8. European Medicines Agency. Connecting the dots towards global knowledge of the international medicine regulatory landscape: mapping of international initiatives. Available at: www.ema.europa.eu/en/documents/leaflet/connecting-dots-towards-global-knowledge-international-medicine-regulatory-landscape-mapping_en.pdf (accessed January 2021).

9. Food and Drug Administration. 21st Century Cures Act. Available at: www.fda.gov/regulatory-information/selected-amendments-fdc-act/21st-century-cures-act (accessed January 2021).

10. European Medicines Agency. EU Medicines Agencies network strategy to 2020, working together to improve health. Available at: www.ema.europa.eu/en/documents/other/eu-medicines-agencies-network-strategy-2020-working-together-improve-health_en.pdf (accessed January 2021).

11. European Medicines Agency. Regulatory science strategy 2025. Available at: www.ema.europa.eu/en/about-us/how-we-work/regulatory-science-strategy#regulatory-science-strategy-to-2025-section (accessed January 2021).

12. National Medical Products Administration (NMPA). http://english.nmpa.gov.cn/drugs.html (accessed January 2021).

13. Engen S. The improving Japanese pharmaceutical regulatory environment. Available at: Locustwalk.com/the-improving-japanese-pharmaceutical-regulatory-environment/ (accessed January 2021).

14. Food and Drug Administration. Investigational new drug (IND) application. Available at: www.fda.gov/drugs/types-applications/investigational-new-drug-ind-application (accessed January 2021).

15. Food and Drug Administration. Formal meetings between the FDA and sponsors or applicants of PDUFA products guidance for industry, December 2017. Available at: www.fda.gov/regulatory-information/search-fda-guidance-documents/formal-meetings-between-fda-and-sponsors-or-applicants-pdufa-products-guidance-industry (accessed January 2021).

16. Food and Drug Administration. Special protocol assessment guidance for industry, April 2018. Available at: www.fda.gov/regulatory-information/search-fda-guidance-documents/special-protocol-assessment-guidance-industry (accessed January 2021).

17. Food and Drug Administration. Expedited programs for serious conditions: drugs and biologics, May 2014. Available at: www.fda.gov/regulatory-information/search-fda-guidance-documents/expedited-programs-serious-conditions-drugs-and-biologics (accessed January 2021).

18. European Medicines Agency. Clinical trial regulation. Available at: www.ema.europa.eu/en/human-regulatory/research-development/clinical-trials/clinical-trial-regulation (accessed January 2021).

19. European Medicines Agency. Scientific advice and protocol assistance. Available at: www.ema.europa.eu/en/human-regulatory/research-development/scientific-advice-protocol-assistance (accessed January 2021).

20. European Medicines Agency. Adaptive pathways. Available at: www.ema.europa.eu/en/human-regulatory/research-development/adaptive-pathways (accessed January 2021).

21. European Medicines Agency. PRIME: priority medicines. Available at: www.ema.europa.eu/en/human-regulatory/research-development/prime-priority-medicines (accessed January 2021).

22. European Medicines Agency. Conditional marketing authorization. Available at: www.ema.europa.eu/en/human-regulatory/marketing-authorisation/conditional-marketing-authorisation (accessed January 2021).

23. European Medicines Agency. Exceptional circumstances. Available at: www.ema.europa.eu/en/glossary/exceptional-circumstances (accessed January 2021).

24. Japan Pharmaceutical Manufacturers Association. Pharmaceutical Administration and Regulations in Japan. Available at: www.jpma.or.jp/english/parj/ (accessed January 2021).

25. Kajiwara E, Shikano M. Considerations and regulatory challenges for innovative medicines in expedited approval programs: breakthrough therapy and Sakigake designation. *Ther Innov Regul Sci* 2020; **54**: 814–20.

26. Kondo H, Sugita T, Ida N, Fukushima H, Yasuda N. A comparison of PMDA and EMA consultations for regulatory and scientific matters in drugs and regenerative medicine products. *Ther Innov Regul Sci* 2017; **51**: 355–9.

27. Zhuxing Y, Haixue W. The regulatory requirements and critical points of drug clinical trials registration in China. Available at: www.appliedclinicaltrialsonline.com/view/regulatory-requirements-and-key-points-drug-clinical-trials-registration-china (accessed January 2021).

28. Jianqing C. What's new for conditional approval of drugs in China? *Tigermed Insight*. Available at: https://tigermedgrp.com/whats-new-for-conditional-approval-of-drugs-in-china/ (accessed January 2021).

29. Covington and Burling. China promulgates revised drug registration regulation, August 2020. Available at: www.cov.com/-/media/files/corporate/publications/2020/04/china-promulgates-revised-drug-registration-regulation.pdf (accessed January 2021).

30. Centre for Innovation and Regulatory Science. CIRS RD Briefing 77: new drug approvals in six major authorities, June 2020. Available at: www.cirsci.org/publications/cirs-rd-briefing-77-new-drug-approvals-in-six-major-authorities/ (accessed January 2021).

31. Xu W, Yuanyuan D. New drug approvals in China in 2019. Available at: https://globalforum.diaglobal.org/issue/may-2020/new-drug-approvals-in-china-in-2019/ (accessed January 2021).

32. Food and Drug Administration. Qualification process for drug development tools guidance for industry and FDA staff, November, 2020. Available at: www.fda.gov/regulatory-information/search-fda-guidance-documents/qualification-process-drug-development-tools-guidance-industry-and-fda-staff (accessed January 2021).

33. European Medicines Agency. Qualification of novel methodologies for medicine development. Available at: www.ema.europa.eu/en/human-regulatory/research-development/scientific-advice-protocol-assistance/qualification-novel-methodologies-medicine-development-0 (accessed January 2021).

34. Food and Drug Administration. About biomarkers and qualification. Available at: www.fda.gov/drugs/biomarker-qualification-program/about-biomarkers-and-qualification (accessed January 2021).

35. European Medicines Agency. Opinions and letters of support on the qualification of novel methodologies for medicine development. Available at: www.ema.europa.eu/en/human-regulatory/research-development/scientific-advice-protocol-assistance/novel-methodologies

-biomarkers/opinions-letters-support-qualification-novel-methodologies-medicine-development (accessed January 2021).

36. Arnerić SP, Batrla-Utermann R, Beckett L, et al. Cerebrospinal fluid biomarkers for Alzheimer's disease: a view of the regulatory science qualification landscape from the Coalition Against Major Diseases CSF Biomarker Team. *J Alzheimers Dis* 2017; **55**: 19–35.

37. Sauer JM, Porter AC; Biomarker Programs, Predictive Safety Testing Consortium. Preclinical biomarker qualification. *Exp Biol Med (Maywood)* 2018; **243**: 222–7.

38. Pacifici E, Bain S (eds.). *An Overview of FDA Regulated Products: From Drugs and Cosmetics to Food and Tobacco*. Cambridge, MA: Academic Press; 2018.

39. Van Norman GA. Drugs and devices: comparison of European and US approval processes. *J Am Coll Cardiol Basic Transl Sci* 2016; **1**: 399–412.

40. Food and Drug Administration. Benefit–risk assessment in drug regulatory decision making.

Draft PDUFA VI implementation plan (FY 2018-2022). Available at: www.fda.gov/files/about%20fda/published/Benefit-Risk-Assessment-in-Drug-Regulatory-Decision-Making.pdf (accessed January 2021).

41. Juhaeri J. Benefit–risk evaluation: the past, present and future. *Ther Adv Drug Saf* 2019; **10**: 2042098619871180;DOI: http://doi.org/10.1177/2042098619871180.

42. European Medicines Agency. Benefit–risk methodology. Available at: www.ema.europa.eu/en/about-us/support-research/benefit-risk-methodology (accessed January 2021).

43. Morant AV, Vestergaard HT, Blædel-Lassen A, Navikas V. US, EU, and Japanese regulatory guidelines for development of drugs for treatment of Alzheimer's disease: implications for global drug development. *Clin Transl Sci* 2020; **13**: 652–64.

44. Cummings J, Lee G, Ritter A, Sabbagh M, Zhong K. Alzheimer's disease drug development pipeline: 2020. *Alzheimers Dement (N Y)* 2020; **6**: e12050.

Alzheimer's Disease Clinical Trial Study Partners

Joshua Grill

29.1 Introduction

Alzheimer's disease (AD) is a healthcare crisis that is increasing in prevalence and cost at unsustainable rates. Nearly 6 million Americans and 50 million people worldwide are living with dementia. Yet, AD rarely affects just one person. Unrelenting disease progression will render patients with AD dependent upon others and 16 million Americans endure tremendous physical, emotional, and financial burden of providing care to an afflicted loved one. In fact, the burden of informal caregiving is a main driver of the economic impact of this progressive fatal disorder [1]. The current and future economic implications of AD have resulted in a societal investment in research, with a main goal of identifying treatments capable of slowing or stopping disease progression. These investments have spurred new avenues of basic research to elucidate disease pathophysiology and identify promising treatment targets. The ultimate path to improved care of the millions of people living with AD and reduced burden for their caregivers will be through randomized controlled clinical trials of candidate interventions.

Family caregivers play an invaluable role in AD clinical trials; they serve as study partners to participants [2]. Trial success hinges on the contributions made by these vital stakeholders. They are essential to enrollment decisions, trial compliance, outcome measurements, and completion or dropout. The work performed by study partners must not be overlooked; it must be studied to improve trial designs and practices. In this chapter, I will overview the study partner role, the scientific evidence for how this role can impact trial outcomes, and how the role has changed as AD trials have expanded to include earlier disease stages (Table 29.1).

29.2 The Role of Study Partners in AD Clinical Trials

29.2.1 History and Terminology

AD is the single most common cause of dementia, that is, cognitive impairment that hinders activities of daily living. Accordingly, the majority of AD trials have enrolled patients who meet criteria for dementia using protocol-defined requirements, such as those outlined in the National Institute on Neurological and Communicative Disorders and Stroke–Alzheimer's Disease and Related Dementias Association. These trials, to date, have been the only ones to successfully demonstrate adequate safety and efficacy for treatment approval by the US Food and Drug Administration (FDA). Trials in AD dementia typically enroll patients with mild-to-moderate or moderate-to-severe disease. On a more limited basis, trials have

Table 29.1 Study partner roles across the spectrum of AD trials (minor, moderate, major)

Role	AD dementia trials	MCI/prodromal AD trials	Preclinical AD trials
Recruitment	Major	Major	Major
Informed consent	Major	Moderate	Minor
Transportation/visit compliance	Major	Moderate	Minor
Treatment compliance	Major	Moderate	Minor
Adverse-event reporting	Major	Moderate	Minor
Outcome measurement	Major	Major	Major
Retention	Major	Major	?

Abbreviations: AD, Alzheimer's disease; MCI, mild cognitive impairment.

focused on severe disease and non-cognitive symptoms such as agitation and other neuropsychiatric symptoms. While trials in dementia remain prominent, especially for symptomatic therapies, trials of putative disease-modifying therapies have increasingly included earlier disease stages.

With the development of clinical criteria for mild cognitive impairment (MCI) in the 1990s, AD trials began enrolling patients who did not meet criteria for dementia but had demonstrable cognitive decline. An explosion of AD biomarker research in the 2000s led to MCI trials that incorporated positron emission tomography (PET) imaging and cerebrospinal fluid (CSF) protein analysis to confirm abnormalities in amyloid beta as evidence of "MCI due to AD" or "prodromal AD." Longitudinal observational studies in cognitively unimpaired participants revealed that biomarker changes precede even mild cognitive symptoms, leading to the proposal of biomarker-based research diagnostic criteria for asymptomatic or "preclinical" AD, primarily for use in interventional studies. Numerous trials, including some large registration studies, have enrolled preclinical AD participants.

Through this evolution and since the first AD trials performed in the 1980s and 1990s, one common feature has been the requirement of co-enrollment of a participant–study-partner dyad. In early dementia trials, the role of patient caregivers was essential – patients could not transport themselves to study sites and often needed assistance with managing study medications, some of which required multiple daily doses. Though the very first trials did not incorporate informant reports as protocol-defined assessments of efficacy, experts quickly recognized the need to do so, leading to the consistent use of informant-based outcome measures of patient functional performance [3]. Essentially every AD trial since, regardless of the diagnostic category of the participants enrolled (dementia, MCI/prodromal AD, preclinical AD), has similarly required dyadic enrollment.

With the movement to pre-dementia disease stages, AD trials required a transition in nomenclature. In contrast to the early trials of the 1980s and 1990s, which were highly reliant on caregivers to achieve success, MCI trials enrolled patients who were by definition functionally independent. Thus, referring to the co-enrolling individual as "caregiver" was inaccurate and inappropriate. Therein the terminology "study partner" was coined. This important change in nomenclature has been used consistently for the last two decades, including now in preclinical AD trials.

29.2.2 Trial Recruitment

Recruitment of participants to AD trials is frequently inadequate [4]. Few trials complete accrual on schedule; fewer still enroll samples that are representative of the larger disease-suffering population. Recruitment to AD trials is challenging for myriad reasons, including the following: the condition is underdiagnosed; awareness of trials remains suboptimal; and trials are carefully designed, often with strict enrollment criteria to protect the integrity of the study and the safety of those enrolled, resulting in exclusion of most patients [5]. Criteria are typically outlined in trial protocols for the study partner as well. Most specify a minimal level of contact with the participant, and this is true for trials in each diagnostic category. Dyads are rarely excluded due to the available study partner's qualifications. However, systematic evaluation of the impact of differing criteria for study partners has not been performed.

Compared to trials in other areas of medicine, recruitment to AD trials could be said to be *twice as difficult*. AD trialists need to recruit not one but two individuals. Trial enrollment decisions have been compared to a "balance sheet"; participants must weigh the potential benefits of participation against the potential risks and burdens. In AD trials, the burden falls both on the patient participant who will be randomly assigned to drug or placebo, and the study partner who may attend every visit, manage transportation, oversee or administer the study treatment, and monitor for and report adverse events. Given all of this, the role of the study partner in the decision about whether to enroll is critical.

AD patients and their study partners engage in shared decision making when considering enrollment in clinical trials [6]. Even in mild AD dementia, the caregiver's role in the decision is prominent and may actually assume "veto" power, as an unwilling caregiver may preclude trial participation for most dyads. Dyadic decision making changes over the course of the disease. When examining medical decision making, Karlawish and colleagues found that roughly half of dyads in the mildest disease stages engaged in shared decision making and the role of the caregiver increased substantially with greater dementia severity [7]. When deciding about trials, caregivers may feel compelled to project the desires and belief systems of their loved one living with dementia, while also incorporating their own beliefs, desires, and concerns [6]. One reason caregivers cite for enrolling in trials is the hope that effective therapy could reduce the burden of care. Alternatively, the risks may include an added burden of care if the participant were to suffer untoward health events as a result of participation [6]. The physical, emotional, and financial burden faced would also understandably make the added burden of trial participation unappealing for many caregivers.

What about trials in pre-dementia populations? Even in MCI, where patients are functionally independent, most patient–partner dyads indicate that they make trial decisions in partnership [8]. The perceived facilitators and barriers to participation are largely similar to those observed in dementia trials, with the participant's potential direct benefit and safety risks most frequently cited. A notable addition to the desires of MCI patients and partners, however, is to learn more about the patient's condition [8]. This likely results from the uncertainty associated with the MCI syndrome, and the potential implications of biomarker testing in the setting of trials as a means to gain more information about disease etiology and prognosis.

While the role of study partners in preclinical AD trials is less critical than in trials enrolling symptomatic patients, it is still the case that participants must have a study partner to be eligible. In local recruitment registries, relatively new tools to aid trial recruitment, one-quarter of cognitively unimpaired older participants indicate that they do not have a person who could fill the required study-partner role [2], potentially precluding their participation. In one study of potential preclinical AD trial participants, 18% of participants acknowledged that the study-partner requirement was a barrier to participation [9]. While participants more frequently affirmed the positive aspects of enrolling in preclinical AD trials with a study partner (e.g., 76% indicated they would want their study partner present when they learned their biomarker eligibility results), 59% felt reluctance toward inconveniencing the person who would be their partner and 5% felt reluctant to share their biomarker results [9].

29.2.3 Informed Consent

AD is a progressive neurodegenerative disorder, ultimately affecting all domains of cognition, including executive function (reasoning and decision making). The essential ethical principles of informed consent include that an individual is given adequate information to make an informed decision, that they are able to make that decision free of coercion or undue influence, and that they have the capacity to make the decision whether to enroll. Capacity is specific to a decision; it is not an all-or-none concept. A person living with dementia may have the capacity to make some decisions (e.g., which candidate to vote for), but lack the capacity to make an enrollment decision for a complex clinical trial. A variety of tools have been developed to assist investigators in assessing an individual's capacity to provide informed consent in a research study. A review of these tools is beyond the scope of this chapter except to clarify that each tool aims to establish whether the potential participant can demonstrate that they are making a choice, that they understand the study and appreciate its requirements and risks, and that they apply reasoning to their decision.

Inclusion of individuals who lack the capacity to provide informed consent in research is essential to advances in a wide variety of neurological conditions, including AD. The Declaration of Helsinki originally laid the ethical foundation for research in persons unable to provide informed consent, but numerous surveys of researchers and the public support the practice. People living with AD dementia frequently lack the capacity to provide informed consent for AD trials [10]. In these cases, surrogate consent is needed. Guidelines for who can serve as a surrogate provider of informed consent vary from state to state (and nation to nation), but legally authorized representatives and legal spouses most often fulfill this role. Except in unique circumstances, a surrogate provider of consent cannot enroll a participant against their will. That is, the person living with dementia must still provide assent, agreeing to participate despite not having capacity to provide consent. Even if a person with dementia maintains capacity, they may look to the study partner to assist in understanding the trial obligations and support in arriving at the decision about whether to participate.

Not surprisingly, research assessments of people with MCI find that they perform better than patients with AD dementia and worse than healthy controls on standardized instruments examining capacity [11]. Patients with MCI rarely have trouble demonstrating a choice, but may exhibit impairment on measures of reasoning or understanding. This impairment may be related to the severity of cognitive decline, especially executive function [12] and may worsen over time [13]. These observations emphasize the importance of study partners in MCI/prodromal AD trials. Though most patients with MCI will have the capacity to provide informed consent at baseline, this could change over the course of the trial. Though reassessment of capacity is typically reserved for situations that require re-consent, these situations may in fact bring challenging decisions regarding whether to continue participation, for example in light of new information or protocol amendments that substantially alter the safety or burden of participation.

29.2.4   Trial Conduct

Once participants are enrolled, study partners play vital roles in the conduct of AD trials. In trials enrolling patients with moderate and severe dementia, compliance may be completely dependent upon the study partner. Scheduling and attending visits, adherence to oral medications, providing medical history, and reporting of adverse events all rely on the study partner. In mild-to-moderate dementia, the degree to which study compliance is dependent upon the partner may be reduced, but the role is no less important to trial success. Even in MCI trials, partners may play key roles in fulfilling trial requirements.

In addition to ensuring the successful completion of study visits, study partners play a pivotal role in whether participants complete the study overall. One review found that 19 of 29 examined AD clinical trials failed to achieve 80% completion (a common assumption for study power calculations) [4]. The importance of retention in AD trials cannot be overstated. A greater than expected drop-out can harm trial integrity, lowering the statistical power, and risking bias or error [14]. Just as the decision to enroll in a study may hinge upon the study partner's desire to see the patient with dementia or MCI participate, so too does the decision to continue in a study. A multitude of interventions to enhance AD research participant retention exist [15, 16]. Retention interventions have been broadly categorized into 12 strategies, with most focused on communicating the importance of a study, reducing its burden, or otherwise offering means to facilitate continued participation. In symptomatic populations, many of these interventions could

be interpreted to target study partners as much as participants. Perhaps the most compelling evidence to suggest the importance of study partners in trial retention comes from observations related to differential retention frequencies among varying study partner types (see Section 29.3).

In essentially all AD trials, study partners will be asked to serve as the source of information that assesses clinical efficacy, be it related to cognitive performance, activities of daily living (function), or neuropsychiatric symptoms. Until recently [17], the only path to FDA approval in AD was to demonstrate efficacy on dual co-primary outcome measures, including a measure of cognition and a measure of function [18]. Therefore, most trials – and necessarily all registration trials – included a scale suitable for demonstrating a clinically meaningful benefit on function. Though early trials used the Clinicians Global Impression of Change (CGIC), a categorical assessment of the expert investigator's evaluation of the patient's change from baseline, this soon gave way to versions of the scale that incorporated study-partner input (CGIC-Plus) [3]. Ultimately, validated scales such as the Clinical Dementia Rating Scale – sum of boxes (CDR-sb) and the Alzheimer's Disease Cooperative Study (ADCS) Activities of Daily Living (ADL) scale came to predominate as functional co-primary outcomes. The CDR, like the CGIC-Plus, incorporates input from the study partner with direct observations of the participant. The ADCS ADL, as well as versions adapted for severe dementia and MCI, are exclusively reliant upon partner completion. Recent guidance from the FDA established a pathway to approval based on a single global outcome measure, with the CDR-sb offered as an example of an acceptable single primary [17]. Thus, for the foreseeable future, study-partner reporting of patient outcomes seems likely to remain essential for demonstrating efficacy of putative therapies sufficient for FDA approval.

In preclinical AD, cognitively unimpaired participants may be unlikely to demonstrate functional decline during the course of a trial. This makes traditional approaches to demonstrating clinically meaningful benefits inappropriate for these trials. Outcomes proposed as potentially assessing clinical meaningfulness, such as the Cognitive Function Instrument [19], intriguingly include patient and study partner versions, permitting exploration of who is the better informant in preclinical AD trials – the study partners or the cognitively unimpaired participants themselves. When comparing to objective measures of cognition, studies repeatedly find that participants' reports better correlate early in a study, but give way to stronger associations with informant reports with greater-duration follow-up [19, 20]. Thus, even in these trials enrolling cognitively intact and functionally independent participants, study partners may be essential to producing the highest integrity data for trial outcomes [21].

29.3 Study Partner Types

29.3.1 Disparities in Participation

More than 16 million Americans provide care to a person living with AD dementia [22]. Most are unpaid. Most are women. And most are family members. Two-thirds of unpaid caregivers are caring for a parent living with dementia. The prevalence of adult-child caregivers is the result of several factors. Women are at higher risk for AD, due in part (but not entirely) to their greater longevity, and most people with AD being over the age of 75. Despite the higher disease risk among women, wives are more likely than husbands to be caregivers. But the modal caregiver–patient relationship in the United States is an adult daughter caring for a parent.

In AD trials, most study partners are the primary caregiver of the participant. Yet a stark contrast exists in the demography of AD trial study partners compared to AD caregivers. Whereas spouses make up only a fraction of all caregivers

to people with AD, they make up a preponderance of AD trial study partners. An assessment of six trials performed by the ADCS found remarkable consistency in the dyadic composition of trial populations. Across these trials, 67% of participants enrolled with a spouse study partner, compared to 26% who enrolled with an adult-child study partner [23]. The trial-to-trial variation was minimal; the range of the proportions of spouse study partners was 62–74% (Figure 29.1). Similar results have been observed in other trials. In four Phase 3 trials sponsored by Eli Lilly and company – two of the gamma-secretase inhibitor semagacestat and two of the monoclonal antibody solanezumab – 64% of more than 3,000 participants enrolled with a spouse study partner [24]. This differed somewhat by global region in these multinational trials, but in North America more than 70% of 1,884 participants enrolled with a spouse partner. Even in MCI trials, in which the burden of caregiving should be reduced if present at all, similar disparities in participation exist. In the ADCS MCI trial of donepezil and vitamin E, for example, 73% of participants enrolled with a spouse partner, compared to 14% who enrolled with an adult child.

29.3.2 Dyadic Recruitment

Enrolling in trials is more difficult for adult children caring for a parent with AD than it is for spouses. Adult-child study partners are younger, more likely to be working, and more likely to have other dependents, than are spouse study partners [23]. Dyadic recruitment may also shape

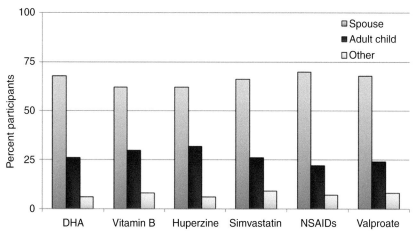

Figure 29.1 Frequency of study-partner types across six mild-to-moderate AD trials conducted by the ADCS. Trials included studies of docosahexaenoic acid (DHA), high-dose B vitamin supplementation (vitamin B), huperzine, simvastatin, the non-steroidal anti-inflammatory drugs (NSAIDs) rofecoxib and naproxen, and valproate. Data taken from Grill et al. [23].

the demographics of trial participant samples. Compared to participants who enroll with a spouse, participants who enroll with a non-spouse study partner are older, more often male, and are more likely to be from a minority race or ethnicity. In short, participants who enroll with a non-spouse partner may better represent the greater disease-suffering population than do those with a spouse. These associations may be especially important for efforts to improve diversity in trials. In the six ADCS trials noted above, only 11% of participants were from any minority race or ethnicity. Adult–child dyads accounted for 46% of all diverse participants.

Why are non-spousal dyads under-represented in AD trials? AD participants lacking a spouse may less frequently be eligible for AD trials [25]. This difference is due in part to differences in age, but many trials do not, and should not [26], apply an upper age limit. A larger driver of disparities in participation could in fact be attitudinal. Adult-child caregivers are more likely than spouses to feel that their caregiving burden is overwhelming [27]. Yet burden may not drive decisions about whether or not to enroll. In a study balanced for spouse vs. adult-child caregivers, 35% of caregivers said that they "probably" or "definitely" would enroll with their loved one in a hypothetical trial of a disease-modifying therapy. Spouses were 2.5 times more likely than adult children to indicate willingness to participate in the hypothetical trial. Other significant predictors of willingness included older study-partner age and higher scores on the Research Attitude Questionnaire (RAQ) scale. In contrast, no measure of caregiving burden (including logistical burden associated with participation, financial burden, caregiver depression, or measures of patient functional impairment or behavioral symptoms) was associated with willingness to participate [28]. The RAQ has been shown to predict willingness to participate and study completion and may therefore serve as an ideal outcome measure for interventional studies to improve attitudes and increase participation in AD trials, especially in adult-child caregivers. Determining how best to do so remains an area of great need, but could have major implications to trial generalizability.

The approach to trial enrollment decisions in MCI may similarly differ for spousal and non-spousal dyads. In a small study of MCI dyads, most MCI patients and study partners agreed that they would make trial decisions in partnership. The

apparent exception, however, was patients who lacked a spouse. These patients more frequently indicated that they would make an enrollment decision unilaterally, even though their partners often indicated that the dyad would decide together [8].

Even in preclinical AD trials, the role of study partners seems to impact on who participates. Compared to Whites, African American/Blacks more frequently rated the study-partner requirement as an important barrier to participation (79% vs. 57%) in one hypothetical study [29]. Attitudes toward the requirement differ based on who fills the study partner role [9], and this appears to differ by ethnoracial group. In the first ever preclinical AD trial, the Anti-Amyloid treatment in Asymptomatic AD (A4) study [30], 58% of White participants enrolled with a spouse study partner, compared to 46% for Asians, 45% for Hispanics, and 27% for African American/Blacks. Thus, across the spectrum of AD trials, improving enrollment of participants with non-spousal study partners may represent an important opportunity to diversify trial samples.

29.3.3 Differential Rates of Trial Completion among Partner Types

In addition to decisions about enrolling in trials, study partners may play key roles in decisions to remain in trials. In ADCS trials, differential completion rates were apparent among dyad types. Among participants with spouse study partners, 75% completed trials, compared to 68% for adult–child dyads, and 66% for non-spouse–non-adult-child ("other") dyads [23]. In multivariable analyses, these differences remained significant when controlling for covariates such as age and disease severity. The differences translated into a 30% and 70% increased risk of drop-out for adult–child and other dyads, respectively, compared to spousal dyads. In the Phase 3 semagacestat trials, 35%, 38%, and 36% of spousal, adult–child, and other dyads, respectively, dropped out prior to protocol-defined study completion. Though significant in unadjusted models, the difference among dyad types was not significant in models adjusting for potential confounding factors (p-value 0.928). Instead, participant age was identified as the primary characteristic to explain the relationship between study-partner type and the risk of failing to complete the trial in exploratory models [31]. In the ADCS MCI trial of donepezil and vitamin E, unmarried participants dropped out more frequently than married ones [32]. Given the relatively low number of completed preclinical AD trials, formal assessments of predictors of completion have not yet been performed.

29.3.4 Differential Impact of Partner Types on Trial Outcome Measures

Adult-child and spouse caregivers may view the disease differently. This may lead to differential interest or motivation to participate in research but it may also have ramifications to trial measurements. For example, adult-child caregivers rate patient quality of life lower than do spouse caregivers [33]. The type of study partner may also be associated with the accuracy and consistency of reporting [34]. In natural history studies, non-spousal partners more frequently provide discrepant measures of memory, orientation, and problem solving than do spouses [34–36]. In ADCS trials, measures of disease progression may have differed among dyad types [23]. Trends were observed toward slower decline among ADCS trial participants with adult-child partners for the Mini Mental State Examination (MMSE) and CDR-sb. Variance in trial outcome measures also differed. Together, the amount of change in an outcome measure and the variance of that change in a population determine the effect size and associated power of a trial. Table 29.2 provides estimated effect sizes for commonly used co-primary outcome measures in AD registration trials for studies enrolling only particular dyad types, based on ADCS trial data [23]. Estimated effect sizes are reduced for non-spousal dyad groups. Thus, increasing enrollment of these dyads, which is clearly needed, could come at a cost to trials. More work is needed to fully understand these risks and how to mitigate potential negative implications to trial power.

One thing that can likely increase outcome-measure variance is the need to replace the study partner mid-study. In the National Alzheimer's Coordinating Center longitudinal observational study, study-partner replacement was a frequent occurrence: 15.5% of participants experienced study-partner replacement at least once [37]. Replacement was more frequent among participants with adult-child (24%) and other study partners (38%) at baseline, compared to those with spouse partners (10%). Spouse dyads accounted for the most absolute cases of replacement, however, due to their prevalence in the study [37]. Older age, male sex, and minority race and ethnicity were associated with replacing a spouse partner. In contrast, only younger partner age was associated with replacing an adult-child partner. For non-spouse, non-adult child partners, lower education and Latino ethnicity were associated with being replaced. Most importantly, replacement affected between-visit outcome-measure scores for the CDR-sb, Neuropsychiatric Inventory, and the Functional Assessment Questionnaire (FAQ). FAQ change scores were greater in participants who replaced their partner, compared to a matched group with stable partners. The variance of the change in each scale was higher in those who replaced partners, compared to a matched group with no partner replacement. The extent to which these results generalize to trials is not yet known, though work is ongoing. For example, in four Phase 3 industry-sponsored AD dementia trials (two of semagacestat and two of solanezumab), the rates of study-partner replacement ranged from 3% to 7%, potentially having a meaningful impact on trial data.

Table 29.2 Effect sizes for 18-month change in outcomes by dyad group from six ADCS mild-to-moderate AD trials

Group	ADCS ADL scale		CDR-sb scale	
	Mean change +/– SD	Effect size	Mean change +/– SD	Effect size
Spousal dyads	−11.6 +/– 11.40	1.02	3.10 +/– 2.91	1.06
Adult–child dyads	−9.74 +/– 12.95	0.75	2.81 +/– 2.69	1.04
Other dyads	−9.22 +/– 13.40	0.69	2.36 +/– 2.46	0.95

Abbreviations: ADCS ADL, Alzheimer's Disease Cooperative Study Activities of Daily Living; CDR-sb, Clinical Dementia Rating Scale – sum of boxes; SD, standard deviation.

The relationship of the study partner to the participant can affect outcome measurements in preclinical AD trials as well. Identifying the onset of cognitive decline is among the most critical roles of study partners in these trials [21]. With longer durations, the strength of associations between subjective scales and objective performance will favor the partner over the participant themselves [19, 20]. Examinations of data from the ADCS Prevention Instruments (PI) project, a large trial planning project, however, explored whether the relationship between the participant and their partner affected this association [38]. In the ADCS PI, regardless of study-partner type, participants were better than study partners at predicting future cognitive status. In cross-sectional assessments over time, however, the results differed substantially by dyad type. Spousal partners outperformed participants in predicting current cognitive performance later in the study. Participants with non-spouse study partners, in contrast, outperformed their partners in assessing cognition at later times [38]. Therefore, even in preclinical AD trials, study-partner characteristics may affect the integrity of trial data, and efforts to increase the validity of assessments may be needed.

29.4 The Role of Study Partners in the AD Drug-Development Ecosystem

Efforts are needed to make it easier for participant–study-partner dyads to participate in AD trials. This could include providing respite or other forms of education and support to caregivers of people living with dementia, especially in the burdensome moderate-to-severe stages. The burden of participation must be reduced as much as possible. Offering home visits, transportation, and other means of removing hassles for study partners can make it easier for them to accept invitations to participate [39]. To make it easier for non-spouse study partners, specifically, this may mean offering visits during non-traditional times, such as evenings and weekends. Remote study visits, collecting adverse-event and functional outcome-measure data through telephone or teleconferences may be essential to enable working caregivers to participate in trials.

Study partners do work. This contribution cannot be overlooked. In fact, it should be compensated. Few investigators perform clinical trials

without compensation for their efforts. Why should we expect anything different for participants and their study partners? Gelinas and colleagues provide an important structure for considering financial payments to research participants [40]. At minimum, participation should be cost neutral – participants should be *reimbursed* for their incurred costs while participating in research. It is offensive that these essential contributors to the greater research agenda should also be expected to pay to park or pay for public transportation in order to provide this unique service. In fact, they deserve *compensation*, a fair wage, for providing this service, just as expert investigators and their teams do. But if the field truly wants to accelerate research advances and to diversify research samples (that is, recruit currently under-represented dyads), financial *incentivization* may be needed – offering more than a fair wage – in an effort to facilitate dyads making a decision they otherwise would not. Aside from financial incentives, investigators should do everything in their power to make it easier for dyads to say yes to trials and to conduct studies to instruct the field on how best to accelerate trials and improve their conduct. Failure to do so risks unacceptable delays or, worse, failed trials.

29.5 Lessons Learned from Studying Study Partners for AD Drug Development

My hope is that this chapter has provided compelling support for the importance of study partners in the AD drug-development ecosystem. Despite this importance, study partners are often overlooked in research to improve trial design, efforts to accelerate or improve recruitment, and trial conduct. A stronger focus on study partners across the spectrum of AD trials could meaningfully accelerate drug development, increase trial power (possibly permitting shorter and smaller studies), and improve trial integrity and generalizability. What more rationale could be needed to invest in research on the study-partner role and resources to facilitate their contributions to the field?

References

1. Hurd MD, Martorell P, Delavande A, Mullen KJ, Langa KM. Monetary costs of dementia in the United States. *N Engl J Med* 2013; **368**: 1326–34.

2. Largent EA, Karlawish J, Grill JD. Study partners: essential collaborators in discovering treatments

for Alzheimer's disease. *Alzheimers Res Ther* 2018; **10**: 101.

3. Knopman DS. Clinical trial design issues in mild to moderate Alzheimer disease. *Cogn Behav Neurol* 2008; **21**: 197–201.

4. Grill JD, Karlawish J. Addressing the challenges to successful recruitment and retention in Alzheimer's disease clinical trials. *Alzheimers Res Ther* 2010; **2**: 34.

5. Schneider LS, Olin JT, Lyness SA, Chui HC. Eligibility of Alzheimer's disease clinic patients for clinical trials. *J Am Geriatr Soc* 1997; **45**: 923–8.

6. Karlawish JH, Casarett D, Klocinski J, Sankar P. How do AD patients and their caregivers decide whether to enroll in a clinical trial? *Neurology* 2001; **56**: 789–92.

7. Karlawish JH, Casarett D, Propert KJ, James BD, Clark CM. Relationship between Alzheimer's disease severity and patient participation in decisions about their medical care. *J Am Geriatr Soc Neurol* 2002; **15**: 68–72.

8. Cox CG, Ryan BAM, Gillen DL, Grill JD. A preliminary study of clinical trial enrollment decisions among people with mild cognitive impairment and their study partners. *Am J Geriatr Psychiatry* 2019; **27**: 322–32.

9. Cox CG, Ryan MM, Gillen D, Grill JD. Is reluctance to share Alzheimer's disease biomarker status with a study partner a barrier to preclinical trial recruitment? *J Prev Alzheimers Dis* 2021; **8**: 52–8.

10. Karlawish JH, Casarett DJ, James BD. Alzheimer's disease patients' and caregivers' capacity, competency, and reasons to enroll in an early-phase Alzheimer's disease clinical trial. *J Am Geriatr Soc* 2002; **50**: 2019–24.

11. Okonkwo O, Griffith HR, Belue K, et al. Medical decision-making capacity in patients with mild cognitive impairment. *Neurology* 2007; **69**: 1528–35.

12. Jefferson AL, Lambe S, Moser DJ, et al. Decisional capacity for research participation in individuals with mild cognitive impairment. *J Am Geriatr Soc* 2008; **56**: 1236–43.

13. Okonkwo OC, Griffith HR, Copeland JN, et al. Medical decision-making capacity in mild cognitive impairment: a 3-year longitudinal study. *Neurology* 2008; **71**: 1474–80.

14. National Research Council (US) Panel on Handling Missing Data in Clinical Trials. *The Prevention and Treatment of Missing Data in Clinical Trials*. Washington, DC: National Academies Press; 2010.

15. Grill JD, Kwon J, Teylan MA, et al. Retention of Alzheimer disease research participants. *Alzheimer Dis Assoc Disord* 2019; **33**: 299–306.

16. Robinson KA, Dinglas VD, Sukrithan V, et al. Updated systematic review identifies substantial number of retention strategies: using more strategies retains more study participants. *J Clin Epidemiol* 2015; **68**: 1481–7.

17. Kozauer N, Katz, R. Regulatory innovation and drug development for early-stage Alzheimer's disease. *N Engl J Med* 2013; **368**: 1169–71.

18. Leber P. Observations and suggestions on antidementia drug development. *Alzheimer Dis Assoc Disord* 1996; **10**: 31–5.

19. Amariglio RE, Donohue MC, Marshall GA, et al. Tracking early decline in cognitive function in older individuals at risk for Alzheimer disease dementia: the Alzheimer's Disease Cooperative Study Cognitive Function Instrument. *JAMA Neurol* 2015; **72**: 446–54.

20. Ryan MM, Grill JD, Gillen DL, Alzheimer's Disease Neuroimaging Initiative. Participant and study partner prediction and identification of cognitive impairment in preclinical Alzheimer's disease: study partner vs. participant accuracy. *Alzheimers Res Ther* 2019; **11**: 85.

21. Grill JD, Karlawish J. Study partners should be required in preclinical Alzheimer's disease trials. *Alzheimers Res Ther* 2017; **9**: 93.

22. Alzheimer's Association. 2020 Alzheimer's disease facts and figures. *Alzheimers Dement* 2020; **16**: 391–460.

23. Grill JD, Raman R, Ernstrom K, Aisen P, Karlawish J. Effect of study partner on the conduct of Alzheimer disease clinical trials. *Neurology* 2013; **80**: 282–8.

24. Grill JD, Raman R, Ernstrom K, et al. Comparing recruitment, retention, and safety reporting among geographic regions in multinational Alzheimer's disease clinical trials. *Alzheimers Res Ther* 2015; **7**: 39.

25. Grill JD, Monsell S, Karlawish J. Are patients whose study partners are spouses more likely to be eligible for Alzheimer's disease clinical trials? *Dement Geriatr Cogn Disord* 2012; **33**: 334–40.

26. Bernard MA, Clayton JA, Lauer MS. Inclusion across the lifespan: NIH policy for clinical research. *JAMA* 2018; **320**: 1535–6.

27. Conde-Sala JL, Garre-Olmo J, Turro-Garriga O, Vilalta-Franch J, Lopez-Pousa S. Differential features of burden between spouse and adult-child caregivers of patients with Alzheimer's disease: an exploratory comparative design. *Int J Nurs Stud* 2010; **47**: 1262–73.

28. Cary MS, Rubright JD, Grill JD, Karlawish J. Why are spousal caregivers more prevalent than nonspousal caregivers as study partners in AD dementia clinical trials? *Alzheimer Dis Assoc Disord* 2015; **29**: 70–4.

29. Zhou Y, Elashoff D, Kremen S, et al. African Americans are less likely to enroll in preclinical Alzheimer's disease clinical trials. *Alzheimers Dement (N Y)* 2017; **3**: 57–64.

30. Sperling RA, Rentz DM, Johnson KA, et al. The A4 study: stopping AD before symptoms begin? *Sci Transl Med* 2014; **6**: 228fs13.

31. Berstein OM, Grill JD, Gillen DL. Recruitment and retention of participant and study partner dyads in two multinational Alzheimer's disease registration trials. *Alzheimers Res Ther* 2021; **13**: 16.

32. Edland SD, Emond JA, Aisen PS, Petersen RC. NIA-funded Alzheimer centers are more efficient than commercial clinical recruitment sites for conducting secondary prevention trials of dementia. *Alzheimer Dis Assoc Disord* 2010; **24**: 159–64.

33. Conde-Sala JL, Garre-Olmo J, Turro-Garriga O, Vilalta-Franch J, Lopez-Pousa S. Quality of life of patients with Alzheimer's disease: differential perceptions between spouse and adult child caregivers. *Dement Geriatr Cogn Disord* 2010; **29**: 97–108.

34. Grill JD, Karlawish J. Consider the source: the implications of informant type on outcome assessments. *Alzheimer Dis Assoc Disord* 2015; **29**: 364.

35. Ready RE, Ott BR, Grace J. Validity of informant reports about AD and MCI patients' memory. *Alzheimer Dis Assoc Disord* 2004; **18**: 11–16.

36. Cacchione PZ, Powlishta KK, Grant EA, Buckles VD, Morris JC. Accuracy of collateral source reports in very mild to mild dementia of the Alzheimer type. *J Am Geriatr Soc* 2003; **51**: 819–23.

37. Grill JD, Zhou Y, Karlawish J, Elashoff D. Frequency and impact of informant replacement in Alzheimer disease research. *Alzheimer Dis Assoc Disord* 2015; **29**: 242–8.

38. Nuno MM, Gillen DL, Grill JD, et al. Study partner types and prediction of cognitive performance: implications to preclinical Alzheimer's trials. *Alzheimers Res Ther* 2019; **11**: 92.

39. Karlawish J, Cary MS, Rubright J, Tenhave T. How redesigning AD clinical trials might increase study partners' willingness to participate. *Neurology* 2008; **71**: 1883–8.

40. Gelinas L, Largent EA, Cohen IG, et al. Framework for ethical payment to research participants. *N Engl J Med* 2018; **378**: 766–71.

Chapter 30

From Trials to Practice: Are We Ready for a Disease-Modifying Treatment?

Soeren Mattke

30.1 Introduction

The COVID-19 pandemic has certainly taught us that even well-resourced and sophisticated health systems can be overwhelmed by a new challenge in the absence of proper advance planning. And, less dramatically, other case studies illustrate the difficulty of systems to adapt to new treatments that affect large numbers of patients. The first direct-acting antiviral drugs for hepatitis C, for example, not only created a fiscal shock because of the high unit cost of the treatments and the large number of prevalent patients but also resulted in wait times because of a lack of specialists who could correctly identify treatment eligible patients, as initial treatments were only effective in certain subtypes of the disease. A similar case was sacubitril/valsartan, the first novel drug for congestive heart failure in many years. In spite of evidence for reduction of over 20% in mortality and hospital admission rates, adoption was slower than expected initially. An important reason was that primary care clinicians, who manage most heart failure patients, found the drug's complex uptitration and monitoring process to be incompatible with their workflow.

Against this background, the chapter explores the implications of making an Alzheimer's disease (AD) treatment accessible to the large number of potentially eligible patients, in particular when it first becomes available, because of the large backlog of prevalent cases. It looks at the expected patient journey, discusses resources required at each step of the journey, analyzes how well available resources match the expected demand for several countries, and explores solutions to capacity constraints.

30.2 The Context of Emerging Therapeutics

30.2.1 Highly Prevalent Disease

In recent years, our understanding of AD has evolved from a symptom-oriented toward a biology-defined condition, the so-called amyloid, tau, and neurodegeneration (A/T/N) framework [1]. It is now seen as a continuum that starts with the pathological hallmarks of the disease and no symptoms, the preclinical stage, progresses to mild cognitive impairment (MCI), and finally to dementia due to AD. The preclinical stage may last for years and even decades. Because of that long prodromal phase, the true prevalence of the disease itself is unknown. Estimates do exist, however, for prevalence of the symptomatic phases of the disease. Of note, epidemiological data that are based on symptoms do not necessarily differentiate based on the underlying etiology. In other words, while AD is the most frequent cause of cognitive decline, other conditions account for 25–45% of cases.

The confluence of population aging and increasing burden of risk factors for dementia, such as hypertension, hypercholesterolemia, and diabetes, means that cognitive decline has become very common, in particular in developed economies. Peterson et al. reported MCI prevalence rates of 6.7% for ages 60–64, 8.4% for ages 65–69, 10.1% for ages 70–74, 14.8% for ages 75–79, and 25.2% for ages 80–84 [2]. Translated to country populations, it was estimated that 13.8 million individuals in the USA [3] and 20 million individuals in the European Union (EU) countries plus the UK [4] today live with MCI due to any cause.

An estimated 5.5 million patients live with AD-related dementia in the USA and 3.6 million in Japan today, a number that is projected to increase to 11.6 million by 2040 for the USA [5] and to 8 million by 2050 for Japan [6]. In spite of the enormous burden, cognitive decline remains substantially underdiagnosed, particularly in early stages. For example, a recent meta-analysis suggested a pooled rate of 61.7% of undetected dementia [7].

30.2.2 Preventive Paradigm

There is unambiguous evidence that AD dementia cannot be reversed, as multiple clinical trials have failed to show an effect at that stage. This result appears biologically plausible because complex organs are known to have some degree of redundancy and plasticity but no regenerative potential. Like myocytes, neurons have lost their ability to divide and their loss is irreversible. Consequently, treatment of AD has shifted to a preventive paradigm, under which drugs are being used at early symptomatic and maybe even in preclinical stages to halt the progression to dementia. Most current trials enroll patients with MCI and mild dementia. Obviously, identifying patients at such mild stages is considerably more difficult than finding highly symptomatic cases, not to mention finding patients in preclinical stages as some current prevention trials do [8].

30.2.3 Complexity of Diagnostic and Treatment Process

The preventive paradigm creates enormous capacity challenges for healthcare systems, because prevention in the case of AD has little in common with typical preventive measures that tend to be cheap, simple, and scalable, such as statin treatment and flu shots. As I will explain below, prevention of AD dementia is more akin to high-end oncology care than to our traditional connotations of prevention. Moreover, determining treatment eligibility requires a complex differential diagnosis because the typical elderly patients commonly suffer from reversible and irreversible co-morbid conditions that may contribute to cognitive impairment, such as depression and vascular disease. Disentangling those competing etiologies to find patients who are likely to benefit from an expensive treatment, with potential side effects, requires skill, patience, and experience.

30.3 The Patient Journey toward a Treatment

30.3.1 Initial Evaluation

Systematic screening would be the logical approach to find an early-stage disease with mild or no symptoms, just like screening programs for cancer and cardiovascular risk factors. However, screening for cognitive decline is currently not recommended for lack of evidence for net clinical benefit and, consequently, it is not covered in any country that the University of Southern California (USC) Brain Health Observatory has reviewed so far. While this

assessment might change with the introduction of a disease-modifying treatment, for now patients will get identified serendipitously during an office visit for other reasons – a general geriatric assessment or because they present with a subjective memory complaint. This initial evaluation typically occurs in the primary care setting or, as in the case of South Korea, dementia centers that offer walk-in cognitive testing. It can be unstructured or based on a brief instrument, such as the Mini-Mental State Examination (MMSE) or the Montreal Cognitive Assessment (MoCA).

30.3.2 Confirmatory Diagnosis

Patients with suspected cognitive decline are usually referred to a dementia specialist for confirmatory neurocognitive testing and determination of the etiology, ideally after ruling out addressable causes such as substance use, depression, and vitamin B_{12} deficiency and detecting possible structural causes such as a past stroke. In patients with confirmed cognitive decline, biomarker testing is required to ascertain the pathological hallmarks of AD, either with an amyloid positron emission tomography (PET) scan or with examination of cerebrospinal fluid (CSF).

30.3.3 Treatment Delivery and Monitoring

With a confirmed treatment indication, patients will start treatment, which in many cases consists of monthly or biweekly intravenous infusions. The treatment also requires regular MRI for amyloid-related imaging abnormalities (ARIA) and repeated specialist visits to monitor effectiveness and safety, as well as to apply stopping rules.

30.4 Assessment of Preparedness

The combination of a prevalent disease, a large pool of undiagnosed patients, and a complex diagnostic and monitoring process is what makes access to a disease-modifying treatment so challenging from a capacity standpoint, particularly when the treatment initially becomes available. Once the backlog of prevalent cases has been handled, capacity tends to be sufficient for the much smaller number of incident cases. The initial surge in demand for services also makes planning decisions difficult. On the one hand, the progressive nature of the disease means that wait times should be minimized; on the other, investing into dedicated capacity to scale for that initial surge would not be efficient. The USC Brain Health Observatory analyzes how well the infrastructure of countries matches the initial demand for services, looks into the institutional preparedness of countries to adapt to this challenge, and assesses promising solutions.

30.4.1 Capacity Simulation

To date, we have simulated the capacity to provide timely access to a disease-modifying treatment for Australia [9], Canada [10], France [4], Germany, Italy, Japan [11], South Korea [12], Spain, Sweden, Taiwan [13], the UK, and the USA [3]. For these analyses, we use estimates for the age structure of a country's population and the resulting burden of disease and estimates for the capacity of dementia specialists to conduct confirmatory testing, for capacity to perform biomarker testing, and for capacity for infusion delivery. We use a simulation model to project how well supply and demand for services match and what the implications for wait times are, assuming that the treatment becomes available in 2021.

As shown in Table 30.1, wait times are projected to differ substantially even among high-income countries. Initial average wait times range from 5 months and 9 months in Germany and Sweden, respectively, to 28 months in Canada. In France, Canada, and Taiwan, we project that it will take over a decade to clear the backlog of prevalent cases and to make a treatment accessible with little delay.

The number of dementia specialists (geriatricians, geriatric psychiatrists, and neurologists) relative to the population turns out to be the most salient main bottleneck. As shown in Figure 30.1, the number varies by a factor of five. Countries, in which psychiatrists are more involved in dementia care, such as Germany, Japan, and Sweden, tend to have a higher density of specialists, since psychiatry is a much larger specialty than neurology and geriatrics, and consequently shorter wait times.

The second most important bottleneck is the capacity for biomarker testing to confirm the presence of the AD pathology. As this diagnosis can be made based on amyloid PET scans or examination of CSF, two factors determine the capacity. The first is the number of PET scanners relative to population size. As shown in Figure 30.2, this statistic varies by a factor of ten between the UK and the USA, with most countries having between 1.5 and 3 devices per 1 million population. However, these numbers disguise important differences in access to PET scanners within countries, particularly geographically vast countries, as those devices tend to be located in densely populated areas. Further, the short half-life of the amyloid ligand means that PET scans can only be performed in reasonable proximity to a cyclotron to produce said ligand, again limiting access in rural areas.

The second factor is the cultural differences of patients' willingness to undergo a lumbar puncture. While patients in continental Europe

Table 30.1 Projected wait times for access to a disease-modifying treatment in high-income countries

Country	Peak wait time (months)	Year of peak wait time	First year with wait <12 months	Year in which backlog has cleared
Australia	10	2021	2021	2024
Canada	28	2021	2033	2050
France	19	2021	2025	2032
Germany	5	2023	2021	2021
Italy	10	2023	2021	2023
Japan	15	2021	2022	2025
South Korea	14	2022	2023	2029
Spain	12	2022	2021	2025
Sweden	9	2023	2021	2022
Taiwan	24	2021	2042	>2050
UK	14	2022	2024	2027
US	19	2022	2026	2026

Note: Assuming that evaluation for eligibility to receive a disease-modifying treatment starts in 2021.

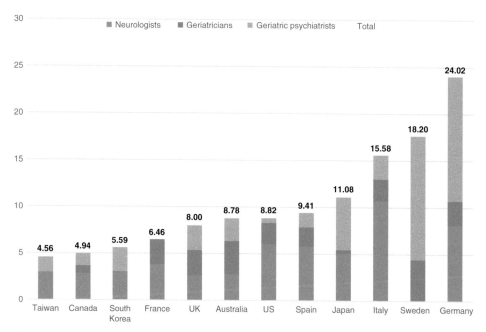

Figure 30.1 Estimated number of dementia specialists per 100,000 population in high-income countries. (Note: neurologists are not involved in dementia care in Sweden and psychiatrists are not involved in France. South Korea and Taiwan only recently established geriatrics as a separate specialty and thus have only a negligible number of those specialists for now.)

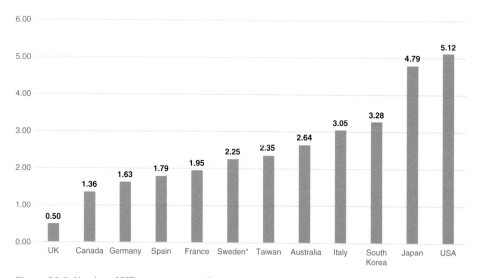

Figure 30.2 Number of PET scanners per 1 million population in high-income countries. (Note: *Sweden only reports hospital-based PET scanners.)

are reportedly quite accepting of this procedure, patients in North America and East Asia are fearful of pain and complications. Experts estimated the share of patients who would be willing to undergo a diagnostic lumbar puncture for confirmatory biomarker testing to be as high as 90% in the EU countries and as low as 5% in South Korea. As lumbar punctures do not require dedicated infrastructure, we assume capacity to be unconstrained

in high-income countries, which allows for rapid scaling and also extension of diagnostic services to less populated areas, and overcomes potential constraints on PET capacity.

There are several other potential constraints for which the impact on access to a disease-modifying treatment is harder to quantify. Several treatments are delivered intravenously and robust data on capacity of infusion sites do not exist. However, experts in most countries took the position that capacity could easily be scaled to accommodate demand. Other bottlenecks might be capacity to conduct MRI scans and availability of specialized medical personnel such as neuroradiologists.

Figure 30.3 illustrates the combined effects of the capacity limits on the trajectories of projected wait times for the G7 countries. Canada, as a country with low specialist density, limited number of PET scanners, and cultural aversion to lumbar punctures, is projected to have long and lasting wait times. Even though wait times are initially long in the USA because of a limited number of specialists, the ample availability of PET scan capacity allows clearing the backlog quickly. Germany, with a high number of specialists, is projected to see minimal

wait times, as a willingness to use CSF diagnostics compensates for the low density of PET scanners.

Figure 30.4 illustrates that the predicted wait times are not merely an inconvenience to patients. Because of the progressive nature of the disease, there is a risk that cognitive decline reaches a point at which the treatment is no longer expected to be effective, while patients queue for specialist care. We estimate that between 1% (Germany) and 22% (Canada) of AD dementia cases could be avoided with timely access.

30.4.2 Institutional Preparedness

It is important to keep in mind that capacity alone is an imperfect measure of how well a country's health system is prepared for the advent of a

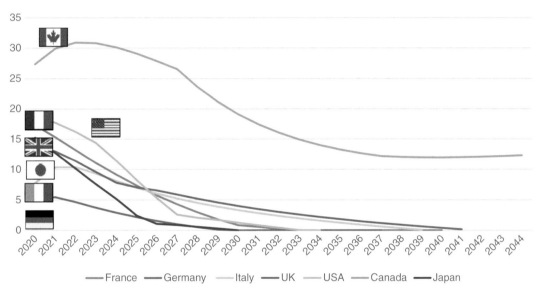

Figure 30.3 Projected average wait times in months in G7 countries.

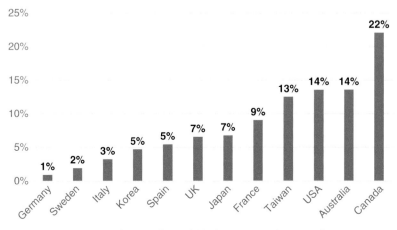

Figure 30.4 Proportion of potentially avoidable dementia cases because of wait times.

disease-modifying treatment. Equally important are planning decisions, funding, system-immanent incentives, regulatory and coverage constraints, and provider capabilities. The salience of such considerations is a function of the balance between use of planning and reliance of market forces to set priorities for healthcare systems. In a market-oriented system like that of the USA, government entities have limited (but by no means no) influence over allocation of funds and talent, whereas centrally planned systems, such as those in the UK, are highly dependent on government policy and implementation.

30.4.2.1 Dementia Planning

All countries that we have reviewed so far have crafted or are in the process of crafting a national dementia strategy. In countries with devolved decision making, like Spain and Canada, national plans are often accompanied by regional and/or local guidance for implementation and funding. To date, those plans tend to focus on identification of and care for patients with manifest dementia and support of caregivers. Aside from calling for earlier detection and research into treatment for AD and other dementias, we have not yet seen a strategy that explicitly calls for preparation for a disease-modifying treatment. Non-governmental expert groups, for example the Edinburgh Consensus group in the UK [14] and the MapEA group in Spain [15], have assessed health system preparedness to deliver a disease-modifying treatment, and made explicit recommendations.

Financial Planning

Our analyses show that all countries but the USA functionally operate their healthcare systems under global budgets, either directly, as in tax-funded countries like the UK or Taiwan, or indirectly, through a combination of price regulation and volume controls in social insurance countries like Germany. This approach limits the growth in healthcare spending but makes it difficult for the system to absorb unanticipated substantial increases in demand for services, even if they are temporary and even for high-income countries.

With the likely budget impact of the treatment, a dialog about how to fund access is important but has not received attention in the countries that we have studied. While unknown at this point, the price of the treatment itself will be substantial in light of the manufacturers' need to recoup billions of dollars invested into failed trials. We estimated a price of around $21,000 per year to be cost-effective in the USA [16]. At that price and with an estimated number of around 500,000 patients being identified as treatment eligible each year, annual spending would be over $10 billion. The average annual cost of diagnosing those treatment-eligible patients would add around $7 billion [17].

Capacity Planning: Primary Care

As memory disorders are population-level diseases, afflicted patients will need to access care via the primary care system for initial evaluation, and triage to specialist care. Countries like the UK mandate this pathway via the gatekeeping roles of general practitioners; Canada incentivizes it by paying lower rates for specialist visits without referrals; and others, like France and South Korea, recommend but do not enforce formal referrals. The challenge is that, in all countries of our sample, primary care providers are reluctant to proactively identify cognitive decline and even to investigate memory complaints further because of a combination of workload, skills, and perceptions.

The combination of aging populations and tight finances means that primary care clinicians have to handle growing needs without commensurate growth in resources. Verifying and quantifying a memory complaint requires in-depth conversations with patients and family members as well as initial cognitive testing, tasks that hardly fit into the usual 10–15-minute slot of an office visit. Preconceived notions that cognitive decline is an inevitable consequence of aging, and a perception that diagnosing it formally has no therapeutic consequences, contribute to a lack of willingness to investigate. As a result, primary care clinicians do not develop or maintain skills and workflows for evaluation of memory complaints, resulting in a vicious cycle of underdiagnosis.

There are encouraging signs that more attention is being paid to early detection and diagnosis of memory disorders, as evidence of therapeutic benefit even in the absence of disease-modifying treatment is emerging. Results from the FINGER study [18] suggest that risk-factor management and cognitive training can delay disease progression, and initial findings from the IDEAS study [19] show that an exact diagnosis influences clinical management. At least as important is a realization that patients simply have a right to know about their disease and its prognosis, as strongly advocated in the French national plan for neurodegenerative diseases, just like they would expect for other conditions. Put differently, one would hardly tell a patient with advanced cancer that there is no point in making a formal diagnosis as there are no options to prolong survival.

Capacity Planning: Specialty Care

The likely complexity of the first disease-modifying AD treatments implies that they will remain in the hands of specialists. Formally diagnosing patients and determining whether they are likely to have a net clinical benefit from a treatment requires the integration of findings from a thorough anamnesis with cognitive testing results, biomarkers, and imaging data. Infusion delivery may be necessary, and the safety and efficacy of the treatment will have to be closely monitored. Thus, future memory care models will have to evolve from the current focus on counseling and social care to resemble models in therapeutic areas like oncology and multiple sclerosis. In light of the scarcity of dementia specialists, care models will have to leverage their time efficiently.

A precondition for this evolution will be creating larger-scale memory services. In countries like France and Japan, patients may be referred to specialists in private practice, who work as solo practitioners or in small groups. Memory clinics in Italy and Spain may also be quite small. The patient volume handled in such practice settings will not support a multidisciplinary team and the infrastructure necessary to deliver a disease-modifying treatment, because of its substantial fixed cost.

First and foremost, future models need to be large multispecialty practices with a team of clinical and non-clinical staff to allow task shifting and "top-of-license" practice [20]; that is, delegating tasks that do not require specialist medical training to other clinical staff, and non-clinical tasks to other team members. For example, cognitive tests can be administered by technicians and interpreted by neuropsychologists, leaving only the integration of testing results with biomarkers and imaging results and eventual treatment recommendation to the specialist. Non-clinical tasks, such as coordination with social services, can be delegated to social workers.

Second, future care models will need to be more medicalized to reflect the shift from care to cure. In countries like the UK and Germany, psychiatrists traditionally play an important role in dementia care. As psychiatry is a relatively large specialty, this helps to expand access to care, but many psychiatrists may not have acquired or maintained required skills like lumbar punctures or infusion delivery. Conversely, countries that rely more heavily on the smaller specialty of neurology for dementia care, such as South Korea and Taiwan, have fewer specialists per capita but are better equipped to handle the mechanics of a disease-modifying treatment. Co-location of memory clinics with general hospitals, as in the UK, or inpatient psychiatric facilities, as in Germany, can provide access to the necessary procedural skills and infrastructure, such as recovery beds and fluoroscopy.

Third, memory clinics will need to be differentiated into those that handle routine cases in the community and referral centers that handle complex cases and research, much like in other therapeutic areas. Such centers of excellence have emerged spontaneously, for example in Spain and the USA, or in a planned fashion, such as in France.

30.5 Solutions

30.5.1 Financial Planning

With the expected financial impact of an AD treatment, not just of the treatment itself but also of the diagnostic pathway to determine treatment eligibility, a dialog about resource allocation seems warranted. Given the immediacy of the budget impact and the long latency to realize cost offsets and societal benefits from avoiding or delaying the onset of dementia, creative financing approaches, such as deferred and outcomes-based payment, may become necessary [21]. Such approaches would be particularly attractive for countries with long-term care coverage, as actual cost savings would accrue to these programs in the future [22].

30.5.2 Treatment Models

30.5.2.1 Strengthening the Role of Primary Care

For a population-level disease, primary care clinicians must be an integral part of managing the patient journey, but they will need training and changes to practice models to assume the additional responsibility of detecting and evaluating memory complaints. Making these changes may appear like a daunting task, but experience with conditions such as depression and heart failure have shown that routine management even of complex conditions can be moved into general practice. Encouraging examples are emerging. Countries like Canada and Japan have introduced "geriatrics light" training programs in response to the limited attention that geriatric training typically receives in general medicine programs. Current efforts in many countries to consolidate primary care into larger practices, similar to the general practitioner groups in the UK, create opportunities for within-practice concentration of clinicians on a subset of conditions and task-shifting to clinical and non-clinical support staff. Primary-care-led memory clinics, which require only limited specialist support, have been established in the UK [23], Norway [24], and Canada [25].

30.5.2.2 Training of Other Clinicians
With the long training time for dementia specialists, physicians from other, larger specialties need to be drawn into memory care to fill the gaps in the short run. In South Korea, the Dementia Association and the Association for Geriatric Psychiatry offer a joint training program for physicians with an interest in memory care. The program provides training on screening, diagnosis, treatment, and care of dementia patients, as well as on details of government dementia policy. Japan has trained over 5,000 physicians from various specialties as dementia support doctors, who work at the intersection of primary care, dementia specialists, and specialized medical institutions.

30.5.2.3 Learning from Best Practices
Blueprints for advanced memory care models exist in all countries both within memory care and in other specialties. In particular, oncology has transformed into a specialty that provides complex care in large outpatient treatment centers. Providers, payers, and planners will need to collaborate to codify the lessons learned and best practices from these blueprints into memory care models, with standardized staffing, skill mix, and processes. Such standardization can be achieved through central planning, as in France, or an accreditation scheme, such as in the UK, and clinical trial sites in all countries have acquired the necessary skills and infrastructure. Adequate funding and payment models that reward high-quality care will be crucial.

The experience in other therapeutic areas has shown that such advanced practice models can emerge organically. For example, rheumatology evolved from small clinics to practices with large

infusion centers with the advent of immunomodulating drugs. A similar evolution occurred in multiple sclerosis treatment. However, these specialties had the advantage of long having disease-modifying treatments, albeit of limited effectiveness, and could prioritize non-responders while scaling up. AD is different in that it is one of the last population-level diseases without any disease-modifying treatment, leaving little room for practice models to evolve slowly over time.

30.5.2.4 Tele-care
The COVID-19 pandemic has led to a rapid promulgation of tele-care services, as patients were unable or afraid to seek in-person consultations. The resulting capabilities and funding arrangements could serve as the basis for tele-care-supported memory care models, which would be particularly attractive for vast countries with geographic obstacles to access. In fact, one such model, the Alzheimer's and Dementia Care ECHO Program, is currently being tested in the USA [26]. In this model, dementia specialists provide remote support to primary care practices, with the objective to not only bring specialty care closer to a patient's home but also to train local clinicians in the diagnosis and management of cognitive decline.

30.5.3 Technology
Better technology will be needed urgently for primary care clinicians, who face the daunting task of triaging a potentially large number of patients, ranging from the worried well to those with advanced dementia, hampered by competing priorities and the constraints of tightly scheduled days, with 15-minute intervals for office visits. They will need workflow-compatible tools to identify and prioritize the subset of patients with a likely treatment indication for further evaluation.

30.5.3.1 Cognitive Tests
A recent review [27] suggests that many short cognitive tests for dementia are available but only the MMSE and the MoCA perform reasonably well in the detection of MCI. As both take 10–15 minutes to administer and interpret, however, they may be too long for primary care purposes. Shorter tests and computerized tests, which would also permit the collection of additional clinical variables, such as response time and eye-movement, and facilitate detection of cognitive changes over time, are needed and being developed.

30.5.3.2 Blood Biomarker Tests

Biomarker tests suitable for primary care settings would have two distinct advantages, as they would allow the identification of patients with a reasonable likelihood of having AD. First, this would allow – in combination with a brief cognitive test – the prioritization of patients with a likely treatment indication for specialist referral. Second, they would alleviate the bottlenecks in confirmatory biomarker testing. Recently published results from Palmqvist et al. [28] have shown that a fully automated test for plasma amyloid beta (Aβ) performs well enough for clinical triage. The same group published results that a plasma hyperphosphorylated-tau$_{217}$ (p-tau$_{217}$) test, albeit not yet a fully automated one, performed similarly to PET and CSF biomarkers [29]. Our own analyses suggest that the combination of the above-mentioned plasma Aβ test and the MMSE is the functional equivalent of increasing US specialist and PET capacity by 60% and 40%, respectively, as fewer patients without an eventual treatment indication are referred to further evaluation. The improved triage is estimated to increase correctly identified cases by about 120,000 per year and reduce the average annual cost by $400–700 million [17]. While not yet developed for use in automated systems, plasma tests for p-tau$_{217}$ exhibit similar discriminative accuracy as the plasma Aβ tests [29].

30.5.3.3 Digital Biomarkers

Digital biomarkers, especially those that are continuously and passively collected, have great potential for an early detection of cognitive decline as they are able to identify subtle changes in behavior and activity over time [30]. A recent study, for example, showed that a machine-learning model using digital biomarkers could accurately predict progression risk to dementia within 3 years [31]. Biogen and Apple recently announced a prospective study to monitor cognitive performance over time based on iPhone and smart watch data [32].

30.5.3.4 Prediction Models

Risk equations based on predictive models are a commonly used decision guide for preventive treatment. For example, the American College of Cardiology/American Heart Association Guideline on the Primary Prevention of Cardiovascular Disease distills the underlying evidence into a risk score for treatment decisions [33].

Similar efforts have been launched for AD. The Interceptor project [34] in Italy and the Consortium for the early identification of Alzheimer's disease – Quebec [35] are using a combination of demographic factors, cognitive tests, biomarkers, and imaging results to predict the risk of a patient to progress to manifest dementia, with the objective to prioritize high-risk patients for treatment. A Swedish group recently showed that plasma levels of p-tau$_{181}$ in preclinical AD are predictive of cognitive decline and able to differentiate dementia due to AD from that of other etiologies [36]. While several technical challenges, such as the stability of test performance and definition of cut-offs, need to be addressed before such tests can be introduced into routine practice, they point to a promising approach for triage at the primary care level.

30.6 Lessons Learned for AD Drug Development from the Healthcare System Preparedness Perspective

This chapter has illustrated the magnitude of the challenge of moving a disease-modifying AD treatment from clinical trials into daily practice because of the combination of a highly prevalent disease, a large pool of undiagnosed patients, and a complex diagnostic and monitoring process. The challenges might even be greater in the real world as currently projected, because the assumption on specialist capacity does not account for visits needed to monitor effectiveness and safety of the treatment, and to support patients who will remain in a chronic MCI state. Nor do the estimates account for uneven access based on geography and socioeconomic status. While the experience with other therapies has shown that delivery systems will adapt, the transformation is not likely to occur fast enough in the case of AD treatment.

In an ideal world, we would see drugs developed that can be used in large numbers of patients without complex diagnostics and monitoring, such as statins and selective serotonin reuptake inhibitors, so that we are able to accommodate the new treatment options without fundamental structural changes. Realistically, however, everything that we know about complexity of AD suggests that this hope is unfounded. Treatments might even get more complex as we understand the underlying disease biology better, and move to more personalized and/or combination therapy, in a similar way to the development in oncology.

351

A more promising avenue is to focus on improving the diagnostic technology consisting of biomarkers, cognitive tests, and imaging. Rich data and sophisticated analytical techniques, such as deep learning, might allow us to differentiate disease subtypes with different pathobiological characteristics and prognosis. Such insights may allow us to find patients who may not require treatment, streamline evaluation in specialty care settings, and – maybe – identify subtypes that can be handled in primary care settings. With our limited understanding of brain disorders to date, however, substantial research efforts will have to be devoted to this objective.

In the short run, the lessons learned from the preparedness perspective might have larger implications for how approved drugs are brought to market rather than for drug development. The magnitude of the challenge might imply a different role for manufacturers in making their products accessible. Particularly in less-developed health systems, these lessons could contribute to creating the infrastructure needed to diagnose and treat patients, i.e., offer programs that reduce the risk of cognitive decline as a service and not just a pharmaceutical product [37]. Neither of the above-mentioned solutions are easy to implement, but the response to the COVID-19 epidemic has proven the ability of health systems to adapt rapidly, if there is a sense of urgency. With the first AD treatment now approved in the USA, this very sense of urgency might emerge now and trigger a discussion among patient advocates, policymakers, payers, planners, and providers as to how to make a disease-modifying treatment accessible.

References

1. Jack CR, Bennett DA, Blennow K, et al. NIA–AA Research Framework: toward a biological definition of Alzheimer's disease. *Alzheimers Dement* 2018; **14**: 535–62.

2. Petersen RC, Lopez O, Armstrong MJ, et al. Practice guideline update summary: mild cognitive impairment: report of the Guideline Development, Dissemination, and Implementation subcommittee of the American Academy of Neurology. *Neurology* 2018; **90**: 126–35.

3. Liu JL, Hlávka JP, Hillestad R, Mattke S. Assessing the Preparedness of the U.S. health care system infrastructure for an Alzheimer's treatment. Available at: www.rand.org/pubs/research_reports/RR2272.html (accessed July 9, 2021).

4. Hlavka JP, Mattke S, Liu JL. Assessing the preparedness of the health care system infrastructure in six European countries for an Alzheimer's treatment. *Rand Health Q* 2019; **8**: 2.

5. Hebert LE, Weuve J, Scherr PA, Evans DA. Alzheimer disease in the United States (2010–2050) estimated using the 2010 census. *Neurology* 2013; **80**: 1778–83.

6. Sado M, Ninomiya A, Shikimoto R, et al. The estimated cost of dementia in Japan, the most aged society in the world. *PLoS One* 2018; **13**: e0206508.

7. Lang L, Clifford A, Wei L, et al. Prevalence and determinants of undetected dementia in the community: a systematic literature review and a meta-analysis. *BMJ Open* 2017; **7**: e011146.

8. Sperling RA, Rentz DM, Johnson KA, et al. The A4 study: stopping AD before symptoms begin? *Sci Transl Med* 2014; **6**: 228fs13.

9. Baxi SM, Girosi F, Liu JL. Assessing the preparedness of the Australian health care system infrastructure for an Alzheimer's disease-modifying therapy. Available at: www.rand.org/pubs/research_reports/RR2891.html (accessed July 9, 2021).

10. Liu JL, Hlavka JP, Coulter DT, et al. Assessing the preparedness of the Canadian health care system infrastructure for an Alzheimer's treatment. Available at: www.rand.org/pubs/research_reports/RR2744.html (accessed July 9, 2021).

11. Mattke HJ, Yoong J, Wang M, Goto R. Assessing the preparedness of the Japanese health care system infrastructure for an Alzheimer's treatment. Available at: https://cesr.usc.edu/sites/default/files/CESR%202019-101.pdf (accessed July 9, 2021).

12. Hankyung Jun SKC, Yoong J, Mattke S. Assessing the preparedness of the Korean healthcare system infrastructure for an Alzheimer's treatment. Available at: https://cesr.usc.edu/sites/default/files/Korea_Infrastructure_Projection_final.pdf (accessed July 9, 2021).

13. Hankyung Jun SKC, Yoong J, Mattke S. Assessing the preparedness of the Taiwanese healthcare system infrastructure for an Alzheimer's treatment. Available at: https://cesr.usc.edu/sites/default/files/Taiwan_Infrastructure_Projection_final.pdf (accessed July 9, 2021).

14. Ritchie CW, Russ TC, Banerjee S, et al. The Edinburgh Consensus: preparing for the advent of disease-modifying therapies for Alzheimer's disease. *Alzheimers Res Ther* 2017; **9**: 85.

15. Martínez-Lagea P, Martín-Carrascob M, Arrietad E, Rodrigof J, Formigac F. Map of Alzheimer's disease and other dementias in Spain. MapEA Project. *Rev Esp Geriatr Gerontol* 2018; **53**: 26–37.

16. Jun H, Cho SK, Aliyev ER, Mattke S, Suen S-C. How much value would a treatment for

Alzheimer's disease offer? Cost-effectiveness thresholds for pricing a disease-modifying therapy. *Curr Alzheimer Res* 2020; **17**: 819–22.

17. Mattke S, Cho SK, Bittner T, Hlavka J, Hanson M. Blood-based biomarkers for Alzheimer's pathology and the diagnostic process for a disease-modifying treatment: projecting the impact on the cost and wait times. *Alzheimers Dement (Amst)* 2020; **12**: e12081.

18. Ngandu T, Lehtisalo J, Solomon A, et al. A 2 year multidomain intervention of diet, exercise, cognitive training, and vascular risk monitoring versus control to prevent cognitive decline in at-risk elderly people (FINGER): a randomised controlled trial. *Lancet* 2015; **385**: 2255–63.

19. Rabinovici GD, Gatsonis C, Apgar C, et al. Association of amyloid positron emission tomography with subsequent change in clinical management among Medicare beneficiaries with mild cognitive impairment or dementia. *JAMA* 2019; **321**: 1286–94.

20. Russell-Babin K, Wurmser T. Transforming care through top-of-license practice. *Nurs Manage* 2016; **47**: 24–8.

21. Mattke S, Hoch E. Borrowing for the cure. Available at: www.rand.org/pubs/perspectives/PE141.html (accessed July 9, 2021).

22. Lam J, Jun H, Cho S K, Hanson M, Mattke S. Projection of budgetary savings to US state Medicaid programs from reduced nursing home use due to an Alzheimer's disease treatment. *Alzheimers Dement (Amst)* 2021; **13**: e12159.

23. Greaves I, Greaves N, Walker E, et al. Gnosall Primary Care Memory Clinic: eldercare facilitator role description and development. *Dementia (London)* 2015; **14**: 389–408.

24. Engedal K, Gausdal M, Gjora L, Haugen PK. Assessment of dementia by a primary health care dementia team cooperating with the family doctor: the Norwegian model. *Dement Geriatr Cogn Disord* 2012; **34**: 263–70.

25. Lee L, Hillier LM, Heckman G, et al. Primary care-based memory clinics: expanding capacity for dementia care. *Can J Aging* 2014; **33**: 307–19.

26. Alzheimer's Association. The Alzheimer's and Dementia Care ECHO® Program. Available at: www.alz.org/professionals/professional-providers/echo-alzheimers-dementia-care-program (accessed June 6, 2019).

27. Lam J, Hlávka J, Mattke S. The potential emergence of disease-modifying treatments for Alzheimer disease: the role of primary care in managing the patient journey. *J Am Board Fam Med* 2019; **32**: 931–40.

28. Palmqvist S, Janelidze S, Stomrud E, et al. Performance of fully automated plasma assays as screening tests for Alzheimer disease-related beta-amyloid status. *JAMA Neurol* 2019; **76**: 1060–9.

29. Palmqvist S, Janelidze S, Quiroz YT, et al. Discriminative accuracy of plasma phospho-tau$_{217}$ for Alzheimer disease vs other neurodegenerative disorders. *JAMA* 2020; **324**: 772.

30. Kourtis LC, Regele OB, Wright JM, Jones GB. Digital biomarkers for Alzheimer's disease: the mobile/wearable devices opportunity. *NPJ Digit Med* 2019; **2**: 9.

31. Buegler M, Harms RL, Balasa M, et al. Digital biomarker-based individualized prognosis for people at risk of dementia. *Alzheimers Dement (Amst)* 2020; **12**: e12073.

32. Biogen. Biogen to launch pioneering study to develop digital biomarkers of cognitive health using apple watch and iphone [press release]. Available at: https://investors.biogen.com/news-releases/news-release-details/biogen-launch-pioneering-study-develop-digital-biomarkers (accessed January 2021).

33. Arnett DK, Blumenthal RS, Albert MA, et al. 2019 ACC/AHA guideline on the primary prevention of cardiovascular disease. *J Am Coll Cardiol* 2019; **74**: e177–232.

34. Progetto Interceptor. Interceptor: the project. Available at: www.interceptorproject.com/en/lo-studio-interceptor/ (accessed July 9, 2021).

35. Belleville S, Leblanc AC, Kergoat M-J, et al. The Consortium for the early identification of Alzheimer's disease – Quebec (CIMA-Q). *Alzheimers Dement (Amst)* 2019; **11**: 787–96.

36. Janelidze S, Mattsson N, Palmqvist S, et al. Plasma p-tau$_{181}$ in Alzheimer's disease: relationship to other biomarkers, differential diagnosis, neuropathology and longitudinal progression to Alzheimer's dementia. *Nat Med* 2020; **26**: 379–86.

37. Mattke S, Klautzer L, Mengistu T. Medicines as a service. Available at: www.rand.org/pubs/occasional_papers/OP381.html (accessed July 9, 2021).

Chapter 31

Best Practices for Clinical Trials during COVID-19

Saif-Ur-Rahman Paracha, William Maurice Redden, and
George Grossberg

31.1 Introduction

Over the past few decades, Alzheimer's disease (AD) has emerged as one of the top ten causes of death in the world [1]. The burden of disease on the present healthcare system in the United States has been projected to increase exponentially in the next few decades to approximately 14 million compared to current estimates of 5.8 million [2, 3]. There have been major advances in research related to the mechanisms and treatment of AD, which have led to an improved understanding of the nature of this progressive neurodegenerative illness. The United States Food and Drug Administration (FDA) has approved two groups of medications for the symptomatic treatment of AD. These include the cholinesterase inhibitors and an N-methyl-D-aspartate receptor antagonist. Despite showing promising results as symptomatic therapies in AD, they have not shown preventative or disease-modifying effects [4]. However, on June 7, 2021 the FDA granted "accelerated approval" to the drug aducanumab, a monoclonal antibody targeting amyloid beta, which has disease-modifying potential.

Randomized clinical trials have been the cornerstone of the development of drugs and other therapeutic interventions to improve the quality of life of patients. Unfortunately, 99% of clinical trials in AD drug development have shown no drug–placebo difference [5]. This discouraging failure rate has impeded investment from sponsors and researchers, and in turn delayed emerging treatments from coming to fruition. Several studies from drug-development programs targeting different medical disorders have outlined strategies that can minimize the risk and increase the likelihood of success in drug-development programs. Despite the aforementioned challenges, and rigorous drug-development process, these strategies have provided a template to streamline AD drug development. There has been a call for an increased focus on targeting the appropriate biological processes, disease stages (e.g., preclinical, prodromal, or dementia), and conducting adequately powered studies [6]. These factors, coupled with the increasing burden of disease on a global scale, highlight the importance of drug development for people affected by AD.

31.2 COVID-19 and Clinical Trials

The emergence of COVID-19 as a global pandemic, in March of 2020, caused enormous disruption in planned as well as ongoing clinical trials at the time. Many investigators were asked to assume clinical roles in hospitals due to the overwhelming number of COVID-19 cases [7]. The risk and severity of infection from COVID-19, especially for vulnerable AD subjects, resulted in recommendations to either halt all clinical trials or left it to the discretion of the investigators. According to one estimate, approximately 80% of clinical trials not related to COVID-19 in the United States were shut down or interrupted in response to COVID-19 being designated as a national emergency [8].

31.2.1 Worldwide Impact

As the number of COVID-19 cases increased exponentially, the majority of research dollars and resources were redirected toward prevention and treatment strategies for COVID-19. Financial losses to academic and research institutions, along with the suspension of a large number of clinical trials, translated into massive staff furloughs across the United States [9]. Furthermore, the unknown characteristics of the disease led to fear amongst participants and staff alike of contracting the infection. This in turn led to further disruptions in the clinical trial process, including but not limited to recruitment of participants, follow-up visits, and data processing, threatening the integrity of the trials [10]. Regulatory agencies around the world, including the FDA, the Medicines and Healthcare products Regulatory Agency in the UK, the European Medicines Agency, and the Australian Therapeutic Goods Administration, released guidelines to assist academic programs and clinical investigators in making informed decisions on the conduct of clinical trials during the COVID-19 outbreak [11–14]. These guidelines primarily focused on prioritizing participant safety, and weighing the benefits over risks before resuming trials, with appropriate provisions for infection control.

AD research was particularly impacted during the COVID-19 outbreak. Most of the participant or target population was designated as "high risk" to contract COVID-19 and to have severe or poor outcomes from the infection. Long-term care facilities across the world were reporting major outbreaks and fatalities due to close proximity of residents, and their needs for hands-on care. Over 40% of deaths from COVID-19 were estimated to have occurred in long-term care facilities [15]. Residents of long-term care facilities were kept in isolation, with a growing shortage of staff to care for them. Their relatives were not allowed in-person visitation and were forced to switch to video- or phone-call visits. The concerns and heightened risk of traveling for patients with neurodegenerative conditions further complicated their participation in clinical trials. Naturally, many research projects were halted, with the focus being on prevention of further infections and death.

31.2.2   Patient Perspective

As lockdowns were implemented across the globe in response to the coronavirus epidemic, many clinical trials participants and their families developed a heightened sense of precaution, which was necessary for their own safety. Patients suffering from severe illnesses, despite their eagerness to receive potentially life-saving treatment, were avoiding healthcare facilities due to being designated as high risk for COVID-19 infection.

As we moved further through the pandemic, the effects of prolonged isolation began to show in the community. More patients in clinical practice were complaining of anxiety and depression, as were patients in long-term care facilities. Caregivers of patients with debilitating illnesses such as dementia reported an increase in fatigue and caregiver burden. Psychological interventions were suggested as an appropriate early intervention for this group [16]. One survey indicated that more than 50% of such patients experienced a higher level of stress than pre-pandemic times, and approximately 34% of patients wanted support

from either pastoral care/religious services, support groups, or their families, but were unable to get it. A similar trend was observed in caregivers of these patients [17].

31.2.3   Staff Perspective

The risk of contracting COVID-19, as noted previously, also affected research staff. In accordance with recommendations from the regulatory authorities, many research institutions implemented strict guidelines and adjustments to their trial protocols in order to minimize the risk of transmission of COVID-19 to staff and participants alike. The use of face coverings was mandated across staff and all visitors to healthcare and research facilities. Checkpoints were installed at the main entrance of most facilities to measure visitor temperatures, and screen for COVID-19 symptoms with a checklist that was constantly updated. Most institutions implemented strict guidelines to limit the number of patients or participants allowed in a waiting area at one time. All office areas in contact with visitors were cleaned after each patient or participant visit. Workstations were protected with Plexi-glass partitions to avoid direct spread of secretions between staff and patients. Additionally, remote or virtual protocols were initiated to assist with follow-up visits, and to continue data-gathering practices. Remote access to databases and trial participants enabled research staff to continue work during strict lockdown periods when the risk of infection transmission in the community was high.

As precautionary measures were consolidated, patients and trial participants appeared reassured for their safety, and several trial facilities received affirmative responses when asked if they would visit research facilities for initial or follow-up visits. Many patients cherished these encounters as being their sole social outings in several months. The risk of COVID-19 transmission, however, remained, and patients were asked to sign informed consent forms to display knowledge of the risk despite precautions in place. With more education, research staff and participants were also able to gather adequate follow-up data through virtual visits.

Most sites conducting clinical trials experienced significant delays, impacting timely completion of trials. Although, as of this writing, we can see the "light at the end of the COVID tunnel," future pandemics/public health emergencies will no doubt occur. It is proposed that research institutions can offset future delays/complications by implementing the following best practices:

- Clinical trial protocols of the future should have adequate provisions to adjust for unforeseen circumstances such as COVID-19. At this time, these may include inclusion and validation of virtual visits and data-gathering instruments, including wearables and other monitoring equipment for vital signs. Validation of virtual cognitive and other screening tools as well as virtual administration of efficacy measures needs to be studied and implemented. Extending the duration of recruitment and follow-up for in-depth monitoring of the safety, tolerability, and efficacy of the investigational treatment/intervention may need to be part of revised protocols. All trial participants should be notified whenever a change in protocol takes place.

- Patient education in regard to the risks of infection, and contingency plans to lower the said risk, can not only facilitate continued recruitment but also work toward lowering the rate of attrition from clinical trials. This can be achieved by print and digital media, as well as radio or television advertisements.

- As appointments for initial or follow-up visits are set up, staff should be assigned roles on a rotational schedule to avoid excessive exposure to patients, and to avoid lost time or resources in case staff are exposed to COVID-19.

- Whenever appropriate, in-person visits should be decreased, and virtual visits by video conference should be the initial default option. Consent forms can either be sent to patient homes by mail or electronically and received back as such. If study protocols include questionnaires, these may also be mailed to trial participants, or sent electronically. Additionally, electronic applications can be used for continued follow-up through the trial, since they have an added advantage of having convenient built-in reminders for participants. The investigational product or drug can also be mailed to a participant's home by a contracted courier service. Drug administration can be monitored virtually if needed.

- Needed laboratory work can be obtained by a visiting nurse in the subject's home, thereby obviating the need to travel to a community laboratory or the clinical trial site and minimizing COVID-19 exposure.

- If the trial requires on-site assessments or research staff engagement with subjects, they must be prescreened for COVID-19 contact or symptoms on the day prior to their appointment by a telephone call. If a subject screens positive for any symptom suggestive of COVID-19 infection, they should be directed toward resources to receive expedited COVID-19 testing. Exposure to COVID-19 for trial participants should be minimized by providing low-risk travel options. These may become available by engaging family members or friends in the process. Other alternatives may be home health visits or transportation by staff. Only the trial participants and a caregiver should be allowed to enter the research facility. Accompanying family members or friends should be instructed to return at a specific time to pick them up, or to wait in their motor vehicle in the parking lot. Trial participants with cognitive impairment or physical disabilities are allowed one family member or friend for close assistance during their visit.

- There should be appropriate provisions in place to facilitate safe entrance and exit from the facilities for the trial participants through separate exits while minimizing incidental contact with others.

- On research facility entry, trial participants should be screened for COVID-19 symptoms again, and their temperature should be measured, ideally by an infrared thermometer to avoid close contact between staff and participants. In case of a positive screen, the participant should be returned to their vehicle and recommended testing for COVID-19, as noted previously.

- All workstations should have physical barriers to separate patient and staff space. Disinfection and repeated cleaning of all surfaces at the research site should be ensured to avoid spread of infection between trial participants or staff members [18].

- With COVID-19, or in the event of future infectious disease outbreaks, all research subjects and their caregivers should be required to wear a face covering during visits, and research staff should don masks as well as face shields at all points of contact with research subjects. Disposable gloves should be utilized for hands-on examinations. Appropriate distancing needs to be practiced when possible.

- Given masking protocols, it is important that research staff speak loudly, slowly, and distinctly, making sure that research subjects can hear instructions well.

31.2.4 Sponsor Perspective

The pandemic has had significant impact on sponsors of clinical trials. As noted above, disruptions in trials and financial losses dictated many staff furloughs. This played a major role in the reported difficulty recruiting and maintaining trial participants. Data acquisition and processing was similarly affected, leading to further disruption of trial timelines [19]. Furthermore, in order to maintain the safety of trial participants and research staff, sponsors had to bear the additional expense of personal protective equipment (PPE) at inflated costs. Participant and staff testing requirements stretched budgets further as these became more accessible. While sponsors considered early termination of trials, they faced the possibility of underpowered studies, and potential loss of several months or years of work.

To keep on track, many stakeholders implemented necessary strategies to keep their trials open, with the exception of certain trials that were in challenging geographical locations with intense COVID-19 outbreaks. Resources were shifted to provide for contingency measures as noted above. Success rates were variable, and dependent on several factors, including the geographical area of clinical sites, size of organization, number of COVID-19 cases within study population, and financial reserves/resources. To ensure scientifically and methodologically sound clinical trials, sponsors need to ensure that outcomes are not dictated by COVID-19 risk or infection. Best practices derived from these experiences are listed below:

- As noted previously, research staff should have designated roles on a rotational basis in order to allow for coverage in the event of unplanned absence due to illness or the need to quarantine secondary to COVID-19 exposure.
- Follow-up calls and reminders to trial participants should be listed as an additional responsibility of research staff, to maintain the interest of trial participants in the study, and to ensure adherence to trial protocols. Data gathering and processing should be facilitated by providing staff with remote access to databases in the event of having to work off site.
- To ensure patient safety, there should be provisions for testing of staff and trial participants with symptoms, or with known exposure to COVID-19.
- Adequate PPE should be provided for staff and trial participant use, in case in-person visits are required.
- Pursuant with the recommendations from the FDA, sponsors may increase the duration of follow-up, or increase patient recruitment as the infection rate in the population decreases.
- Sponsors should cite all disruptions caused by COVID-19 in the study manuscript, their impact on data gathering, study design, or results, if any, and the contingency measures taken to counter the impact of COVID-19. All trial participants that were affected by COVID-19 during the study should be identified, along with details of complications they encountered, if any.
- For trials nearing completion, an interim analysis may be implemented in order to extrapolate findings in the study population thus far, and as such terminating the study potentially with a positive or negative result, and reasonable statistical power [18].

31.2.5 Regulatory Perspective

The dwindling number of in-office visits for initial screening and recruitment of trial participants, and in-person follow-up visits for monitoring treatment safety and efficacy, has raised legitimate questions about the reliability of results. Most methods, such as virtual assessments, or remote questionnaire administration, are not well validated, and thus raise concerns for inaccurate results. However, streamlining the process to focus on the primary outcome can provide for a higher reliability. If the primary outcome has been achieved, terminating the study should be prioritized to avoid further exposure of trial participants and research staff to COVID-19. Similarly, if 90% of the expected outcomes have been achieved, the power of the trial cannot be expected to change drastically. Hence, decisions to terminate the study early can be made. Statistical analysis plans should be adjusted or revised according to the anticipated impact of COVID-19 on the study.

Regulators need to encourage sponsors to transition to virtual clinical trial visits when possible, and to develop and validate virtually administered assessment instruments. Further development and validation of remote data-gathering tools such as actigraphy, wearable medical data-gathering devices, and remote observational tools should be fostered and legitimatized.

31.2.6   Long-Term Care Perspective

As mentioned previously, long-term care residents faced a dramatically higher risk of morbidity and mortality from COVID-19 than the general population. As nursing facilities went into "lockdown" and implemented strict isolation protocols, research activities were essentially halted. Under the circumstances, any research unrelated to COVID-19 appeared to have more risks than benefits for this high-risk population. As the impact and volume of COVID-19 cases spread across nursing homes in the United States, staff shortages led to further crises in clinical care and research data acquisition from these facilities. The high incidence of delirium as a consequence of COVID-19 infection in older adults, especially for those suffering from dementia, further complicated follow-up evaluations, and delayed study results or outcome measurements [20].

Virtual visits had an enormous impact in this domain as well. Several studies have highlighted the protective effect of video conferencing on the mental and physical well-being of older adults in long-term care facilities [21]. Tele-health has proven particularly useful in the clinical care of geriatric patients, where it has provided the ability to conference patients and their family members at the same time, while eradicating risk of infection transmission between attendees. These methods can be employed to further ongoing clinical trials in nursing homes. The drugs under study can be mailed to the facility and administered to the patients under the supervision of nursing-home staff. Staff should accordingly be educated relative to study design, and methods of drug administration and monitoring.

Given staff shortages at long-term care facilities, the close proximity of patients, and their needs for hands-on care, it is difficult to estimate how mitigation efforts or contingency plans, enough to minimize the risk of infection transmission from a clinical trials perspective, may begin to occur. While taking into account the effects of COVID-19 infection on study outcomes, trial participants and their surrogate decision makers, if any, should be updated of any change in protocols of clinical studies. Sponsors should be prepared to temporarily halt studies due to the aforementioned challenges and consider an increase in enrollment once the infection rate in facilities drops to safer levels and lockdowns are eliminated.

31.3   Lessons Learned from COVID-19 for AD Drug Development

Ensuring the safety of clinical trial participants during the COVID-19 pandemic has been, rightfully, the highest priority. Organizations that were better prepared for disruptions before the spread of COVID-19 were able to continue working with less disruption, whether they were clinically or research oriented.

Adequate contingency plans should be part of future clinical trial protocols in the event of public health emergencies. The technology forced into widespread clinical use by the COVID-19 pandemic, namely the use of virtual visits, had been available for many years. However, the majority of the industry was caught off guard and had to implement new strategies to make further progress with their projects.

It has become clear from the current pandemic that there is a dire need to remain up to date with ongoing technological advances in order to run clinical trials efficiently. Sponsors and investigators of clinical trials should have open communication to ensure the integrity of the clinical trial process. Additionally, governmental regulatory authorities and institutional review boards should allow necessary technological adaptations and flexibility in study protocols in adapting to emergency situations.

The high number of deaths among older adults in the community secondary to COVID-19, especially those suffering from AD, will have a significant impact on AD clinical research being conducted during this time. The pandemic has highlighted the intense need for rapid and sustained recruitment of patients to clinical trials for AD drug development [22].

References

1. World Health Organization. WHO mortality database. Available at: www.who.int/healthinfo/mortality_data/en/ (accessed June 1, 2021).

2. Alzheimer's Association. 2020 Alzheimer's disease facts and figures. *Alzheimers Dement* 2020; **16**: 391–460.

3. Hebert LE, Weuve J, Scherr PA, et al. Alzheimer disease in the United States (2010–2050) estimated using the 2010 Census. *Neurology* 2013; **80**: 1778–83.

4. Lao K, Ji N, Zhang X, et al. Drug development for Alzheimer's disease: review. *J Drug Target* 2019; **27**: 164–73.

5. Cummings J, Ritter A, Zhong K. Clinical trials for disease-modifying therapies in Alzheimer's disease: a primer, lessons learned, and a blueprint for the future. *J Alzheimers Dis* 2018; 64: S3–22.

6. Cummings J, Feldman HH, Scheltens P, et al. The "rights" of precision drug development for Alzheimer's disease. *Alzheimers Res Ther* 2019; **11**: 76.

7. Tuttle KR. Impact of the COVID-19 pandemic on clinical research. *Nat Rev Nephrol* 2020; **16**: 562–4.

8. Asaad M, Khan Habibullah K, Butler CE, et al. The impact of COVID 19 on clinical trials. *Ann Surg* 2020; **272**: e222–3.

9. Applied Clinical Trials. Findings from a Tufts study examining the effects of COVID-19 on clinical trials. Available at:www.appliedclinicaltrialsonline.com/view/covid-19-and-its-impact-on-the-future-of-clinical-trial-execution (accessed December 20, 2020).

10. Sathian B, Asim M, Banerjee I, et al. Impact of COVID-19 on clinical trials and clinical research: a systematic review. *Nepal J Epidemiol* 2020; **10**: 878–87.

11. Food and Drug Administration. FDA guidance on conduct of clinical trials of medical products during COVID-19 public health emergency. March 2020. Available at: www.fda.gov/regulatory-information/search-fda-guidance-documents/fda-guidance-conduct-clinical-trials-medical-products-during-covid-19-public-health-emergency (accessed May 20, 2020).

12. Medicines and Healthcare products Regulatory Agency Inspectorate. Advice for management of clinical trials in relation to Coronavirus. March 12, 2020. Available at: https://mhrainspectorate.blog.gov.uk/2020/03/12/advice-for-management-of-clinical-trials-in-relation-to-coronavirus/ (accessed June 1, 2021).

13. European Medicines Agency. Guidance on the management of clinical trials during the COVID-19 (Coronavirus) pandemic. *Version* 3. April 28, 2020. Available at: https://ecrin.org (accessed June 1, 2021).

14. Australian Government Agency:Therapeutic goods administration. Clinical trial processes: information relating to COVID-19. March 31, 2020. Available at: www.tga.gov.au/clinical-trial-processes (accessed May 30, 2021).

15. Comas-Herrera A, Zalakain J. Mortality associated with COVID-19 outbreaks in care homes: early international evidence. April 12, 2020. Available at: https://ltccovid.org/2020/04/12/mortality-associated-with-covid-19-outbreaks-in-care-homes-early-international-evidence/ (accessed May 30, 2021).

16. Altieri M, Santangelo G. The psychological impact of COVID-19 pandemic and lockdown on caregivers of people with dementia. *Am J Geriatr Psychiatry* 2021; **29**: 27–34.

17. UsAgainstAlzheimer's. UsAgainstAlzheimer's survey on COVID-19 and Alzheimer's community summary of findings for June 2020 survey (Survey #4). Available at: www.usagainstalzheimers.org/sites/default/files/2020-06/UsA2%20COVID%20Survey%204%20Summary%206.25.20.pdf (accessed June 1, 2021).

18. Anker SD, Butler J, Khan MS, et al. Conducting clinical trials in heart failure during (and after) the COVID-19 pandemic: an Expert Consensus Position Paper from the Heart Failure Association (HFA) of the European Society of Cardiology (ESC). *Eur Heart J* 2020; **41**: 2109–17.

19. Medidata. COVID-19 and clinical trials: the Medidata perspective. Available at: www.medidata.com/wp-content/uploads/2020/08/COVID19-Response8.0_Clinical-Trials_2020824_v1.pdf (accessed Nov 29, 2020).

20. Kennedy M, Helfand BKI, Gou RY, et al. Delirium in older patients with COVID-19 presenting to the emergency department. *JAMA Netw Open* 2020; **3**: e2029540.

21. Lai FH-Y, Yan EW, Yu KK, et al. The protective impact of telemedicine on persons with dementia and their caregivers during the COVID-19 pandemic. *Am J Geriatr Psychiatry* 2020; **28**: 1175–84.

22. Saini KS, de Las Heras B, de Castro J, et al. Effect of the COVID-19 pandemic on cancer treatment and research. *Lancet Haematol* 2020; **7**: e432–5.

Chapter

32

Development of Fluid Biomarkers for Alzheimer's Disease

Kaj Blennow

32.1 Introduction

The field of Alzheimer's disease (AD) clinical research and drug development has witnessed a rapid development of fluid biomarker tests in cerebrospinal fluid (CSF) and blood (plasma and serum). The AD fluid biomarker research field started with using CSF as the matrix, focusing on the development of tests for the key neuropathological changes in AD, today commonly known as the amyloid, tau, and neurodegeneration (A/T/N) classification system [1]. These core AD CSF biomarkers include amyloid beta ($A\beta_{42}$ and $A\beta_{42}/A\beta_{40}$ ratio), hyperphosphorylated tau (p-tau), and total tau (t-tau), and these have been highly validated as diagnostic tests [2]. Based on the development of ultrasensitive immunoassays and mass spectrometry methods, the same biomarkers can today also be measured in blood samples, with recent papers presenting very promising data on their

performance to detect A/T/N pathophysiology. This chapter provides an overview on the state of development and clinical validation of these CSF and blood biomarkers, and how they can be implemented in clinical trials.

32.2 The Core CSF Biomarkers for AD

The typical change in AD is a decrease in CSF $A\beta_{42}$ (and $A\beta_{42}/A\beta_{40}$ ratio) together with increased t-tau and p-tau, the so-called "Alzheimer CSF biomarker profile." These CSF tests for the identification of brain amyloidosis ($A\beta_{42}$ and $A\beta_{42}/A\beta_{40}$ ratio), tau pathology (p-tau), and neurodegeneration (t-tau and neurofilament light chain, NfL), have consistently been shown to be highly accurate in the idenitifcation of AD [3]; for an overview, see Table 32.1.

Table 32.1 The core CSF biomarkers for AD

Asset	Change in AD	Stage of development	Interpretation
$A\beta_{42}$	Low $A\beta_{42}$ is found in AD and prodromal AD Mean change in AD is to around 50% of age-matched controls Sensitivity for AD and prodromal AD >90%	Several validated commercially available immunoassays Reference measurement procedures and certified reference materials available IVD-approved fully automated methods available	Low $A\beta_{42}$ reflects brain amyloid deposition, and shows very high concordance with amyloid PET CSF $A\beta_{42}$ may be an earlier biomarker than amyloid PET to detect brain amyloidosis
$A\beta_{42}/A\beta_{40}$ ratio	Low $A\beta_{42}/A\beta_{40}$ ratio is found in AD and prodromal AD Mean decrease in AD is to around 50% of age-matched controls CSF $A\beta_{42}/A\beta_{40}$ ratio shows a clear bimodal distribution of values in AD and control groups, with higher sensitivity and specificity than for $A\beta_{42}$ alone	Several validated commercially available immunoassays IVD-approved fully automated methods available	The $A\beta_{42}/A\beta_{40}$ ratio is thought to compensate for between-individual variations in "total" $A\beta$ production The $A\beta_{42}/A\beta_{40}$ ratio may be an earlier biomarker than amyloid PET to detect brain amyloidosis

Table 32.1 (cont.)

Asset	Change in AD	Stage of development	Interpretation
p-tau	p-tau$_{181}$ is the most commonly used and clinically validated p-tau variant High p-tau is found in AD and prodromal AD Mean increase in AD is to around 200% of age-matched controls Sensitivity for AD and prodromal AD >90%	Several validated commercially available immunoassays IVD-approved fully automated methods available	High p-tau reflects the phosphorylation state of tau and AD-type tau pathology p-tau is specific for AD; high CSF levels have not been found in other neurodegenerative disorders and are not found in acute brain disorders CSF levels of p-tau$_{181}$, p-tau$_{217}$, and p-tau$_{231}$ correlate tightly
t-tau	High t-tau is found in AD and prodromal AD Mean change in AD is to around 250% of age-matched controls Sensitivity for AD and prodromal AD >90%	Several validated commercially available immunoassays IVD-approved fully automated methods available	High t-tau reflects intensity of neurodegeneration and probably reflects disease progression Very high t-tau is found in disorders with marked neurodegeneration (CJD) and t-tau increases in acute brain disorders (e.g., stroke, trauma) depending on severity of lesions

Abbreviations: Aβ, amyloid beta; AD, Alzheimer's disease; CJD, Creutzfeldt–Jakob disease; CSF, cerebrospinal fluid; IVD, in vitro diagnostics; PET, positron emission tomography; p-tau, hyperphosphorylated tau; t-tau, total tau.

32.2.1 Pathophysiological Considerations for the AD CSF Biomarkers

Several Aβ species of different length are generated from the amyloid precursor protein (APP), and are also secreted to CSF. The 42-amino-acid-long variant (Aβ$_{42}$) is aggregation-prone, and forms amyloid plaques in AD, while Aβ$_{40}$ (having 40 amino acids) is the most abundant form, with around 10 times higher levels than Aβ$_{42}$ [4]. In AD, the CSF level of Aβ$_{42}$ is reduced to around half the level found in cognitively unimpaired elderly people, reflecting the aggregation of Aβ$_{42}$ peptides into plaques, which results in lower amounts of Aβ$_{42}$ being secreted to the extracellular space and the CSF [5]. This hypothesis has been supported by a large number of studies showing very high agreement between lowering of CSF Aβ$_{42}$ levels and amyloid PET positivity [6]. In contrast to Aβ$_{42}$, CSF levels of Aβ$_{40}$ remain within normal ranges in AD. This discrepancy is utilized in the CSF Aβ$_{42}$/Aβ$_{40}$ ratio, in which Aβ$_{40}$ serves as a proxy for "total" Aβ production, thereby normalizing for between-individual differences in basal Aβ production, or CSF dynamics, between individuals [7]. Indeed, the Aβ$_{42}$/Aβ$_{40}$ ratio shows even better concordance with amyloid PET than CSF Aβ$_{42}$ alone [8].

CSF t-tau and p-tau are assumed to come from the basic physiological secretion of tau from neurons to the extracellular fluid and CSF [9]. Indirect support for this hypothesis comes from the knowledge that both t-tau and p-tau are measurable in CSF samples from healthy young individuals, while the secretion of tau from affected neurons is believed to increase in AD [9]. Based on results from animal studies, it has been hypothesized that the increased secretion may be linked to tau spreading between neurons [10]. On the other hand, the secretion of t-tau to the CSF is 10-fold higher in Creutzfeldt–Jakob disease (CJD) than in AD [11]. CJD is a disorder with very intense neurodegeneration, but no tau spreading, which supports CSF t-tau as a "state marker" reflecting the intensity of neurodegeneration [12].

CSF p-tau reflects the phosphorylation state of tau. Several p-tau variants that are phosphorylated at specific amino acids on tau can be measured, including p-tau$_{181}$, p-tau$_{199}$, p-tau$_{217}$, and p-tau$_{231}$ (numbers referring to the amino acid number on the largest tau isoform tau$_{441}$), all show a clear increase in AD, and tight correlation across the p-tau biomarkers [13, 14]. For unknown reasons, CSF t-tau and p-tau levels are highly correlated in normal individuals and within the AD spectrum, while this correlation is lost in disorders with severe neurodegeneration such as CJD [11] and in disorders with acute neuronal damage such as stroke [15], in which t-tau markedly increases but p-tau stays normal. Importantly, CSF p-tau$_{181}$, p-tau$_{217}$, and p-tau$_{231}$ all correlate tightly with each other [16]. These p-tau species also concord well with tau PET, and show increases in cognitively unimpaired individuals with brain amyloidosis also in the stage where brain tau aggregates cannot yet be detected by tau PET [17]. These findings support CSF p-tau as an early biomarker for tau phosphorylation and brain tau pathology.

Interestingly, CSF tau protein has been shown to be present as truncated N-terminal to mid-domain fragments [18], with a major cleavage site in the mid-domain of tau between amino acids 222 and 225 [9], while C-terminal tau fragments have very low abundance. Another potentially important cleavage is in the microtubule-binding domain, after residue 368, which generates a long and aggregation-prone tau fragment which is deposited into tangles [19]. Using an ultrasensitive single-molecule-array (Simoa®) method, a decrease in the tau$_{368}$/t-tau ratio was found along the AD continuum that correlates with the tau pathology load evaluated by tau PET [20]. In contrast to N-terminal and mid-domain p-tau variants such as CSF p-tau$_{181}$ and p-tau$_{217}$, which show increased CSF levels with more extended tau pathology, the decrease in the CSF tau$_{368}$/t-tau ratio with increasing tau pathology load may mirror the decrease in the Aβ$_{42}$/Aβ$_{40}$ ratio found with higher amyloid load.

32.2.2 Diagnostic Performance of the AD CSF Biomarkers

Large prospective studies in memory clinic cohorts also show that the combined used of these CSF biomarkers can identify AD cases at the mild cognitive impairment (MCI) disease stage with accuracy figures around 90% for the differentiation between prodromal AD from stable MCI cases and those developing other dementias [21]. Similar performance figures were found in the Alzheimer's Disease Neuroimaging Initiative (ADNI) study [22].

Importantly, Aβ$_{42}$, which is the most analytically challenging AD CSF biomarker, has undergone extensive standardization efforts, including the production of certified reference materials (CRMs), which are aliquots of a "gold standard"

CSF pool with certified Aβ$_{42}$ levels, set using mass spectrometry-based reference measurement procedures, which are used for harmonization of levels between assay formats, and to assure longitudinal stability across batches [23]. Further, the availability of these biomarker assays on fully automated laboratory instruments has played a pivotal role for the introduction of the core AD CSF biomarkers in clinical diagnostic routine. These instruments involve no manual steps, and have superior performance compared to manual or semi-automated enzyme-linked immunosorbent assay (ELISA) methods. As an example, on the Cobas Elecsys platform, concordance figures for the CSF p-tau/Aβ$_{42}$ ratio with amyloid PET is as high as 0.94–0.96 [24]. Another fully automated platform is the Lumipulse instrument [25], which shows very high performance in the Alzheimer's Association Quality Control program. These fully automated laboratory instruments will assure stable and precise biomarker results across laboratories. Further, the Aβ$_{42}$ CRMs have been used to recalibrate the commercial immunoassays to harmonize levels and allow for the introduction of uniform cut-off levels [26]. This will be important in routine clinical diagnostics, especially in the light of novel disease-modifying drugs. For this purpose, the Alzheimer's Association has published appropriate-use criteria, specific clinical indications for the use of CSF tests in the diagnostic assessment of patients with suspected AD [27].

32.3 Blood Biomarkers for Alzheimer's Disease

While PET and CSF biomarkers work exceptionally well to identify AD pathophysiology, they either need special resources (cyclotrons and PET scanner facilities) – and are therefore expensive and have limited availability – or are regarded as invasive, with potential side effects (some percent of patients get mild headache after a CSF tap). Given the promise of disease-modifying drugs, in the first cases with immunotherapies targeting Aβ pathology, easily accessible and inexpensive biomarkers would be of great value, especially in the first screening of patients with cognitive complaints and suspected AD. Given the extraordinarily low levels of protein biomarkers derived from the brain in blood samples, assays to quantify biomarkers for AD pathophysiologies in plasma or serum require methods with very high analytical sensitivity, and also control of potential interferences, such as heterophilic antibodies, and other potential confounders, such as epitope masking of hydrophobic Aβ peptides by binding to high-abundancy plasma proteins or lipoproteins. Nevertheless, recent developments in analytical techniques have given blood biomarkers that show promise for such applications; for an overview, see Table 32.2.

32.3.1 Brain Amyloidosis: Aβ in Plasma

It has since long been possible to measure $A\beta_{42}$ and $A\beta_{40}$ in plasma, but early studies based on ELISA measurement showed disappointing results, with no or only minor changes and large overlaps in Aβ levels between clinically diagnosed AD cases and controls [3]. This changed with the development of ultrasensitive immunoassays and

Table 32.2 Candidate blood biomarkers for AD

Asset	Change in AD	Stage of development	Interpretation
$A\beta_{42}/A\beta_{40}$ ratio	Low plasma $A\beta_{42}/A\beta_{40}$ ratio is found in AD and prodromal AD Mean plasma $A\beta_{42}/A\beta_{40}$ ratio is 10–15% lower in amyloid-PET-positive MCI/AD cases than in age-matched controls Plasma $A\beta_{42}/A\beta_{40}$ ratio shows an overlap between amyloid-PET-positive and -negative cases without any clear bimodal distribution of values	Several validated commercially available immunoassays Validated immunoprecipitation mass spectrometry assays have been published Fee-for-service testing of plasma $A\beta_{42}/A\beta_{40}$ ratio combined with *APOE* genotype and age (the Amyloid Probability Score) is commercially available	Low plasma $A\beta_{42}/A\beta_{40}$ ratio is associated with brain amyloidosis The fold decrease in $A\beta_{42}/A\beta_{40}$ ratio is much lower in plasma than in CSF, and the correlation between plasma and CSF is poor, suggesting that a large proportion of Aβ in plasma is derived from extra-cerebral sources (e.g., platelets or peripheral tissues)
p-tau	Blood p-tau$_{181}$, p-tau$_{217}$, and p-tau$_{231}$ show a marked increase in AD and prodromal AD, with high AUC values Mean increase in AD compared to age-matched controls is higher for p-tau$_{217}$ than for p-tau$_{181}$	Research grade assays for p-tau$_{181}$, p-tau$_{217}$, and p-tau$_{231}$ are published One Simoa® method for p-tau$_{181}$ in plasma is commercially available	Plasma p-tau increases with larger brain tau pathology load assessed by tau PET Increased p-tau levels are found in the early stages of the AD continuum, when amyloid PET, but not tau PET, is positive Further studies comparing the different p-tau variants (p-tau$_{181}$, p-tau$_{217}$, and p-tau$_{231}$) using the same analytical technology in the same cohorts are needed
t-tau	Plasma t-tau only shows a minor increase in AD, with a massive overlap with control levels	Validated commercial immunoassays are available	Plasma t-tau is a biomarker for acute neuronal injury, but current t-tau assay formats do not work as diagnostic biomarkers for AD The poor correlation between plasma and CSF levels of t-tau suggest a peripheral expression, or that current t-tau assays also may capture the "big tau" isoform produced in peripheral nerves
NfL	High plasma NfL is found in AD and prodromal AD, but with overlap between groups Plasma NfL increases in the presymptomatic phase of AD, as shown in familial-AD-linked mutation carriers	Research grade assays for NfL have been published One Simoa® method for NfL in serum or plasma is commercially available Standardization efforts to develop a certified reference material for serum/plasma NfL is ongoing	Plasma/serum NfL is a general biomarker for neurodegeneration, and is not specific for AD High plasma/serum NfL predicts future rate of cognitive decline and rate of brain atrophy in AD Blood NfL levels higher than those present in AD are found in, for example, FTD, PSP, CBD, and ALS

Abbreviations: Aβ, amyloid beta; AD, Alzheimer's disease; ALS, amyotrophic lateral sclerosis; APOE, apolioprotein E; AUC, area under the curve; CBD, corticobasal degeneration; FTD, frontotemporal dementia; NfL, neurofilament light; PET, positron emission tomography; PSP, progressive supranuclear palsy; p-tau, hyperphosphorylated tau; t-tau, total tau.

immunoprecipitation–mass spectrometry (IP–MS) techniques, combined with the strategy to examine the performance of plasma Aβ in AD and control cohorts classified based on amyloid PET status (as either positive or negative), regardless of clinical diagnosis.

A first study using the Simoa® technique for quantification of Aβ in plasma showed weak but significant associations between the plasma $A\beta_{42}/A\beta_{40}$ ratio and both CSF $A\beta_{42}/A\beta_{40}$ ratio and cortical amyloid PET ligand retention, as well as a significantly lower plasma $A\beta_{42}/A\beta_{40}$ ratio in MCI and AD cases compared to controls [28].

Early studies using the IP–MS technology showed that the Aβ species identified in plasma using matrix-assisted laser desorption/ionization (MALDI) are the same as those in CSF [29, 30], and that selected reaction monitoring methods can be used for quantification of plasma $A\beta_{42}$ and $A\beta_{40}$ [30]. Using a similar IP–MS method involving proteolytic digestion of Aβ peptides before analysis, a significantly lower (14%) $A\beta_{42}/A\beta_{40}$ ratio was found in amyloid-PET-positive cases as compared with those having a negative PET scan, with a high (0.89) receiver-operating-characteristic–area-under-the-curve (AUC) value [31]. Alternative MS techniques based on MALDI, also including the APP fragment APP669-711 together with $A\beta_{42}$ and $A\beta_{40}$ in a composite biomarker, showed very high accuracies to identify brain amyloidosis [32]. Further studies using these MS-based amyloid biomarkers confirm high concordance with both amyloid PET scans and the CSF $A\beta_{42}/A\beta_{40}$ ratio [33], suggesting that plasma Aβ measurement could be an alternative to amyloid PET and CSF tests. Interestingly, similar to what has been found for the CSF $A\beta_{42}/A\beta_{40}$ ratio [34], plasma Aβ may be an earlier indicator of brain amyloidosis than amyloid PET. Results from a recent study suggest that individuals who have a positive amyloid blood test, but a negative PET scan, at baseline have a 15-fold higher risk of being amyloid PET positive at follow-up examination than those with a normal plasma $A\beta_{42}/A\beta_{40}$ ratio at baseline [33].

However, despite these very promising results, some challenges remain that need further study. One is that the correlation between plasma and CSF levels of Aβ is weak, and the reduction in the $A\beta_{42}/A\beta_{40}$ ratio in amyloid-PET-positive cases is only around 10–15% in plasma (as compared with around 50% in CSF), which may be explained by production of Aβ peptides in platelets

and peripheral tissues. The fact that all analytical methods have an inherent variability (often around 10–15%), combined with the very small fold change for the plasma $A\beta_{42}/A\beta_{40}$ ratio (around 10–15%), will introduce difficult challenges to robustly classify patients as being either amyloid positive or negative, especially in those having $A\beta_{42}/A\beta_{40}$ ratios close to the established cut-off. Alternatives may include having a borderline or intermediate zone, with $A\beta_{42}/A\beta_{40}$ values falling in this range being uninterpretable. Further, similar to CSF Aβ tests [23], worldwide efforts are needed to develop CRMs, for harmonization of levels across assay platforms and laboratories. Finally, costs for plasma amyloid tests need to be substantially lower than costs for PET scans to serve as attractive substitutes. The introduction of fully automated instruments for the analysis of plasma $A\beta_{42}/A\beta_{40}$ ratios will likely result in substantially lower cost per sample than technically challenging IP–MS techniques.

32.3.2 Tau Pathology: p-Tau in Plasma

Recent breakthroughs also allow for tau pathology in the brain to be identified by blood biomarkers. A first paper in 2017 presenting data used a Simoa® t-tau assay modified to measure plasma $p\text{-tau}_{181}$ – tau phosphorylated at threonine 181 [35]. Increased plasma $p\text{-tau}_{181}$ was found in AD and also in Down syndrome, and plasma levels correlated well with CSF levels, but the assay lacked sensitivity to measure $p\text{-tau}_{181}$ in many samples, including in some from AD cases [35]. A major step forward came with a paper presenting a new electrochemiluminescence immunoassay developed at Lilly Research laboratories, which is based on the Meso Scale Discovery (MSD) technology [36]. Plasma $p\text{-tau}_{181}$ showed a clear increase in AD dementia, and associations between plasma $p\text{-tau}_{181}$ levels and both amyloid and tau PET [36]. These results were validated in two large studies confirming that plasma $p\text{-tau}_{181}$ is increased in AD, also in the early disease stages, while normal levels are found in several other tauopathies and neurodegenerative disorders, and further that plasma $p\text{-tau}_{181}$ shows a stepwise increase with higher Braak tau stage assessed by tau PET [37, 38].

Another paper presented a new Simoa® sandwich immunoassay for $p\text{-tau}_{181}$, which in IP–MS experiments was shown to specifically capture N-terminal to mid-domain tau fragments phosphorylated at threonine 181, while non-phosphorylated tau species do not react [39]. The Simoa® assay had analytical sensitivity high enough to measure p-tau$_{181}$ in all plasma samples, also from young controls [39]. Again, plasma p-tau$_{181}$ was markedly increased in AD and could differentiate from a wide range of other neurodegenerative disorders and correlated with tau pathology visualized by tau PET [39]. A Simoa® assay for yet another p-tau species, p-tau$_{231}$, has been published confirming a very high performance to identify AD-type tau pathology [40].

A study examining tau species enriched from plasma samples by MS found that the ratio of phosphorylated to non-phosphorylated peptides was higher for p-tau$_{217}$ than for p-tau$_{181}$ in amyloid-PET-positive cases, which may suggest a lower peripheral contribution of p-tau$_{217}$ than of p-tau$_{181}$ to plasma levels [41]. This finding was validated in a larger study, also showing that plasma p-tau biomarkers increase very early in the course of AD, suggesting that plasma p-tau reflects changes in soluble tau metabolism in the stage with only detectable Aβ pathology [42]. A recent large study presented an MSD immunoassay for plasma p-tau$_{217}$ showing a very high performance of p-tau$_{217}$ to identify AD and to separate AD from other neurodegenerative diseases [43].

Results from several papers support p-tau blood biomarkers being positive in the very early phases of AD. Studies examining p-tau in familial AD cohorts found significant increases in MSD p-tau$_{217}$ 20 years before the expected year of onset of cognitive symptoms [43], while similar data were obtained for the Simoa® p-tau$_{181}$ method, with a significant increase 16 years before the expected year of onset in familial AD mutation carriers [44]. The finding that plasma p-tau is increased in amyloid-PET-positive, but tau-PET-negative, cases may suggest that blood p-tau biomarkers reflect abnormal p-tau secretion concomitantly with, or in response to, brain Aβ pathology. However, an alternative explanation is that plasma p-tau increases in early AD cases with both amyloid and tau pathology, but in the phase where tau pathology is not detectable yet by tau PET.

At the other side of the AD continuum, studies comparing the plasma p-tau biomarkers in samples taken during life show close association with AD neuropathology at autopsy. In a cohort of 16 AD and 47 non-AD cases, the MSD p-tau$_{181}$ assay could differentiate AD from non-AD with an AUC

of 0.85 [38], while the MSD p-tau$_{217}$ assay showed a higher AUC of 0.98 [43]. Yet another study using the Simoa® p-tau$_{181}$ method found a very high AUC of 0.97 to differentiate AD from non-AD at autopsy in samples taken 8 years prior to death [45]. These findings are in concert with CSF data, showing that increased p-tau is specifically found in AD, despite p-tau inclusions also being found in neurons or glial cells in other neurodegenerative disorders [46]. The reason why both CSF and plasma p-tau specifically respond to AD-type tau pathology remains elusive.

However, p-tau can also be released to plasma through other mechanisms as well as in response to AD pathology. One study showed that plasma p-tau$_{231}$ showed a very dramatic acute increase in patients with mild traumatic brain injury, with 10 times higher levels than in matched controls [47]. The increase in plasma p-tau was much more marked than that for t-tau and was more pronounced in cases with more severe symptoms or a positive CT scan [47]. The increase in plasma p-tau was still prominent 6 months after the trauma, when t-tau levels had normalized.

A paper examining the trajectories of CSF and plasma biomarkers in relation to amyloid PET positivity showed that Aβ$_{42}$ changed first, closely followed by the Aβ$_{42}$/Aβ$_{40}$ ratio, and then p-tau and t-tau, and not until after the point of amyloid PET positivity was there an evident change in the neurodegeneration biomarker NfL [48]. These findings are consistent with both CSF and plasma being reliable (!) biomarkers of amyloid and tau pathology change before brain amyloidosis can be visualized by PET.

32.3.3 Neurodegeneration: Neurofilament Light Chain and Total Tau

Using ultrasensitive immunoassays, also t-tau can be measured in blood samples [49]. However, an early study on plasma t-tau as an AD biomarker only showed a minor increase in AD dementia, and the correlation between plasma and CSF levels was very poor [50]. Findings were similar in two much larger clinical cohorts [51]. Interestingly, despite plasma t-tau levels being only marginally higher in AD than in controls, longitudinal data indicated that plasma t-tau predicts future cognitive decline, as well as atrophy rate, as measured by MRI and cortical hypometabolism assessed by fluorodeoxyglucose PET [51].

It is unclear why t-tau is an established AD biomarker in CSF, but is not diagnostically useful in plasma, while p-tau works as an AD biomarker both in CSF and plasma. At the same time, plasma t-tau works well to identify neuronal injury in acute brain disorders, such as brain trauma and acute ischemia, in which there is a marked increase, with higher levels predicting poor clinical outcome [52, 53]. A recent MS study could only identify N-terminal to mid-domain (up to amino acid 254) tryptic tau peptides in plasma [41], suggesting a similar tau truncation pattern as in CSF [18]. A possible explanation is that tau in plasma is subjected to more rapid proteolytic degradation in blood [49] than in CSF [9], but this would not explain why p-tau performs well as an AD biomarker in both CSF and plasma. Another possibility is that the t-tau signal in plasma partly comes from tau expressed in peripheral tissues or that current t-tau assays also capture the peripheral nervous system "big tau" isoform, which contains an extra domain encoded by exon 4a, but otherwise is identical to tau in the central nervous system [54], while p-tau has more limited peripheral expression.

The axonal protein NfL can also be quantified in blood using the ultrasensitive Simoa® technology [55]. In the ADNI cohort, plasma NfL showed a marked increase in AD, with an AUC value of 0.87, which is comparable to the core AD CSF biomarkers [56]. In MCI, plasma NfL was highest in cases with evidence of brain amyloidosis by amyloid PET scans, and predicted both faster cognitive deterioration and rate of brain atrophy

[56]. Plasma NfL is also increased in presymptomatic familial-AD gene mutation carriers, before the expected year of symptom onset [57], a finding validated in the Dominantly Inherited Alzheimer's Network study, where the increase in plasma NfL was evident around 7 years before symptom onset in mutation carriers [58], indicating that NfL detects neurodegeneration even in the preclinical stage of the disease. However, plasma NfL is not a specific AD biomarker; instead, it increases in multiple neurological disorders, such as multiple sclerosis and progressive supranuclear palsy, and in acute brain injury such as stroke and brain trauma [59]. Nevertheless, plasma NfL is a most promising neurodegeneration biomarkers in the A/T/N framework and may be useful in tracking disease progression and to monitor effects of disease-modifying drug candidates. A possible future application for plasma NfL is as a screening test in primary care, where it may serve to either identify or rule out neurodegeneration.

32.4 Fluid Biomarkers in Clinical Trials

The AD fluid biomarkers have several applications in clinical trials, including both patient selection (eligibility screening and diagnostic evaluation) and evaluation of drug effects (identification of target engagement and biochemical effects downstream of the pathophysiological drug target); for an overview see Table 32.3. In this context, the

Table 32.3 Applications for fluid biomarkers in AD clinical trials

Application	Principles and methods	Biomarkers	Interpretation and comment
Screening	Eligibility screening for biomarker evidence of brain amyloidosis and/or tau pathology in the initial evaluation of patients Performed in primary care or at the non-specialist clinic Blood tests are optimal for eligibility screening Blood biomarker assays need to be analytically validated for continuous (daily or weekly) use as screening tests The cut-off level for a positive blood test needs to be established before the initiation of the trial	Plasma $A\beta_{42}/A\beta_{40}$ ratio Plasma p-tau	The plasma $A\beta_{42}/A\beta_{40}$ ratio concords with brain amyloidosis assessed by PET, but may lack robustness for repeated screening analyses Plasma p-tau is a sensitive and specific biomarker to identify AD-type tau pathology The preferred performance of a screening test is a very high NPV (above 90%, ideally 95–98%) at an acceptable PPV (50% or preferably higher) Individuals with a negative test are screened out, while those with a positive blood test are admitted to the specialist clinic (clinical trial center) for a detailed diagnostic evaluation before enrollment

Table 32.3 (cont.)

Application	Principles and methods	Biomarkers	Interpretation and comment
Diagnostics	Diagnostic evaluation of patients having a positive test result from eligibility screening before clinical trial enrollment Performed at the specialist clinic (clinical trial center) CSF tests currently preferred given that the CSF tests are highly clinically and analytically validated, have established cut-offs, and CE-marked assays are available on fully automated instruments	CSF $A\beta_{42}$, or better $A\beta_{42}/A\beta_{40}$ ratio CSF p-tau, or p-tau/$A\beta_{42}$ CSF t-tau, or t-tau/$A\beta_{42}$ CSF neurogranin	The CSF $A\beta_{42}/A\beta_{40}$ ratio is the key AD fluid diagnostic biomarker to identify brain amyloidosis An alternative is CSF p-tau/$A\beta_{42}$, which also shows high concordance with amyloid PET CSF t-tau, on its own, or in a ratio with $A\beta_{42}$ (t-tau/$A\beta_{42}$ ratio) works well in AD/control populations, but t-tau may increase due to other causes, e.g., cerebrovascular disease High CSF t-tau and p-tau may also be of value since they predict progression of cognitive deficits during the time window relevant for trials (1–2 years) Increased CSF neurogranin is characteristic for AD, and may add specificity to the diagnostic panel
Theragnostics	Provide evidence of target engagement of a drug candidate in humans CSF or blood samples taken before study initiation, at time points during the trial, and at end of study Blood biomarkers allow for more frequent sampling, but some biomarkers cannot be analyzed in plasma or serum Samples are optimally analyzed in one batch at end of trial	CSF or plasma $A\beta_{42}$, $A\beta_{40}$ CSF sAPPβ, sAPPα CSF or plasma p-tau species (p-tau$_{181}$, p-tau)	Amyloid biomarkers may provide evidence for target engagement of anti-Aβ drug candidates, e.g., BACE1 inhibitor Tau biomarkers may provide evidence for target engagement of an anti-tau drug candidate A change in amyloid or tau biomarker may indicate target engagement also in volunteers, and does thus not predict corresponding downstream effects or symptomatic effects
	Provide evidence of downstream effects on neurodegeneration, synaptic degeneration, and other molecular pathophysiological events, such as glial and microglial activation CSF or blood samples taken at study initiation, at time points during the trial, and at end of study Blood biomarkers allow for more frequent sampling, but some biomarkers cannot be analyzed in plasma or serum Samples can be analyzed in one batch at end of trial, or when indicated during the trial	Neurodegeneration: CSF t-tau, CSF or plasma NfL Synaptic degeneration: CSF neurogranin, CSF SNAP-25, CSF NPTX-2 Tau pathology: CSF or plasma p-tau$_{181}$, p-tau$_{217}$, or p-tau$_{231}$, CSF tau fragments (e.g., tau$_{368}$) Glial/microglial activation: CSF sTREM2, CSF YKL-40 (also known as chitinase-3-like protein 1), plasma GFAP	A change toward normalization in neurodegeneration biomarkers with treatment suggest downstream drug effects on the intensity of the neurodegenerative process A decrease in CSF or plasma p-tau suggests drug effects on tau phosphorylation state or tangle formation Blood tests can be applied more frequently than CSF tests Blood testing will likely have much lower drop-out rates than CSF testing Some biomarkers, e.g., t-tau, synaptic proteins, currently do not work in blood

Note: Anti-Aβ and anti-tau clinical trials are used to exemplify the application of CSF biomarkers in clinical trials; other fluid biomarkers may be relevant for drug candidates with other targets. Abbreviations: Aβ, amyloid beta; AD, Alzheimer's disease; BACE1, beta-site amyloid precursor protein cleaving enzyme 1; CSF, cerebrospinal fluid; GFAP, glial fibrillary acidic protein; NfL, neurofilament light; NPTX-2, neuronal pentraxin 2; NPV, negative predictive value; PPV, positive predictive value; p-tau, phosphorylated tau; sAPP, soluble amyloid precursor protein extracellular domain; SNAP-25, synaptosomal associated protein-25; sTREM2, soluble triggering receptor expressed on myeloid cells 2; t-tau, total tau.

high-accuracy blood tests can be applied more easily and at shorter intervals than CSF tests, and at lower costs than imaging methods. Blood tests therefore have a large potential to revolutionize clinical trial design and accelerate the drug discovery process.

32.4.1 Screening

The implementation of simple, non-invasive, and inexpensive blood tests for eligibility screening in AD clinical trials may dramatically reduce trial costs. Given that AD is defined by brain amyloidosis, the plasma $A\beta_{42}/A\beta_{40}$ ratio is the rational screening biomarker to detect amyloid deposition. The plasma $A\beta_{42}/A\beta_{40}$ ratio concords well with amyloid PET positivity [60], but the change in amyloid-PET-positive individuals in the plasma $A\beta_{42}/A\beta_{40}$ ratio is rather low, around 10–15%, which may introduce difficulties in retaining stability in the dichotomization of individuals into amyloid-positive or -negative cases, especially in those with ratios close to the cut-off.

In contrast, the increase in plasma p-tau in AD is more distinct, with an increase in plasma p-tau in the range of 250–400% across studies (for details see the Alzheimer Research Forum's Alzbiomarker database; www.alzforum.org/alzbiomarker). This results in a very high accuracy in the differentiation [43], which likely will make the dichotomization into positive or negative more robust than for the $A\beta_{42}/A\beta_{40}$ ratio. This supports the use of plasma p-tau as an eligibility screening test. Although it needs to be evaluated, the combination of plasma p-tau and $A\beta_{42}/A\beta_{40}$ in a "tau/amyloid" ratio may be an optimal combination, providing information not only on the presence of pathology but also on the likelihood of future clinical progression.

Plasma NfL may be more difficult to employ as a screening tool in AD clinical trials, given that levels are clearly higher in other neurodegenerative disorders such as frontotemporal dementia and parkinsonian disorders [61, 62], but may serve its purpose in trials on drug candidates for these disorders.

Combining blood biomarker results with apolipoprotein-E (*APOE*) genotype and age in multivariate statistical models may give high AUC values and good separation between AD and control groups in research cohorts [33, 63]. However, when applied in the real-life situation this approach may introduce a bias toward excluding the proportion of AD patients who do not possess the *APOE* ε4 allele, as well as younger (60–70 years of age) AD patients, and instead favor elderly (80–90 years of age) cases.

A blood-based screening tool in primary care could serve as a gatekeeper to the confirmatory diagnostic process at the specialist clinic. A common expert opinion is that a blood biomarker for primary care eligibility screening should have very high negative predictive value, above 90% and ideally 95–98%, and an acceptable positive predictive value, above 50% or preferably higher [64]. This would mean that individuals without the disease are efficiently screened out, which would be ethically correct and save costs for unnecessary second-grade CSF and PET biomarkers in those with a negative test result. Patients with a positive test would be referred to the specialist clinic for more advanced examinations, including either CSF or PET biomarkers, after which those in which brain amyloidosis can be verified can be enrolled in trials with disease-modifying compounds [64].

For clinical trials, the ability to screen large numbers of potential trial participants will reduce the number of late screen failures and thereby reduce costs, decrease enrollment periods, and shorten trial durations. A cost–benefit analysis based on the ADNI data [65] for the employment of plasma p-tau$_{181}$ as a screening biomarker in clinical trials suggested that a trial aiming at recruiting 1,000 amyloid-positive asymptomatic individuals would require around 5,000 PET scans at a cost of $15,000,000 ($3,000 per scan). For comparison, the application of plasma p-tau for eligibility screening would cost $250,000 at $50 per test (or $500,000 at $100 per test) and substantially reduce the number of individuals to be examined by amyloid PET to confirm amyloid positivity for final trial enrollment to less than half, thereby reducing costs substantially. Although these figures are preliminary estimates, the cost saving of $8,300,000 is substantial. Further, the addition of plasma $A\beta_{42}/A\beta_{40}$ to p-tau$_{181}$ may increase the accuracy of prediction, and thereby reduce costs, further [38]. For the future, introducing a simple cognitive test together with blood biomarkers into the triage process in primary care would reduce wait time to, and workload at, the specialist clinic [66].

32.4.2 Diagnostics for Final Clinical Trial Enrollment

It is generally agreed that it is important to use diagnostic biomarkers in AD trials, to increase the number of patients who do have AD pathology, specifically brain amyloidosis and tau pathology. This is essential given the poor accuracy (around 70–80% when related to neuropathology) of a diagnosis based on purely clinical grounds [67, 68]. After eligibility screening, the final verification of amyloid or tau pathology (at the clinical trial center) before clinical trial enrollment is optimally performed by either PET imaging or CSF biomarkers at the specialist clinic. As reviewed above, the combination of CSF Aβ and tau shows excellent agreement with amyloid PET [8] and these CSF biomarkers are available on in vitro diagnostically certified fully automated laboratory analyzers. As an option, CSF neurogranin may be added to the diagnostic biomarker panel to increase specificity [69].

32.4.3 Identifying Target Engagement

Fluid biomarkers are also useful to identify target engagement, that is to provide evidence in humans that a drug candidate engages the intended mechanistic target [2]. While many compounds in early AD trials were taken to clinical testing in patients based on data only from preclinical animal experiments [70], it is now common to evaluate target engagement in Phase 1 studies before entering into Phase 2 and 3. One example is beta-site APP-cleaving enzyme 1 (BACE1) inhibitor treatment, where small short-term Phase 1 trials show a marked and sustained reduction in CSF and plasma levels of $A\beta_{40}$ and $A\beta_{42}$ [71], thereby verifying target engagement of BACE1 inhibitor therapy. However, large Phase 3 clinical trials on BACE1 inhibitors show no clinical benefit, or even cognitive worsening, by this class of compounds [72]. These results indicate that evidence of target engagement in the form of amyloid reductions does not directly translate to an effect on memory disturbances or other cognitive symptoms. Given the uncertainty of a direct mechanistic link between target engagement and clinical benefit, fluid (CSF and blood) biomarkers may provide support of effects on AD pathophysiology downstream of the drug target, as discussed in the section below.

32.4.4 Verifying Downstream Effects

Downstream biomarker evidence of disease modification could hypothetically be obtained in AD trials on anti-amyloid drug candidates by the reductions, toward normalization, of fluid biomarkers for neuronal and synaptic degeneration [73]. While the current lack of clinically available approved disease-modifying treatments (DMT) for AD precludes evaluation of whether this principle holds true, results from other brain disorders where DMT are available indicate that this principle may be possible.

Treatment of children with spinal muscular atrophy with the antisense oligonucleotide drug nusinersen results in a marked decrease in CSF NfL levels, which before treatment are very high, but become normalized after 4–5 doses of the drug, and the reduction correlates with clinical improvements in motor function [74]. Similarly, CSF and serum NfL levels decrease in patients with multiple sclerosis after switching to highly effective disease-modifying therapies [75]. These findings support CSF and blood neurodegeneration biomarkers being applied to monitor downstream effects of effective disease-modifying therapies.

In AD clinical trials, lowering of p-tau levels in CSF or plasma may indicate downstream effects on tau phosphorylation, while lowering of t-tau in CSF or NfL in CSF or blood supports downstream effects on the intensity of neurodegeneration. A published paper with biomarker data from clinical trials of the anti-amyloid antibodies bapineuzumab and gantenerumab, shows reductions in CSF levels of p-tau, t-tau, and neurogranin, suggestive of the downstream effect of Aβ immunotherapy on neurodegeneration, tau pathology, and synaptic degeneration [76–78]. Further, a recent review summarizing unpublished results from the lecanemab (BAN2401) Phase 2 as well as the aducanumab and gantenerumab Phase 3 trials reports significant effects on the neuronal and synaptic degeneration biomarkers CSF NfL and neurogranin, as well as the tau pathology marker CSF p-tau, indicating promising downstream effects of these Aβ immunotherapies [79]. For future trials, the use of blood as an alternative to CSF biomarkers will likely increase the proportion of patients with complete biomarker results. Repeat blood sampling to continuously (e.g., at each antibody infusion or every third month) monitor effects on downstream pathologies might provide important knowledge when assessed throughout the trial.

A prerequisite for the application of biomarker tests as outcome measures in clinical trials is that the biomarker shows low variability during the duration of the trial in patients who are not on treatment. Data on the AD core CSF biomarkers during 6- and 24-month periods show very stable biomarker levels in cases on continuous treatment with acetylcholinesterase inhibitors, with coefficients of variation (CVs) of 4.4–6.6% during 6 months and 7.2–8.7% over 24 months [80, 81]. With regard to blood biomarkers, plasma p-tau$_{181}$ in the ADNI cohort also showed very high longitudinal stability over 24 months with CVs of 7–12% [65], supporting its use in trials to monitor downstream drug effects on tau pathology.

32.4.5 Monitoring Adverse Effects or Events

Amyloid immunotherapy treatments are associated with side effects in the form of amyloid-related imaging abnormalities (ARIA) in a relatively large percentage of cases [82], which necessitates repeated MRI assessments [83]. While most patients with ARIA are asymptomatic, some have more severe symptoms. Hypothetically, the need for repeated MRIs in trials on this class of immunotherapies may be reduced if plasma NfL could serve as a substitute to detect clinically relevant severe ARIA. A sudden increase in plasma NfL compared with pre-treatment levels would in that scenario indicate the need to perform an MRI scan, while stable levels would support further continuous (e.g., monthly) monitoring with plasma NfL levels. The benefit would be, apart from lower costs, the high accessibility of blood sampling, which could be performed even at the patient's primary care unit.

Acknowledgments

Dr. Blennow is supported by the Swedish Research Council (#2017–00915), the Alzheimer Drug Discovery Foundation (ADDF), USA (#RDAPB-201809–2016615), the Swedish Alzheimer Foundation (#AF-742881), Hjärnfonden, Sweden (#FO2017-0243), the Swedish state under the agreement between the Swedish government and the County Councils, the ALF-agreement (#ALFGBG-715986), and European Union Joint Program for Neurodegenerative Disorders (JPND2019-466–236).

Disclosures

Dr. Blennow has served as a consultant, at advisory boards, or at data monitoring committees for Abcam, Axon, Biogen, JOMDD/Shimadzu, Julius Clinical, Lilly, MagQu, Novartis, Roche Diagnostics, and Siemens Healthineers, and is a co-founder of Brain Biomarker Solutions in Gothenburg AB (BBS), which is a part of the GU Ventures Incubator Program.

References

1. Jack CR Jr., Bennett DA, Blennow K, et al. A/T/N: an unbiased descriptive classification scheme for Alzheimer disease biomarkers. *Neurology* 2016; **87**: 539–47.

2. Blennow K. Biomarkers in Alzheimer's disease drug development. *Nat Med* 2010; **16**: 1218–22.

3. Olsson B, Lautner R, Andreasson U, et al. CSF and blood biomarkers for the diagnosis of Alzheimer's disease: a systematic review and meta-analysis. *Lancet Neurol* 2016; **15**: 673–84.

4. Portelius E, Tran AJ, Andreasson U, et al. Characterization of amyloid beta peptides in cerebrospinal fluid by an automated immunoprecipitation procedure followed by mass spectrometry. *J Proteome Res* 2007; **6**: 4433–9.

5. Andreasen N, Minthon L, Vanmechelen E, et al. Cerebrospinal fluid tau and Abeta42 as predictors of development of Alzheimer's disease in patients with mild cognitive impairment. *Neurosci Lett* 1999; **273**: 5–8.

6. Blennow K, Mattsson N, Scholl M, Hansson O, Zetterberg H. Amyloid biomarkers in Alzheimer's disease. *Trends Pharmacol Sci* 2015; **36**: 297–309.

7. Lewczuk P, Lelental N, Spitzer P, Maler JM, Kornhuber J. Amyloid-beta 42/40 cerebrospinal fluid concentration ratio in the diagnostics of Alzheimer's disease: validation of two novel assays. *J Alzheimers Dis* 2015; **43**: 183–91.

8. Janelidze S, Zetterberg H, Mattsson N, et al. CSF Abeta42/Abeta40 and Abeta 42/Abeta 38 ratios: better diagnostic markers of Alzheimer disease. *Ann Clin Transl Neurol* 2016; **3**: 154–65.

9. Sato C, Barthelemy NR, Mawuenyega KG, et al. Tau kinetics in neurons and the human central nervous system. *Neuron* 2018; **98**: 861–4.

10. Mudher A, Colin M, Dujardin S, et al. What is the evidence that tau pathology spreads through prion-like propagation? *Acta Neuropathol Commun* 2017; **5**: 99.

11. Skillback T, Rosen C, Asztely F, et al. Diagnostic performance of cerebrospinal fluid total tau and phosphorylated tau in Creutzfeldt–Jakob disease: results from the Swedish Mortality Registry. *JAMA Neurol* 2014; **71**: 476–83.

12. Blennow K, Hampel H. CSF markers for incipient Alzheimer's disease. *Lancet Neurol* 2003; **2**: 605–13.

13. Hampel H, Buerger K, Zinkowski R, et al. Measurement of phosphorylated tau epitopes in the differential diagnosis of Alzheimer disease: a comparative cerebrospinal fluid study. *Arch Gen Psychiatry* 2004; **61**: 95–102.

14. Hanes J, Kovac A, Kvartsberg H, et al. Evaluation of a novel immunoassay to detect p-tau Thr127 in the CSF to distinguish Alzheimer disease from other dementias. *Neurology* 2020; **95**: e3026–35.

15. Hesse C, Rosengren L, Andreasen N, et al. Transient increase in total tau but not phospho-tau in human cerebrospinal fluid after acute stroke. *Neurosci Lett* 2001; **297**: 187–90.

16. Suarez-Calvet M, Karikari TK, Ashton NJ, et al. Novel tau biomarkers phosphorylated at T181, T217 or T231 rise in the initial stages of the preclinical Alzheimer's continuum when only subtle changes in Abeta pathology are detected. *EMBO Mol Med* 2020; **12**: e12921.

17. Mattsson-Carlgren N, Andersson E, Janelidze S, et al. Abeta deposition is associated with increases in soluble and phosphorylated tau that precede a positive tau PET in Alzheimer's disease. *Sci Adv* 2020; **6**: eaaz2387.

18. Meredith JE Jr., Sankaranarayanan S, Guss V, et al. Characterization of novel CSF tau and p-tau biomarkers for Alzheimer's disease. *PloS One* 2013; **8**: e76523.

19. Zhang Z, Song M, Liu X, et al. Cleavage of tau by asparagine endopeptidase mediates the neurofibrillary pathology in Alzheimer's disease. *Nat Med* 2014; **20**: 1254–62.

20. Blennow K, Chen C, Cicognola C, et al. Cerebrospinal fluid tau fragment correlates with tau PET: a candidate biomarker for tangle pathology. *Brain* 2020; **143**: 650–60.

21. Hansson O, Zetterberg H, Buchhave P, et al. Association between CSF biomarkers and incipient Alzheimer's disease in patients with mild cognitive impairment: a follow-up study. *Lancet Neurol* 2006; **5**: 228–34.

22. Shaw LM, Vanderstichele H, Knapik-Czajka M, et al. Cerebrospinal fluid biomarker signature in Alzheimer's Disease Neuroimaging Initiative subjects. *Ann Neurol* 2009; **65**: 403–13.

23. Kuhlmann J, Andreasson U, Pannee J, et al. CSF Abeta 1–42: an excellent but complicated Alzheimer's biomarker – a route to standardisation. *Clin Chim Acta* 2017; **467**: 27–33.

24. Hansson O, Seibyl J, Stomrud E, et al. CSF biomarkers of Alzheimer's disease concord with amyloid-beta PET and predict clinical progression: a study of fully automated immunoassays in BioFINDER and ADNI cohorts. *Alzheimers Dement* 2018; **14**: 1470–81.

25. Kaplow J, Vandijck M, Gray J, et al. Concordance of Lumipulse cerebrospinal fluid t-tau/Abeta 42 ratio with amyloid PET status. *Alzheimers Dement* 2020; **16**: 144–52.

26. Boulo S, Kuhlmann J, Andreasson U, et al. First amyloid beta 1–42 certified reference material for re-calibrating commercial immunoassays. *Alzheimers Dement* 2020; **16**:1493–503.

27. Shaw LM, Arias J, Blennow K, et al. Appropriate use criteria for lumbar puncture and cerebrospinal fluid testing in the diagnosis of Alzheimer's disease. *Alzheimers Dement* 2018; **14**: 1505–21.

28. Janelidze S, Stomrud E, Palmqvist S, et al. Plasma beta-amyloid in Alzheimer's disease and vascular disease. *Sci Rep* 2016; **6**: 26801.

29. Kaneko N, Yamamoto R, Sato TA, Tanaka K. Identification and quantification of amyloid beta-related peptides in human plasma using matrix-assisted laser desorption/ionization time-of-flight mass spectrometry. *Proc Jpn Acad Ser B Phys Biol Sci* 2014; **90**: 104–17.

30. Pannee J, Tornqvist U, Westerlund A, et al. The amyloid-beta degradation pattern in plasma: a possible tool for clinical trials in Alzheimer's disease. *Neurosci Lett* 2014; **573**: 7–12.

31. Ovod V, Ramsey KN, Mawuenyega KG, et al. Amyloid beta concentrations and stable isotope labeling kinetics of human plasma specific to central nervous system amyloidosis. *Alzheimers Dement* 2017; **13**: 841–9.

32. Nakamura A, Kaneko N, Villemagne VL, et al. High performance plasma amyloid-beta biomarkers for Alzheimer's disease. *Nature* 2018; **554**: 249–54.

33. Schindler SE, Bollinger JG, Ovod V, et al. High-precision plasma beta-amyloid 42/40 predicts current and future brain amyloidosis. *Neurology* 2019; **93**: e1647–59.

34. Palmqvist S, Mattsson N, Hansson O, Alzheimer's Disease Neuroimaging Initiative. Cerebrospinal fluid analysis detects cerebral amyloid-beta accumulation earlier than positron emission tomography. *Brain* 2016; **139**: 1226–36.

35. Tatebe H, Kasai T, Ohmichi T, et al. Quantification of plasma phosphorylated tau to use as a biomarker for brain Alzheimer pathology: pilot case–control studies including patients with Alzheimer's disease and Down syndrome. *Mol Neurodegener* 2017; **12**: 63.

36. Mielke MM, Hagen CE, Xu J, et al. Plasma phospho-tau 181 increases with Alzheimer's

disease clinical severity and is associated with tau- and amyloid-positron emission tomography. *Alzheimers Dement* 2018; **14**: 989–97.

37. Thijssen EH, La Joie R, Wolf A, et al. Diagnostic value of plasma phosphorylated tau 181 in Alzheimer's disease and frontotemporal lobar degeneration. *Nat Med* 2020; **26**: 387–97.

38. Janelidze S, Mattsson N, Palmqvist S, et al. Plasma p-tau$_{181}$ in Alzheimer's disease: relationship to other biomarkers, differential diagnosis, neuropathology and longitudinal progression to Alzheimer's dementia. *Nat Med* 2020; **26**: 379–86.

39. Karikari TK, Pascoal TA, Ashton NJ, et al. Blood phosphorylated tau 181 as a biomarker for Alzheimer's disease: a diagnostic performance and prediction modelling study using data from four prospective cohorts. *Lancet Neurol* 2020; **19**: 422–33.

40. Ashton NJ, Pascoal TA, Karikari TK, et al. Plasma p-tau231: a new biomarker for incipient Alzheimer's disease pathology. *Acta Neuropathol* 2021; **141**: 709–24.

41. Barthelemy NR, Horie K, Sato C, Bateman RJ. Blood plasma phosphorylated-tau isoforms track CNS change in Alzheimer's disease. *J Exp Med* 2020; **217**;DOI: http://doi.org/10.1084/jem.20200861.

42. Barthelemy NR, Bateman RJ, Hirtz C, et al. Cerebrospinal fluid phospho-tau T217 outperforms T181 as a biomarker for the differential diagnosis of Alzheimer's disease and PET amyloid-positive patient identification. *Alzheimers Res Ther* 2020; **12**: 26.

43. Palmqvist S, Janelidze S, Quiroz YT, et al. Discriminative accuracy of plasma phospho-tau 217 for Alzheimer disease vs other neurodegenerative disorders. *JAMA* 2020; **24**: 772–81.

44. O'Connor A, Karikari TK, Poole T, et al. Plasma phospho-tau 181 in presymptomatic and symptomatic familial Alzheimer's disease: a longitudinal cohort study. *Mol Psychiatry* 2020;DOI: https://doi.org/10.1038/s41380-020-0838-x.

45. Lantero Rodriguez J, Karikari TK, Suarez-Calvet M, et al. Plasma p-tau$_{181}$ accurately predicts Alzheimer's disease pathology at least 8 years prior to post-mortem and improves the clinical characterisation of cognitive decline. *Acta Neuropathol* 2020; **140**: 267–78.

46. Kovacs GG. Invited review: neuropathology of tauopathies: principles and practice. *Neuropathol Appl Neurobiol* 2015; **41**: 3–23.

47. Rubenstein R, Chang B, Yue JK, et al. Comparing plasma phospho tau, total tau, and phospho tau–total tau ratio as acute and chronic traumatic

brain injury biomarkers. *JAMA Neurol* 2017; **74**: 1063–72.

48. Palmqvist S, Insel PS, Stomrud E, et al. Cerebrospinal fluid and plasma biomarker trajectories with increasing amyloid deposition in Alzheimer's disease. *EMBO Mol Med* 2019; **11**: e11170.

49. Randall J, Mortberg E, Provuncher GK, et al. Tau proteins in serum predict neurological outcome after hypoxic brain injury from cardiac arrest: results of a pilot study. *Resuscitation* 2013; **84**: 351–6.

50. Zetterberg H, Wilson D, Andreasson U, et al. Plasma tau levels in Alzheimer's disease. *Alzheimers Res Ther* 2013; **5**: 9.

51. Mattsson N, Zetterberg H, Janelidze S, et al. Plasma tau in Alzheimer disease. *Neurology* 2016; **87**: 1827–35.

52. Mattsson N, Zetterberg H, Nielsen N, et al. Serum tau and neurological outcome in cardiac arrest. *Ann Neurol* 2017; **82**: 665–75.

53. Shahim P, Tegner Y, Wilson DH, et al. Blood biomarkers for brain injury in concussed professional ice hockey players. *JAMA Neurol* 2014; **71**: 684–92.

54. Vacchi E, Kaelin-Lang A, Melli G. Tau and alpha synuclein synergistic effect in neurodegenerative diseases: when the periphery is the core. *Int J Mol Sci* 2020; **21**: 5030.

55. Gisslen M, Price RW, Andreasson U, et al. plasma concentration of the neurofilament light protein (NfL) is a biomarker of CNS injury in HIV infection: a cross-sectional study. *EBioMedicine* 2016; **3**: 135–40.

56. Mattsson N, Andreasson U, Zetterberg H, Blennow K. Association between longitudinal plasma neurofilament light and neurodegeneration in patients with Alzheimer disease. *JAMA Neurol* 2019; **76**: 791–9.

57. Weston PSJ, Poole T, Ryan NS, et al. Serum neurofilament light in familial Alzheimer disease: a marker of early neurodegeneration. *Neurology* 2017; **89**: 2167–75.

58. Preische O, Schultz SA, Apel A, et al. Serum neurofilament dynamics predicts neurodegeneration and clinical progression in presymptomatic Alzheimer's disease. *Nat Med* 2019; **25**: 277–83.

59. Khalil M, Teunissen CE, Otto M, et al. Neurofilaments as biomarkers in neurological disorders. *Nat Rev Neurol* 2018; **14**: 577–89.

60. Schindler SE, Bollinger JG, Ovod V, et al. High-precision plasma beta-amyloid 42/40 predicts current and future brain amyloidosis. *Neurology* 2019; **93**: e1647–59.

61. Hansson O, Janelidze S, Hall S, et al. Blood-based NfL: a biomarker for differential diagnosis of parkinsonian disorder. *Neurology* 2017; **88**: 930–7.

62. Illan-Gala I, Lleo A, Karydas A, et al. Plasma tau and neurofilament light in frontotemporal lobar degeneration and Alzheimer's disease. *Neurology* 2021; **96**: e671–83.

63. Palmqvist S, Janelidze S, Stomrud E, et al. Performance of fully automated plasma assays as screening tests for Alzheimer disease-related β-amyloid status. *JAMA Neurol* 2019; **76**: 1060–9.

64. Hampel H, O'Bryant SE, Molinuevo JL, et al. Blood-based biomarkers for Alzheimer disease: mapping the road to the clinic. *Nat Rev Neurol* 2018; **14**: 639–52.

65. Karikari TK, Benedet AL, Ashton NJ, et al. Diagnostic performance and prediction of clinical progression of plasma phospho-tau 181 in the Alzheimer's disease neuroimaging initiative. *Mol Psychiatry* 2020; **26**: 429–42.

66. Mattke S, Cho SK, Bittner T, Hlavka J, Hanson M. Blood-based biomarkers for Alzheimer's pathology and the diagnostic process for a disease-modifying treatment: projecting the impact on the cost and wait times. *Alzheimers Dement (Amst)* 2020; **12**: e12081.

67. Beach TG, Monsell SE, Phillips LE, Kukull W. Accuracy of the clinical diagnosis of Alzheimer disease at National Institute on Aging Alzheimer Disease Centers, 2005–2010. *J Neuropathol Exp Neurol* 2012; **71**: 266–73.

68. Knopman DS, DeKosky ST, Cummings JL, et al. Practice parameter: diagnosis of dementia (an evidence-based review). Report of the Quality Standards Subcommittee of the American Academy of Neurology. *Neurology* 2001; **56**: 1143–53.

69. Portelius E, Olsson B, Hoglund K, et al. Cerebrospinal fluid neurogranin concentration in neurodegeneration: relation to clinical phenotypes and neuropathology. *Acta Neuropathol* 2018; **136**: 363–76.

70. Blennow K, de Leon MJ, Zetterberg H. Alzheimer's disease. *Lancet* 2006; **368**: 387–403.

71. Kennedy ME, Stamford AW, Chen X, et al. The BACE1 inhibitor verubecestat (MK-8931) reduces CNS beta-amyloid in animal models and in Alzheimer's disease patients. *Sci Transl Med* 2016; **8**: 363ra150.

72. Wessels AM, Lines C, Stern RA, et al. Cognitive outcomes in trials of two BACE inhibitors in Alzheimer's disease. *Alzheimers Dement* 2020; **16**: 1483–92.

73. Masters CL, Bateman R, Blennow K, et al. Alzheimer's disease. *Nat Rev Dis Primers* 2015; **1**: 15056.

74. Olsson B, Alberg L, Cullen NC, et al. NfL is a marker of treatment response in children with SMA treated with nusinersen. *J Neurol* 2019; **266**: 2129–36.

75. Piehl F, Kockum I, Khademi M, et al. Plasma neurofilament light chain levels in patients with MS switching from injectable therapies to fingolimod. *Mult Scler* 2018; **24**: 1046–54.

76. Blennow K, Zetterberg H, Rinne JO, et al. Effect of immunotherapy with bapineuzumab on cerebrospinal fluid biomarker levels in patients with mild to moderate Alzheimer disease. *Arch Neurol* 2012; **69**: 1002–10.

77. Ostrowitzki S, Lasser RA, Dorflinger E, et al. A Phase III randomized trial of gantenerumab in prodromal Alzheimer's disease. *Alzheimers Res Ther* 2017; **9**: 95.

78. Salloway S, Sperling R, Fox NC, et al. Two Phase 3 trials of bapineuzumab in mild-to-moderate Alzheimer's disease. *N Engl J Med* 2014; **370**: 322–33.

79. Tolar M, Abushakra S, Hey JA, Porsteinsson A, Sabbagh M. Aducanumab, gantenerumab, BAN2401, and ALZ-801-the first wave of amyloid-targeting drugs for Alzheimer's disease with potential for near term approval. *Alzheimers Res Ther* 2020; **12**: 95.

80. Blennow K, Zetterberg H, Minthon L, et al. Longitudinal stability of CSF biomarkers in Alzheimer's disease. *Neurosci Lett* 2007; **419**: 18–22.

81. Zetterberg H, Pedersen M, Lind K, et al. Intra-individual stability of CSF biomarkers for Alzheimer's disease over two years. *J Alzheimers Dis* 2007; **12**: 255–60.

82. Sevigny J, Chiao P, Bussiere T, et al. The antibody aducanumab reduces Abeta plaques in Alzheimer's disease. *Nature* 2016; **537**: 50–6.

83. Sperling RA, Jack CR Jr., Black SE, et al. Amyloid-related imaging abnormalities in amyloid-modifying therapeutic trials: recommendations from the Alzheimer's Association Research Roundtable Workgroup. *Alzheimers Dement* 2011; **7**: 367–85.

Chapter 33

Brain Imaging for Alzheimer's Disease Clinical Trials

Dawn C. Matthews and Mark E. Schmidt

33.1 Introduction

Imaging biomarkers have assumed an increasingly important role in the diagnosis and evaluation of treatment effect in Alzheimer's disease (AD). In pharmaceutical clinical trials, imaging can help to address key hurdles by confirming pathology for patient inclusion/exclusion, enabling analysis stratification based on the likely rate of clinical decline, detecting treatment effects with fewer subjects, characterizing treatment responders, and elucidating the neurological basis for the clinical response. This chapter aims to provide clinical trialists and others with an understanding of how imaging data that appear in the clinical literature are generated, some of the technical issues that can influence the reliability and interpretability of the data, and how these biomarkers can be incorporated to support clinical trials.

Imaging data sets acquired in large-scale trials such as the Alzheimer's Disease Neuroimaging Initiative (ADNI) have greatly increased our understanding of the pathological, neurodegenerative, and functional course of AD. In 2011, these findings led to a substantial revision of AD diagnostic criteria by the National Institute on Aging–Alzheimer's Association (NIA–AA) that related directly to therapeutic trials. The historical clinical–pathological definition was shifted to a three-stage clinical–biological definition of AD (preclinical, prodromal/mild cognitive impairment [MCI] due to AD, and clinical), which specially identified criteria for use in AD clinical trials based upon imaging and cerebrospinal fluid (CSF) biomarkers [1]. More recently, the NIA–AA again updated AD diagnostic criteria for clinical trial use to a solely biological continuum of disease defined by an "A/T/N" framework, where "A" is amyloid as measured by positron emission tomography (PET) or CSF amyloid beta (Aβ), "T" is tau as measured by PET or CSF hyperphosphorylated tau (p-tau), and "N" is neurodegeneration or neuronal injury as measured by volumetric MRI, glucose metabolism,

or total tau [2]. The A/T/N framework is notably focused on those disease characteristics known to be measurable using imaging or CSF biomarkers. The US Food and Drug Administration (FDA) and the European Medicines Agency (EMA) have recognized this diagnostic paradigm shift and have supported the use of imaging and other biomarkers in clinical trials.

Several key clinical development questions that can be addressed using imaging are listed below. The primary imaging modalities used in AD trials are then briefly described, followed by an overview of AD progression and the associated changes observed in several key imaging biomarkers. Specific imaging approaches to address the clinical development questions are then discussed, organized by imaging modality.

33.2 Incorporation of Imaging Biomarkers into Clinical Trials

To obtain imaging benefit in AD clinical trials, an important starting point is to define the questions to be addressed, which may include:

- **Patient enrollment**: (a) Does this patient have AD pathology? (b) Does this patient have co-morbidities or risk factors that merit exclusion? (c) Is this patient at a stage of pathology progression that is targeted by this treatment?
- **Patient safety**: (a) Does this treatment cause adverse vasogenic edema or hemorrhage effects? (b) Does this treatment cause functional effects linked to adverse clinical effects?
- **Target engagement**: (a) Does this drug engage and/or affect the target (pathology, receptor, process) as intended? (b) What is the dose response?
- **Treatment effect (downstream)**: (a) Does treatment slow the functional and/or neurodegenerative consequences of disease

progression? (b) Does treatment introduce any potential symptomatic effects or side effects? (c) What are the characteristics of patients in whom a treatment effect is observed?

- **Patient stratification for analysis:** (a) Is this patient likely to accumulate pathology at a particular rate? (b) Is this patient likely to worsen in cognitive and/or functional endpoints at a particular rate?

33.2.1 Imaging Modalities

The primary imaging modalities used in clinical trials to address the above questions are MRI and PET. MRI provides high-resolution digital representations of brain tissue by applying magnetic field pulses and radio waves to affect the behavior of protons in brain tissue, and detecting information as these protons return to their resting states. Its most established use is in depicting the volume and integrity of brain tissue, but a variety of more exploratory MRI sequences can produce information regarding white-matter-tract integrity, cerebral blood flow, and chemistry. Benefits include high spatial resolution, lack of radiation, no injection or contrast agent (optional), and the ability to acquire multiple different types of sequences in a single session of around an hour or less.

PET imaging detects the amount and spatial location of molecular targets of interest by using an injected molecular entity (ligand) that has been labeled with a positron-emitting isotope with a relatively short half-life (110 minutes in the case of [^{18}F]fluorine). After the ligand labeled with a radioactive isotope crosses the blood–brain barrier and as the isotope decays, it emits a positron that is rapidly annihilated by an electron, emitting two gamma rays, detected by the PET scanner. The timing and spatial locations of these many events are mathematically reconstructed using software to produce an image of the tracer distribution and concentration throughout the brain. By using ligands that have selective binding affinity for particular targets, PET is able to visualize and quantify the amount and spatial location of a wide range of targets including amyloid, tau, glucose metabolism (a primary energy source for neuronal activity, reflecting neuronal function [3]), inflammation, neuroreceptors, radiolabeled investigational drugs, and other entities or processes. Examples of MRI, fluorodeoxyglucose (FDG) PET, amyloid PET, and tau PET images are shown in Figure 33.1.

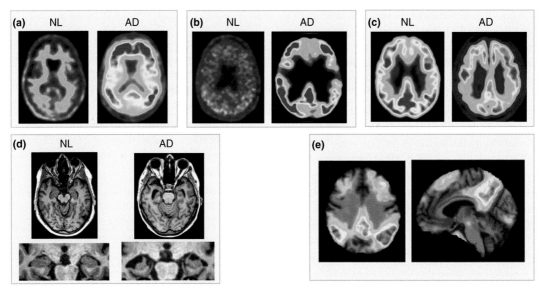

Figure 33.1 Images from cognitively normal, amyloid-negative (NL) patients and patients with AD: (a) NAV-4694 amyloid PET scans (data: Meilleur/Enigma) showing accumulation in frontal, temporal, and parietal cortices in AD, (b) MK-6240 tau PET scans demonstrating accumulation in temporoparietal and frontal cortices in AD (data: Cerveau/Enigma), (c) FDG PET scans showing reduced temporoparietal glucose metabolism with some frontal involvement in AD (data: ADNI, Cleveland Clinic), (d) T1-weighted MRI scans demonstrating reduced medial temporal volume and increased ventricle size in AD, and (e) the fusion (spatial alignment and overlay) of a PI-2620 tau PET scan on the same patient's MRI scan (data: Life Molecular Imaqinq). Scans shown in (a), (b), and (d) are from the same normal 76-year-old female and the same 77-year-old female with a clinical diagnosis of AD.

33.2.2 Imaging Biomarkers across the AD Spectrum

A representation of AD progression and changes observed in several imaging biomarkers is illustrated in Figure 33.2. It is now understood that the AD timeline begins 20 or more years prior to symptom onset as soluble Aβ oligomers accumulate and then aggregate into fibrillar plaques measurable with amyloid PET imaging. The amyloid burden ("A" in A/T/N) and associated amyloid PET values increase steadily during preclinical and early prodromal (MCI) stages, approaching a plateau by late MCI or early dementia. Inflammation is an early factor that may be caused by and contributory to toxic amyloid [4], and is measurable using PET imaging on an exploratory basis. Soluble p-tau isoforms such as p-tau$_{217}$ increase in parallel with fibrillar amyloid, prior to and continuing beyond the point at which amyloid PET

positivity is reached. With an apparent lag relative to amyloid accumulation, tau aggregates into neurofibrillary tangles (NFTs; "T" in A/T/N) [5]. This time lag may be less than originally hypothesized, as recently developed tau PET tracers have revealed tau in subjects with amyloid levels at or below quantitative thresholds for amyloid positivity [6]. Early tau deposition is observed in the transentorhinal cortex (Braak stage 1), followed by the hippocampus in typical cases (Braak stage 2) and/or amygdala, with subsequent progressive expansion to the lateral temporal cortices and functionally, rather than spatially, connected neocortical regions. This spatial sequence of tau differs from that of amyloid, which is first observed in the neocortex (particularly precuneus, posterior cingulate, and orbitofrontal regions) and only later observed in medial temporal tissue [7]. Tau PET patterns correspond to clinical phenotype [8] and show a relationship to age, with greater posterior

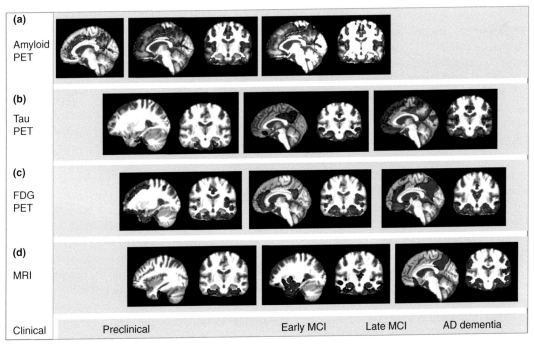

Figure 33.2 Imaging biomarkers in an example of typical evolution across the AD spectrum. (a) Amyloid plaques measured with florbetapir PET (Avid Radiopharmaceuticals) appear in the cingulate and frontal cortex, spreading pervasively throughout the temporal and parietal cortex, with variable occipital accumulation and less intensity in medial temporal regions (ADNI data); (b) Neurofibrillary tangles measured using MK-6240 tau PET (Cerveau Technologies) appear in the transentorhinal cortex expanding to other medial temporal cortex, and spreading to the neocortex after sufficient amyloid accumulation; (c) Reductions in glucose metabolism measured with FDG PET are observed early on in the hippocampus and posterior cingulate, expanding to the temporoparietal cortices with variable frontal and occipital decline (ADNI data); (d) Atrophy is observed on MRI in the medial temporal cortices, progressing to the neocortex (ADNI data). Image positions reflect a sequential order between modalities but time-related relationships are still under study by the field. Patterns of tau, glucose metabolism, and atrophy vary with phenotype and individual. Analyses by ADMdx.

Clinical diagnosis AD, 61 years, FMMSE 13, ADAS-cog 52

Clinical diagnosis AD, 71 years, MMMSE 23, ADAS-cog 24

Clinical diagnosis AD, 79 years, MMMSE 23, ADAS-cog 20

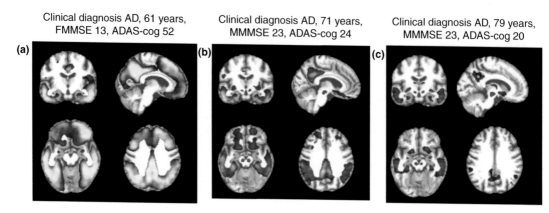

Figure 33.3 Comparison of tau burden (orange-red, superimposed on MRI template) in younger vs. older patients with a clinical diagnosis of AD (Cleveland Clinic, flortaucipir provided by Avid Radiopharmaceuticals). ADAS-cog, Alzheimer's Disease Assessment Scale – cognitive subscale; FMMSE, Folstein Mini-Mental State Examination; MMMSE, modified Mini-Mental State Examination.

and frontal burden in younger patients compared to predominantly medial-lateral temporal regions and lower total burden in the oldest patients [9] (Figure 33.3).

The "N" (neuronal damage) effects of AD also begin very early in the disease process. The soluble amyloid oligomers, mediated by soluble p-tau oligomers, degrade synaptic plasticity and neuronal connectivity [10, 11]; oligomeric forms have been imaged experimentally in animal models. Regional cerebral glucose metabolism, measured with FDG PET, is tightly coupled to synaptic function and begins to decrease in hippocampus and posterior cingulate at least 13 years prior to symptom onset [12]. As the disease progresses, an FDG PET pattern of temporoparietal hypometabolism worsens and correlates with clinical decline. Varying degrees of asymmetry and frontal and occipital involvement are present, and pattern variations correspond to clinical phenotype and with tau distribution. As neuronal loss occurs, tissue progressively atrophies, resulting in reductions in volume and cortical thickness that can be measured with volumetric MRI. Tissue loss begins with transentorhinal and hippocampal reductions at least 5 years prior to symptom onset, continuing to worsen and expand to patterns that correlate with those of tau [13, 14] and FDG PET, and with clinical decline. Temporal atrophy is dominant in older patients corresponding to the temporal-dominant tau topology observed in this age group. In younger patients, parietal and frontal atrophy become more pronounced, consistent with the more pervasive tau seen in these patients. Throughout the disease,

other related effects occur including reductions in regional blood flow, disruption in correlated networks of neuronal activity, and deficits in white-matter-tract integrity, which can all be measured using MRI and/or PET.

33.2.3 Imaging Biomarker Value in Clinical Trials

The changes observed in various imaging biomarkers with disease progression provide opportunity to use this information to support clinical trials. Biomarkers offer increased diagnostic accuracy over clinical assessment alone, as illustrated by clinical trials of bapineuzumab and solanezumab in which 36% of enrolled apolipoprotein-E ε4 (*APOE-4*) non-carriers diagnosed as AD were found to lack amyloid pathology [15]. Longitudinal treatment effects on imaging endpoints can be measured with fewer participants than would be typically required to detect clinical endpoint changes, reducing required patient numbers by an order of magnitude and excluding those for whom the therapeutic would bring no benefit. Despite efforts to develop cognitive tests sensitive to preclinical changes [16], biomarkers remain essential to measure disease progression in this stage. As predictors of cognitive decline, imaging biomarkers can also reduce the number of participants required to detect clinical endpoint effects. In general, imaging can help to transform the historical "black box" of clinical worsening to a well-characterized, patient-specific stage of pathology, function, and neurodegeneration for therapeutic targeting.

33.3 MRI in AD Drug Development

MRI diagnostic and volumetric sequences have been established in AD trials and are discussed below. Additional sequences are then described that are considered exploratory as they have not yet achieved the necessary standardization for consistently reliable clinical trial use across multiple sites and vendors.

33.3.1 Diagnostic MRI for Exclusion from Patient Enrollment

MRI is often used during enrollment screening to rule out alternate sources of cognitive decline such as tumor, infarct(s), overt vascular dementia, abnormal pressure, and hemorrhage. A T1-weighted scan showing gray, white, and CSF tissue can be used to check for potential abnormalities such as tumors, stroke or bleeds, ventricular enlargement consistent with normal-pressure hydrocephalus, and other conditions. White-matter lesions are assessed using fluid-attenuated inversion recovery (FLAIR) or T2-weighted scans. The extent of white-matter disease can be graded according to the Fazekas scale of 0 to 3 [17] (Figure 33.4). Since moderate-to-severe white-matter disease can be a contributor to cognitive status and decline [18], excessive lesions may prompt exclusion or, alternatively, this information may be used as a covariate in analysis. Diffusion-weighted imaging is used to detect infarctions and also aids in evaluation for tumor, infection, and demyelination. Gradient recalled echo T2* (T2*GRE)- or susceptibility-weighted imaging (SWI) sequences can be used to detect macro and microhemorrhages. Screening sequences are often read visually by the local radiologist for each site but may also be read centrally. It is useful to provide a guide regarding the exclusion criteria and what should be included in the radiology report, in order to reduce variability across sites. Trials may combine the basic screening sequences with more advanced specifications and/or additional sequences that will be used for other purposes in the trial, reducing the total number of imaging visits for enrolled patients.

33.3.2 Diagnostic MRI for Patient Safety Monitoring

MRI-based safety monitoring has become an important component of anti-amyloid clinical trials. This need became particularly evident when 6% of patients treated with the immunotherapy AN1792 developed meningoencephalitis [19]. At the request of the FDA, recommendations for safety monitoring were developed by the Alzheimer's Association Research Roundtable Workgroup [20]. Terminology for amyloid-related imaging abnormalities (ARIA) was developed to include ARIA-E (vasogenic edema) and ARIA-H (microhemorrhages defined as parenchymal hemosiderin deposits with a maximum diameter that is less than a threshold typically in the range of 5–10 mm, large hemosiderin deposits ≥10 mm, or superficial hemosiderosis in leptomeninges) [21]. ARIA-E is measurable with a FLAIR MRI scan, while ARIA-H is detectable with T2*GRE or SWI sequences. ARIA-E and ARIA-H abnormalities were subsequently reported in 35% and 18% of patients treated with aducanumab and 28–42% and 15–25% of patients treated with gantenerumab, respectively [22].

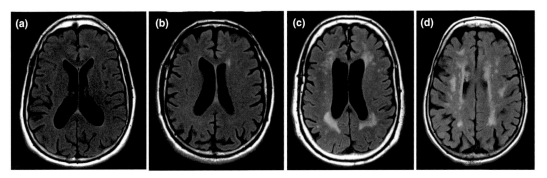

Figure 33.4 Examples of white-matter disease in mild-to-moderate late-onset AD patients illustrating the range of potentially confounding disease that may be present in clinical trial recruits at this stage, with Fazekas scores of (a) 0, (b) 1, (c) 2, d) 3. (Image source: Cleveland Clinic.)

When developing safety imaging protocols for clinical trials, some technical and logistical factors should be considered. A greater number of microhemorrhages and smaller sizes are detectable using higher-field-strength scanners and when using a SWI sequence as compared to GRE, although GRE has often been used due to its broad availability and practical implementation [20]. Thresholds for safety reads should be consistent with the scanners and sequences used. Centralized reads and standardization of protocols, thresholds, and documentation are important to assure consistency of evaluation across sites. Evaluation is typically done on a visual basis, although some algorithms are in development to aid in the detection of microhemorrhages.

33.3.3 Volumetric MRI for Patient Enrollment, Stratification, and Endpoint Measurement

33.3.3.1 Diagnostic Support for Patient Inclusion
Atrophy measured with MRI has been identified by the NIA–AA diagnostic criteria as a marker for the "N" aspect of the A/T/N criteria for clinical trials [2]. Hippocampal atrophy has received particular focus due to its early and ongoing progression throughout AD. In the literature, volume is typically expressed as either cubic centimeters (cm³) or else as a percentage of total intracranial volume (unitless) to normalize for head size. As a reference point, hippocampal volumes in prodromal (MCI) and mild AD average around 1–2 standard deviations below age- and sex-matched normal reference values. In preclinical and early MCI stages, entorhinal cortical thickness and hippocampal subfield measures provide greater sensitivity as the earliest changes occur in these regions. Several different software packages have been developed that can accurately and reproducibly measure these structures, making this feasible in large-scale trials. Since algorithms differ in their delineation and detection of anatomical boundaries, it is important to make comparisons of statistical power, rates of change, and deviations from reference norms using consistent methods and relative change rather than attempting to compare absolute values across different algorithms.

Hippocampal atrophy by itself is not specific to AD. By combining information from multiple regions, and/or different attributes using multivariate machine-learning algorithms (classifiers), specificity in diagnosis can be increased. For example, classifiers that combine hippocampal volume with shape features have predicted amyloid positivity in MCI patients and cognitively normal individuals with accuracies of 89% and 79–82% respectively [23]. Classifiers using combinations of anatomical structures have been demonstrated to differentiate AD, frontotemporal dementia (FTD), and other dementias, as well as variants within AD [24, 25]. Multivariate classification of volumetric data can be predictive of tau burden, and can be combined with information such as APOE-4 carrier status and amyloid, to further increase accuracy [26].

33.3.3.2 Stratification for Analysis
Volumetric MRI can also be used as a predictor to stratify patient populations for expected rate of clinical decline. This stratification can help to ensure that comparisons between arms are made using populations that are adequately matched, and it can reduce variability within an analysis group that would otherwise reduce statistical power. Trial design involves determining what tissue to measure, what threshold(s) to use for stratification, and required sample size. Numerous published studies have focused on hippocampal volume, which is predictive of the subsequent rate of clinical progression in AD. In late-MCI patients from ADNI, use of a hippocampal volume cut point for patient selection reduced sample sizes required to detect a treatment effect over 2 years in the Mini-Mental State Examination (MMSE), Clinical Dementia Rating – sum of boxes (CDR-sb), and Alzheimer's Disease Assessment Scale – cognitive subscale (ADAS-cog) by approximately 40–60%. The projected reduction in trial costs, taking into account the cost of screening out excluded patients, was approximately 30–40% [27]. For preclinical and early prodromal stages, entorhinal cortical thickness, perirhinal volume, and certain hippocampal subfields used in multivariate approaches may provide the most sensitive predictors of decline [28, 29]. Data from ADNI and other studies can be used to estimate required sample sizes using each approach.

33.3.3.3 Detection of Disease-Modifying Effect
Since slowing neurodegeneration should slow the rate of atrophy, volumetric MRI can be used in AD clinical trials as an endpoint for disease

modification. The number of subjects required per arm to detect a slowing of atrophy depends upon the structure measured, the quantitation method applied, disease stage, whether or not the study population is first enriched for amyloid and/or tau positivity, and whether a correction for aging is applied. Without enrichment, estimated sample sizes of approximately 170 for AD and 285 for MCI have been reported to detect a 25% reduction in the rate of hippocampal atrophy over 12 months (two-tailed $p < 0.05$, 80% power) [30]. Treatment-related slowing of hippocampal atrophy in AD patients has been observed in association with some therapeutics including donepezil [31], nilotinib (a tyrosine kinase inhibitor) [32], and tramiprosate (a soluble amyloid anti-aggregation agent) [33]. Favorable clinical treatment effects were also observed in those trials. Conversely, an increase in the rate of hippocampal atrophy was observed in early and mild AD patients with the beta-site APP-cleaving enzyme inhibitor lanabecestat over a period of 18–24 months, as well as adverse clinical effects [34]. Other anatomical structures and use of multivariate classifiers or regression models have potential to provide sensitivity and statistical power beyond that of hippocampal volume.

Some caution is merited in selecting anatomical structures as disease-modification endpoints. Treatment-related ventricular enlargement and brain volume reductions not correlated with clinical status have been observed in some studies of anti-amyloid immunotherapies [35, 36], suggesting against their use for this drug class. The impact of therapeutic inflammation reduction in AD upon brain volume has not been determined, but transient inflammatory episodes in multiple sclerosis increase brain volume [37] and significant reductions might have an opposite effect, confounding atrophy measurement.

33.3.3.4 Technical Considerations in Volumetric MRI

Brain volumes, though not cortical thicknesses, correlate with head size, and therefore measurement and correction for intracranial volume is important. The volumes and thicknesses of most anatomical structures in the brain vary to different degrees with age, sex, scanner field strength, and scanner manufacturer. Erroneous conclusions may be drawn in comparing groups unless adjustments are made for these covariates. Regional atrophy

rates differ between younger, early-onset AD and late onset; an imbalance in these ages within or across arms can impact data interpretation. For longitudinal measurement, the same scanner and sequence should always be used for any given participant. Minimizing patient head motion during image acquisition is also very important during the trial, as motion produces numerous types of artifact that can reduce biomarker accuracy.

The selection of the measurement and analysis approach also affects accuracy and required sample sizes. Reproducibility and accuracy also vary across different measurement approaches (for example, hippocampal segmentation vs. the boundary shift integral [BSI]), and across permutations of a particular measurement approach (for example, which hippocampal segmentation approach is used, or what additional steps are applied after use of the BSI). In addition, some automated software packages are able to take all serial scans into account to eliminate bias toward any one time point ("longitudinal" vs. "cross-sectional" pipelines); this can improve reproducibility and accuracy relative to the small changes (a few percent) that are being measured [38, 39]. The statistical power of longitudinal measurement may also be increased by adding time points, such as a third imaging session rather than only two.

33.3.4 Practical Implementation of MRI in AD Clinical Trials

Successful MRI implementation in a clinical trial typically involves collaboration between the clinical trialist and an imaging contract research organization (CRO), and also benefits from input or published findings from academic researchers. Several steps are involved in trial preparation and execution. As a starting point, the imaging application(s) (e.g., diagnostic evaluation for exclusion and/or safety, stratification, endpoint measurement) is identified. Decisions should take into account whether the study must be conducted at multiple sites, and the feasibility of standardizing and executing the imaging protocols. For volumetric applications, a next step is to specify the anatomical structure or atrophy pattern to be measured. This is the "N" in the case of diagnostic confirmation, the predictive measure in the case of stratification, or the endpoint if for a longitudinal assessment of disease modification. For diagnostic confirmation or stratification, an appropriate deviation (threshold) from the reference mean must also be determined. An estimated number of required participants per arm can be calculated based upon data from sources such as ADNI, other studies, or proof-of-concept trials. An imaging charter, imaging technical manual, and imaging source documents (documenting protocol execution, deviations, or issues for each imaging session) are then typically developed, along with the imaging sections of the statistical analysis plan. The software that will be used (e.g., by the imaging CRO) to process and measure volumes must also be identified and should have been validated for performance.

Standardization across multiple imaging sites is critical in order to pool data and for trial success. Imaging sites must be qualified with regard to their ability to properly execute protocols and deliver high-quality images in a timely manner, which requires appropriate equipment, staff, and procedures. As part of qualification, sites should provide images acquired using a phantom (object with grid or other characteristics that test resolution, contrast, and other characteristics) as well as a human volunteer/deidentified research subject. Scanner issues such as inadequate gray/white contrast, white artifact, spatial distortion, or other artifacts must be identified and addressed prior to the study. Data-transfer logistics should be tested prior to study initiation. During the trial, phantom scans should be acquired periodically, as scanners can drift or develop issues over time. Visual quality control as well as other checks should be performed on all image segmentations (identifying the anatomical boundaries of the tissue to be measured) used to produce volumetric values.

33.3.5   Additional Exploratory MRI Applications

MRI can also provide information regarding white-matter integrity, blood flow, and function. However, common to all of these are substantial challenges in the standardization of image acquisitions, vendor differences, and analysis. Therefore, these are considered exploratory approaches but have been incorporated into various trials on that basis.

33.3.6   White-Matter-Integrity Diffusion Tensor Imaging

Diffusion tensor imaging (DTI) provides information regarding white-matter-tract integrity by measuring the directionality of water-molecule travel at each spatial location in the brain. DTI uses paired electromagnetic pulses to impose a directional shift on the molecules, followed by a pulse to reverse the shift. Molecules that are unconstrained to move ("diffuse") in a particular direction will change location. The degree of diffusion gradient applied is called a b-value. In an intact axon, white-matter travel has high directionality (fractional anisotropy [FA] value typically normalized to a range of 0 to 1), restricted by axonal structure and the myelin sheath. With loss of integrity, the directionality of flow decreases and measures of radial diffusivity (RD) and mean diffusivity (MD) (normalized range of 0 to 1) increase. In addition to the numerical values, colored FA maps are used to convey the directional integrity of the various tracts, while tractograms show a three-dimensional representation of the fibers (Figure 33.5). Although

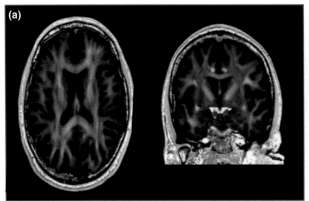
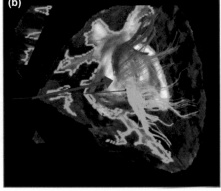

Figure 33.5 DTI: (a) FA image and (b) tractogram showing fibers associated with the white matter of the thalamus. Images generated using BrainSuite (www.brainsuite.org).

DTI findings across studies and sites have been historically variable, recent studies have demonstrated multi-site clinical trial feasibility [40]. Longitudinal changes in DTI have been measured in AD and FTD patients with reasonable effect sizes regarding disease progression for clinical trials [41].

Technical considerations for DTI include the sequence specification and correction for "free water." The signal measured at a particular voxel consists of an intracellular signal related to axonal integrity plus free-water contributions from extracellular space, which can be caused by vessel disease, inflammation, vasogenic edema, and other factors. A correction algorithm to separate free water from other signals has been developed, which requires only one b-value [42], but estimation is improved with acquisition of multiple b-values [43], as adopted in ADNI 3 and the Human Connectome project. Scanners with multi-band capability (the ability to excite multiple slices in parallel for increased efficiency) are preferable as they are able to acquire multiple b-values for free-water correction within a reasonable time. An additional consideration is that DTI values can vary between scanner models, and these differences must be reconciled for use in multi-center trials.

33.3.7 Perfusion (Cerebral Blood Flow) Measurement with Arterial Spin Labeling

Arterial spin labeling (ASL) MRI enables measurement of perfusion, which correlates closely with blood flow and provides a biomarker for the progressive reductions in blood flow that are associated with AD. ASL patterns of reduced blood flow have been demonstrated to differentiate AD, FTD, and Lewy body disease patients [44]. It therefore has potential use for disease and/or phenotype characterization. In measuring symptomatic treatment response, ASL has shown correlation with dopamine-transporter responses to several different medications [45], and some studies of acetylcholinesterase inhibitors have found treatment associated increases in cerebral blood flow in AD-relevant regions [46]. For measurement of longitudinal disease-modifying effects, achieving sufficient statistical power with reasonable sample sizes has not yet been demonstrated.

Technical considerations matter greatly with ASL. In brief, radiofrequency pulses are applied to magnetically label water protons in blood that will flow to tissue to be imaged. After a specified time delay to allow the protons to travel to capillary beds in the tissue of interest, the tissue is imaged and subtracted from an image of the same tissue without labeling, creating a perfusion image. ASL is challenged by a low signal-to-noise ratio, and factors such as cerebrovascular disease can confound blood-transit-time estimation. However, pseudo-continuous ASL (PCASL) sequences acquired in three-dimensional mode and arterial-transit-time maps to reduce flow rate confounds have produced quality similar to PET imaging (see Zhang et al. for a review [47]). The successful applications described above used PCASL acquisition sequence. Hematocrit levels can also affect ASL measures and should be taken into account [48].

33.3.8 Measurement of Neuronal Connectivity with Resting-State Functional MRI

A second type of functional MRI (fMRI) is blood-oxygen-level-dependent (BOLD) fMRI, which detects signal changes associated with the replenishment of oxygenated blood to support neuronal energy demands. Resting-state BOLD fMRI measures the correlation between spontaneous low-frequency fluctuations (<0.1 Hz) in a detected signal across various brain regions, and can be acquired within a 10-minute period. The default mode network (DMN), comprised of regions that are actively correlated when the brain is not engaged in cognitive or other activity, is strikingly similar to the characteristic posterior cingulate and temporoparietal pattern of tau accumulation and glucose hypometabolism in AD. DMN connectivity becomes abnormal in prodromal AD and decreases in AD dementia providing a marker of decline [49]. BOLD fMRI has been used to study the effects of donezepil, rivastigmine, galantamine, memantine, and other medications in AD. Treatment-related increases in connectivity have been observed in AD-relevant regions but reported results have varied with regard to which regions are affected [46]. BOLD fMRI can be subject to image artifact, and various processing pipelines have been developed to optimize the signal-to-noise ratios and useful information [50].

33.3.9 Measurement of Chemical Concentrations with MRS

Magnetic resonance spectroscopy (MRS) imaging provides information regarding the relative concentrations of certain metabolites in imaged tissue. In brief, application of electromagnetic energy causes protons to emit radio waves at frequencies that, because of influence by their surrounding molecular structure electrons, are specific to the chemical entity in which the proton is located. The area under each frequency peak translates to relative concentration. In clinical trials, MRS can provide confirmation of biochemical mechanisms, complementing other information. For example, in a 6-month Phase 2 study of 42 AD patients, MRS data showed that riluzole, a glutamate modulator, was associated with an increase in glutamine in the posterior cingulate as compared to placebo [51]. This confirmed mechanism of action and was consistent with study outcomes relating to a favorable effect on posterior cingulate glucose metabolism and clinical endpoints. A consistent finding across MRS studies in AD has been the reduction of N-acetylaspartate (NAA), a marker related to neuronal integrity, in the posterior cingulate and in other AD-relevant regions [52]. However, while cross-sectional measurement is significant, longitudinal measurement of NAA in AD and amyotrophic lateral sclerosis has not shown statistical group differences, which has been attributed to technical variability.

33.4 PET in AD Drug Development

The primary PET modalities applied in AD clinical trials measure amyloid, tau, and glucose metabolism, and their applications are described below. Additional exploratory PET modalities are then summarized. First, some background is presented regarding how to interpret PET measurements, and overall considerations.

33.4.1 Acquisition and Measurement of PET Data

The signal intensity at each point within a PET scan represents the amount of the molecular entity (e.g., amyloid, tau, or glucose uptake) present at a particular spatial location in the brain. The values seen in clinical literature for AD that quantify these intensities are often expressed as standardized uptake value ratios (SUVRs) and sometimes may be expressed as distribution value ratios (DVRs).

These both represent the amount of the molecular entity in a region or voxel (three-dimensional pixel) of interest, but they are derived in different ways as follows. When a radiotracer is injected, it crosses from the blood into brain tissue, where it is taken up at a rate that correlates with blood flow. This is followed by a transition period during which tracer amounts decline and reach a "pseudo-equilibrium" state associated with binding to the target of interest (such as tau). Over time, the tracer will leave (clear) the tissue, but depending upon how much of the entity to which it binds is present in the tissue, it will stay in the tissue for longer and with higher signal. The rise and fall of signal over time, when measured by the scanner and plotted, is referred to as a time activity curve (Figure 33.6). The pseudo-equilibrium time window is referred to as the "late timeframe."

SUVR refers to the ratio of the value in the tissue of interest compared to (divided by) the value in the "reference" tissue that does not contain the molecular entity and will have a lower value, both measured during the late timeframes. For practical reasons, patients are often only imaged during those late timeframes, rather than lying on the scanner table for what may be 60–90 or more minutes. However, changes in blood flow or tracer clearance can contribute to changes in the SUVR, producing error [53]. This is relevant for patients in later stages of disease during which blood flow may be decreasing more rapidly, or when the treatment causes blood-flow changes. Error due to blood-flow changes can be eliminated by imaging the patient from the time of injection through the late timeframes, or by acquiring a two-part scan with the earliest time window (e.g., the first 20 minutes) and the late timeframe window (on the order of from 50–70 minutes or 80–100 minutes post-injection, depending on the tracer), and a break in between. In either case, a series of simultaneous mathematical equations are used to determine the contributions of blood flow and tracer binding to the overall signal intensity, producing a distribution volume ratio (DVR) comparable to but typically lower in value than an SUVR. Methods are also in development to obtain sufficient information from the first 30 minutes of the scan, avoiding the need for late timeframes. When comparing values, it is important to confirm whether a DVR or SUVR has been used, as they should not be compared directly.

One of the most important considerations in longitudinal PET measurement (whether FDG,

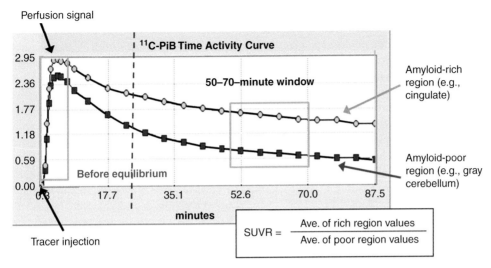

Figure 33.6 Plot of time activity curve, in this case for [¹¹C]PiB amyloid PET. The "late timeframe" window, shown as a rectangle, identifies the post-injection time window during which the SUVR is calculated, as the average signal over that time period in the amyloid-rich (target) region divided by the average signal over that time period in the reference region.

amyloid, tau, or other) is which reference region to use. A reference region is used to normalize values in target regions because the signal strength in each scan varies by injected dose, individual blood–brain-barrier penetration, and other factors. Dividing by a reference region can help to cancel out these influences, and creates the "R" (ratio), in SUVR. Ideally, a reference region remains stable during disease progression and exposure to treatment. In AD, the cerebellum and/or pons have often been selected because they do not typically accumulate AD pathology or decline as quickly as other regions in glucose metabolism. However, technical factors can cause variability in the cerebellum from a few percent to around 30%, overwhelming the small annual changes from which a slowing of progression is to be detected (often 1–5% depending upon the imaging modality). The variability is due to the combination of its low signal intensity (such that technical noise causes large swings in value), vulnerability to head motion, and location in slices other than those with the regions of interest, across which scanner sensitivity may vary. Selecting a reference region that is from similar slices of the brain as the target regions, such as subcortical white matter or unaffected cortical tissue, can be useful as a reference. Examples of the impact on statistical power and required sample sizes are included in Sections 33.4.2.1 and 33.4.4, on amyloid and on glucose metabolism, respectively. Regardless of the regions measured, the same scanner should always

be used for all longitudinal visits for a given study participant.

Other considerations include whether to smooth the images, whether to measure tissue in "template" (common head shape and size) or "native" (individualized) space, which atlas (probabilistic region of interest boundaries) to use, and whether to correct for "partial volume effects." Smoothing refers to applying a numerical filter to each voxel to blur higher-resolution images to be comparable to images of lower resolution, so that images from different scanners can be pooled and/or compared. Partial volume effects relate to the contamination (e.g., dilution or amplification) of measured tissue intensity by neighboring voxels of different tissue.

33.4.2 Amyloid PET for Diagnostic Confirmation and Evaluation of Treatment Effects on Fibrillar Amyloid

33.4.2.1 Diagnostic Confirmation and Evaluation of Treatment Effects on Fibrillar Amyloid

One of the primary applications of PET in AD clinical trials has been to confirm amyloid positivity (the "A" in A/T/N) for patient enrollment. In some trials, this has been done using a "visual read" of an amyloid PET scan based upon tracer-specific methods approved for clinical use, while in others a quantitative value has been compared to a pre-set threshold. Amyloid PET also serves as a key biomarker to quantify treatment effects upon fibrillar amyloid burden, enabling demonstration of dose-dependent reductions in amyloid burden in clinical trials of aducanumab [54] and gantenerumab [55].

When incorporating amyloid PET into a trial, one decision to be made is which tracer to use. The first amyloid-specific tracer was ^{11}C-Pittsburgh compound B ([11C]PiB), which is still used in some academic settings. Several ^{18}F tracers have since been developed and approved for clinical use, including florbetapir (Amyvid™, Avid Radiopharmaceuticals), flutemetamol (Vizamyl™, GE Healthcare), florbetaben (Neuraceq™, Life Molecular Imaging), and NAV-4964 (Enigma Biomedical Group, not yet FDA cleared). These tracers all measure amyloid-plaque burden but differ in how many minutes after tracer injection the image is acquired, their signal ranges in response to amyloid binding, and their white-matter signal intensity. For a discussion of the history of PET and information regarding tracer chemistries, see Schmidt et al. [56].

In addition to tracer selection, decisions are required regarding which target regions (regions of interest) or voxel-based pattern to measure and which reference region. Because amyloid tends to accumulate in a rather generalized manner across cortical tissue, a cortical average that includes frontal, cingulate, parietal, and temporal regions is often used. For diagnostic confirmation, a threshold SUVR is typically pre-specified to determine which persons are amyloid positive. It is important to note that this number varies depending upon which tracer, which regions of interest, and which reference region have been used. To reconcile differences between tracers and methods, the Centiloid scale was developed [57]. This regresses values obtained from different tracers, regions of interest, and analysis methods to a common measure that can be referenced to a common threshold value. Some clinical trials have allowed use of either CSF Aβ or amyloid PET to determine amyloid status. It should be noted that while the diagnostic accuracy of these has been found to be comparable in some studies, decreases in CSF Aβ corresponding to amyloid positivity have been found to occur prior to associated increases in amyloid PET SUVR [7].

For longitudinal measurement, selecting target regions where accumulation is earliest and/or most rapid may help to increase the statistical power. However, the selection of reference region has an even greater impact. Results from several studies suggest that inclusion of white matter in the reference region offers a major benefit due to higher signal and less vulnerability to technical noise. For example, the number of subjects required to detect a 25% slowing in the rate of amyloid accumulation measured with florbetapir PET at 80% power in amyloid-positive MCI patients was 8,076 using the whole cerebellum as the reference region, 2,718 using the pons, and 325 using subcortical white matter (located in overlapping slices with regions of interest) [58]. The numerous technical considerations that can impact the quality of amyloid PET measurements are described in Schmidt et al. [59] and in the Amyloid PET Profile developed by the Quantitative Imaging Biomarker Alliance working group (https://qibawiki.rsna.org/index.php/Profiles).

33.4.2.2 Early-Frame Amyloid

There is additional information regarding brain function that can be obtained from an amyloid PET scan. The first few minutes following tracer injection of an amyloid or tau PET scan produce an image that correlates with blood flow and with FDG PET (Figure 33.7). This image can provide functional and disease-pattern information, differentiating between AD, FTD, and other dementias [60]. It should be noted that although blood flow is typically correlated with glucose metabolism (with decoupling observed in later disease), it is not the same as FDG PET, and while there is overlapping information, there are also some differences. These include greater variability and lower sensitivity to longitudinal changes associated with disease progression than observed using FDG PET. However, early-frame amyloid can provide a relatively efficient means, using a single PET visit, to obtain (a) information on functional status and dementia type, (b) blood flow to correct for amyloid burden, and (c) amyloid burden itself.

33.4.3 Tau PET

Applications of Tau PET in AD clinical trials include diagnostic confirmation of AD, patient inclusion based upon tau positivity or a certain Braak/other defined stage, identification of different AD variants likely to have different clinical phenotypes, stratification for likely clinical worsening, and measurement of treatment effect on NFT accumulation and/or removal.

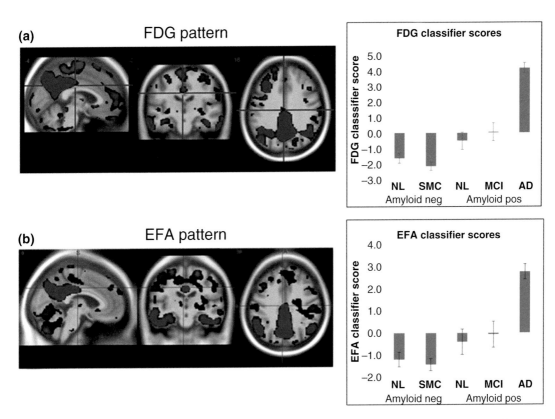

Figure 33.7 Comparison of the patterns associated with AD progression from cognitively normal amyloid-negative subjects through amyloid positive MCI and AD dementia for (a) FDG PET (*n* = 56) and (b) early-frame amyloid (EFA) (*n* = 62). Classifiers were developed using scans from the same subjects as available and the same time points. Canonical variate scores quantify each individual's degree of expression of the pattern of hypometabolism (blue) or "perfusion" (blue) or preservation (orange-red) relative to whole brain. The higher the score on the *y*-axis, the greater the pattern expression. Error bars = standard error of the mean. NL, cognitively normal; SMC, subjective memory complaint; MCI, mild cognitive impairment; AD, AD dementia. Data from ADNI (www.adni-info.org); analysis by ADMdx.

As with amyloid, a decision to be made in trial design is which tracer to use. However, in contrast to amyloid, tau tracers have an even more diverse set of characteristics. The first tracer specific for tau was flortaucipir (AV-1451/T807, Avid Radiopharmaceuticals), followed by multiple "second-generation" tau tracers including MK-6240 (Cerveau Technologies), PI-2620 (Life Molecular Imaging), GTP1 (Genentech), and ^{18}F-PM-PBB3 (Aprinoia). These tracers have differences in sensitivity, specificity, and off-target binding. Flortaucipir and MK-6240 have shown greater specificity for the 3R + 4R paired helical filament tau found in AD as compared to isoforms found in other dementias. PI-2620 has shown binding to AD-like tau and to structures affected by 4R tau such as in progressive supranuclear palsy [61]. ^{18}F-PM-PBB3 binds to tau in multiple forms of dementia [62]. MK-6240 has

demonstrated greater sensitivity and signal-to-noise ratios for early-stage medial temporal tau, elevating the field's understanding of the temporal relationship between amyloid and tau [6]. These and other tracers also exhibit off-target binding in sinuses and/or meninges to varying degrees, discriminated through visual and/or quantitative approaches. MK-6240 exhibits a high dynamic range (range of signal intensity) from low to high tau burden [63].

As with other PET imaging, key decisions in implementing tau PET are the selection of tracer, target regions, and reference region. Since the spatial distribution of tau is more variable and clinically meaningful than with amyloid, the relatively simple five regions of interest composite may not be optimal. Methods under investigation to optimize detection include various tau-focused target-region combinations [64], voxel-based

387

comparisons, and machine-learning-derived pattern measurement.

Tau PET involves some additional technical considerations. Off-target binding and white-matter uptake can create confounds in tau PET to varying degrees depending on the tracer. Flortaucipir shows high signal uptake in the striatum and choroid plexus, as well as in other regions not observed to the same extent with second-generation tracers. Uptake in the meninges and/or sinuses by second-generation or other tracers may spill into cortical regions, discriminated through visual or quantitative methods. Tau tracers can also exhibit considerable binding in the cerebellar vermis and/or other clusters within the cerebellum, another SUVR reference region. Erosion of region borders, limitation to certain slices, and thresholding to remove high signal clusters have been applied to address these confounds [65]. To reduce the influence of spill-in from high-tau-burden cortical regions into subcortical white tissue that may be used as a SUVR reference, the parametric estimation of reference signal intensity (PERSI) method was developed using the tracer AV-1451 that employs a two-part Gaussian decomposition [66].

Another consideration with currently available tau tracers is that they do not achieve steady-state equilibrium over time in regions of moderate to high NFT density, even over several hours. This may be due to rebinding of the tracer in the intraneuronal space (for intracellular NFTs), as it is not observed in regions of high amyloid burden where the target is extracellular. This makes it critical to start each scan, particularly serial scans, at the same time point following tracer injection, and to measure over the same time window. Differences in start time can be mathematically corrected but these are approximations.

Similar to amyloid, the early frames of the scan or the R1 image from a dynamic scan can be used to evaluate disease patterns [67].

33.4.4   FDG PET Imaging of Glucose Metabolism

33.4.4.1 Differentiation of Dementias and Prediction of Amyloid and AD Tau Pathology

FDG PET offers an alternate biomarker for the "N" in A/T/N, and brings unique value by reflecting functional change that occurs prior to and with tissue loss, as well as downstream effects of changes in tau pathology that do not affect all patients in the

same way. The different patterns of regional hypometabolism associated with AD and other dementias make FDG PET a useful approach to detect and differentiate these diseases [68]. Multivariate classifiers that take into account relationships between regions have provided increased accuracy, enabling differentiation of AD, FTD, Lewy body disease, vascular disease, and variants of AD and FTD [69]. In participants of a clinical trial of rasagiline, tau PET findings were consistent with the presence of an AD-like pattern determined using an FDG PET dementia differentiation classifier [70].

33.4.4.2 Stratification for Clinical Progression

Reductions in glucose metabolism measured by FDG PET are predictive of clinical worsening in preclinical, early and late prodromal, and dementia stages of AD. In ADNI data, FDG showed the greatest effect size for predicting conversion from MCI to AD as well as worsening ADAS-cog scores compared to amyloid burden, entorhinal cortical thickness, hippocampal volume, CSF biomarkers, and other volumetric measures [71]. Using a pattern of hypometabolism and relative preservation derived from machine learning, FDG PET was also the most significant predictor of worsening in the Logical Memory Delayed score and conversion to a clinical diagnosis of MCI in amyloid-positive preclinical ADNI subjects as compared to baseline clinical scores, hippocampal volume, and standard region of interest FDG PET measures (ADNI data).

33.4.4.3 Detection of Disease-Modifying and Symptomatic Effects

Longitudinal glucose metabolism measurement can be used to detect treatment-related disease modification. Using a statistical (composite) region of interest developed by Chen et al., FDG PET is projected to require approximately 66 participants per arm to detect a 25% slowing of decline over 12 months (two-tailed $p < 0.05$, 80% power) in AD, or 217 participants per arm for MCI [72]. This demonstrates the importance of reference region and target region combinations, as these sample sizes are considerably lower than those projected using other SUVR approaches. Depending upon treatment-effect size, statistical power can be demonstrated with smaller groups. For example, in a 6 month study of the glutamate modulator riluzole in 42 AD patients (20 placebo, 22 riluzole), treatment-related mitigation of decline in FDG PET signal was observed in the posterior cingulate ($p <$ 0.001, 97% power) and temporoparietal regions ($p < 0.05$), as well as in an AD-like pattern of hypometabolism. FDG PET pattern scores correlated significantly with baseline ADAS-cog and with longitudinal changes in ADAS-cog [70]. Importantly, FDG detects functional changes that are independent of or occur prior to changes in tissue volume, enabling detection of treatment effects within 6–9-month proof-of-concept study timeframes.

FDG PET can also be used to measure symptomatic effects that may not involve disease modification. For example, in a 6-month study of the monoamine oxidase B inhibitor rasagiline in 50 mild-to-moderate AD patients, a significant treatment effect on FDG PET was observed in frontostriatal networks consistent with rasagiline's dopamine-preserving mechanism of action. Favorable effects on glucose metabolism were consistent with directional clinical outcomes. Baseline FDG PET, volumetric MRI, and tau PET thresholds were also identified beyond which clinical endpoint treatment effects could be best detected [70] (Figure 33.8). As another example, FDG PET showed favorable effects upon glucose metabolism associated with phenserine in AD patients, correlating with clinical benefit [73].

33.4.4.4 Additional Technical Considerations

Because FDG PET measures all neuronal activity, it reflects energy utilization associated with any physical, cognitive, or affective activity. In AD, the first 30–45 minutes during which tracer uptake occurs are typically spent in a dimly lit room, at rest but with eyes and ears open, and without audiovisual distraction. Patient compliance to this protocol is critical as the signal associated with activation exceeds the typically few percent change associated with disease-related decline and drug effect. If the patient is compliant in one scan but

cognitively challenged, physically active, or experiencing mood changes in the next scan, the change in FDG PET will reflect those changes rather than the drug effect.

33.4.5 Other PET Imaging Modalities

33.4.5.1 Inflammation

Inflammation has become a highly attractive target for discovery of AD therapeutics given its evident role in disease. Despite its importance, there is not currently an "I" for inflammation in the A/T/N schema due to several factors that have precluded having an established biomarker for it. These include a lack of consensus on a tracer, limitations of observation of differences to group rather than individual level, the need to perform full dynamic scans (rather than acquiring only late timeframes), no clear mechanism for multi-site imaging because of the lack of consensus on methods, difficulty in interpreting the data, and different findings in different stages of disease. To date, PET imaging has been applied to measure inflammation using tracers that bind to the translocator protein (TSPO), an outer-mitochondrial-membrane protein that is upregulated in neuroinflammation. This first of these, [^{11}C]PK-11195, is still in use but has a very low signal-to-noise ratio, due to factors including low brain penetration, high non-specific binding, and a lack of affinity for the polymorphism-induced A147 T subtype of TSPO. The lack of affinity may also be viewed as an advantage in certain cases. Several second-generation tracers including [^{18}F]PBR-28 have been developed but also bind with lower affinity to the A147 T TSPO. To address this, genotyping and classification of imaged participants as high-affinity binders (HABS), medium-affinity binders (MABS, heterozygous), or low-affinity binders (LABS, homozygous for A147 T TSPO) is used in order

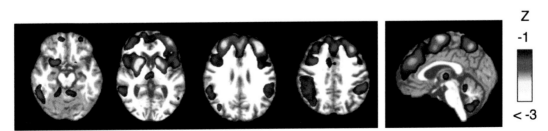

Figure 33.8 Effects of rasagiline upon cerebral glucose metabolism as compared to placebo in mild-to-moderate AD patients, measured using FDG PET. Voxels in which rasagiline-treated patients declined in glucose metabolism at a lesser rate than placebo-treated patients are shown in orange overlaid on a template MRI, illustrating rasagiline's frontostriatal effects.

to either include only HABS or to stratify groups for comparison. Third-generation tracers such as [^{18}F]GE-180 have improved binding to both types of TSPO, but blood–brain-barrier penetration has been low. A new derivative of PK-11195 that is less susceptible to low-affinity binding is also being tested. Interpretability of TSPO PET has some uncertainty due to the finding that TSPO can be present in activated astrocytes and endothelial cells, such that signal cannot be solely attributed to microglial activation. Given attention to these considerations and to the analysis approach used, TSPO PET with associated genotyping provides an endpoint for use in exploratory trials (see Kreisl et al. for a review [74]).

33.4.5.2 Other Targets

Other relevant PET tracers are in development. The tracer [^{18}F]AV-133, which is specific for the vesicular monoamine transporter 2, provides a measure of dopamine transporters when evaluated in the striatum as a potential indicator of Lewy body disease. The signal-to-noise level exceeds that of the single-photon emission computed tomography DATscan used to determine dopamine deficit, with a reduced uptake time compared to the 3–6 hours required for a DATscan. The tracer [^{11}C]UCB-J, which binds to synaptic vesicle glycoprotein 2A, has been developed as a measure of synaptic density [75]. Discovery efforts for tracers for alpha-synuclein and transactive response DNA-binding protein 43 kDa (TDP-43) are ongoing. TDP-43 is associated with frontotemporal dementia, AD, and hippocampal sclerosis, and has been found to accelerate the rate of hippocampal atrophy and memory decline beyond that due to other AD pathology [76]. PET imaging can be used to label an investigational compound to study kinetics and distribution.

33.4.6 Practical Implementation of PET in Clinical Trials

Successful implementation of PET in a clinical trial, as with MRI, involves collaboration between the clinical trialist and an imaging CRO, with input or published findings from academic researchers. The implementation steps that were described for MRI are also involved in PET, with additional factors mentioned here. First, the modalities and tracers must be selected. Thresholds for study inclusion and/or for analysis stratification need

to be selected. A series of measurement decisions must also be made, often by the imaging CRO but with agreement by the study sponsor. These include whether a region of interest, pattern-based, or other voxel-based approach will be used for measurement, how to define the boundaries for any regions of interest, whether to combine region of interest values using a simple average or a volume-weighted average, whether to use template space (all brains spatially warped into the same anatomical map) or native space, whether or not to correct for partial volume effects associated with scanner resolution and tissue atrophy, and whether or not to smooth the image. An imaging charter, PET manual, and source documents need to be developed, along with the imaging portion of the statistical analysis plan. As with MRI, site qualification involves an assessment of equipment, staff, and procedures, and a review of phantom scans. In PET AD clinical trials, a Hoffman phantom that replicates brain anatomy has often been used to demonstrate white/gray contrast and scanner resolution. However, this can be difficult to fill with the radioactive solution used for the scan, and does not capture all issues. Evaluation of other phantoms and a healthy volunteer are therefore desirable. During the trial, inspection of headers, protocol implementation, visual image, and subject motion must be performed, and appropriate analyses conducted.

33.5 Regulatory Guidance Related to Imaging

The FDA and EMA have both expressed recognition of the shift in diagnostic criteria to a clinical–biological paradigm, and the value of imaging and other biomarkers to drug development. The FDA draft guidance document "Early Alzheimer's disease: developing drugs for treatment" [77] and the EMA "Clinical investigation of medicines for the treatment of Alzheimer's disease" [78] provide their perspectives. The FDA guidance supports the use of biomarkers (including imaging) to inform diagnosis for patient inclusion, clinical trial enrichment, and pre-specified stratification in all clinical trial phases. For "Stage 1" preclinical patients, given that clinical decline is not readily observed, the use of biomarkers as endpoints to demonstrate slowing of disease is supported as a path to accelerated approval, with the caveat that a clinical study would follow. For "Stage 2," where clinical decline is observable, clinical endpoints are required for pivotal trials. However, the guidance expresses support for biomarkers in early trials to establish endpoints and sample sizes required. Imaging biomarkers that correlate with clinical endpoints, such as FDG PET and MRI, can offer particular benefit.

33.6 Imaging in Context with CSF and Plasma Biomarkers

CSF assays, and more recently plasma assays, have become capable of measuring abnormal amyloid as well as multiple isotopes of phosphorylated tau [5]. Plasma assays in particular can reduce the patient burden and potential cost and are likely to become a method of choice to screen for disease pathology. In this case, imaging can be focused on those applications in which it provides unique information. The first of these is by quantifying the functional effects of disease and treatment-related modification that correspond with the clinical benefit required for drug approval. Functional and volumetric imaging have also shown greater statistical power than fluid biomarkers in predicting subsequent clinical decline [71]. Imaging is required to obtain spatial distribution information regarding aggregated tau, atrophy, and functional loss that correspond to clinical phenotype. It is also essential to directly quantify insoluble target engagement and impact. Imaging will continue to be necessary as part of screening and safety monitoring to rule out confounds and adverse events that are not characterized by abnormal proteins. Combinations of fluid and imaging biomarkers can enable well-characterized, interpretable clinical trials with controlled patient burden and cost.

33.7 Summary

The costs of conducting failed large-scale trials in variable patient populations without proof of target engagement or a well-defined relationship between biology and clinical effect have been immense. Imaging, though an added cost to study design, can aid greatly in the successful implementation and value obtained from clinical trials. Exploratory proof-of-concept studies can reasonably include multiple imaging biomarkers in order to establish effect sizes and needed sample sizes. By identifying affected brain networks, appropriate clinical endpoints can be selected. Imaging characterization of subjects in which treatment effects are observable can also guide patient selection or stratification for treatment-effect detection in larger populations. In conjunction with advances in fluid and other biomarkers, imaging can provide unique, clinically relevant insights to the functional, neurodegenerative, and target-engagement aspects of AD and therapeutic intervention, supporting clinical trial success.

References

1. Khachaturian ZS. Revised criteria for diagnosis of Alzheimer's disease: National Institute on Aging–Alzheimer's Association diagnostic guidelines for Alzheimer's disease. *Alzheimers Dement* 2011; 7: 253–6.

2. Jack CR Jr., Bennett DA, Blennow K, et al. A/T/N: an unbiased descriptive classification scheme for Alzheimer disease biomarkers. *Neurology* 2016; **87**: 539–47.

3. Magistretti PJ, Pellerin L. Cellular mechanisms of brain energy metabolism and their relevance to functional brain imaging. *Philos Trans R Soc Lond B Biol Sci* 1999; **354**: 1155–63.

4. Minter MR, Taylor JM, Crack PJ. The contribution of neuroinflammation to amyloid toxicity in Alzheimer's disease. *J Neurochem* 2016; **136**: 457–74.

5. Janelidze S, Mattsson N, Palmqvist S, et al. Plasma p-tau$_{181}$ in Alzheimer's disease: relationship to other biomarkers, differential diagnosis, neuropathology and longitudinal progression to Alzheimer's dementia. *Nat Med* 2020; **26**: 379–86.

6. Rogers MB. Tau PET scans turn positive when amyloid does; symptoms follow. AlzForum series: Clinical Trials on Alzheimer's Disease 2019, Part 8 of 9. January, 2020. Available at: www.alzforum.org/news/conference-coverage/tau-pet-scans-turn-positive-when-amyloid-does-symptoms-follow (accessed November 15, 2020).

7. Palmqvist S, Schöll M, Strandberg O, et al. Earliest accumulation of β-amyloid occurs within the default-mode network and concurrently affects brain connectivity. *Nat Comm* 2017; **8**: 1214.

8. Ossenkoppele R, Schonhaut DR, Schöll M, et al. Tau PET patterns mirror clinical and neuroanatomical variability in Alzheimer's disease. *Brain* 2016; **139**: 1551–67.

9. Koychev I, Gunn RN, Firouzian A, et al. PET tau and amyloid-β burden in mild Alzheimer's disease: divergent relationship with age, cognition, and cerebrospinal fluid biomarkers. *J Alzheimers Dis* 2017; **60**: 283–93.

10. Guerrero-Muñoz MJ, Gerson J, Castillo-Carranza DL. Tau oligomers: the toxic player at synapses in Alzheimer's disease. *Front Cell Neurosci* 2015; **9**: 464.

11. Vargas LM, Cerpa W, Muñoz FJ, Zanlungo S, Alvarez AR. Amyloid-β oligomers synaptotoxicity: the emerging role of EphA4/c-Abl signaling in Alzheimer's disease. *Biochim Biophys Acta Mol Basis Dis* 2018; **1864A**: 1148–59.

12. Insel PS, Ossenkoppele R, Gessert D, et al. Time to amyloid positivity and preclinical changes in brain metabolism, atrophy, and cognition: evidence for emerging amyloid pathology in Alzheimer's disease. *Front Neurosci* 2017; **11**: 281.

13. La Joie R, Visani AV, Baker SL, et al. Prospective longitudinal atrophy in Alzheimer's disease correlates with the intensity and topography of baseline tau-PET. *Sci Transl Med* 2020; **12**: eaau5732.

14. Timmers T, Ossenkoppele R, Wolters EE, et al. Associations between quantitative [^{18}F] flortaucipir tau PET and atrophy across the Alzheimer's disease spectrum. *Alzheimers Res Ther* 2019; **11**: 60.

15. Salloway S, Sperling R, Fox NC, et al. Two phase 3 trials of bapineuzumab in mild-to-moderate Alzheimer's disease. *N Engl J Med* 2014; **370**: 322–33.

16. Weintraub S, Carrillo MC, Farias ST, et al. Measuring cognition and function in the preclinical stage of Alzheimer's disease. *Alzheimers Dement (N Y)* 2018; **4**: 64–75.

17. Fazekas F, Chawluk JB, Alavi A, et al. MR signal abnormalities at 1.5 T in Alzheimer's dementia and normal aging. *AJR Am J Roentgenol* 1987; **149**: 351–6.

18 Mirza SS, Saeed U, Knight J, et al. *APOE* ε4, white matter hyperintensities, and cognition in Alzheimer and Lewy body dementia. *Neurology* 2019; **93**: e1807–19.

19. Orgogozo JM, Gilman S, Dartigues JF. Subacute meningoencephalitis in a subset of patients with AD after Abeta42 immunization. *Neurology* 2003; **61**: 46–54.

20. Sperling RA, Jack CR Jr., Black SE, et al. Amyloid-related imaging abnormalities in amyloid-modifying therapeutic trials: recommendations from the Alzheimer's Association Research Roundtable Workgroup. *Alzheimers Dement* 2011; **7**: 367–85.

21. Greenberg SM, Vernooij MW, Cordonnier C, et al. Cerebral microbleeds: a guide to detection and interpretation. *Lancet Neurol* 2009; **8**: 165–74.

22. Tolar M, Abushakra S, Hey JA, Porsteinsson A, Sabbagh M. Aducanumab, gantenerumab, BAN2401, and ALZ-801-the first wave of amyloid-targeting drugs for Alzheimer's disease with potential for near term approval. *Alzheimers Res Ther* 2020; **12**: 95.

23. Wu J, Dong Q, Gui J, et al. Predicting brain amyloid using multivariate morphometry statistics, sparse coding, and correntropy: validation in 1,125 individuals from the ADNI and OASIS database. *bioRxiv* 2020;DOI: http://doi.org/10.1101/2020.10.16.343137.

24. Lukic AS, Andrews RD, Bourakova V, et al. MRI, FDG, and early frame amyloid image classifiers to characterize and differentiate Alzheimer's disease variants and non-AD dementias. *Alzheimers Dement* 2018; **14**: P1429–30.

25. Davatzikos C, Resnick SM, Wu X, Parmpi P, Clark CM. Individual patient diagnosis of AD and FTD via high-dimensional pattern classification of MRI. *Neuroimage* 2008; **41**: 1220–7.

26. Giorgio J, Jagust WJ, Baker S, et al. Predicting future regional tau accumulation in asymptomatic and early Alzheimer's disease. *bioRxiv* 2020;DOI: http://doi.org/10.1101/2020.08.15.252601.

27. Yu P, Sun J, Wolz R, et al. Operationalizing hippocampal volume as an enrichment biomarker for amnestic mild cognitive impairment trials: effect of algorithm, test-retest variability, and cut point on trial cost, duration, and sample size. *Neurobiol Aging* 2014; **35**: 808–18.

28. Rabin JS, Neal TE, Nierle HE, et al. Multiple markers contribute to risk of progression from normal to mild cognitive impairment. *Neuroimage Clin* 2020; **28**: 102400.

29. Woodard JL, Bellaali Y, Dricot L, et al. Multivariate prediction of rate of decline in memory functioning over six years using imaging biomarkers. *Alzheimers Dement* 2020; **16**: e045645.

30. Leung KK, Barnes J, Ridgway GR, et al. Alzheimer's Disease Neuroimaging Initiative. Automated cross-sectional and longitudinal hippocampal volume measurement in mild cognitive impairment and Alzheimer's disease. *Neuroimage* 2010; **51**: 1345–59.

31. Hashimoto M, Kazui H, Matsumoto K, et al. Does donepezil treatment slow the progression of hippocampal atrophy in patients with Alzheimer's disease? *Am J Psychiatry* 2005; **162**: 676–82.

32. Turner RS, Hebron ML, Lawler A, et al. Nilotinib effects on safety, tolerability, and biomarkers in Alzheimer's disease. *Ann Neurol* 2020; **88**: 183–94.

33. Gauthier S, Aisen PS, Ferris SH. Effect of tramiprosate in patients with mild-to-moderate Alzheimer's disease: exploratory analyses of the MRI sub-group of the Alphase study. *J Nutr Health Aging* 2009; **13**: 550–7.

34. Wessels AM, Tariot PN, Zimmer, JA, et al. Efficacy and safety of lanabecestat for treatment of early and mild Alzheimer disease: the AMARANTH

and DAYBREAK-ALZ randomized clinical trials. *JAMA Neurol* 2020; **77**: 199–209.

35. Novak G, Fox N, Clegg S, et al. Changes in brain volume with bapineuzumab in mild to moderate Alzheimer's disease. *J Alzheimers Dis* 2016; **49**: 1123–34.

36. Fox NC, Black RS, Gilman S, et al. Effects of Abeta immunization (AN1792) on MRI measures of cerebral volume in Alzheimer disease. *Neurology* 2005; **64**: 1563–72.

37. Cheriyan J, Kim S, Wolansky LJ, Cook SD, Cadavid D. Impact of inflammation on brain volume in multiple sclerosis. *Arch Neurol* 2012; **69**: 82–8.

38. Reuter M, Schmansky NJ, Rosas HD, Fischl B. Within-subject template estimation for unbiased longitudinal image analysis. *Neuroimage* 2012; **61**: 1402–18.

39. Iglesias JE, Van Leemput K, Augustinack J, et al. Bayesian longitudinal segmentation of hippocampal substructures in brain MRI using subject-specific atlases. *Neuroimage* 2016; **141**: 542–55.

40. Teipel SJ, Kuper-Smith JO, Bartels C, et al. Multicenter tract-based analysis of microstructural lesions within the Alzheimer's disease spectrum: association with amyloid pathology and diagnostic usefulness. *J Alzheimers Dis* 2019; **72**: 455–65.

41. Elahi FM, Marx G, Cobigo Y, et al. Longitudinal white matter change in frontotemporal dementia subtypes and sporadic late onset Alzheimer's disease. *Neuroimage Clin* 2017; **16**: 595–603.

42. Pasternak O, Sochen N, Gur Y, Intrator N, Assaf Y. Free water elimination and mapping from diffusion MRI. *Magn Reson Med* 2009; **62**: 717–30.

43. Hoy AR, Ly M, Carlsson CM, et al. Microstructural white matter alterations in preclinical Alzheimer's disease detected using free water elimination diffusion tensor imaging. *PloS One* 2017; **12**: e0173982.

44. Binnewijzend MA, Kuijer JP, van der Flier WM, et al. Distinct perfusion patterns in Alzheimer's disease, frontotemporal dementia and dementia with Lewy bodies. *Eur Radiol* 2014; **24**: 2326–33.

45. Dukart J, Holiga Š, Chatham C, et al. Cerebral blood flow predicts differential neurotransmitter activity. *Sci Rep* 2018; **8**: 4074.

46. Guo H, Grajauskas L, Habash B, D'Arc RC, Song X. Functional MRI technologies in the study of medication treatment effect on Alzheimer's disease. *Aging Med (Milton)* 2018; **1**: 75–95.

47. Zhang N, Gordon ML, Goldberg TE. Cerebral blood flow measured by arterial spin labeling MRI at resting state in normal aging and Alzheimer's disease. *Neurosci Biobehav Rev* 2017; **72**: 168–75.

48. Smith LA, Melbourne A, Owen D, et al. Cortical cerebral blood flow in ageing: effects of haematocrit, sex, ethnicity and diabetes. *Eur Radiol* 2019; **29**: 5549–58.

49. Greicius MD, Srivastava G, Reiss AL, Menon V. Default-mode network activity distinguishes Alzheimer's disease from healthy aging: evidence from functional MRI. *Proc Natl Acad Sci USA* 2004; **101**: 4637–42.

50. Churchill NW, Spring R, Afshin-Pour B, Dong F, Strother SC. An automated, adaptive framework for optimizing preprocessing pipelines in task-based functional MRI. *PLoS One* 2015; **10**: e0131520.

51. Matthews DC, Mao X, Dowd K, et al. Riluzole, a glutamate modulator, slows cerebral glucose metabolism decline in patients with Alzheimer's disease: a pilot multimodal neuroimaging study. *Brain* 2021; Jun 18: awab222.

52. Maul S, Giegling I, Rujescu D. Proton magnetic resonance spectroscopy in common dementias: current status and perspectives. *Front Psychiatry* 2020; **11**: 769.

53. van Berckel BN, Ossenkoppele R, Tolboom N, et al. Longitudinal amyloid imaging using ¹¹C-PiB: methodologic considerations. *J Nucl Med* 2013; **54**: 1570–6.

54. Sevigny J, Chiao P, Bussière T, et al. The antibody aducanumab reduces Aβ plaques in Alzheimer's disease. *Nature* 2016; **537**: 50–6.

55. Ostrowitzki S, Lasser RA, Dorflinger E, et al. A Phase III randomized trial of gantenerumab in prodromal Alzheimer's disease. *Alzheimers Res Ther* 2017; **9**: 95.

56. Schmidt ME, Matthews DC, Andrews RD, Mosconi L. Positron emission tomography in Alzheimer disease: diagnosis and use as biomarker endpoints. In *Translational Neuroimaging*, McArthur RA (ed.). New York: Academic Press; 2013: 131–74.

57. Klunk WE, Koeppe RA, Price JC. The Centiloid project: standardizing quantitative amyloid plaque estimation by PET. *Alzheimers Dement* 2015; **11**: 1–15.e154.

58. Chen K, Roontiva A, Thiyyagura P, et al. Alzheimer's Disease Neuroimaging Initiative. Improved power for characterizing longitudinal amyloid-β PET changes and evaluating amyloid-modifying treatments with a cerebral white matter reference region. *J Nucl Med* 2015; **56**: 560–6.

59. Schmidt ME, Chiao P, Klein G, et al. The influence of biological and technical factors on quantitative analysis of amyloid PET: points to consider and

393

recommendations for controlling variability in longitudinal data. *Alzheimers Dement* 2015; **11**: 1050–68.

60. Rostomian AH, Madison C, Rabinovici GD, Jagust WJ. Early ^{11}C-PIB frames and ^{18}F-FDG PET measures are comparable: a study validated in a cohort of AD and FTLD patients. *J Nucl Med* 2011; **52**: 173–9.

61. Brendel M, Barthel H, van Eimeren T, et al. Assessment of ^{18}F-PI-2620 as a biomarker in progressive supranuclear palsy. *JAMA Neurol* 2020; **77**: 1408–19.

62 Tagai K, Ono M, Kubota M, et al. High-contrast in vivo imaging of tau pathologies in Alzheimer's and non-Alzheimer's disease tauopathies. *Neuron* 2020; **109**: 42–58;DOI: http://doi.org/10.1016/j.neuron.2020.09.042.

63. Betthauser TJ, Cody KA, Zammit MD, et al. In vivo characterization and quantification of neurofibrillary tau PET radioligand ^{18}F-MK-6240 in humans from Alzheimer disease dementia to young controls. *J Nucl Med* 2019; **60**: 93–9.

64. Maass A, Landau S, Baker SL, Alzheimer's Disease Neuroimaging Initiative. Comparison of multiple tau-PET measures as biomarkers in aging and Alzheimer's disease.*Neuroimage* 2017; **157**: 448–63.

65. Baker SL, Maass A, Jagust WJ. Considerations and code for partial volume correcting [^{18}F]-AV-1451 tau PET data. *Data Brief* 2017; **15**: 648–57;DOI: http://doi.org/10.1016/j.dib.2017.10.024.

66. Southekal S, Devous MD Sr., Kennedy I, et al. Flortaucipir F 18 quantitation using parametric estimation of reference signal intensity. *J Nucl Med* 2018; **59**: 944–51.

67. Beyer L, Nitschmann A, Barthel H, et al. Early-phase [^{18}F]PI-2620 tau-PET imaging as a surrogate marker of neuronal injury. *Eur J Nucl Med Mol Imaging* 2020; **47**: 2911–22.

68. Foster NL, Heidebrink JL, Clark CM, et al. FDG-PET improves accuracy in distinguishing frontotemporal dementia and Alzheimer's disease. *Brain* 2007; **130**: 2616–35.

69. Xia Y, Lu S, Wen L, et al. Automated identification of dementia using FDG-PET imaging. *Biomed Res Int* 2014; **2014**: 421743.

70. Matthews DC, Ritter A, Thomas RG, et al. Rasagiline effects on glucose metabolism, cognition, and tau in Alzheimer's dementia. *Alzheimers Dement (N Y)* 2021; 7: e12106.

71. Beckett L, Harvey D, Donohue M, et al. Biostatistics Core ADNI 2 summary and ADNI 3 plans. Available at https://slideplayer.com/slide/12666696/ (accessed November 20, 2020).

72. Chen K, Langbaum JB, Fleisher AS, et al. Alzheimer's Disease Neuroimaging Initiative. Twelve-month metabolic declines in probable Alzheimer's disease and amnestic mild cognitive impairment assessed using an empirically pre-defined statistical region-of-interest: findings from the Alzheimer's Disease Neuroimaging Initiative. *Neuroimage* 2010; **51**: 654–64.

73. Kadir A, Andreasen N, Almkvist O, et al. Effect of phenserine treatment on brain functional activity and amyloid in Alzheimer's disease. *Ann Neurol* 2008; **63**: 621–31.

74. Kreisl WC, Kim MJ, Coughlin JM, et al. PET imaging of neuroinflammation in neurological disorders. *Lancet Neurol* 2020; **19**: 940–50.

75. Mecca AP, Chen MK, O'Dell RS, et al. In vivo measurement of widespread synaptic loss in Alzheimer's disease with SV2A PET. *Alzheimers Dement* 2020; **16**: 974–82.

76. Josephs KA, Dickson DW, Tosakulwong N, et al. Rates of hippocampal atrophy and presence of post-mortem TDP-43 in patients with Alzheimer's disease: a longitudinal retrospective study. *Lancet Neurol* 2017; **16**: 917–24.

77. US Department of Health and Human Services, Food and Drug Administration, Center for Drug Evaluation and Research (CDER), and Center for Biologics Evaluation and Research (CBER). Early Alzheimer's disease: developing drugs for treatment. Guidelines for industry. Available at: www.fda.gov/downloads/Drugs/GuidanceComplianceRegulatoryInformation/Guidances/UCM596728.pdf (accessed November 15, 2020).

78. European Medicines Agency. Clinical investigation of medicines for the treatment of Alzheimer's disease/ CPMP/EWP/553/1995. Available at: www.ema.europa.eu/en/documents/scientific-guideline/guideline-clinical-investigation-medicines-treatment-alzheimers-disease-revision-2_en.pdf (accessed November 20, 2020).

Chapter 34

Sharing of Alzheimer's Disease Research Data in the Global Alzheimer's Association Interactive Network

Cally Xiao, Scott C. Neu, and Arthur W. Toga

34.1 Introduction

Data sharing is becoming more common in scientific research, providing transparency, aiding reproducibility, and promoting meta-analysis studies [1]. Meta-analyses aggregate existing data sets together in order to estimate an overall mean effect with higher accuracy, as well as to reach broad generalizations about different phenomena. Meta-analysis studies have become increasingly more prevalent and are essential to the progression of science by efficiently reusing primary studies, quantifying what is already known, and identifying the unknown [2].

Alzheimer's disease (AD) is prevalent worldwide and its incidence over the coming decades is expected to increase along with aging populations and advances in medicine that prolong life [3]. Thus, it is ever more important and urgent to determine the causes of and find therapeutic options for AD. Recent technological advances in imaging, biomarkers, proteomics, and genetics have contributed significant amounts of AD research data [4, 5]. However, these advancements along with individual studies from isolated institutions present only a fraction of the story, calling for a need to unite separate efforts into a central hub to manage data on AD and dementia. The Global Alzheimer's Association Interactive Network (GAAIN) was established in 2015 to address this need and to build a global virtual community for sharing AD and dementia research data [6].

34.2 GAAIN Overview

34.2.1 Background

The first of its kind, GAAIN (www.gaain.org) is a federated network connecting independently operated AD and dementia-related data repositories from around the world. GAAIN is a collaboration between the Alzheimer's Association and the Laboratory of Neuro Imaging (LONI) at the University of Southern California. Half a decade after its inception, the GAAIN platform has achieved much coverage worldwide, linking together over 50 data partners from 17 different countries into a network consisting of over 500,000 subjects and over 30,000 data attributes.

The GAAIN platform offers flexibility to accommodate new and updated data sets and is highly sensitive to data ownership and privacy concerns. At the time of writing, GAAIN features 54 data partners and is currently onboarding more than 50 additional studies that are in various stages of recruitment. Data partners always retain full ownership of their data and have the freedom to choose the data attributes they would like to link to the network. Data-access processes remain unchanged in GAAIN and researchers can only access entire data sets through the data partners themselves.

34.2.2 Tools

The flagship tool of the GAAIN platform is the GAAIN Interrogator, which allows for cohort discovery, data-set aggregation, data visualization, and preliminary data analysis [7]. Over 1,400 researchers have registered to use the GAAIN Interrogator. Researchers can choose one or more data sets, define their own variables, and create custom cohorts. Analysis results include odds ratios from logistic regressions, correlations from linear regressions, survival fractions from Cox regressions, and in the case of pooled data sets, weighted odds ratios from Mantel–Haenszel meta-analyses.

The Cohort Scout, another tool available in GAAIN, is an interactive interface for cohort building and sharing that does not require a registered account. Researchers can quickly search across all data sets for attributes and then visualize trends within individual attributes. After constructing a cohort based on attributes of interest, the cohort can be saved and referenced under a permanent URL that can be shared and returned to at any time.

GAAIN tools are free for all researchers and data partners can also freely share their data with the scientific community through GAAIN.

34.2.3   Protecting Privacy

GAAIN provides a resource for researchers to discover and explore studies to use in secondary analyses while protecting the data ownership concerns of its data partners.

In order to use the GAAIN Interrogator, researchers must first agree to the terms of use that state that they will not use analysis results from the Interrogator for publication purposes and that they will establish formal collaborations with data partners of interest before publishing results. As an incentive to further protect data partners, the analysis methods used by the Interrogator and the underlying analytical models are not made publicly available.

Data partners are required to remove any type of information that could potentially be used to identify subjects from collected data sets before linking to the GAAIN platform. Scatterplots are not used by the GAAIN Interrogator to prevent the identification of outliers, and cohorts cannot be created with five or less subjects to protect subject identity.

34.3   GAAIN Data-Sharing Platform

34.3.1   Architecture

Many studies are required by their funding agencies to share their results and some already have data-application protocols in place to grant access to authorized researchers. However, data sharing by individual organizations may be technologically and labor intensive. GAAIN aims to address these needs of our data partners by simplifying the data linking process. After a formal agreement between LONI and the data partner is established, the data partner first exports the data they wish to share into one or more comma-separated values (CSV) files, which are then loaded into a data partner client (DPC) that links to GAAIN.

The DPC is a lightweight Java executable file, which is individually modified for each data partner based upon sampled rows of their data set and

a data dictionary. Using the data dictionary, data attributes are mapped in their native schema to GAAIN. This way, data partners may follow any naming conventions for their attributes and values. Once prepared, each data partner downloads its DPC and then loads its CSV files into it, which also contain a web-based administration page to control their on-/offline status. When online, the DPC communicates with the GAAIN central servers as researchers make queries using GAAIN tools (Figure 34.1). As a policy, the partner data set is never written to disk anywhere outside of the partner's institution. The DPC is designed to not interfere with local production systems and partners may periodically update their linked data by loading updated data sets. Data partners can request that LONI host their DPCs, in which case their data sets are securely stored at LONI while they retain full data-access control.

34.3.2   Data Partners

We currently have 54 data partners participating in GAAIN from 17 countries across North and South America, Europe, Asia, and Australia (Figure 34.2a). The majority (39) are longitudinal studies, with nine cross-sectional studies, four clinical trials, and two multi-project repositories (Figure 34.2b).

Data partners can share as many attributes as they wish with researchers who use GAAIN tools, provided the data can be stored in a spreadsheet following certain rules. Attributes in GAAIN generally fall into the following categories: demographic (age, sex, marital status, etc.), cognitive (Mini-Mental State Examination [MMSE] scores, global Clinical Dementia Rating [CDR] scores, Trails A and B, etc.), diagnosis (clinical diagnosis of AD, mild cognitive impairment [MCI], or other pathologies), genetic (apolipoprotein-E ε4 [APOE-4] genotype, various single nucleotide polymorphisms [SNPs]), imaging-derived (hippocampal volume from MRI scans, amyloid status based on positron emission tomography [PET] scans, etc.), lifestyle (living situation, whether or not the subject exercises, smokes, etc.), family history (whether a parent or sibling has been diagnosed with dementia), medical history (whether the subject takes any medication, has hypertension, diabetes, etc.), and laboratory (blood and cerebrospinal fluid [CSF] tests for biomarkers and health indicators). Figure 34.2c depicts the breadth and depth of data available in GAAIN.

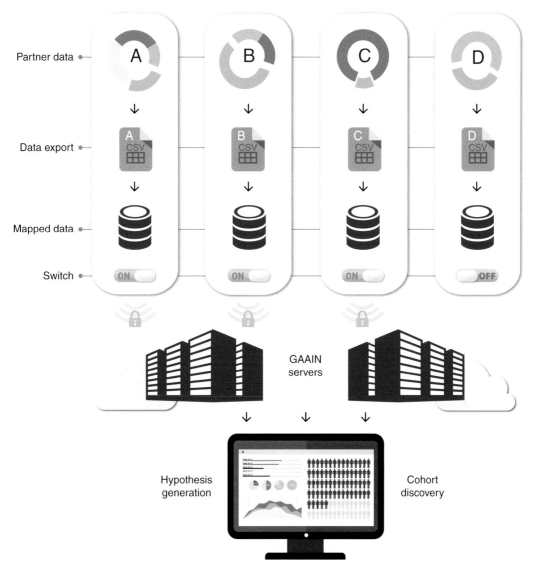

Partner data

Data export

Mapped data

Switch

GAAIN
servers

Hypothesis
generation

Cohort
discovery

Figure 34.1 GAAIN architecture workflow. Individual data partners prepare their data set for export into a CSV file. The GAAIN team maps the data and prepares a DPC for each data partner. Data partners then load their CSV files into the DPC and control their on-/offline status. When online, the DPC communicates with the GAAIN servers to facilitate hypothesis generation and cohort discovery. Image designed by and used with permission from Caroline O'Driscoll.

34.3.3   Clinical Trials in GAAIN

As mentioned previously, there are currently four clinical trials linked to the GAAIN platform. The Comprehensive Assessment of Long-term Effects of Reducing Intake of Energy (CALERIE) is a clinical trial that compared a test group of participants who followed a diet with 25% fewer calories for 2 years to a control group of participants who sustained their normal diets, and found that the caloric restriction group improved on multiple cardiometabolic risk factors including hypertension and hypercholesterolemia [8]. This finding is significant for the AD research community because hypertension and hypercholesterolemia are both risk factors for developing AD [9]. The three other clinical trials in GAAIN examined the safety and efficacy of monoclonal anti-amyloid antibodies: crenezumab, solanezumab, and gantenerumab [10]. The Alzheimer's Prevention Initiative (API) Colombia trial recruited nondemented individuals with high genetic risk for developing AD to test the safety and efficacy of

397

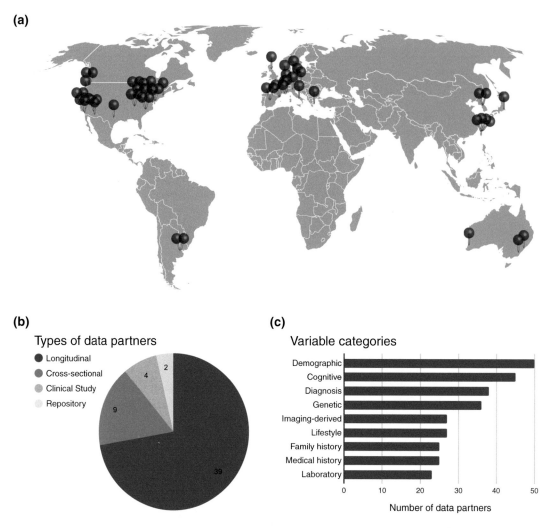

Figure 34.2 Overview of GAAIN data partners. (a) Pinned locations of GAAIN data partners. (b) Types of data sets provided by GAAIN data partners. (c) Categories of attributes available for analysis in the GAAIN Interrogator along with the number of data partners providing attributes in each category.

crenezumab in preventing AD symptoms [11]. The study is projected to finish by 2022. The multi-center Dominantly Inherited Alzheimer's Network Trials Unit (DIAN-TU) study, which also tested solanezumab and gantenerumab in participants at high genetic risk of developing AD, has recently been completed [12]. The Anti-Amyloid Treatment in Asymptomatic Alzheimer's Disease (A4) study is examining the effects of solanezumab on slowing the progression of memory problems in clinically normal older individuals with high amyloid brain burden, and is ongoing until 2023 [13]. The API and DIAN-TU studies have preliminarily shared baseline demographic data with GAAIN, and the A4 study has shared more extensive baseline data. Once the studies are ready to share their final trial

results, we have mechanisms in place to readily allow them to update their data sets.

34.3.4 Analyses

In the GAAIN Interrogator, researchers can analyze both individual and pooled data sets. Before analyzing pooled data sets, researchers first search for attributes of interest using key words in the top right of the Interrogator interface.

Pooling together multiple data sets for analysis in the GAAIN Interrogator involves the following steps: (1) new categorical or binary variables are defined (Figure 34.3a) and attributes from data sets are mapped to the newly defined variables, (2) cohorts are created from pooled variables (Figure 34.3b), and (3) the cohorts and variables are

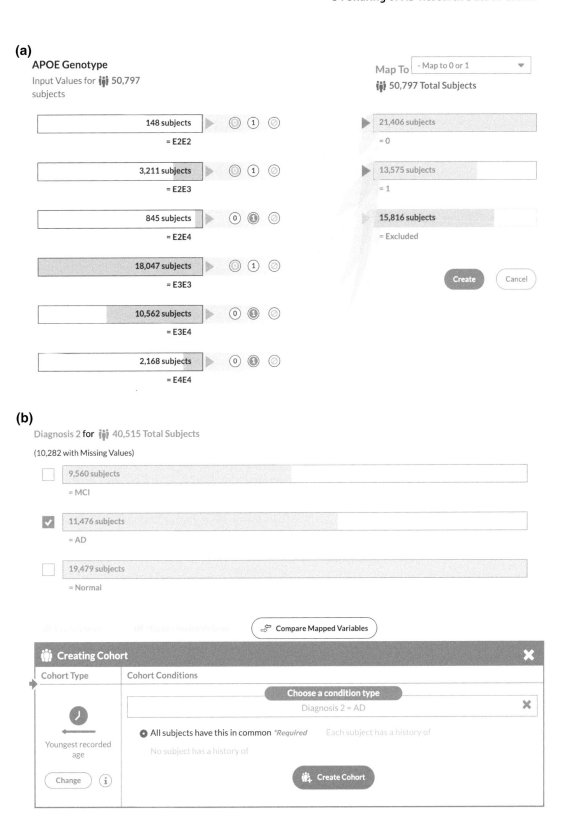

Figure 34.3 Pooling data in the GAAIN Interrogator. (a) Attributes of interest are mapped to categorial or binary variables. (b) Cohorts are created from one or more variables.

used in analyses. When constructing analyses with individual data sets, researchers can define new variables as well as directly use the attributes provided by the data partner.

34.3.4.1 Logistic Regression

In a logistic-regression example, we can see that having one or two copies of the *APOE-4* allele, a history of hypertension, and stroke are all risk factors for developing a case outcome, which is defined here as either MCI or AD (Figure 34.4a). However, the risks differ between Hispanic subjects and non-Hispanic White (NHW) subjects.

Combining studies from the Alzheimer's Disease Neuroimaging Initiative (ADNI) and the National Alzheimer's Coordinating Center (NACC), including over 22,000 NHW subjects and over 2,000 Hispanic subjects, we see that having the *APOE-4* allele or a prior stroke contribute to a case outcome more for NHW subjects than for Hispanic subjects, but having a history of hypertension contributes to a case outcome more for Hispanic subjects than for NHW subjects. The difference in case outcome risk between NHW subjects and Hispanic subjects with the *APOE-4* allele is statistically significant, and has been previously reported [14], and may

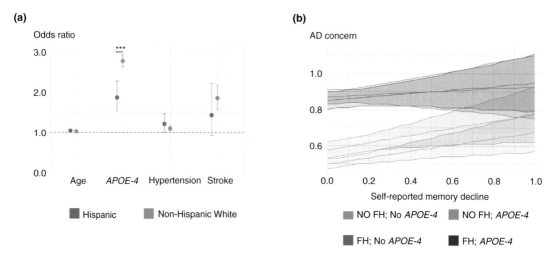

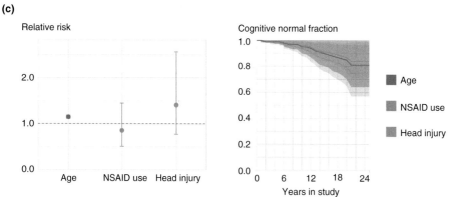

Figure 34.4 Analyzing trends in the GAAIN Interrogator. (a) Logistic regression depicting the odds ratios of age, presence of the *APOE-4* allele, hypertension, and stroke contributing to a case outcome (MCI or AD), comparing Hispanic and non-Hispanic White (NHW) populations. This analysis includes more than 22,000 NHW subjects and more than 2,000 Hispanic subjects pooled from NACC and ADNI studies. The difference of odds ratios for the *APOE-4* allele between the two populations is statistically significant ($p \leq 0.001$). (b) Linear regression depicting the correlation between self-reported memory decline and concern for developing AD in nearly 2,500 subjects from the A4 study. The subjects are further divided into groups with or without a family history (FH) of AD, and with or without the *APOE-4* allele. The self-reported memory decline and concern for developing AD attributes are converted into binary variables. (c) Cox regression depicting the relative risks and cognitive normal fraction of age, NSAID use, and prior head injury of more than 700 subjects pooled from CBAS and the APOE4 Gene Dose Program.

be explained by differences in amyloid burden between Hispanic and non-Hispanic *APOE-4* carriers [15].

34.3.4.2 Linear Regression

In a linear-regression example, including nearly 2,500 subjects from the A4 clinical trial, we see that self-reported memory problems over the past year are positively correlated with concerns for developing AD in those without a family history of AD, with or without the *APOE-4* allele, though the y-intercept is higher in those with *APOE-4* (Figure 34.4b). There is no correlation between self-reported memory problems and concern for developing AD in those with a family history of AD, with or without *APOE-4*, because the concern is already high. Here, the self-reported memory decline and concern for developing AD attributes are converted into binary variables to analyze the correlation.

34.3.4.3 Cox Regression

In a Cox-regression example, including more than 700 subjects from the Czech Brain Aging Study (CBAS) and the APOE4 Gene Dose Program, we see that current history of taking non-steroidal anti-inflammatory drugs (NSAIDs) slightly prevents cognitive decline over time, whereas having a history of head injury slightly contributes to cognitive decline. Here, cognitive decline was defined in the CBAS group as having MMSE scores decrease from above 25 to below 24 over the course of the study, and in the APOE4 Gene Dose Program, as clinician-diagnosed cognitive decline over the course of the study. Although not statistically significant, these trends follow those reported in the literature for NSAIDs [16] and head injury [17]. A closer look at the full data sets while using a consistent definition of cognitive decline would reveal more specific trends.

34.3.5 Applying for Data Access

After a researcher has used GAAIN tools to explore and gain insight into one or more data sets, the researcher may then apply for full access to the data sets. We have made this process easier for researchers by providing a direct link to the data partners' data application web pages with an "Apply" link displayed below each partner logo. In addition, each partner also has their own web page within GAAIN where researchers can find out

more information and email data partners through a contact form. We request that all publications resulting from data discovery using GAAIN to cite GAAIN in their acknowledgments section.

34.4 GAAIN Applications

34.4.1 Meta-Analysis Studies

Researchers who have used GAAIN for their meta-analysis studies were able to leverage and combine existing data to answer questions that would not be possible when analyzing one data set alone. For example, in a meta-analysis study using data sets discovered in GAAIN, researchers found that women with the *APOE-3/4* genotype had an increased risk of developing AD compared to men between 65 and 75 years of age but had similar risks overall between 55 and 85 years of age [18]. In another study, researchers used two data sets available in GAAIN to find that, surprisingly, alcohol use was associated with better cognitive performance, with the effect more prominent in the United States than in Taiwan [19]. Combining data sets also gives the advantage of pooling subjects with characteristics that have low prevalence in the population, such as those diagnosed with MCI plus suspected non-amyloid pathology (SNAP–MCI). Researchers examined MRI scans of SNAP–MCI subjects combined from four data sets in GAAIN and discovered that SNAP–MCI subjects had faster atrophy rates in the frontal cortex than MCI subjects, although there appeared to be no differences in cortical thickness between the two groups after correcting for site-related variations [20].

34.4.2 GAAIN Community

GAAIN plays an important role in the global effort to advance AD and dementia research. As many data partners have extensive imaging data from MRI, PET, and CT scans, imaging data attributes such as hippocampal volume from MRI scans and amyloid status from PET scans have been made available for exploration and analysis in GAAIN. Many GAAIN data partners also share raw and processed image files in the LONI Image and Data Archive (IDA; ida.loni.usc.edu), which is a global resource for storing and sharing imaging, clinical, bio-specimen, and genetic data for AD and other neurodegenerative diseases [21]. This cross representation of data between GAAIN and the IDA provides a cohesive link between preliminary data analysis and imaging file analysis for researchers as well as for greater visibility for data partners.

Some GAAIN data partners have themselves collected data across multiple institutions. For example, ADNI has standardized data-acquisition protocols for multiple sites across the United States [22] and now contributes more than 3,000 subjects to GAAIN. NACC maintains a national database of 29 studies across the United States [23] and contributes more than 42,000 subjects to GAAIN. Similarly, the French National Alzheimer Database (Banque Nationale Alzheimer; BNA) consolidates data from memory units and independent specialists across France and its overseas territories [24], which adds more than 200,000 subjects to GAAIN. By connecting multiple national collaborative projects such as ADNI, NACC, and BNA internationally, GAAIN provides a central hub for exploring data from AD and dementia studies from around the world.

GAAIN is funded by the Alzheimer's Association and participates in activities sponsored by the Alzheimer's Association, such as webinars and its annual Alzheimer's Association International Conference. Our growing presence on social media platforms has allowed us to onboard more data partners and attract new researchers to GAAIN.

34.5 Future Directions

GAAIN provides data analysis tools, enables pooling of data sets, and has brought together data from longitudinal studies, cross-sectional studies, and clinical trials. We plan to onboard many more data partners, especially from studies of under-represented groups in AD and dementia research. We are also constantly improving the GAAIN platform using feedback from researchers and data partners. Our vision for the future of GAAIN involves more widespread usage and awareness, where researchers interested in a particular question related to AD and dementia first look to GAAIN to explore trends in linked data sets, and then design meta-analysis studies and new clinical trials. We hope this will increase collaborations in the global community of researchers that are working toward effective treatments and preventative options for those suffering from AD and dementia.

References

1. Conrado DJ, Karlsson MO, Romero K, et al. Open innovation: towards sharing of data, models and workflows. *Eur J Pharm Sci* 2017; **109**: S65–71.

2. Gurevitch J, Koricheva J, Nakagawa S, et al. Meta-analysis and the science of research synthesis. *Nature* 2018; **555**: 175–82.

3. Alzheimer's Association. 2020 Alzheimer's disease facts and figures. *Alzheimers Dement* 2020; **16**: 391–460.

4. Villa C, Lavitrano M, Salvatore E, et al. Molecular and imaging biomarkers in Alzheimer's disease: a focus on recent insights. *J Pers Med* 2020; **10**: 1–32.

5. Sancesario GM, Bernardini S. Alzheimer's disease in the omics era. *Clin Biochem* 2018; **59**: 9–16.

6. Toga AW, Neu SC, Bhatt P, et al. The Global Alzheimer's Association Interactive Network. *Alzheimers Dement* 2016; **12**: 49–54.

7. Neu SC, Crawford KL, Toga AW. Sharing data in the global Alzheimer's Association Interactive Network. *Neuroimage* 2016; **124**: 1168–74.

8. Kraus WE, Bhapkar M, Huffman KM, et al. 2 years of calorie restriction and cardiometabolic risk (CALERIE): exploratory outcomes of a multicentre, Phase 2, randomised controlled trial. *Lancet Diabetes Endocrinol* 2019; **7**: 673–83.

9. Silva MVF, Loures CDMG, Alves LCV, et al. Alzheimer's disease: risk factors and potentially protective measures. *J Biomed Sci* 2019; **26**: 1–11.

10. Rygiel K. Novel strategies for Alzheimer's disease treatment: an overview of anti-amyloid beta monoclonal antibodies. *Indian J Pharmacol* 2016; **48**: 629–36.

11. Tariot PN, Lopera F, Langbaum JB, et al. The Alzheimer's Prevention Initiative Autosomal-Dominant Alzheimer's Disease Trial: a study of crenezumab versus placebo in preclinical *PSEN1 E280A* mutation carriers to evaluate efficacy and safety in the treatment of autosomal-dominant Alzheimer's disease. *Alzheimers Dement (N Y)* 2018; **4**: 150–60.

12. Mills SM, Mallmann J, Santacruz AM, et al. Preclinical trials in autosomal dominant AD: implementation of the DIAN-TU trial. *Rev Neurol* 2013; **169**: 737–43.

13. Sperling RA, Donohue MC, Raman R, et al. Association of factors with elevated amyloid burden in clinically normal older individuals. *JAMA Neurol* 2020; **77**: 735–45.

14. Tang MX, Stern Y, Marder K, et al. The *APOE-ε4* allele and the risk of Alzheimer disease among African Americans, whites, and Hispanics. *JAMA* 1998; **279**: 751–5.

15. Duara R, Loewenstein DA, Lizarraga G, et al. Effect of age, ethnicity, sex, cognitive status and *APOE* genotype on amyloid load and the threshold for amyloid positivity. *Neuroimage Clin* 2019; **22**: 101800.

16. O'Bryant SE, Zhang F, Johnson LA, et al. A precision medicine model for targeted NSAID therapy in Alzheimer's disease. *J Alzheimers Dis* 2018; **66**: 97–104.

17. Li Y, Li Y, Li X, et al. Head injury as a risk factor for dementia and Alzheimer's disease: a systematic review and meta-analysis of 32 observational studies. *PLoS One* 2017; **12**: e0169650.

18. Neu SC, Pa J, Kukull W, et al. Apolipoprotein E genotype and sex risk factors for Alzheimer disease: a meta-analysis. *JAMA Neurol* 2017; **74**: 1178–89.

19. Funk-White M, Moore AA, McEvoy LK, et al. Alcohol use patterns and cognitive impairment: a cross-country comparison. Alzheimer's Association International Conference, July 26–30, 2020.

20. Rane S. Detecting cortical signatures of suspected non-amyloid pathology using large harmonized datasets. Alzheimer's Association International Conference, July 26–30, 2020.

21. Crawford KL, Neu SC, Toga AW. The Image and Data Archive at the Laboratory of Neuro Imaging. *Neuroimage* 2016; **124**: 1080–3.

22. Weiner MW, Aisen PS, Jack CR, et al. The Alzheimer's Disease Neuroimaging Initiative: progress report and future plans. *Alzheimers Dement* 2010; **6**: 202–11.

23. Beekly DL, Ramos EM, van Belle G, et al. The National Alzheimer's Coordinating Center (NACC) Database: an Alzheimer disease database. *Alzheimer Dis Assoc Disord* 2004; **18**: 270–7.

24. Anthony S, Pradier C, Chevrier R, et al. The French national Alzheimer database: a fast growing database for researchers and clinicians. *Dement Geriatr Cogn Disord* 2014; **38**: 271–80.

Chapter 35

Pharmacogenetics in Alzheimer's Disease Drug Discovery and Personalized Treatment

Ramon Cacabelos

35.1 Introduction

Genomic defects, epigenetic aberrations, cerebrovascular dysfunction, and multiple environmental conditions are the major risk factors that precipitate pathogenic cascades leading to the clinical phenotype of Alzheimer's disease (AD) [1]. The main focus of pharmacological research over the past 50 years has been the identification of cognitive enhancers. The identification of a selective cholinergic dysfunction in the basal forebrain and cortical neuronal loss led to the introduction of acetylcholinesterase inhibitors (AChEIs) as an option to restore cholinergic neurotransmission in the late 1970s. Tacrine was the first AChEI introduced in 1993 followed by a new generation of AChEIs (donepezil, galantamine, rivastigmine, huperzine A) and memantine, an N-methyl-D-aspartate (NMDA) glutamate receptor partial inhibitor. No new US Food and Drug Administration (FDA)-approved drugs for AD had been reported in 18 years before aducanumab was approved on June 6, 2021 [2]. Pharmacological treatment represents about 10–20% of AD direct costs depending on disease stage and country [2].

Common co-morbidities in AD require the coadministration of AChEIs with other drugs (>6–10 drugs/day). There is also abuse of psychotropic drugs and anticholinergics, which can potentially interact with AChEIs in AD, contributing to severe drug–drug interactions (DDIs) and variable adverse drug reactions (ADRs) [3]. In order to prevent DDIs and ADRs in AD, the first pharmacogenetic (PGx) studies with AChEIs and combination treatments were performed in the late 1990s and early 2000s. Fewer than 100 studies have been published on the pharmacogenetics of AD treatment for the past 3 decades. About 80% of the variability in drug pharmacokinetics and pharmacodynamics is attributed to PGx factors [4].

Most PGx studies in AD have used the apolipoprotein-E (APOE) gene and genes of the cytochrome P450 family (CYPs) as reference genes; however, the gene network that integrates the PGx apparatus consists of at least five categories of genes: pathogenic, mechanistic, metabolic, transporter, and pleiotropic genes. Furthermore, the pharmacological outcome is highly influenced by components of the PGx machinery, the chemical properties of each drug, and other diverse factors (e.g., compliance, nutrition, metabolic conditions, concomitant drugs) [4, 5].

This chapter summarizes (i) the most important components of the PGx apparatus in AD, (ii) the pharmacogenetics (also known as pharmacogenomics) of anti-dementia drugs currently available, and (iii) the potential benefits that the use of pharmacogenetics could bring in the development of new forms of therapeutic intervention in AD.

35.2 Structure of the Pharmacogenetic Machinery in AD

The PGx machinery is composed of a network of gene clusters coding for proteins and enzymes responsible for drug targeting and processing, as well as critical components of the epigenetic machinery that regulates gene expression [6]. The pharmagenes involved in the PGx response to drugs can be classified into five major categories (Figure 35.1): (i) pathogenic genes which are associated with disease pathogenesis; (ii) mechanistic genes coding for components of enzymes, receptor subunits, transmitters, and messengers associated with the mechanism of action of drugs; (iii) metabolic genes of different categories that encode Phase I–II reaction enzymes responsible for drug metabolism; (iv) transporter genes coding for drug transporters; and (v) pleiotropic genes which encode proteins and enzymes involved in a

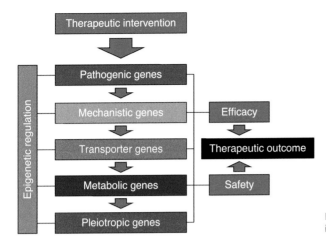

Figure 35.1 Basic structure of the PGx machinery involved in drug efficacy and safety.

great variety of metabolic cascades and metabolomic networks [4–6]. Rare variants contribute to approximately 30–40% of functional variability in 146 pharmagenes with clinical relevance. Over 240 pharmagenes are potentially associated with ADRs, and over 400 genes and their products influence drug efficacy and safety [7, 8].

The expression or repression of all these genes and their products are regulated in a redundant and promiscuous fashion by the epigenetic machinery (DNA methylation/demethylation, histone/chromatin remodeling, microRNA regulation), configuring the pharmacoepigenetic apparatus [6, 9, 10]. The same enzyme/protein/transporter can process a multitude of drugs, and the same drug can be processed by different gene products in an orchestrated manner to operate as a security system against xenobiotic intruders [10].

35.2.1 Pathogenic Genes

AD is characterized by (i) the extracellular accumulation of aggregated amyloid beta (Aβ) in amyloid plaques resulting from the abnormal amyloidogenic processing of the amyloid precursor protein (APP) by beta-site APP-cleaving enzyme 1 (BACE1) and gamma-secretase; (ii) intracellular neurofibrillary tangles formed by hyperphosphorylation of tau proteins; (iii) selective neuronal loss in the forebrain, hippocampus, and neocortical regions; (iv) widespread desarborization of neurons in circuits associated with higher activities of the central nervous system (CNS); (iv) neuroinflammatory reactions in amyloidogenic foci; (v) region-specific, selective neurotrophic and neurotransmitter deficits

(acetylcholine, norepinephrine, dopamine, serotonin, neuropeptides); (vi) epigenetic dysregulation of over 100 pathogenic genes; and (vii) cerebrovascular insufficiency and/or damage in selective strategic brain regions [1, 11]. Over 600 genes are potentially involved in the pathogenic cascades leading to AD-related neurodegeneration [1, 12, 13]. Mutations in the *APP*, presenilin 1 (*PSEN1*), presenilin 2 (*PSEN2*), and microtubule associated protein tau (*MAPT*) genes are present in less than 5% of AD cases. These mutations are important for three main reasons: (i) highly pathogenic influence leading to early-onset (familial) AD cases; (ii) reference genes for transgenic models currently used in drug development, either conventional drugs or immunotherapy; and (iii) PGx modifiers.

The presence of the ε4 allele in the *APOE* gene is the most important risk factor among top pathogenic genes; *APOE-4* is the major risk factor for AD, rapid cognitive decline, and poor response to treatment [1, 14, 15]. Many other single nucleotide polymorphisms (SNPs) in diverse genes may contribute to AD-related neurodegeneration and premature neuronal death, including genes encoding components of the PGx machinery [16].

35.2.2 Mechanistic Genes

Mechanistic genes are those that encode proteins, enzymes, and receptor subunits related to the mechanism of action of drugs. Key elements in the cholinergic neurotransmission include acetylcholine (ACh) precursors (choline, acetyl coenzyme A [acetyl-CoA]), ACh synthesis (choline acetyltransferase) and degradation enzymes (acetylcholinesterase, butyrylcholinesterase), choline transporter, vesicular ACh transporter, and cholinergic receptors (nicotinic, muscarinic).

Cholinergic neurons of the basal forebrain (basocortical cholinergic pathway, septohippocampal cholinergic pathway), where the nucleus basalis of Meynert is located, and cortical cholinergic projections are the brain territories mainly affected in AD, with 60–80% depletion of cholinergic markers in severe cases [16].

35.2.2.1 Choline Acetyltransferase

Choline acetyltransferase (ChAT), the enzyme responsible for the biosynthesis of ACh from choline and acetyl-CoA, is encoded in the *CHAT* gene located at 10q11.23. At least seven polymorphic forms of *CHAT* result from the alternative splicing of three 5′ exons named R, N, and M to exon 1, containing the ATG initiation codon. The first intron of the *CHAT* gene encompasses the open reading frame encoding the vesicular acetylcholine transporter (VAChT), which is responsible for the transportation of ACh from the cytoplasm into the synaptic cleft. Mutations in *CHAT* and/or the solute carrier family 18 (vesicular actylcholine), member 3 (*SLC18A3*) gene, which encodes for VAChT, may represent potential susceptibility to AD [16].

35.2.2.2 Acetylcholinesterase

Acetylcholinesterase (AChE) is a serine hydrolase that hydrolyzes ACh to yield choline and acetate in the synaptic cleft where residual choline is recycled by the choline transporter to be available at the presynaptic level for *de novo* synthesis of ACh. The AChE gene (*ACHE*)(7q22.1) contains six exons and spans about 7 kb, coding for a protein of 583 amino acids. *ACHE* variants with catalytic activity include synaptic *ACHE* (*ACHE-S*) or tailed *ACHE* (*ACHE-T*)(exon 6), the most frequent variant in the brain; erythrocyte *ACHE* (*ACHE-E*) or hydrophobic *ACHE* (*ACHE-H*) (exon 5); and read-through *ACHE* (*ACHE-R*) (intron 4-exon 5). The Yt erythrocyte blood group antigen system is inserted in the AChE molecule (*ACHE*, His322Asn). A 4-bp deletion located 17 kb upstream of the transcription start site that abolishes one of the two adjacent hepatocyte nuclear factor-3 (HNF3) binding sites causes hypersensitivity to AChEIs and severe CNS symptoms under low-dose exposure to pyridostigmine. AChE activity is decreased in AD brains and APP is involved in the regulation of AChE [16, 17].

35.2.2.3 Butyrylcholinesterase

Human serum cholinesterase (acylcholine acylhydrolase) or butyrylcholinesterase (BuChE) is a serine hydrolase that catalyzes the hydrolysis of ACh and choline esters, such as the muscle relaxants succinylcholine and mivacurium. BuChE is a 574-amino acid protein encoded by the *BCHE* gene (four exons, 64 kb) located at 3q26.1. Over 30 genetic variants of *BCHE* have been described. In AD cases, the allelic frequency of the K variant is >0.2 (vs. 0.09 in controls); and the risk for AD in carriers of the K variant increases in the presence of the *APOE-4* allele in most studies. In mild cognitive impairment (MCI) cases, the presence of *BCHE-K* and *APOE-4* accelerates cognitive decline, hippocampal volumetric loss, and progression to AD [18].

35.2.2.4 Choline Transporter

The choline transporter (CHT) is encoded by the solute carrier family 5 (choline transporter), member 7 (*SLC5A7*) gene (2q12.3), with nine exons spanning 25 kb. CHT is a Na^+- and Cl^--dependent high-affinity 580-amino acid protein (63.2 kD) with 12 transmembrane (TM) domains responsible for the uptake of choline for ACh synthesis in cholinergic neurons. An A-to-G transition at nucleotide 265, resulting in an Ile89-to-Val substitution (I89 V) within the third TM domain causes a reduction in the maximum rate of choline uptake by about 40%. The high-affinity CHT expressed in cholinergic neurons represents a rate-limiting step for ACh synthesis. Disruption of CHT function leads to decreased choline uptake and ACh synthesis, with the consequent impairment in cholinergic neurotransmission. CHT dysfunction may contribute to AD pathology. Aβ decreases choline uptake activity and cell surface CHT protein levels. CHT trafficking is different in wild-type APP (*APPwt*) and in Swedish mutant APP (*APPswe*) SHSY5Y human neuroblastoma cells. The APP–CHT interaction is decreased in *APPswe* [19].

Mutations in *PSEN1* may regulate cholinergic signaling via CHT. Cortical neurons express active CHT1, and CHT1-mediated choline uptake activity is reduced in *PSEN1* M146V mutant knock-in mice [20]. In a mouse model of scopolamine-induced amnesia, scopolamine decreases ChAT, CHT, VAChT, and muscarinic ACh receptor M1 (M1 R) in the septum and hippocampus [16].

35.2.2.5 Vesicular Acetylcholine Transporter

VAChT is encoded in the *SLC18A3* gene (10q11.23). This gene encodes a transmembrane protein that transports ACh into presynaptic secretory vesicles to be released at cholinergic terminals in the CNS and peripheral nervous system. The *SLC18A3* gene is located within the first intron of the *CHAT* gene. Mutations in the *SLC18A3* gene cause presynaptic congenital myasthenic syndrome-21. Nitrosylation of VAChT is increased in the frontal cortex and hippocampus of *APP–PSEN1* mice [21]. B6.eGFPChAT congenic mice with multiple gene copies of VAChT exhibit high VAChT protein expression in the hippocampal formation, accompanied by enhanced ACh release [22]. Mice with a targeted mutation in the *SLC18A3* gene show a 40% reduction in transporter expression, with memory deficits which can be reversed with AChEIs. Decreased expression of the splicing regulator hnRNPA2/B1BACE1 causes abnormal splicing in *BACE1*, increased APP processing and accumulation of soluble $A\beta_{42}$ together with increases in glycogen synthase kinase-3, tau hyperphosphorylation, caspase-3, and neuronal death. In human brains, there is correlation between decreased levels of VAChT and hnRNPA2/B1 levels with increased tau hyperphosphorylation [23]. There is a selective loss of cholinergic terminals in the neocortex and hippocampus of double transgenic (*APP*-K670 N/M671 L + *PSEN1*-M146 L) mice, with relevant alterations in VAChT. The levels of ChAT, AChE, and BuChE are similar in the hippocampus of young *apoE-4* and *apoE-3* mice. ChAT levels tend to decrease more in the *apoE-4* than in *apoE-3* mice. The levels of muscarinic receptors are also higher in the *apoE-4* mice. ACh release from hippocampal slices is reduced in old *apoE-4* mice in parallel with reduced VAChT levels [24].

The distribution of VAChT in early AD shows a decrease of about 47–62% in the cingulate cortex and parahippocampal-amygdaloid complex. The number of ChAT and VAChT neurons correlates with the severity of dementia and shows no relationship with *APOE* status. Cholinergic basocortical and septo-hippocampal pathways are particularly damaged in AD as reflected by PET studies of the VAChT [25].

35.2.2.6 Cholinergic Receptors

Nicotinic and muscarinic ACh receptors are the final effectors of cholinergic neurotransmission.

Nicotinic acetylcholine receptors (nAChRs) play an important role in the prefrontal cortex where cortical and subcortical inputs are integrated to execute higher activities of the CNS (learning, attention, working memory planning, decision making, perception of reality). Mutations in the *CHRNB2* or *CHRNA7* genes that encode the nicotinic receptor β2 and α7 subunits can lead to brain disorders, including AD [26]. α7nAChR, encoded by the *CHRNA7* gene, is involved in AD pathogenesis connected to hypocholinergic neurotransmission and Aβ deposition. Carriers of the *CHRNA7* rs7179008 variant showed decreased risk of dementia. α7nAChR is a putative receptor of Aβ and the α7nAChR–Aβ complex is found in neuritic plaques in the neocortex. This α7nAChR–Aβ interaction might lead to receptor activation. α7nAChR binds to soluble Aβ with a high affinity, and Aβ activates p38 mitogen-activated protein kinase (MAPK) and extracellular signal-regulated kinase 1/2 signaling pathways via α7nAChR, resulting in internalization of $A\beta_{42}$. SNPs in the *CHRNA7* gene or in the fusion gene containing *CHRNA7* partial duplication (*CHRFAM7A*) may represent a susceptibility trait to AD. *CHRFAM7A*-2-bp deletion or *CHRNA7* SNPs (rs1514246, rs2337506, rs8027814) might be protective for AD [16, 27].

Loss of basal forebrain cholinergic neurons correlates with cognitive decline in AD. Exposure to Aβ upregulates neuronal α7nAChRs and increases neuronal excitability; and α7nAChRs mediate, in part, Aβ-induced neurotoxicity, which is prevented by either the α7nAChR antagonist methyllycaconitine or by α7 subunit gene deletion. In contrast, it appears that α7nAChR selective agonists (e.g., PHA-543613) and galantamine ameliorate Aβ-impaired working and reference memory, suggesting that α7nAChR activation reduces Aβ-induced cognitive deficits whereas receptor blockage increases Aβ toxicity and cognitive impairment [28].

α7nAChR gene silencing demonstrates that both the anti-inflammatory and neuroprotective effects of ACh rely on α7nAChR pathways in which microglial cells are involved; and the activation of α7nAChR alleviates $A\beta_{42}$-induced neurotoxicity via downregulation of p38 and JNK MAPKs. The JAK2/STAT3 and PI3 K/AKT signaling pathways influence the neuroprotective and anti-inflammatory effects of α7nAChR [29].

In the TgCRND8 mouse model, downregulation of over 80% cholinergic-related transcripts, and upregulation of transcripts related to axon guidance, glutamatergic synapses, kinase activity, and AD-related genes (*Sorl1*, *Ptk2b*) have been demonstrated [30].

35.2.3 Metabolic Genes

Metabolic genes encode enzymes involved in Phase I–II reactions in the liver and other tissues. Phase-I reaction enzymes include alcohol dehydrogenases, aldehyde dehydrogenases, aldo-keto reductases, amine oxidases, carbonyl reductases, cytidine deaminases, CYPs of monooxygenases, cytochrome b5 reductase, dihydropyrimidine dehydrogenase, esterases, epoxidases, flavin-containing monooxygenases, glutathione reductase/peroxidases, peptidases, prostaglandin endoperoxide synthases, short-chain dehydrogenases, reductases, superoxide dismutases, and xanthine dehydrogenase. The most relevant Phase-II reaction enzymes include the following: amino acid transferases, dehydrogenases, esterases, glucuronosyl transferases, glutathione transferases, methyl transferases, *N*-acetyl transferases, thioltransferase, and sulfotransferases [4–6, 9].

Most PGx studies with AChEIs in AD are related to CYPs. Nearly 30% of AD cases are deficient for CYP2D6 and CYP3A4/5 enzymes associated with the metabolism of AChEIs. However, approximately 80% of patients are deficient metabolizers for the tetragenic cluster integrated by *CYP2D6, 2C19, 2C9*, and *3A4/5* variants which encode enzymes responsible for the metabolism of 60–80% of drugs of current use, showing ontogenic-, age-, sex-, circadian-, and ethnic-related differences. CYP geno-phenotypes differentiate extensive (EM; normal, NM), intermediate (IM), poor (PM), or ultra-rapid metabolizers (UM) with great geographic and ethnic variability worldwide [4–6].

35.2.4 Transporter Genes

The most important categories of transporters include the following: ATPase (P-type subfamily), V-type (vacuolar H+-ATPase subunit), and ATPase (F-type subfamily); ATP-binding cassette transporters: subfamily A (ABC1), subfamily B (MDR/TAP), subfamily C (CFTR/MRP), subfamily D (ALD), subfamily E (OABP), subfamily F (GCN20), and subfamily G (WHITE); and solute carriers: high-affinity glutamate and neutral amino acid transporter family (SLC)[6].

Polymorphic variants in ABC and SLC transporters may affect AD pathogenesis and response to over 1,000 drugs, including AChEIs and memantine [4–6]. Many other transporters are associated with AD pathogenesis [16]. Defective transporters are attractive candidates for therapeutic intervention in AD and their mutations should be taken into account in PGx strategies [16, 31].

35.2.5 Pleiotropic Genes

Over 6,000 different genes involved in metabolomic networks may be affected by pharmacological treatment and epigenetic changes, with practical consequences from a pharmacogenomic and pharmacoepigenetic perspective [6].

35.3 Pharmacogenetics of Acetylcholinesterase Inhibitors

35.3.1 Donepezil

Donepezil is the most prescribed AChEI for the treatment of AD [32–34](Table 35.1). Donepezil is a selective AChEI with a long elimination half-life ($T_{1/2}$) of 70 h and is metabolized in the liver [35]. Donepezil clearance is 7.3 l/h with gender- and inter-individual variability (30%) [36]. Donepezil increases brain ACh levels by 35% and decreases AChE activity by 40–90%, with no effect on ChAT, VAChT, CHT, or muscarinic receptors. Donepezil might also exert some beneficial effects against $A\beta_{40}$-induced neurotoxicity. Donepezil is a major substrate of CYP2D6, CYP3A4, AChE, and UGTs, inhibits AChE and BuChE, and is transported by ABCB1 [35, 37] (Table 35.1). Individual variation in metabolic genes (*CYP2D6*) and pathogenic genes (*APOE*) modulates the response to donepezil treatment [38]. Several *CYP2D6* variants may modify donepezil efficacy and safety in AD [32, 33]; and *APOE* and *CYP2D6* variants are determinant in the effects of donepezil [32, 33, 37, 38].

APOE-4 carriers tend to be the worst responders and *APOE-3* carriers are the best responders to donepezil in either monotherapy or drug combination regimes; *CYP2D6*-EMs are the best responders and *CYP2D6*-PMs are the worst responders [1, 4, 5, 32, 33, 37, 39].

CYP2D6-PMs show a 32% slower elimination and *CYP2D6*-UMs show a 67% faster elimination [36]. Carriers of the mutant *CYP2D6*10* allele responded better (58% responders) than

Table 35.1 Pharmacological properties and pharmacogenetics of conventional anti-dementia drugs

Drug	Properties	Pharmacogenetics
Cl—H	**Name: donepezil hydrochloride,** aricept, 120011-70-3, donepezil HCl, BNAG, E-2020, E2020 **IUPAC name:** 2-[(1-benzylpiperidin-4-yl)methyl]-5,6-dimethoxy-2,3-dihydroinden-1-one hydrochloride **Molecular formula:** $C_{24}H_{30}ClNO_3$ **Molecular weight:** 415.9529 g/mol **Category:** cholinesterase inhibitor **Mechanism:** centrally active, reversible acetylcholinesterase inhibitor; increases the acetylcholine available for synaptic transmission in the CNS **Effect:** nootropic agent, cholinesterase inhibitor, parasympathomimetic effect	**Pathogenic genes:** *APP, APOE, CHAT* **Mechanistic genes:** *ACHE, BCHE, CHAT, CHRNA7* **Drug metabolism-related genes:** • **substrate:** *CYP2D6* (major), *CYP3A4* (major), *UGTs, ACHE* • **inhibitor:** *ABCB1, ACHE, BCHE, ERG* **Transporter genes:** *ABCB1, ABCA1, ABCG2, SCN1A* **Pleiotropic genes:** *APOE, PLP, MAG, MBP, CNPase, MOG*
Br —H	**Name: galantamine hydrobromide**, galanthamine hydrobromide, 1953-04-4, nivalin, razadyne, UNII-MJ4PTD2VVW, nivaline **IUPAC name:** (1S,12S,14R)-9-methoxy-4-methyl-11-oxa-4-azatetracyclo[8.6.1.0^{1,12}.0^{6,17}]heptadeca-6,8,10(17),15-tetraen-14-ol **Molecular formula:** $C_{17}H_{22}BrNO_3$ **Molecular weight:** 368.26548 g/mol **Category:** Cholinesterase inhibitor **Mechanism:** Reversible and competitive acetylcholinesterase inhibition leading to an increased concentration of acetylcholine at cholinergic synapses; modulates nicotinic acetylcholine receptor; may increase glutamate and serotonin levels **Effect:** nootropic agent, cholinesterase inhibitor, parasympathomimetic effect	**Pathogenic genes:** *APOE, APP* **Mechanistic genes:** *ACHE, BCHE, CHRNA4, CHRNA7, CHRNB2, SLC18A3* **Drug metabolism-related genes:** • **Substrate:** *ABCB1, CYP2D6* (major), *CYP3A4* (major), *UGT1A1* • **Inhibitor:** *ACHE, BCHE* **Transporter genes:** *ABCB1, SLC18A3*

Table 35.1 (cont.)

Drug	Properties	Pharmacogenetics
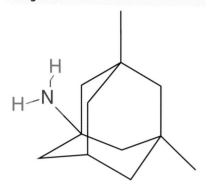	**Name: memantine hydrochloride**, 41100-52-1, namenda, memantine HCL, axura, 3,5-mimethyl-1-adamantanamine hydrochloride, 3,5-dimethyladamantan-1-amine hydrochloride **IUPAC name:** 3,5-dimethyladamantan-1-amine hydrochloride **Molecular formula:** $C_{12}H_{22}ClN$ **Molecular weight:** 215.76278 g/mol **Category:** N-methyl-D-aspartate (NMDA) receptor antagonist **Mechanism:** binds preferentially to NMDA receptor-operated cation channels; may act by blocking actions of glutamate, mediated in part by NMDA receptors **Effect:** dopamine agent, antiparkinson agent, excitatory amino acid antagonist, antidyskinetic	**Pathogenic genes:** *APOE, MAPT, PSEN1* **Mechanistic genes:** *CHRFAM7A, DLGAP1, FOS, GRIN2A, GRIN2B, GRIN3A, HOMER1, HTR3A* **Drug metabolism-related genes:** • **Inhibitor:** *CYP1A2* (weak), *CYP2A6* (weak), *CYP2B6* (strong), *CYP2C9* (weak), *CYP2C19* (weak), *CYP2D6* (strong), *CYP2E1* (weak), *CYP3A4* (weak), *NR1I2* **Transporter genes:** *NR1I2* **Pleiotropic genes:** *APOE, MAPT, MT-TK, PSEN1*
	Name: rivastigmine tartrate, 129101-54-8, SDZ-ENA 713, rivastigmine hydrogentartrate, rivastigmine hydrogen tartrate, ENA 713, ENA-713 **IUPAC name:** (2*R*,3*R*)-2,3-dihydroxybutanedioic acid;[3-[(1*S*)-1-(dimethylamino)ethyl]phenyl] *N*-ethyl-*N*-methylcarbamate **Molecular formula:** $C_{18}H_{28}N_2O_8$ **Molecular weight:** 400.42352 g/mol **Category:** cholinesterase inhibitor **Mechanism:** increases acetylcholine in CNS through reversible inhibition of its hydrolysis by acetylcholinesterase **Effect:** neuroprotective agent, cholinesterase inhibitor, cholinergic agent	**Pathogenic genes:** *APOE, APP, CHAT* **Mechanistic genes:** *ACHE, BCHE, CHAT, CHRNA4, CHRNB2, SLC18A3* **Drug metabolism-related genes:** • **Substrate:** *UGT1A9, UGT2B7* • **Inhibitor:** *ACHE, BCHE* **Transporter genes:** *SLC18A3* **Pleiotropic genes:** *APOE, MAPT*

Table 35.1 (cont.)

Drug

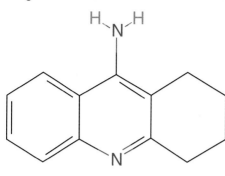

Properties

Name: tacrine hydrochloride, tacrine HCl, 1684-40-3, hydroaminacrine, 9-amino-1,2,3,4-tetrahydroacridine hydrochloride, tenakrin

IUPAC name: 1,2,3,4-tetrahydroacridin-9-amine hydrochloride

Molecular formula: $C_{13}H_{15}ClN_2$

Molecular weight: 234.7246 g/mol

Category: cholinesterase inhibitor

Mechanism: elevates acetylcholine in cerebral cortex by slowing degradation of acetylcholine

Effect: nootropic agent, cholinesterase inhibitor, parasympathomimetic effect

Pharmacogenetics

Pathogenic genes: *APOE*
Mechanistic genes: *ACHE, BCHE, CHRNA4, CHRNB2*

Drug metabolism-related genes:
- **Substrate:** *CYP1A2 (major), CYP2D6 (minor), CYP3A4 (major), CES1, GSTM1, GSTT1*
- **Inhibitor:** *ACHE, BCHE, CYP1A2 (weak)*

Transporter genes: *ABCB4, SCN1A*

Pleiotropic genes: *APOE, LEPR, MTHFR*

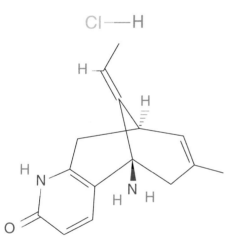

Name: (-)-huperazine A, huperzine A; huperzine-A; 102518-79-6; (+/−)-huperzine A

IUPAC name: (1R,9R,13E)-1-amino-13-ethylidene-11-methyl-6-azatricyclo[7.3.1.02,7]trideca-2(7),3,10-trien-5-one

Molecular formula: $C_{15}H_{18}N_2O$

Molecular weight: 242.32 g/mol

Category: neuroprotectant, cholinesterase inhibitor

Mechanism: increases acetylcholine in the brain by inhibiting acetylcholinesterase and slowing acetylcholine hydrolysis

Effect: neuroprotective, acetylcholinesterase inhibitor, cognitive enhancer, anti-epileptic

Pathogenic genes: *APP, APOE*
Mechanistic genes: *ACHE*
Drug metabolism-related genes:
- **Substrate:** *ABCB1, CYP1A2, CYP3A1, CYP3A2, CYP2C11, CYP2E1, CES1, CES2*
- **Inhibitor:** *ACHE*
- **Inducer:** *CYP1A2*

Transporter genes: *ABCB1, ABCG2*

Pleiotropic genes: *APOE, BDNF*

Gene abbreviations: ABCA1: ATP-binding cassette, subfamily A, member 1; ABCB1: ATP-binding cassette, subfamily B, member 1; ABCB4: ATP-binding cassette, subfamily B, member 4; ABCG2: ATP-binding cassette, subfamily G, member 2; ACHE: acetylcholinesterase; APOE: apolipoprotein E; APP: amyloid precursor protein; BCHE: butyrylcholinesterase; BDNF: brain-derived neurotrophic factor; CES1: carboxylesterase 1; CES2: carboxylesterase 2; CHAT: choline acetyltransferase; CHRFAM7A: CHRNA7 (exons 5-10) and FAM7A (exons A-E) fusion; CHRNA4: cholinergic receptor, neuronal nicotinic, alpha polypeptide 4; CHRNA7: cholinergic receptor, neuronal nicotinic, alpha polypeptide 7; CHRNB2: cholinergic receptor nicotinic beta 2 subunit; CNPase: cyclic nucleotide phosphodiesterase; CYP1A2: cytochrome P450, family 1, subfamily A, polypeptide 2; CYP2A6: cytochrome P450, family 2, subfamily A, polypeptide 6; CYP2B6: cytochrome P450, family 2, subfamily B, polypeptide 6; CYP2C9: cytochrome P450, family 2, subfamily C, polypeptide 9; CYP2C11: cytochrome P450, family 2, subfamily C, polypeptide 11; CYP2C19: cytochrome P450, family 2, subfamily C, polypeptide 19; CYP2D6: cytochrome P450, family 2, subfamily D, polypeptide 6; CYP2E1: cytochrome P450, family 2, subfamily E, polypeptide 1; CYP3A1: cytochrome P450, family 3, subfamily A, polypeptide 1; CYP3A2: cytochrome P450, family 3, subfamily A, polypeptide 2; CYP3A4: cytochrome P450, family 3, subfamily A, polypeptide 4; DLGAP1: discs, large (*Drosophila*) homolog-associated protein 1; ERG: ETS transcription factor; FOS: FBJ murine osteosarcoma viral oncogene homolog; GRIN2A: glutamate receptor, ionotropic, *N*-methyl-D-aspartate, subunit 2A; GRIN2B: glutamate receptor, ionotropic, *N*-methyl-D-aspartate, subunit 2B; GRIN3A: glutamate receptor, ionotropic, *N*-methyl-D-aspartate, subunit 3A; GSTM1: glutathione S-transferase mu 1; GSTT1: glutathione S-transferase theta 1; HOMER1: homer homolog 1 (*Drosophila*); HTR3A: 5-hydroxytryptamine receptor 3; LEPR: leptin receptor; MAG: myelin associated glycoprotein; MAPT: microtubule-associated protein tau; MBP: myelin basic protein; MOG: myelin-oligodendrocyte glycoprotein; MTHFR: 5,10-methylenetetrahydrofolate reductase; MT-TK: mitochondrially encoded tRNA lysine; NR1I2: nuclear receptor subfamily 1, group I, member 2; PLP: proteolipid protein; PSEN1: presenilin 1; SCN1A: sodium voltage-gated channel, alpha subunit 1; SLC18A3: solute carrier family 18 (vesicular acetylcholine), member 3; UGT1A1: UDP glucuronosyltransferase 1 family, polypeptide A1; UGT1A9: UDP glucuronosyltransferase 1 family, polypeptide A9; UGT2B7: UDP glucuronosyltransferase 2 family, polypeptide B7; UGTs: UDP glucuronosyltransferase family.

carriers of the wild-type *CYP2D6*1* allele [40]. The *CYP2D6*10* variant strongly affects steady-state plasma concentration of donepezil and therapeutic outcome in Asian populations [41]. The concomitant use of memantine increases donepezil plasma concentrations; and co-medication with antidepressants attenuates the clinical response. The co-administration of ketoconazole and donepezil alters donepezil plasma concentration, suggesting a compromise of the CYP3A4–CYP2D6 metabolizing pathways.

*CYP3A5*3, ABCB1* 3435C>T, *ABCB1* 1236C>T, and *APOE-4* genotypes do not affect steady-state plasma concentrations of donepezil [41]. Studies in China showed that *CYP2D6*10* carriers treated with donepezil/galantamine have lesser side effects and respond better to AChEIs [41].

ABCA1 regulates cholesterol transport and ApoE metabolism. AD patients with the *ABCA1* rs2230806 G/G genotype respond better to donepezil than carriers of the A/A and A/G genotypes; and *ABCA1* rs2230806 G/G-*APOE-3* non-carriers tend to show a better clinical response to donepezil. Lower plasma donepezil concentration-to-dose ratios and better clinical response to donepezil have been reported in patients homozygous for the T/T/T genotype in the *ABCB1* haplotypes 1236 C/2677 G/3435C (46%) and 1236 T/2677 T/3435 T (41%). Donepezil may inhibit ABCB1 [16].

*APOE-4/BCHE-K** carriers show an earlier age of onset, an accelerated cognitive decline, and a differential response to donepezil therapy. In patients with MCI, donepezil accelerates cognitive decline in homozygous *BCHE-K* and *APOE-4* carriers. The *BCHE-K* variant is associated with lower AChE hydrolyzing activity, and BuChE activity increases in parallel with disease progression. These results suggest that *BCHE-K* and *APOE-4* carriers should not be prescribed donepezil for MCI and, consequently, donepezil is not recommended in AD patients with the *BCHE-K* and/or *APOE-4* variants [42].

Donepezil may induce upregulation of α7nAChR protein levels, potentially protecting neurons against neurodegeneration. *CHRNA7* rs8024987 (C/G) and rs6494223 (C/T) tend to respond better to donepezil. Donepezil-induced α7nAChR upregulation is higher in T/T carriers (7–15%) than in C/C or C/T carriers [43].

Donepezil treatment tends to increase APP forms in *APOE-4* non-carriers and interacts with many drugs causing cardiotoxicity [16].

35.3.2   Galantamine

Galantamine is a reversible, competitive AChEI and an allosteric modulator of nAChRs. This drug is rapidly absorbed (T_{max} = 1 h), with low protein binding (28.3–33.8%), a steady-state volume of distribution (V_{ss}) of 193 l, and an elimination half-life of 7–8 h (20–25% is excreted unchanged in urine) [35]. Median clearance in male and female patients with AD is 14.8 and 12.4 l/h, respectively, probably due to body weight differences rather than a real gender effect. Metabolic clearance is reduced by 60% in patients with liver dysfunction. Galantamine increases the levels of brain VAChT.

Galantamine is a major substrate of CYP2D6, CYP3A4, ABCB1, and UGT1A1, and an inhibitor of AChE and BuChE. *APOE, APP, CHRNA4, CHRNA7,* and *CHRNB2* variants may also affect galantamine efficacy and safety [16, 35, 37] (Table 35.1). Galantamine is mainly metabolized by CYP2D6 and CYP3A4 enzymes. Major metabolic pathways are glucuronidation, *O*-demethylation, *N*-demethylation, *N*-oxidation, and epimerization. *CYP2D6* variants are major determinants of galantamine pharmacokinetics, with *CYP2D6*-PMs presenting 45% and 61% higher dose-adjusted galantamine plasma concentrations than heterozygous and homozygous *CYP2D6*-EMs [35, 44]; however, these pharmacokinetic changes might not substantially affect pharmacodynamics.

Galantamine induces fewer side effects in Chinese *CYP2D6*10* carriers. Caution should be taken when administering galantamine with agents which affect CYP2D6 and CYP3A4 metabolic enzymes. Co-administration of galantamine with strong CYP2D6 inhibitors (e.g., paroxetine) or strong CYP3A4 inhibitors (e.g., ketoconazole) increases galantamine bioavailability by 40% and 30%, respectively [16].

There is no linear correlation between galantamine concentration and cognitive response in AD patients. Galantamine bioavailability and its therapeutic effects may be modified by interaction with foods and nutritional components [16].

Several studies indicate that galantamine in AD may show better results in *APOE-4* non-carriers. Patients with MCI treated with galantamine for 1 year also showed a lower rate of whole brain atrophy, preferentially among *APOE-4* carriers. Others suggest no major influence of *APOE* variants in the effects of galantamine in AD. *CHRNA7* rs8024987 variants may also affect galantamine in females [16].

35.3.3 Rivastigmine

Rivastigmine is a dual AChEI with brain-region selectivity (>40% AChE inhibition) and a long-lasting effect. Rivastigmine also inhibits peripheral BuChE (>10%).

Saturable first-pass metabolism leads to 35% bioavailability of the administered dose and non-linear short half-life pharmacokinetics, with renal elimination. Rivastigmine is a pseudo-irreversible dual inhibitor of AChE and BChE with a very short $T_{1/2}$ (1–2 h) and longer duration of action due to blockade of AChE and BChE for around 8.5 and 3.5 h, respectively.

Rivastigmine increases VAChT and ChAT expression in the frontal cortex, hippocampus, striatum, and cerebellum, providing additional effects on cholinergic neurotransmission. Rivastigmine metabolism is mediated by esterases in the liver and in the intestine [35, 37, 45]. *APOE, APP, CHAT, ACHE, BCHE, CHRNA4, CHRNB2, SLC18A3*, and *MAPT* variants may affect rivastigmine pharmacokinetics and pharmacodynamics (Table 35.1). Rivastigmine is more effective in *APOE-4* non-carriers in different ethnic groups: *APOE-3* carriers are the best responders and *APOE-4* carriers are the worst responders. CYP enzymes are not involved in the metabolism of rivastigmine. *UGT2B7*-PMs show higher rivastigmine levels with a poor response to treatment. In combination treatments with memantine, carriers of *CYP2D6*3, UGT2B7*, and *UGT1A9*5* variants show differential responses to treatment. Two SNPs in the intronic region of *CHAT* (rs2177370 and rs3793790) and *CHRNA7* variants may influence the response to AChEIs.

The *BCHE-K* variant (rs1803274) causes reduced enzyme activity and lower response to rivastigmine. Other SNPs outside the coding sequence (5′UTR [rs1126680] and/or intron 2 [rs55781031]) of the *BCHE* gene, in addition to the K-variant (p.A539 T), may also be responsible for reduced enzyme activity. Carriers of these deleterious SNPs should receive lower doses of rivastigmine or start treatment with a different AChEI.

Females with the *BCHE-wt/wt* show a better benefit with rivastigmine than males, and *BCHE-K* male carriers show a faster cognitive decline than females. The progression of cognitive decline in male *BCHE-K* and in female *BCHE-wt/wt* may be attenuated by rivastigmine. *BCHE-K–APOE-4* carriers show a poor cognitive response to rivastigmine patch or memantine add-on therapy [16].

35.3.4 Huperzine A

Huperzine A, a natural *Lycopodium* sesquiterpene alkaloid extracted from the Chinese medicinal plant *Huperzia serrata*, is a reversible and highly selective second-generation AChEI for AD approved in China in 1994 [46]. Huperzine A shows different pharmacokinetic features in elderly and young healthy subjects. In elderly subjects, the plasma concentration–time profile of huperzine A follows a one-compartment model with first-order absorption and elimination. Age is a covariate with significant influence on huperzine A clearance.

In rat liver microsomes, huperzine A metabolism is mediated primarily by CYP1A2, with a secondary contribution of CYP3A1/2 and negligible involvement of CYP2C11 and 2E1. Huperzine A is excreted unchanged by kidney rather than metabolized by human liver, with no apparent involvement of CYP enzymes (CYP1A2, 2A6, 2C9, 2C19, 2D6, 2E1 and 3A4) [47] (Table 35.1). At a toxicological dose in rats, huperzine A may induce CYP1A2 by transcription enhancement. Carboxylesterases (CESs; CES1 and CES2) are enzymes catalyzing the hydrolysis of ester, amide, and carbamate chemicals. CESs might be tangentially involved in huperzine A metabolism.

Huperzine A penetrates the brain and interacts with ABCB1 and ABCG2 efflux transporters. Huperzine A is a substrate of ABCB1. In *Abcb1a−/−* mice, the brain to plasma concentration ratio of huperzine A is higher than in wild-type animals [16].

35.3.5 Memantine

Memantine is a non-competitive low-affinity NMDA receptor antagonist which binds preferentially to NMDA receptor-operated cation channels. Its long $T_{1/2}$ is about 70 h and it is eliminated unchanged via the kidneys; however, several genes can influence its efficacy and safety [35]. Memantine inhibits the actions of glutamate via NMDA receptors, and antagonizes GRIN2A, GRIN2B, GRIN3A, HTR3A, and CHRFAM7A. *APOE, PSEN1*, and *MAPT* are pathogenic genes which might influence the effects of memantine in AD;

413

and variants in some mechanistic genes (*GRIN2A*, *GRIN2B*, *GRIN3A*, *HTR3A*, *CHRFAM7A*, *FOS*, and *HOMER1*) may also modify its therapeutic effects. CYP2B6 and CYP2D6 are strongly inhibited by memantine. In contrast, CYP1A2, CYP2A6, CYP2C9, CYP2C19, CYP2E1, and CYP3A4 are weakly inhibited [35, 37, 48]. Studies in human liver microsomes show that memantine inhibits CYP2B6 and CYP2D6, decreases CYP2A6 and CYP2C19, and has no effect on CYP1A2, CYP2E1, CYP2C9, or CYP3A4. Its co-administration with CYP2B6 substrates decreases memantine metabolism by 65%. *NR1I2* rs1523130 is the only genetic covariate for memantine clearance in clinical studies. *NR1I2* rs1523130 CT/TT carriers show a slower memantine elimination than carriers of the CC genotype [48].

Memantine transport across the blood–brain barrier might be facilitated by proton-coupled organic cation antiporters. Memantine can be used alone or in combination with AChEIs in AD. Proteomic studies in the hippocampus and the cerebral cortex of AD-related transgenic mice (3×Tg-AD) treated with memantine revealed alterations in the expression of 233 and 342 proteins, respectively. In *APP23* transgenic mice with cerebral amyloid angiopathy, memantine reduces cerebrovascular Aβ and hemosiderin deposits by enhancing Aβ-cleaving insulin-degrading enzyme expression. Memantine increases histamine neuron activity, as reflected by a 60% increase in brain tele-methylhistamine levels and an increase in hypothalamic H_3 autoreceptors, where histamine neurons are located [16].

35.4 Pharmacogenetics of Multifactorial Treatments

Most studies in which AD patients are treated with multifactorial combinations reveal that *APOE-3* carriers are the best responders and *APOE-4* carriers are the worst responders. Concerning CYP-related PGx outcomes, *CYP2D6*-EMs are the best responders, *CYP2D6*-PMs are the worst responders, and *CYP2D6*-IMs and *CYP2D6*-UMs show an intermediate response [1, 4–6, 32, 33]. Interactions between ApoE and translocase of outer mitochondrial membrane 40 (TOMM40) affect the risk of AD and the response to drugs. *TOMM40* poly T-S/S carriers are the best responders, VL/VL and S/VL carriers are intermediate responders, and

L/L carriers are the worst responders to treatment. *TOMM40*-L/L and -S/L carriers in haplotypes with *APOE-4* are the worst responders to treatment. *TOMM40*-S/S carriers, and to a lesser extent *TOMM40*-S/VL and *TOMM40*-VL/VL carriers, in haplotypes with *APOE-3* are the best responders to treatment. The *TOMM40*-L/L genotype is exclusively associated with the *APOE-4/4* genotype in 100% of the cases, and this haplotype (4/4–L/L) might be responsible for premature neurodegeneration and consequent early onset of the disease, a faster cognitive deterioration, and a limited response to conventional treatments [49].

35.5 Pharmacoepigenetics

Epigenetic factors are important in AD pathogenesis and response to treatment [11, 16]. Sirtuin (*SIRT*) variants may alter the epigenetic machinery, contributing to AD pathogenesis. The *SIRT2*-C/T genotype (rs10410544) (50.92%) has been associated with AD susceptibility in the *APOE-4*-negative population (*SIRT2*-C/C, 34.72%; *SIRT2*-T/T 14.36%). *SIRT2–APOE* bigenic clusters yield 18 haplotypes that influence the PGx outcome. *APOE-3/4* and *APOE-4/4* genotypes accumulate in *SIRT2*-T/T > *SIRT2*-C/T > *SIRT2*-C/C carriers, and *SIRT2*-T/T and *SIRT2*-C/T genotypes accumulate in *APOE-4/4* carriers. *SIRT2*-C/T carriers tend to be the best responders, *SIRT2*-T/T carriers are intermediate responders, and *SIRT2*-C/C carriers are the worst responders to a multifactorial treatment. PGx outcomes related to *APOE–SIRT2* bigenic clusters show that 3/3–C/C carriers respond better than 3/3–T/T and 3/4–C/T carriers, whereas 3/4–C/C and 4/4–C/C carriers are the worst responders. *SIRT2*-C/T–*CYP2D6*-EMs are the best responders [50].

35.6 Future Trends

Since AD-related neurodegeneration starts 20–30 years before the onset of the disease, new forms of intervention should be addressed to interfere with disease progression in very early (presymptomatic) stages of the disease. In animal models, this is technically feasible with immunotherapy (vaccines), multi-target interventions, and neural stem-cell transplantation [2, 18].

The implantation of prophylactic strategies and/or early pharmacological intervention in the presymptomatic population at risk or in cases with MCI (who in 20% of the cases will evolve into dementia) would require (i) a clear identification of susceptibility to dementia with genomic, epigenetic, and other presymptomatic biomarkers (most of them still unspecific), and (ii) suitable drugs chronically administered under strict PGx protocols. Unfortunately, neither condition exists at the present time; and, particularly, the available drugs are contraindicated for this purpose due to inefficacy and/or unwanted effects.

Over the past decade, the most prevalent pharmacological categories currently investigated as candidate strategies for the treatment of AD include neurotransmitter enhancers (more than 2,000 novel AChEIs), anti-amyloid agents, multi-target drugs, anti-tau agents, and diverse natural products. Some novel drugs, novel targets, revised old drugs, anti-inflammatory drugs, neuroprotective peptides, stem-cell therapy, nano-carriers/nanotherapeutics, and others (combination treatments, cognitive enhancers/nootropics, neurotrophic factors, polyunsaturated fatty acids, hormone therapy, epigenetic drugs, RNA interference/gene silencing, microRNAs, gene therapy) have also been investigated in exploratory studies for the treatment of AD, with uneven results and poor PGx information [2].

Based on current experience, with obvious limitations, the implementation of pharmacogenomic procedures can bring the following benefits: (i) accelerate the development of new therapeutic strategies aimed at combating specific pathogenic factors; (ii) improve the recruitment of patients with homogeneous genomic characteristics for clinical trials; (iii) more efficiently differentiate aspects related to the efficacy and safety of anti-dementia treatments; (iv) avoid high-risk drug interactions in patients receiving multiple treatments for concomitant diseases; (v) reduce specific ADRs of commonly used anti-dementia agents in the daily clinic; and (vi) reduce time in drug development and costs associated with pharmacological toxicity.

Acknowledgments

I would like to thank my collaborators at the International Center of Neuroscience and Genomic Medicine EuroEspes, Corunna, Spain, for technical assistance. This article was funded by EuroEspes Biomedical Research Center and IABRA (International Agency for Brain Research and Aging), Corunna, Spain.

Disclosure

Dr. Cacabelos is president and stockholder of EuroEspes (Biomedical Research Center), EuroEspes Biotechnology (Ebiotec), IABRA, and EuroEspes Publishing Co. He has no other relevant affiliations or financial involvement with any other organization or entity with a financial interest in or financial conflict with the subject matter or materials discussed, apart from those disclosed.

References

1. Cacabelos R, Fernández-Novoa L, Lombardi V, et al. Molecular genetics of Alzheimer's disease and aging. *Meth Find Exp Clin Pharmacol* 2005; **27**: 1–573.

2. Cacabelos R. Have there been improvement in Alzheimer's disease drug discovery over the past 5 years? *Expert Opin Drug Discov* 2018; **13**: 523–38.

3. Cacabelos R, Cacabelos N, Carril JC. The role of pharmacogenomics in adverse drug reactions. *Expert Rev Clin Pharmacol* 2019; **12**: 407–42.

4. Cacabelos R, Cacabelos P, Torrellas C, et al. Pharmacogenomics of Alzheimer's disease: novel therapeutic strategies for drug development. *Methods Mol Biol* 2014; **1175**: 323–556.

5. Cacabelos R, Carril JC, Cacabelos P, et al. Pharmacogenomics of Alzheimer's disease: genetic determinants of phenotypic variation and therapeutic outcome. *J Genomic Med Pharmacogenomics* 2016; **1**: 151–209.

6. Cacabelos R, Carril JC, Sanmartín A, et al. Pharmacoepigenetic processors: epigenetic drugs, drug resistance, toxicoepigenetics, and nutriepigenetics. In *Pharmacoepigenetics*, Cacabelos R (ed.). San Diego, CA: Academic Press/ Elsevier; 2019: 191–424.

7. Kozyra M, Ingelman-Sundberg M, Lauschke VM. Rare genetic variants in cellular transporters, metabolic enzymes, and nuclear receptors can be important determinants of interindividual differences in drug response. *Genet Med* 2017; **19**: 20–9.

8. Zhou ZW, Chen XW, Sneed KB, et al. Clinical association between pharmacogenomics and adverse drug reactions. *Drugs* 2015; **75**: 589–631.

9. Cacabelos R, Tellado I, Cacabelos P. The epigenetic machinery in the life cycle and pharmacoepigenetics. In *Pharmacoepigenetics*, Cacabelos R (ed.). San Diego, CA: Academic Press/ Elsevier; 2019: 1–100.

10. Cacabelos R. Pleiotropy and promiscuity in pharmacogenomics for the treatment of Alzheimer's disease and related risk factors. *Future Neurol* 2018; **13**.

11. Cacabelos R. Epigenomic networking in drug development: from pathogenic mechanisms to pharmacogenomics. *Drug Dev Res* 2014; **75**: 348–65.

12. Dorszewska J, Prendecki M, Oczkowska A, et al. Molecular basis of familial and sporadic Alzheimer's disease. *Curr Alzheimer Res* 2016; **13**: 952–63.

13. Jamal S, Goyal S, Shanker A, et al. Computational screening and exploration of disease-associated genes in Alzheimer's disease. *J Cell Biochem* 2017; **118**: 1471–9.

14. Zhou L, Li HY, Wang JH, et al. Correlation of gene polymorphisms of *CD36* and *ApoE* with susceptibility of Alzheimer disease: a case–control study. *Medicine (Baltimore)* 2018; **97**: e12470.

15. Davies G, Harris SE, Reynolds CA, et al. A genome-wide association study implicates the APOE locus in nonpathological cognitive ageing. *Mol Psychiatry* 2014; **19**: 76–87.

16. Cacabelos R. Pharmacogenetic considerations when prescribing cholinesterase inhibitors for the treatment of Alzheimer's disease. *Expert Opin Drug Metab Toxicol* 2020; **16**: 673–701.

17. Shapira M, Tur-Kaspa I, Bosgraaf L, et al. A transcription-activating polymorphism in the *ACHE* promoter associated with acute sensitivity to anti-acetylcholinesterases. *Hum Mol Genet* 2000; **9**: 1273–81.

18. Lane R, Feldman HH, Meyer J, et al. Synergistic effect of apolipoprotein E epsilon4 and butyrylcholinesterase K-variant on progression from mild cognitive impairment to Alzheimer's disease. *Pharmacogenet Genomics* 2008; **18**: 289–98.

19. Cuddy LK, Seah C, Pasternak SH, et al. Amino-terminal β-amyloid antibody blocks β-amyloid-mediated inhibition of the high-affinity choline transporter CHT. *Front Mol Neurosci* 2017; **10**: 361.

20. Payette DJ, Xie J, Guo Q. Reduction in CHT1-mediated choline uptake in primary neurons from presenilin-1 M146V mutant knock-in mice. *Brain Res* 2007; **1135**: 12–21.

21. Wang Y, Zhou Z, Tan H, et al. Nitrosylation of vesicular transporters in brain of amyloid precursor protein/presenilin 1 double transgenic mice. *J Alzheimers Dis* 2017; **55**:1683–92.

22. Nagy PM, Aubert I. Overexpression of the vesicular acetylcholine transporter increased acetylcholine release in the hippocampus. *Neuroscience* 2012; **218**: 1–11.

23. Kolisnyk B, Al-Onaizi MA, Xu J, et al. Cholinergic regulation of hnRNPA2/B1 translation by M1 muscarinic receptors. *J Neurosci* 2016; **36**: 6287–96.

24. Dolejší E, Liraz O, Rudajev V, et al. Apolipoprotein E4 reduces evoked hippocampal acetylcholine release in adult mice. *J Neurochem* 2016; **136**: 503–9.

25. Albin RL, Bohnen NI, Muller MLTM, et al. Regional vesicular acetylcholine transporter distribution in human brain: A [^{18}F] fluoroethoxybenzovesamicol positron emission tomography study. *J Comp Neurol* 2018; **526**: 2884–97.

26. Wallace TL, Bertrand D. Importance of the nicotinic acetylcholine receptor system in the prefrontal cortex. *Biochem Pharmacol* 2013; **85**: 1713–20.

27. Ma KG, Qian YH. Alpha 7 nicotinic acetylcholine receptor and its effects on Alzheimer's disease. *Neuropeptides* 2019; **73**: 96–106.

28. Sadigh-Eteghad S, Talebi M, Mahmoudi J, et al. Selective activation of α7 nicotinic acetylcholine receptor by PHA-543613 improves Aβ25–35-mediated cognitive deficits in mice. *Neuroscience* 2015; **298**: 81–93.

29. Li L, Liu Z, Jiang YY, et al. Acetylcholine suppresses microglial inflammatory response via α7nAChR to protect hippocampal neurons. *J Integr Neurosci* 2019; **18**: 51–6.

30. McKeever PM, Kim T, Hesketh AR, et al. Cholinergic neuron gene expression differences captured by translational profiling in a mouse model of Alzheimer's disease. *Neurobiol Aging* 2017; **57**: 104–19.

31. Vauthier V, Housset C, Falguières T. Targeted pharmacotherapies for defective ABC transporters. *Biochem Pharmacol* 2017; **136**:1–11.

32. Cacabelos R, Llovo R, Fraile C, et al. Pharmacogenetic aspects of therapy with cholinesterase inhibitors: the role of CYP2D6 in Alzheimer's disease pharmacogenetics. *Curr Alzheimer Res* 2007; **4**: 479–500.

33. Cacabelos R. Donepezil in Alzheimer's disease: from conventional trials to pharmacogenetics. *Neuropsychiatr Dis Treat* 2007; **3**: 303–33.

34. Brewster JT, Dell'Acqua S, Thach DQ, et al. Classics in chemical neuroscience: donepezil. *ACS Chem Neurosci* 2019; **10**: 155–67.

35. Noetzli M, Eap CB. Pharmacodynamic, pharmacokinetic and pharmacogenetic aspects of drugs used in the treatment of Alzheimer's disease. *Clin Pharmacokinet* 2013; **52**: 225–41.

36. Noetzli M, Guidi M, Ebbing K, et al. Population pharmacokinetic approach to evaluate the effect of CYP2D6, CYP3A, ABCB1, POR and NR1I2 genotypes on donepezil clearance. *Br J Clin Pharmacol* 2014; **78**: 135–44.

37. Cacabelos R. *World Guide for Drug Use and Pharmacogenomics*. Corunna: EuroEspes Publishing; 2012.

38. Xiao T, Jiao B, Zhang W, et al. Effect of the *CYP2D6* and *APOE* polymorphisms on the efficacy of donepezil in patients with Alzheimer's disease: a systematic review and meta-analysis. *CNS Drugs* 2016; **30**: 899–907.

39. Cacabelos R, Martínez R, Fernández-Novoa L, et al. Genomics of dementia: *APOE*- and *CYP2D6*-related pharmacogenetics. *Int J Alzheimers Dis* 2012; **2012**: 518901.

40. Zhong Y, Zheng X, Miao Y, et al. Effect of *CYP2D6*10* and *APOE* polymorphisms on the efficacy of donepezil in patients with Alzheimer's disease. *Am J Med Sci* 2013; **345**: 222–6.

41. Yaowaluk T, Senanarong V, Limwongse C, et al. Influence of *CYP2D6, CYP3A5, ABCB1, APOE* polymorphisms and nongenetic factors on donepezil treatment in patients with Alzheimer's disease and vascular dementia. *Pharmgenomics Pers Med* 2019; **12**: 209–24.

42. Sokolow S, Li X, Chen L, et al. Deleterious effect of butyrylcholinesterase K-variant in donepezil treatment of mild cognitive impairment. *J Alzheimers Dis* 2017; **56**: 229–37.

43. Russo P, Kisialiou A, Moroni R, et al. Effect of genetic polymorphisms (SNPs) in *CHRNA7* gene on response to acetylcholinesterase inhibitors (AChEI) in patients with Alzheimer's disease. *Curr Drug Targets* 2017; **18**: 1179–90.

44. Noetzli M, Guidi M, Ebbing K, et al. Relationship of *CYP2D6, CYP3A, POR*, and *ABCB1* genotypes with galantamine plasma concentrations. *Ther Drug Monit* 2013; **35**: 270–5.

45. Birks JS, Grimley Evans J. Rivastigmine for Alzheimer's disease. *Cochrane Database Syst Rev* 2015; **10**: CD001191.

46. Gul A, Bakht J, Mehmood F. Huperzine-A response to cognitive impairment and task switching deficits in patients with Alzheimer's disease. *J Chin Med Assoc* 2019; **82**: 40–3.

47. Lin PP, Li XN, Yuan F, et al. Evaluation of the in vitro and in vivo metabolic pathway and cytochrome P450 inhibition/induction profile of huperzine A. *Biochem Biophys Res Commun* 2016; **480**: 248–53.

48. Noetzli M, Guidi M, Ebbing K, et al. Population pharmacokinetic study of memantine: effects of clinical and genetic factors. *Clin Pharmacokinet* 2013; **52**: 211–23.

49. Cacabelos R, Goldgaber D, Vostrov A, et al. APOE-TOMM40 in the pharmacogenomics of dementia. *J Pharmacogenomics Pharmacoproteomics* 2014; **5**: 135.

50. Cacabelos R, Carril JC, Cacabelos N, et al. Sirtuins in Alzheimer's disease: SIRT2-related genophenotypes and implications for pharmacoepigenetics. *Int J Mol Sci* 2019; **20**: E1249.

Chapter 36

The Role of Electroencephalography in Alzheimer's Disease Drug Development

Willem de Haan and Niels Prins

36.1 Introduction

It took the inventor of the human EEG, Hans Berger, only a few years after his invention to describe EEG abnormalities in dementia, including an autopsy-proven case of Alzheimer's disease (AD) [1, 2]. Since then, thousands of research papers and a few hundred reviews have been published on EEG research in dementia, showing increasingly robust and reproducible neurophysiological changes during the AD disease course. EEG changes in normal aging and (preclinical) AD, as well as their potential pathophysiological substrates, are now fairly well known. One might therefore expect that the clinical role of EEG in AD is now well defined. Surprisingly, this turns out not to be the case. As opposed to dementia with Lewy bodies or Creutzfeldt–Jakob disease, EEG is not a part of official research/clinical criteria in AD, and opinions on the usefulness of EEG still vary.

Several reasons for the ambiguous role of EEG in AD can be offered. First of all, methodological problems are one source of controversy between various studies. Many early studies suffer from various problems such as small group size; bad matching of groups in terms of age, gender, and disease duration; and the influence of centrally acting drugs. Second, there has been a lack of consensus about which EEG measures to use, and varying evidence on the reproducibility of these measures.

In recent years, however, there is a notable trend moving away from the use of EEG exclusively for ruling out other conditions and toward identifying AD-specific abnormalities. This is nicely illustrated by a recent position paper by the Electrophysiology Professional Interest Area of the Alzheimer's Association International Society to Advance Alzheimer's Research and Treatment, claiming that the supporting evidence for the application of electrophysiology in AD clinical research as well as drug discovery pathways warrants the inclusion of EEG and magnetoencephalography

(MEG) biomarkers in the main multicentric projects planned in AD patients [3].

From a more fundamental research perspective, the prominent role of abnormal patterns of cerebral activity in very early-phase AD is becoming increasingly evident [4]. In particular, hippocampal amyloid-induced neuronal hyperexcitability and -activity is reported, but also more widespread excitation/inhibition disbalance [5]. This not only makes neurophysiological data in AD interesting from a diagnostic or prognostic perspective, but it may also have direct therapeutic consequences [6].

In this chapter we first discuss the neurophysiological basis of EEG and its relation to AD pathology, then present a brief overview of the literature on EEG in normal aging and the AD spectrum, including pharmaco-EEG outcomes in AD trials and their relation to other disease markers. We conclude with a section on best practices for EEG in clinical trials.

36.2 EEG Assessment of Brain Activity

36.2 1 The Physiological Basis of EEG

Electrophysiology is a multiscale methodology suited to probing the effects of AD neuropathological processes (e.g., amyloid beta 1–42 [$A\beta_{42}$], hyperphosphorylated tau, neurodegeneration of cholinergic systems, dysregulation of glutamate homeostasis) and disease-modifying drugs on synchronization/desynchronization and coupling/decoupling of brain neural activity in preclinical research. However, direct assessment of individual neurons or neuronal circuits requires invasive techniques. Of the more patient-friendly, non-invasive techniques suitable for clinical trials, EEG and MEG are the closest representation of neuronal activity. Since the EEG signal reflects the electrical field generated by summed post-synaptic potentials of

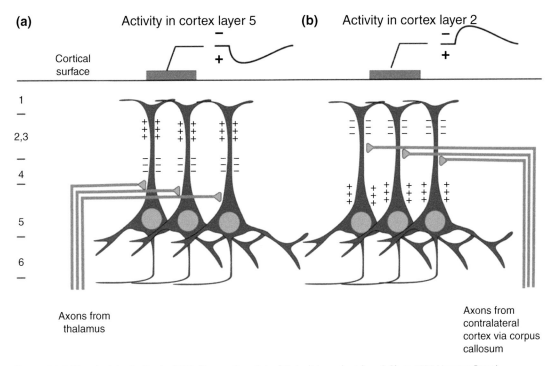

(a) Activity in cortex layer 5

(b) Activity in cortex layer 2

Cortical surface

1

2,3

4

5

6

Axons from thalamus

Axons from contralateral cortex via corpus callosum

Figure 36.1 The physiological basis of EEG. (Source: *Essentials of Clinical Neurophysiology*, S. Blum, 2007, Humana Press.)

thousands of aligned cortical pyramidal neurons, it is a relatively direct measure of regional neuronal – including synaptic – function (Figure 36.1). This is relevant for AD, where synaptic failure is considered to be one of the key features [7]. The high temporal resolution of EEG captures the relevant frequencies used in cognitive processing, mainly occurring within the millisecond range (1–45 Hz). Its spatial resolution on the other hand is relatively low (±6 cm² per electrode), and limited to cortical activity, although it is good to realize that oscillations are often generated by the reciprocal influence of cortical and subcortical structures such as the thalamus. Hippocampal activity is therefore hard to capture directly with scalp EEG, but is within reach using invasive EEG electrodes, or MEG with source reconstruction. The exact relationship between cellular AD pathophysiology and oscillatory EEG changes over time is certainly not fully elucidated yet, but with the help of translational and computational studies, our understanding is steadily improving [8]. It appears that in early-phase AD, amyloid-induced neuronal hyperexcitability disturbs the natural excitation/inhibition balance of neural circuits, leading to disrupted synchronization between distant neuronal assemblies, subsequently impairing cognitive processing. Excitotoxicity also leads to cell and synapse loss, destroying brain connectivity.

36.2.2   EEG Analysis

Despite the unclear exact relationship between cellular-level AD pathophysiology and the macro-scale EEG signal, from a century of dementia EEG research a robust pattern of brain activity changes in AD has emerged, which is useful for both research and clinical practice. In this chapter, we will focus on task-free© resting-state© EEG analysis, since this has produced the most robust results so far and does not require more challenging study paradigms in this cognitively impaired population.

36.2.2.1 Visual Analysis

Traditionally, EEG is evaluated visually by trained neurophysiologists. This has led to a considerable body of knowledge about brain activity abnormalities in various conditions, including AD. Today, visual inspection of the (digital) EEG is still a cornerstone of the clinical evaluation, but it is increasingly complemented by quantitative methods that can be found in nearly every EEG software package. The reason that visual inspection is still the standard is that neurophysiological data are noisy and filled with artifacts. An observed sharp wave can be a sign of epilepsy, but can also be an EKG artifact. The experienced eye can differentiate between the two by considering the context of the signal (e.g., spread to surrounding channels)

419

and by altering settings (e.g., different montages, filter settings). More relevant to AD, slowing of the posterior dominant rhythm is associated with cognitive decline, but can also just be a sign of drowsiness, which should already be corrected during the recording process by the EEG technician. In short, for optimal data acquisition, selection, and interpretation, visual inspection remains of vital importance.

36.2.2.2 Quantitative Analysis

Most EEG acquisition software packages offer quantitative analysis options, and they can also be found in independent, freely available programs like Matlab toolboxes or standalone applications. To obtain reliable results, appropriate data segment selection is required. For typical, good-quality resting-state© EEG, around 1–2 minutes (the exact length depends on the used sample frequency) of clean data is sufficient. Quantitative EEG outcome measures have been increasingly used over the previous years in AD trials [9]. To evaluate resting-state brain activity, several types of analysis can be employed:

36.2.2.3 Regional Oscillatory Activity: Spectral Analysis

The most established type of analysis is description of oscillatory power in the time–frequency domain for all relevant regions, or averaged over multiple regions. The power spectrum gives an impression of the oscillatory frequencies that can be observed in the data. These are usually binned in frequency bands, ranging from slow delta (0.5–4 Hz) and theta (4–8 Hz) activity, to fast alpha (8–13 Hz), beta (13–30 Hz), and gamma (30–45 Hz) activity. The relative share of these bands is expressed as "relative power," and gives a good impression of the regional neurophysiological performance of the subject. For AD, the dominant posterior peak frequency (around 10 Hz in healthy adults), and the relative theta and alpha power are the most informative measures.

36.2.2.4 Interregional Communication: Functional Connectivity

Clinical symptoms may be due, to a considerable extent, to disrupted communication between distributed brain areas, justifying a description of AD as a disconnection syndrome [10]. In addition to local oscillatory activity, communication between brain regions can be examined neurophysiologically by comparing EEG signals from different regions. Amplitude and phase-based coupling can be described with a large array of "functional connectivity" measures, and can demonstrate changes in interregional communication, which is known to deteriorate in AD. Functional connectivity can then also be compared to structural connectivity patterns, using for example diffusion tensor imaging. Reproducibility of EEG functional connectivity measures has shown to be acceptable [11].

36.2.2.5 System-Level Communication: Functional Network Analysis

When pairwise functional connectivity between regions has been described, a large-scale "functional network" can be assembled, and subsequently analyzed with modern network analysis tools. This recent development has shown that system-level activity patterns correlate to cognition, and can help to better understand the coordination of cognitive processes in the brain [12]. Like functional connectivity measures, network analysis has not yet produced stronger markers than the "traditional" spectral analysis measures, but at present can be included as exploratory, secondary outcome measures for further development.

The three main types of resting-state© EEG analysis are shown in Figure 36.2.

36.3 EEG Changes across the AD Spectrum

In the past decades, a large body of evidence has mounted, illustrating that, in AD, neurophysiological activity as assessed by human EEG shows changes in pre-dementia AD, progressing over time. Here, we provide a brief overview of oscillatory changes, starting with normal aging across the AD spectrum.

36.3.1 Normal Aging

Compared to the extensive EEG changes that occur in the earliest years of life, reflecting developmental processes in the brain, the EEG remains relatively stable after the age of 18. However, EEG changes do occur with normal aging, especially after the age of 60, and it is important to delineate these from the earliest signs of pathology. EEG changes with normal aging have been described extensively [13]. The physiological "posterior dominant rhythm" or "alpha rhythm" of awake, healthy adults

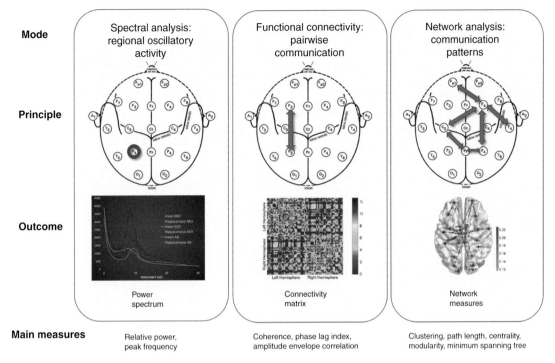

Figure 36.2 The three main types of resting-state© EEG analysis.

is characterized by prominent oscillatory activity in the frequency range of 8–13 Hz, a posterior temporal and parieto-occipital dominance, and a clear suppression to eye-opening ("reactivity"). The characteristics of the alpha rhythm, and in particular the alpha peak frequency, are very stable properties within a person and have a strong genetic basis. Several of these characteristics have been reported to change with normal aging, most notably the alpha peak frequency, relative power, and reactivity. However, even in the very old, the peak frequency is not expected to drop below 7.5–8 Hz. In a single subject, slowing of the alpha peak frequency over time by more than 1 Hz is also a sign of pathology. Focal abnormalities, especially in the anterior temporal areas, are quite prevalent, occurring in over one-third of subjects over 60 years, often with a preference for the left temporal areas. At present, it cannot be excluded that focal temporal theta and delta may be early biomarkers of temporal lobe dysfunction of neurodegenerative origin.

36.3.2 Subjective Cognitive Decline

EEG may predict future cognitive decline in subjects who have subjective cognitive decline (SCD), but do not fulfill criteria for mild cognitive impairment (MCI) [14]. Baseline EEG in 44 normal elderly subjects with subjective complaints was able to predict future cognitive decline during an impressive 7-year follow-up. Decliners were characterized by increased theta power, slowing of the mean frequency, and abnormal functional connectivity, especially in the right hemisphere in their baseline EEGs. These very early changes were confirmed in a more recent study, where an increase in delta and, again, particularly in theta power, as well as a decrease in peak frequency and alpha power, predicted cognitive decline [15].

36.3.3 Mild Cognitive Impairment

EEG changes in subjects with MCI compared to healthy elderly subjects have been described in many studies, indicating an increase in theta power and connectivity in MCI subjects compared to healthy controls. This increase is often interpreted as a compensatory reaction, but is more likely to be a sign of pathological hyperexcitation. An important question is whether the EEG changes in MCI predict conversion to dementia. Several studies have found that decreased alpha power and increased and more anterior-located theta power proved to be reliable predictors for conversion to AD [16, 17]. A significant association between temporal focal abnormalities and MCI has been reported, which suggests a link with hippocampal dysfunction, but this needs to be investigated further [18].

36.3.4 Alzheimer's Disease

There is general agreement that the EEG in AD is characterized by a relatively non-specific, stage-dependent pattern of diffuse slowing (Figure 36.3) [19]. In the earliest phase of the disease the EEG can be normal, especially in late-onset cases. After the theta power increase already mentioned in the SCD and MCI phases, power decreases in the beta and alpha band, and further increases in the theta and delta band. The alpha peak frequency decreases, and the reactivity of the alpha rhythm of eye-opening also diminishes. So, an increase in theta and decrease in beta power are probably the first and most sensitive EEG changes in AD. Multiple and/or extensive focal abnormalities are not typical, and may be related to the frequent occurrence of vascular pathology in AD. Epileptiform abnormalities are also rare, while AD is associated with a significantly increased risk of epilepsy, especially in early-onset and severe AD. Mortality in patients with early AD was predicted by a decrease in alpha and beta activity determined by spectral analysis of the EEG [20].

EEG abnormalities pointing to abnormal functional interactions between brain regions have been reported consistently in AD, showing patterns of reduced functional connectivity in AD [21]. Moving beyond pairwise interactions, in recent years studies of the dynamical processes in neural networks underlying the EEG in AD have reported a loss of structure, hierarchy, and complexity [22–24].

36.3.4.1 Diagnostic Accuracy

The diagnostic accuracy of EEG, based upon measures of EEG slowing or disturbed functional connectivity, fluctuates around 80% [3]. Although sensitivity to early changes is generally good, the typical diffuse EEG slowing is not very specific for AD, and no specific EEG phenomena are pathognomonic [25]. Novel machine-learning-based approaches, often combining multiple EEG-based measures, claim to improve classification performance quite spectacularly, but need further replication [26–28]. Nevertheless, we can conclude that the test characteristics of EEG do not compare unfavorably with those of some other biomarkers [29, 30]. In addition, it should be remembered that these results can be obtained with relatively simple, semi-quantitative visual assessment of the EEG [31].

36.3.5 Relation of EEG with Other AD Disease Markers

Apart from their diagnostic and prognostic value, EEG changes may shed light on the underlying

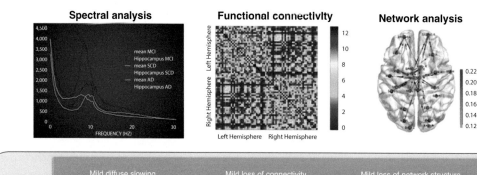

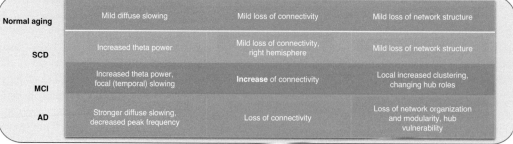

Figure 36.3 Main resting-state© EEG changes across the AD spectrum.

pathology that influences brain function and cognition in AD.

36.3.5.1 Cognitive Status and Disease Severity

As expected from the reported studies above, oscillatory slowing correlates with cognitive decline. The most consistent findings are the more anterior localization of alpha and beta rhythms, higher delta and theta power, and lower alpha band power and reactivity [3]. In addition, loss of functional connectivity in the fast frequencies relates to impaired performance on neuropsychological tests [32].

36.3.5.2 Metabolic Change

There is considerable evidence for a loss of central cholinergic function in AD. This cholinergic loss is presumably due to a loss of neurons in the nucleus basalis of Meynert, which projects to medial temporal and neocortical brain areas. In fact, the general slowing of the EEG in AD has been interpreted as mainly a cholinergic effect [33]. Therefore, we might expect that treatment with drugs that stimulate the central cholinergic system will reverse the EEG slowing, and that EEG changes might predict which patients will show the best response to cholinergic treatment; studies have confirmed these expectations [34, 35].

36.3.5.3 Structural Pathology

The relation between functional EEG changes and the underlying structural pathology is technically difficult to assess, and incompletely understood. While amyloid deposition is a hallmark of AD, not many studies have examined its relation to EEG. On the other hand, a correlation between abnormally phosphorylated tau protein in the cerebrospinal fluid and the alpha/delta ratio of the EEG was reported as early as 1988 [36]. Links between EEG and atrophy are consistent, where mainly a negative correlation between theta power and hippocampal volume has been observed [37]. The relation between apolipoprotein-E genotype and EEG phenomena is complex, and depends upon the study conditions, the EEG measure investigated, and the presence or absence of AD pathology [38].

36.4 Pharmaco-EEG in Clinical AD Trials

A modest number of randomized controlled trials have incorporated EEG-based measures as a secondary outcome marker. Various aspects of AD pathophysiology have been targeted in clinical trials with EEG as an outcome measure; here we present a representative selection.

36.4.1 Cholinesterase Inhibitors and N-methyl-D-aspartate Antagonists

The restorative effect of cholinesterase inhibitors on oscillatory activity in the EEG has been repeatedly demonstrated [39]. After a few weeks of treatment, delta (0.4–4 Hz) or theta (4–8 Hz) rhythms decrease, dominant alpha rhythms (8–13 Hz) increase. Beneficial effects are mainly found in "responders," that is, those with objective cognitive improvement. In contrast, only one study has explored the long-term effects of memantine, a non-competitive N-methyl-D-aspartate channel blocker, on resting-state$^{©}$ EEG in AD, showing a theta rhythm reduction.

36.4.2 Anti-Amyloid Drugs

Up till now, amyloid-targeting treatment strategies have shown disappointing clinical efficacy, despite massive effort. In the SAPHIR study, a randomized controlled trial in biomarker-supported AD patients on a 12-week regimen of PQ912, a glutaminyl cyclase inhibitor that blocks the formation of toxic amyloid oligomers, a significant reduction of theta power was observed [40]. Spectral analyses of the oscillatory EEG activity showed a difference in mean change in global relative theta power (4–8 Hz) in the PQ912 group compared to placebo in the intention to treat ($p = 0.002$, Cohen's $d = 0.29$), modified intention to treat ($p < 0.001$, $d = 0.32$), and per protocol ($p = 0.002$, $d = 0.37$) populations. Global functional connectivity and measures reflecting functional network topology did not show differences between treatment groups. However, a significant increase in the alpha band functional connectivity as assessed with the amplitude envelope correlation (AEC) was shown in the active group [41]. A significant increase in global AEC with leakage correction in the alpha frequency band was found with PQ912 treatment compared to placebo ($p = 0.004$, $d = 0.58$); see Figure 36.4. The effect remained significant when corrected for sex, country, apolipoprotein-E ε4 gene carriage, age, baseline value, and change in relative alpha power.

36.4.3 Nutritional Supplements

Resting-state functional connectivity improvements have been described in studies with the

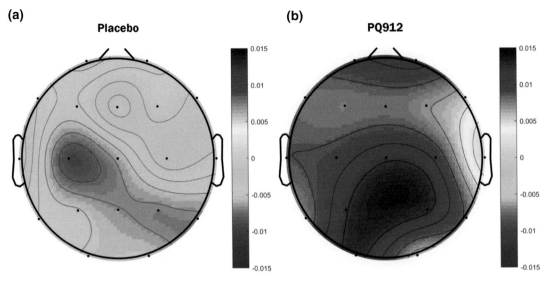

(a) Placebo **(b) PQ912**

Figure 36.4 Headplots of the observed change in AEC-c of the alpha band in the placebo group (a) and intervention group (b) in the PQ912 study. Red indicates an increase, green no change, and blue a decrease. The scales next to each plot represent which value corresponds with which color in the concurrent plot. The placebo group shows a global decrease with the lowest values in parietal areas, whereas the intervention group shows a global increase, which is predominant in the parietal areas. (For interpretation of the references to color in this figure legend, the reader is referred to the web version of this article.) (Source: https://doi.org/10.1016/j.clinph.2019.09.014.)

nutritional supplement Souvenaid®, consisting of higher delta band connectivity and more stable beta network measures in the active group, as opposed to a decline in the placebo group [42, 43].

To conclude, EEG has been used mainly in cholinesterase inhibitor trials, where oscillatory improvements go hand in hand with temporary cognitive improvement/stabilization. In the present, dominant, amyloid-targeting trials, far fewer applications of EEG have been reported, but the appreciation for EEG as measure of connectivity/synaptic function is growing. EEG outcomes have shown meaningful improvements when cognitive or other outcome measures did not. Overall, the reduction of resting-state theta (4–8 Hz) power seems to be the most robust result, confirming the pathological nature of this oscillatory change. More EEG-related results are expected to come out within the next few years, as several clinical AD trials that involve EEG outcome measures are underway.

36.5 Best Practices in Multi-center Trial EEG Analysis

When designing and conducting trials with EEG-based outcome measures, many practical choices can have a substantial effect on the reliability of the results. Here we offer various practical lessons learned from previous trials.

36.5.1 EEG Timing

When choosing EEG as outcome measure, there are many different options, as discussed above; resting-state, task-related, event-related potential, spectral measures, connectivity, and so on. What to choose? Although this does depend on the specific tested compound and expected mechanism of action, in general the acquisition of resting-state© EEG data is preferred. Resting-state, eyes-closed conditions produce robust oscillatory patterns that correlate with disease, and simplify the data acquisition process in these cognitively impaired patients.

The traditional visual analysis requires trained physicians, but is still the most important way to assure the data quality. Artifacts, drowsiness, or other unexpected conditions (signs of epilepsy or metabolic encephalopathy) should be identified, and automated detection algorithms (e.g., independent component analysis) are less reliable and involve arbitrary choices. Visual analysis also gives a first impression of the neurodegenerative abnormalities expected in AD (slowing of the posterior dominant rhythm).

Quantitative analysis should at least include spectral analysis (peak frequency, relative power in common frequency bands), since these are the most robust measures to capture AD. In early-phase, pre-clinical AD, theta power (4–8 Hz) is the most used marker. Spectral analysis is routinely performed by most clinics, and available in most software packages. Functional connectivity and network analysis are more advanced and experimental measures, for which specific expertise should be sought in an experienced research group. The specific choice of markers for a trial should be decided in advance, for example a batch consisting of the main spectral outcome measures, a solid functional connectivity measure, and, for more exploratory purposes, several network measures. With good data selection, the quantitative EEG analysis can be performed in a matter of days.

EEG timing of course depends on the expected compound mechanism, but commonly consists of a baseline EEG and one or two study EEGs at later time points, for example, halfway through and at the end of the study. For long-term effects, EEGs could also be repeated weeks to months after study termination. The baseline EEG should preferably be close to the randomization and study start data, but since the EEG quality has to be checked, an intermittent period of 1–2 weeks is optimal.

36.5.2 EEG Recording

Pharmacological AD trials usually involve multiple recruitment sites, such as hospitals or clinics. Since EEG is routinely performed and available in many neurological clinics, no new equipment or specific expertise is required. However, standardization of EEG recordings is necessary, as many different EEG machines with pre-set parameters are in use. Uniformity is achieved through the following precautions: thorough site instruction and technical support, a test phase in which sample EEG data are checked by the central analysis team, and the use of a common EEG data format to which all recordings must be converted.

Clinical neurophysiology technicians should work according to local standard operating procedures to obtain uniform EEG recordings with a minimum of artifacts. A clinical neurophysiologist/neurologist should preferably be responsible for the department, supervision of the technicians, and EEG recording procedures. For international guidelines of the International Federation of Clinical Neurophsiology (IFCN), please visit: www.clinph-journal.com/content/guidelinesIFCN. Participating sites should receive a detailed EEG site manual including all practical information, such as how to store and send the data. To ensure optimal quality during the study, EEG technicians should be present during the recording, and they should work with a standard operating procedure for the study. Data recording, conversion, and storage should be performed in the same manner and with the same equipment for the length of the study, preferably by the same people. To maximize data quality before study commencement, it is advisable to let every site provide a sample "dummy run" recording using the required study settings, to make sure that all sites can deliver data that can be combined for further analysis. This usually requires a few rounds of technical communication between the sites and EEG analysis center, but has a very positive impact on the data quality. Nonetheless, every study EEG should still be quality checked by the analysis team (within a few days). If the quality of an EEG is for some reason insufficient for analysis, it could then still be repeated within a 1–2-week time window without consequences. In practice, the need to re-record an EEG is rare: usually clean segments can be found in the data.

To obtain good-quality EEG data, there is no need for very elaborate, unusual set-ups or procedures. During the resting-state recording, no additional activities such as hyperventilation or flashlight stimulation are needed. At least 15 minutes of resting-state with alternated eyes-open and eyes-closed data is sufficient. The technical settings (e.g., channels, sample frequency, filter settings) required are also common, but should nevertheless be strictly adhered to. Preferably, all patients should be recorded on the same EEG system and all recording parameters should be kept unchanged across patients and visits! An alternative is to temporarily provide all participating sites with similar equipment and software, but this does require additional on-site training. Planning the EEGs in the morning when the patient is well rested helps to prevent drowsiness. A note of all current medication of the patient should be made, as drugs affecting the central nervous system (e.g., benzodiazepines, antipsychotics, antidepressants, and anti-epileptic drugs) can influence the EEG signals. During recording, the patient should

425

be in a supine position, as this position leads to less muscle artifacts than an upright position. The room should be illuminated but deprived of ambient noise. The technician should monitor the EEG recording and make all efforts to minimize artefacts and drowsiness during the recording. Note that these requirements are almost all standard EEG practice.

36.5.3   EEG Data Processing

EEG trial data should be exported in a convenient general format, and for multi-center trials a good standard file format is EDF or ASCII, since most systems will be able to convert the data to this format. Anonymized data should then be uploaded to a secure online data portal, along with a checklist of the used settings and other details of the recording. After the quality check, sites should receive timely confirmation of the data quality, or technical support to solve issues. When a study data set is complete, batch analysis of the desired outcome measures can be performed, before entering the final phase of statistical analysis to describe treatment effects.

36.6   Conclusion

The role of EEG in pharmacological AD trials is modest but growing. Practical benefits of EEG such as its non-invasiveness, widespread use, and cost-efficiency make EEG a suitable treatment-monitoring technique. The relative direct representation of neuronal and synaptic function is relevant for AD in both early and advanced stages. Empirical knowledge about AD-related neurophysiological changes can be summarized by a gradual diffuse oscillatory slowing (mainly posterior), coupled with a loss of functional connectivity and functional network topology. These changes start to happen early in the AD disease process, are sensitive to different types of treatment, and therefore may lead to the development of potent treatment-monitoring markers. At present, resting-state theta power (4–8 Hz) is the most robust marker of AD. Given the recent findings on the prominent role of early-phase abnormal neuronal excitability in AD, and recent improvements in non-pharmacological treatment options (e.g., deep brain stimulation, deep transcranial magnetic stimulation), accurately capturing neurophysiological change in AD becomes relevant from multiple angles. The

main challenges in using EEG for (multi-center) trials are reaching a consensus on most effective outcome measures, and obtaining consistent data quality [44].

Acknowledgments

The authors wish to express their gratitude to Dr. Alida Gouw for providing valuable comments on the content of this chapter.

References

1. Berger H. Über das Elektrenkephalogramm des Menschen. Dritte Mitteilung. *Arch Psychiatr Nervenkr* 1931; **94**: 16–60.

2. Berger H. Über das Elektrenkephalogramm des Menschen. Fünfte Mitteilung. *Arch Psychiatr Nervenkr* 1932; **98**: 231–54.

3. Babiloni C, Blinowska K, Bonanni L, et al. What electrophysiology tells us about Alzheimer's disease: a window into the synchronization and connectivity of brain neurons. *Neurobiol Aging* 2020; **85**: 58–73.

4. Palop JJ, Mucke L. Network abnormalities and interneuron dysfunction in Alzheimer disease. *Nat Rev Neurosci* 2016; **17**: 777–92.

5. Styr B, Slutsky I. Imbalance between firing homeostasis and synaptic plasticity drives early-phase Alzheimer's disease. *Nat Neurosci* 2018; **21**: 463–73.

6. Canter RG, Penney J, Tsai LH. The road to restoring neural circuits for the treatment of Alzheimer's disease. *Nature* 2016; **539**: 187–96.

7. Selkoe DJ. Alzheimer's disease is a synaptic failure. *Science* 2002; **298**: 789–91.

8. D'Amelio M, Rossini PM. Brain excitability and connectivity of neuronal assemblies in Alzheimer's disease: from animal models to human findings. *Prog Neurobiol* 2012; **99**: 42–60.

9. van Straaten EC, Scheltens P, Gouw AA, Stam CJ. Eyes-closed task-free electroencephalography in clinical trials for Alzheimer's disease: an emerging method based upon brain dynamics. *Alzheimers Res Ther* 2014; **6**: 86.

10. Delbeuck X, Van der Linder M, Colette F. Alzheimer's disease as a disconnection syndrome? *Neuropyschol Rev* 2003; **13**: 79–92.

11. Briels CT, Schoonhoven DN, Stam CJ, et al. Reproducibility of EEG functional connectivity in Alzheimer's disease. *Alzheimers Res Ther* 2020; **12**: 68.

12. Stam CV, Van Straaten ECW. The organization of physiological brain networks. *Clin Neurophysiol* 2012; **123**: 1067–87.

13. Rossini PM, Rossi S, Babiloni C, Polich J. Clinical neurophysiology of aging brain: from normal aging to neurodegeneration. *Prog Neurobiol* 2007; **83**: 375–400.

14. Prichep LS, John ER, Ferris SH, et al. Prediction of longitudinal cognitive decline in normal elderly with subjective complaints using electrophysiological imaging. *Neurobiol Aging* 2006; **27**: 471–81.

15. Gouw AA, Alsema AM, Tijms BM, et al. EEG spectral analysis as a putative early prognostic biomarker in nondemented, amyloid positive subjects. *Neurobiol Aging* 2017; **57**: 133–42.

16. Jelic V, Johansson S-E, Almkvist O, et al. Quantitative electroencephalography in mild cognitve impairment: longitudinal changes and possible prediction of Alzheimer's disease. *Neurobiol Aging* 2000; **21**: 533–40.

17. van der Hiele K, Bollen EL, Vein AA, et al. EEG markers of future cognitive performance in the elderly. *J Clin Neurophysiol* 2008; **25**: 83–9.

18. Liedorp M, van der Flier WM, Hoogervorst EL, Scheltens P, Stam CJ. Associations between patterns of EEG abnormalities and diagnosis in a large memory clinic cohort. *Dement Geriatr Cogn Disord* 2008; **27**: 18–23.

19. Jeong J. EEG dynamics in patients with Alzheimer's disease. *Clin Neurophysiol* 2004; **115**: 1490–505.

20. Claus JJ, Ongerboer de Visser BW, Walstra GJM, et al. Quantitative spectral electroencephalography in predicting survival in patients with early Alzheimer disease. *Arch Neurol* 1998; **55**: 1105–11.

21. Stam CJ. Nonlinear dynamical analysis of EEG and MEG: review of an emerging field. *Clin Neurophysiol* 2005; **116**: 2266–301.

22. Stam CJ. Modern network science of neurological disorders. *Nat Rev Neurosci* 2014; **15**: 683–95.

23. Stam CJ, Jones BF, Nolte G, Breakspear M, Scheltens P. Small-world networks and functional connectivity in Alzheimer's disease. *Cereb Cortex* 2007; **17**: 92–9.

24. Sun J, Wang B, Niu Y, et al. Complexity analysis of EEG, MEG, and fMRI in mild cognitive impairment and Alzheimer's disease: a review. *Entropy* 2020; **22**: 239.

25. Dauwels J, Vialatte F, Cichocki A. Diagnosis of Alzheimer's disease from EEG signals: where are we standing? *Curr Alzheimer Res* 2010; **7**: 487–505.

26. Simpraga S, Alvarez-Jimenez R, Mansvelder HD, et al. EEG machine learning for accurate detection of cholinergic intervention and Alzheimer's disease. *Sci Rep* 2017; **7**: 1–11.

27. Vecchio F, Miraglia F, Alù F, et al. Classification of Alzheimer's disease with respect to physiological aging with innovative EEG biomarkers in a machine learning implementation. *J Alzheimers Dis* 2020; **75**: 1253–61.

28. Dauwan M, van der Zande JJ, van Dellen E, et al. Random forest to differentiate dementia with Lewy bodies from Alzheimer's disease. *Alzheimers Dement (Amst)* 2016; **4**: 99–106.

29. Van der Flier WM, Scheltens P. Use of laboratory and imaging investigations in dementia. *J Neurol Neurosurg Psychiatry* 2005; **76**: v45–52.

30. Drago V, Babiloni C, Bartrés-Faz D, et al. Disease tracking markers for Alzheimer's disease at the prodromal (MCI) stage. *J Alzheimers Dis* 2011; **26**: 159–99.

31. Rossini PM, Di Iorio R, Vecchio F, et al. Early diagnosis of Alzheimer's disease: the role of biomarkers including advanced EEG signal analysis. Report from the IFCN-sponsored panel of experts. *Clin Neurophysiol* 2020; **131**: 1287–310.

32. Stam CJ, van der Made Y, Pijnenburg YAL, Scheltens Ph. EEG synchronization in mild cognitive impairment and Alzheimer's disease. *Acta Neurol Scand* 2003; **108**: 90–6.

33. Riekkinen P, Buzsaki G, Riekkinen P Jr., Soininen H, Partanen J. The cholinergic system and EEG slow waves. *Electroenceph Clin Neurophysiol* 1991; **78**: 89–96.

34. Babiloni C, Cassetta E, Dal Forno G, et al. Donepezil effects on sources of cortical rhythms in mild Alzheimer's disease: responders vs. non-responders. *Neuroimage* 2006; **31**: 1650–65.

35. Adler G, Brassen S, Chwalek K, Dieter B, Teufel M. Prediction of treatment response to rivastigmine in Alzheimer's dementia. *J Neurol Neurosurg Psychiatry* 2004; **75**: 292–4.

36. Jelic V, Blomberg M, Dierks T, et al. EEG slowing and cerebrospinal fluid tau levels in patients with cognitive decline. *Neuroreport* 1988; **9**: 157–60.

37. Grunwald M, Hensel A, Wolf H, Weiss T, Gertz HJ. Does the hippocampal atrophy correlate with the cortical theta power in elderly subjects with a range of cognitive impairment? *J Clin Neurophysiol* 2007; **24**: 22–6.

38. Ponomareva NV, Korovaitseva GI, Rogaev EI. EEG alterations in non-demented individuals related to apolipoprotein E genotype and to risk of Alzheimer disease. *Neurobiol Aging* 2008; **29**: 819–27.

39. Babiloni C, Del Percio C, Bordet R, et al. Effects of acetylcholinesterase inhibitors and memantine on resting-state electroencephalographic rhythms in Alzheimer's disease patients. *Clin Neurophysiol* 2013; **124**: 837–50.

40. Scheltens P, Hallikainen M, Grimmer T, et al. Safety, tolerability and efficacy of the glutaminyl cyclase inhibitor PQ912 in Alzheimer's

disease: results of a randomized, double-blind, placebo-controlled Phase 2a study. *Alzheimers Res Ther* 2018; **10**: 107.

41. Briels CT, Stam CJ, Scheltens P, et al. In pursuit of a sensitive EEG functional connectivity outcome measure for clinical trials in Alzheimer's disease. *Clin Neurophysiol* 2020; **131**: 88–95.

42. de Waal H, Stam CJ, Lansbergen MM, et al. The effect of Souvenaid on functional brain network organisation in patients with mild Alzheimer's

disease: a randomised controlled study. *PLoS One* 2014; **9**: e86558.

43. Scheltens P, Twisk JW, Blesa R, et al. Efficacy of Souvenaid in mild Alzheimer's disease: results from a randomized, controlled trial. *J Alzheimers Dis* 2012; **31**: 225–36.

44. Cassani R, Estarellas M, San-Martin R, Fraga FJ, Falk TH. Systematic review on resting-state EEG for Alzheimer's disease diagnosis and progression assessment. *Dis Markers* 2018; **2018**: 5174815.

Chapter

37

Institutional Review Boards and Oversight of Alzheimer's Disease Trials

Emily A. Largent and Joshua Grill

37.1   Introduction

Clinical research and care have long been considered distinct activities. Central to the research/care distinction is the idea that the purpose of research – the creation of generalizable knowledge to benefit future patients – is fundamentally different than the purpose of clinical care – the delivery of personalized therapy to benefit the current patient. Other defining characteristics of research will be readily familiar to those involved in trials of novel interventions to prevent or treat Alzheimer's disease (AD). These include methodologies such as randomization, blinding, and use of placebo controls that would be anathema in care because they sacrifice personalization of care to the pursuit of scientific validity and methodological rigor. Employment of such methods, as well as the inclusion of procedures that offer no prospect of direct medical benefit to participants, is justified by the pursuit of socially valuable information – such as a disease-modifying therapy for AD [1]. Although trial participants may receive excellent care in the course of their research participation, the fact is that there are often aspects of research participation that are not in the participants' best interests.

Due to the differences between them, clinical research and care are governed by distinct ethical and regulatory frameworks. While there are many facets to these frameworks, the focus of this chapter is the requirement for an independent review of research. Research participants' needs and interests may be in tension with the needs and interests of the investigators or sponsors who conduct AD trials and other research. Investigators "inherently have multiple, legitimate interests – interests to conduct high-quality research, complete the research expeditiously, protect research subjects, obtain funding, and advance their careers" [2]. However thoughtful and well-intentioned investigators are, their multiplicity of interests can

generate conflicts and may result in an inability to objectively reflect on their own studies. Therefore, investigators may need someone unaffiliated with their study to "check their work" and to ensure that they comply with ethical and regulatory standards for human subjects research.

Independent review is intended to offer an impartial assessment of proposed research and is, therefore, considered a requirement of ethical research [2]. Done well, independent review ensures that the research is socially valuable and scientifically rigorous, that ethical principles are followed, and that adequate and appropriate safeguards are in place to protect the rights and welfare of participants. Independent review also serves as a check on investigators – for instance, by checking their qualifications to conduct and supervise AD trials or by scrutinizing conflicts of interest (COIs).

In the United States, institutional review boards (IRBs) occupy a crucial independent oversight role and are, therefore, a familiar part of the AD research landscape. IRB is a generic term used to refer to an appropriately constituted group that has been formally designated to review and to monitor human subjects research. An IRB has authority to approve, require modifications to, or disapprove study protocols. Thus, IRB review serves an important role in protecting the rights and welfare of research participants. Review by an IRB is required for human subjects research funded by US government agencies (as outlined by the United States Department of Health and Human Services Code of Federal Regulations [CFR] regulation 45 CFR 46), as well as for clinical investigations of interventions – such as drugs, biologics, and devices – under the jurisdiction of the US Food and Drug Administration (FDA) (21 CFR 56). Institutions engaged in federally funded human subjects research must formalize their commitment to protecting human subjects and to complying with the requirements set forth at 45

CFR 46. In addition, they may voluntarily extend this commitment to cover all of the human subjects research conducted under their auspices, regardless of the source of support, for their own compliance purposes. Thus, IRB review may be necessary to satisfy ethical, regulatory, and institutional oversight requirements regardless of the funding source or the nature of the intervention.

In this chapter, we first look at the composition and role of IRBs. Next, we consider how to manage COIs. Finally, we highlight a number of ethical issues that IRBs might confront when reviewing AD trials.

37.2 Composition and Role of Institutional Review Boards

The term "institutional review board" was introduced in 1974 [3]. At that time, single-site research was the norm. Yet, in the intervening decades, the research enterprise has changed significantly. There has been a growth in public and private spending on research. The majority of trials are now multi-site, and many are multinational. Moreover, science is evolving. These trends are all readily apparent in AD research, as in research more broadly.

In light of these trends, "the number of, investment in, and responsibilities of IRBs have continued to increase" [3]. Additionally, concern about the bureaucracy, expansive role, and questionable efficacy of IRBs has grown.

37.2.1 Types of IRBs

As noted previously, IRB is a generic term used to refer to a group that has been formally designated to review and monitor human subjects research. In discussions, people may refer more specifically to local, independent, or single IRBs. These terms refer to different models of IRB oversight. There is an ongoing debate over which model is best; here, we briefly identify relevant considerations.

A *local IRB* is the IRB established by an institution – for example, at research universities, academic medical centers, and healthcare institutions – for the purpose of reviewing research conducted at the institution or with institutional support. A purported strength of local IRB review is that the IRB is well positioned to provide meaningful consideration of various local factors in assessing research activities. These might include the cultural backgrounds of prospective subjects, community attitudes about research, and the

institutional and investigator capacity to conduct or support a proposed study. A weakness is that local variation can result in slow and inconsistent reviews [4, 5]. This can impede research, add expense, and introduce delays – particularly in multi-center trials [6]. There is also concern that local IRBs may lack objectivity about research that brings their institution funding and prestige. Moreover, local IRBs may be "more concerned with protection of the institution than the protection of human research participants" [7].

Independent IRBs are not owned or operated by the organizations for which they provide oversight. Rather, an independent IRB conducts reviews on behalf of many different investigators, institutions, and organizations. Independent IRBs are subject to the same regulatory requirements applicable to all IRBs, and a significant percentage are accredited by the Association for the Accreditation of Human Research Protection Programs, a non-profit accrediting program. Independent IRBs are not necessarily commercial IRBs. For example, the National Cancer Institute (NCI) has a Central Institutional Review Board that serves institutions across the country that are conducting NCI-sponsored research.

Nevertheless, independent IRBs often are also *commercial IRBs* that receive payment for their services. Opponents of this model worry that for-profit IRBs are prone to the conflicts inherent in being paid. For example, will they approve a study in order to please their customers and keep them coming back [8–10]? There is also a concern that, when investigators use IRBs not affiliated with their own institution, they may "shop around" for approval. At the same time, independent IRBs might do a better job on average than local IRBs because they have the resources to do high-quality, responsive, expert reviews or because their paid business model demands high-quality work. They also eliminate redundancy when applied to multi-site studies. Unfortunately, data comparing the performance of independent IRBs and local IRBs are not readily available.

As of January 2018, the National Institutes of Health (NIH) has required that all sites participating in multi-site studies involving non-exempt human subjects research funded by the NIH use a *single IRB* (sIRB) to conduct the ethical review required for the protection of human subjects (81 FR 40325). Under the NIH sIRB policy, all local research sites rely on the approval and oversight of the sIRB of record, rather than conducting their own reviews (though nothing in the policy prohibits sites from duplicating the sIRB). The NIH policy is consistent with the revised Common Rule, which requires sIRB review for all covered research (45 CFR 46.114). A chief goal of sIRB requirements is to eliminate duplicative IRB review and reduce unnecessary administrative burdens without diminishing human subjects protections; however, some individuals have expressed concerns that sIRB review will itself raise additional administrative burdens as sites determine how best to work together. It is worth noting that sIRBs can be local or independent.

37.2.2 Membership

IRB composition is generally dictated by the relevant research regulations. For instance, Under the Federal Policy for the Protection of Human Subjects (or "Common Rule") an IRB must have "at least five members, with varying backgrounds to promote complete and adequate review of research activities commonly conducted by the institution" (45 CFR 46.107). Additionally, the Common Rule requires that IRBs include "at least one member whose primary concerns are in scientific areas and at least one member whose primary concerns are in nonscientific areas," as well as "at least one member who is not otherwise affiliated with the institution." IRBs often combine the roles of non-scientific and non-affiliated member and call the individual in this joint role the "community member." The perspectives of community members should be valued because, ideally, they reflect the views and concerns of potential research participants [11].

Collectively, the members of an IRB should be qualified to review the scientific, clinical, and ethical aspects of research. The members should also be diverse. Diversity of race, gender, and cultural backgrounds introduces multiple perspectives to the review process and promotes complete evaluation of research activities. Ideally, the combination of competence and diversity fosters investigators' respect and society's trust.

37.2.3 Scope of Review

IRBs act as gatekeepers. They review study protocols and related materials – such as informed consent documents and recruitment materials – to ensure the adequacy of human subject protections.

Initial review and approval of a study protocol, before a study is initiated, is followed by ongoing review and monitoring of research activities. In addition, "IRBs are often responsible for review of scientific merit, conflicts of interest, and compliance with privacy regulations," though other committees or bodies may be convened to fill these important roles [12]. We discuss COIs at greater length below.

37.2.4 IRB Efficacy

Research activities undergo independent review in order to protect human subjects. It remains unclear, however, whether – and if so, to what extent – IRBs achieve this goal. A frequent critique of IRBs is that they focus their attention on completing paperwork and ensuring bureaucratic compliance at the expense of thoughtful review. Thus, the system has been criticized for "simultaneous overregulation and underprotection" [13]. At present, it is unclear to what extent IRBs actually protect research participants, or how we would measure whether they do so [12, 14, 15]. This is an area where further work is needed.

37.3 Conflicts of Interest

As noted in the introduction, investigators can have a multiplicity of interests. While their primary professional interest is in creating generalizable knowledge, they can have many secondary interests, such as obtaining funding, publishing, gaining prestige, and advancing their careers. COIs arise in situations in which an investigator's "professional judgment concerning a primary interest is at risk of being biased by a secondary interest, resulting in possible harm to … the integrity of research" [16]. On this understanding, there are no *potential* or *perceived* COIs. Rather, "A COI describes a situation in which there is a risk of bias and resulting harm, not a situation in which bias or harm necessarily occurs. Thus, a situation marked by risk of bias from a secondary interest is no less a COI because it does not result in bias or harm" [16]. Although secondary interests can be financial or non-financial, attention is often focused on financial interests.

COIs are worrisome "because of their potential effect on the quality, outcome, and dissemination of research, as well as their effects on the public's perception of and trust in researchers and universities" [17]. These concerns may be heightened in the

431

context of clinical trials both due to the increasing complexity and frequency of academic–industry ties as well as evidence suggesting that COIs may negatively affect the quality of clinical studies and also the ethical obligation to protect research participants [18].

37.3.1 Strategies for Managing Conflicts of Interest

Conflict management can take the form of disclosure and peer review or, in some cases, prohibition of the arrangement or activity [19]. Here, we provide a high-level overview of key stakeholders and strategies they might employ to manage COIs.

Investigators. Investigators should disclose their financial and non-financial COIs – including but not limited to grant funding, personal financial payments, intellectual property (IP), or stock – in a consistent, transparent manner. A challenge, of course, is that individuals may not always agree that a particular relationship creates a COI. Thus, it is better to err on the side of disclosing too much than too little – whether in publications, in presentations, or to other stakeholders. Additionally, investigators should avoid entering agreements that impede their access to relevant data, interfere with their ability to analyze or interpret data, or that inhibit their independent preparation and publication of manuscripts [20].

Funders. Some funders have policies regarding COIs. For instance, the NIH requires that institutions seeking or receiving NIH funding have a written, enforced policy for identifying and managing financial COIs. The NIH Director, Francis Collins, has observed that managing financial COIs in biomedical research "can prove to be a major challenge because of the complex relationships among government, academia, and industry. Partnerships between NIH-funded researchers and industry are often essential to the process of moving discoveries from the bench to the bedside" [21].

Academic Institutions. Academic institutions have heterogeneous policies for disclosing, reviewing, and managing COIs [17]. Whereas some institutions require disclosure by all faculty members, others require disclosure only from individuals engaged in research, for instance, as a principal investigator. Institutional strategies for managing disclosed COIs might include oversight of research activities or divestiture of financial interests. Because approximately one-third of life sciences

faculty engage in industry consulting, institutions may also review consulting agreements on an optional or a mandatory basis [22, 23].

Institutional Review Boards. Many, though not all, academic institutions inform their local IRB of known COIs [24]. Additionally, IRBs may have distinct strategies for managing COIs. For instance, an IRB may ask if the principal investigator has interests related to the study. If the answer is "yes," this will generally need to be disclosed to prospective participants as part of the recruitment and informed consent process. IRB members may also have financial ties to industry that constitute COIs [25]. Therefore, IRB members should determine whether a particular role, relationship, or other interest could constitute a COI for a particular protocol, and manage their own conflict as appropriate.

Journals. Journals encourage authors to provide a "complete and broad disclosure," allowing readers to decide for themselves whether there is a COI relevant to their assessment of an article [26]. Similarly, editors and peer reviewers have a responsibility to disclose their own COIs and to recuse themselves as appropriate [20].

37.3.2 Managing Conflicts in AD Trials

Within the AD research community, there are multiple examples of how to deal with COIs. The Alzheimer's Disease Cooperative Study (ADCS) was formed in 1991 as part of National Institute on Aging (NIA) efforts to facilitate discovery, development, and testing of new drugs for the treatment of AD. The ADCS Internal Ethics Committee has a "Disclosure and Conflict of Interest Management Policy" that was first adopted in 2000, though it has subsequently been revised. The policy acknowledges the increasing number of relationships between academic investigators and industry while also seeking to ensure that ADCS research is not compromised by these relationships. The policy requires regular disclosure of financial interests and relationships, stock and ownership interests, and intellectual property interests for the individual ADCS members and their first-degree relatives. The Internal Ethics Committee monitors compliance with the policy and, in situations where COIs arise, works with the ADCS member to clarify, modify, or eliminate the COI. The policy also requires disclosure of relevant information in ADCS publications. A similar policy has been adopted for the recently funded AD Clinical Trials Consortium.

37.4 Other Ethical Considerations for AD Drug Development

When reviewing research, there are a number of other ethical issues of which IRBs must be mindful; here, we consider three that are of particular relevance to AD trials.

37.4.1 Capacity and Consent

Informed consent is widely recognized as an ethical and regulatory requirement in human subjects research. Yet, as a matter of scientific necessity, some AD trials enroll adults who lack capacity to grant informed consent from the outset. Participants also may have capacity at the time of enrollment only to have it erode as the trial progresses. Thus, investigators must have – and IRBs must review – a plan for assessing capacity and securing valid informed consent.

Capacity is the task-specific ability to make a sufficiently informed decision [27]. It encompasses a combination of decisional abilities, including the ability to understand, appreciate, and rationally manipulate information and to communicate a consistent decision. An individual's cognition or diagnoses can be proxies for capacity, but they are not the same thing as capacity. Tests that measure overall cognition, such as the Mini-Mental State Examination or the Montreal Cognitive Assessment, may be useful to predict the likelihood that a person will have diminished capacity, but these tests cannot substitute for an assessment of decisional abilities. Similarly, a diagnosis or label such as "dementia" is, by itself, insufficient grounds for concluding that an individual has diminished capacity.

How then, might investigators assess capacity? A common strategy is to disclose key facts about a study and then assess through conversation whether the prospective participant understands that information. For example, the prospective participant might then be asked to "teach back," or explain in their own words, what was disclosed about the purpose of the study, how participation will or will not benefit them, or how participation in the study will affect their daily life. The accuracy of the prospective participant's answers informs the final determination of capacity or incapacity.

Some structured tools are also available for capacity assessment [28, 29].

Adults with capacity are empowered decision makers. One way that we respect the autonomy of adults with capacity is by seeking their informed consent. The consent process allows them to decide for themselves if participation in a particular study is consistent with their preferences, values, and interests. When adults lack the capacity to make their own research-related decisions, others must make decisions on their behalf. These individuals are often referred to as *surrogate decision makers*. Yet, even if an adult lacks decisional capacity, they may retain one or more of its constituent abilities – understanding, appreciation, reasoning, and evincing a choice – to a meaningful extent. As a result, there may be strategies short of consent – sometimes called "partial-involvement strategies" – that investigators can employ. *Assent*, perhaps the most well-known partial-involvement strategy, has been defined as "the agreement to participate in research based on less than full understanding" [30]. The goal of assent is to provide a prospective participant with information and to allow them to determine whether they want to participate in a particular study [31]. To give assent, a prospective participant should have at least a minimal level of understanding of what participation entails and also the ability to express a choice. Assent should generally be paired with consent from the appropriate surrogate decision maker. *Dissent*, which can be verbal or non-verbal, is an objection to research participation. Generally, individuals don't have to demonstrate any understanding of a study for their dissent to be respected. Seeking assent and allowing for dissent are means of involving individuals with diminished capacity in research-related decision making and demonstrating respect for them as persons. These concepts can, however, be somewhat vague, and investigators should indicate to the IRB what standards they will use when making such assessments [32].

37.4.2 Dual-Role Consent

In large, multi-site AD trials, individuals will often be recruited from a clinical population. Site investigators may also be clinicians who have pre-existing relationships with prospective research participants. Classic statements of research ethics advise against permitting physician-investigators to obtain consent for study participation from patients with whom they have a pre-existing treatment relationship, though US human subjects research regulations do not prohibit it [33]. Rather, IRBs are encouraged to use their discretion.

Reticence about "dual-role" consent reflects the view, outlined in the introduction, that clinical research and care are normatively different. These normative differences extend to the nature of the physician–patient as compared to the investigator–participant relationship. There is concern that allowing dual-role consent – and blurring the boundary between clinical research and care – could lead to ethical transgressions. Concerns that patients could feel obligated to participate in studies for which their physician is also the investigator predominate. Yet, while this fear seems reasonable, empirical evidence also suggests that at least some patients prefer to discuss research participation with their treating physician [34, 35].

Thus, investigators and IRBs need to consider the appropriateness of dual-role consent in AD research. For example, IRBs might condition their approval of dual-role consent on identifying someone other than the treating physician with whom the patient can discuss the trial, allowing patients not to make an immediate decision, and having a research team member other than the treating physician obtain the patient's signature on the informed consent document. Notably, a team-based approach, reflective of both the clinical context and research practice, will often have ethical advantages and may be ethically necessary, depending on trial features.

37.4.3   Early Trial Closure

Early trial closure has, unfortunately, been a common occurrence in AD drug development. In 2019, Roche discontinued Phase 3 studies of crenezumab; Merck terminated its Phase 3 trial of verubecestat; Novartis, Amgen, and the Banner Alzheimer's Institute discontinued Phase 2/3 studies of umibecestat; and Eisai and Biogen halted Phase 3 studies of both aducanumab and elenbecestat. These trials were stopped early after interim analyses suggested that the potential benefits of proceeding no longer outweighed the risks, due either to futility or safety concerns. (We note, however, that aducanumab was subsequently approved by the FDA.)

The decision to stop an AD trial – or any trial – early because of futility or harm is complex and requires weighing statistical and ethical considerations. It also highlights the critical independent oversight role of data safety monitoring boards (DSMBs). Statistical stopping guidelines – pre-specified rules about what results would trigger a recommendation to stop the trial – can serve as objective guidelines for DSMB decisions. However, they must be carefully designed at the outset to account for the possibility of harm and also to guard against too readily consigning potentially promising drugs to the rubbish bin. A crucial challenge is to balance the well-being of individual participants enrolled in the trial with the broader social interest in generating reliable data for the benefit of future patients. In the context of AD, there is a critical need for effective disease-modifying therapies. If a trial is erroneously stopped early, a potentially valuable treatment may be lost. If a trial continues too long, participants may be adversely affected.

Once the extraordinarily difficult decision to stop a trial early is reached, there are numerous logistical challenges. An entire infrastructure has been built over years to advance the trial and, in a moment, it must grind to a halt. Chief among the logistical challenges is the rapid notification of hundreds or even thousands of trial participants [36]. Questions about how best to communicate with and offer support to research participants after trials stop early have recently attracted increased attention. Strategies might include addressing the potential for a trial to stop early in informed consent documents, working with IRBs to speed notification so that participants learn their trial has stopped from the site rather than via the news or social media, making information about DSMBs and stopping rules readily available to participants, working to connect participants to services and supports, and improving post-trial communication [36, 37].

37.5   Conclusion

AD trials are critically important. Conducting them well requires careful attention to ethical and regulatory issues. IRBs fill a necessary role by providing independent oversight; IRBs must attend to the relevant human subjects research regulations and must also be mindful of issues such as COIs, capacity, and consent. Ensuring that AD trials are conducted in accordance with ethical principles and regulatory requirements allows investigators, sponsors, regulatory authorities, persons with AD, their care partners – and ultimately society – to have confidence in the results of AD trials.

References

1. Largent EA, Joffe S, Miller FG. Can research and care be ethically integrated? *Hastings Cent Rep* 2011; **41**: 37–46.

2. Emanuel EJ, Wendler D, Grady C. What makes clinical research ethical? *JAMA* 2000; **283**: 2701–11.

3. Grady C. Institutional review boards: purposes and challenges. *Chest* 2015; **148**: 1148–55.

4. Silverman H, Hull SC, Sugarman J. Variability among institutional review boards' decisions within the context of a multicenter trial. *Crit Care Med* 2001; **29**: 235–41.

5. Hirshon JM. Variability in institutional review board assessment of minimal-risk research. *Acad Emerg Med* 2002; **9**: 1417–20.

6. Cummings J, Aisen PS, DuBois B, et al. Drug development in Alzheimer's disease: the path to 2025. *Alzheimers Res Ther* 2016; **8**: 39.

7. Fost N, Levine RJ. The dysregulation of human subjects research. *JAMA* 2007; **298**: 2196.

8. Lynch HF, Rosenfeld S. Institutional review board quality, private equity, and promoting ethical human subjects research. *Ann Intern Med* 2020; **173**: 558–62.

9. Emanuel EJ, Lemmens T, Elliot C. Should society allow research ethics boards to be run as for-profit enterprises? *PLoS Med* 2006; **3**: e309.

10. Lemmens T, Freedman B. Ethics review for sale? Conflict of interest and commercial research review boards. *Milbank Q* 2000; **78**: 547–84.

11. Klitzman R. Institutional review board community members: who are they, what do they do, and whom do they represent? *Acad Med* 2012; **87**: 975–81.

12. Grady C. Do IRBs protect human research participants? *JAMA* 2010; **304**: 1122–3.

13. Gunsalus CK. Mission Creep in the IRB World. *Science* 2006; **312**: 1441.

14. Lynch HF, Nicholls SG, Meyer M, Taylor HA. Of parachutes and participant protection: moving beyond quality to advance effective research ethics oversight. *J Empir Res Hum Res Ethics* 2019; **14**:190–6.

15. Tsan M-F. Measuring the quality and performance of institutional review boards. *J Empir Res Hum Res Ethics* 2019; **14**: 187–9.

16. McCoy MS, Emanuel EJ. Why there are no "potential" conflicts of interest. *JAMA* 2017; **317**: 1721–2.

17. Cho MK, Ryo S, Schissel A, Drummond R. Policies on faculty conflicts of interest at US universities. *JAMA* 2000; **284**: 2203.

18. Ahn R, Woodbridge A, Abraham A, et al. Financial ties of principal investigators and randomized controlled trial outcomes: cross sectional study. *BMJ* 2017; **356**: i6770.

19. Institute of Medicine. *Patient Outcomes Research Teams (PORTS): Managing Conflict of Interest*. Washington, DC: The National Academies Press; 1981.

20. International Committe of Medical Journal Editors. Disclosure of financial and non-financial relationships and activities, and conflicts of interest. Available at: www.icmje.org/recommendations/ browse/roles-and-responsibilities/author-responsibilities--conflicts-of-interest.html (accessed November 22, 2020).

21. Rockey SJ. Managing financial conflict of interest in biomedical research. *JAMA* 2010; **303**: 2400.

22. Morain SR, Joffe S, Campbell EG, Mello MM. Institutional oversight of faculty–industry consulting relationships in U.S. medical schools: a Delphi study. *J Law Med Ethics* 2015; **43**: 383–96.

23. Mello MM, Murtagh L, Joffe S. Beyond financial conflicts of interest: institutional oversight of faculty consulting agreements at schools of medicine and public health. *PLoS One* 2018; **13**: e0203179.

24. Ehringhaus SH. Responses of medical schools to institutional conflicts of interest. *JAMA* 2008; **299**: 665.

25. Campbell EG, Weissman JS, Vogeli C. Financial relationships between institutional review board members and industry. *N Engl J Med* 2006; **355**: 2321–9.

26. Bauchner H, Fontanarosa PB, Flanagin A. Conflicts of interests, authors, and journals: new challenges for a persistent problem. *JAMA* 2018; **320**: 2315.

27. Appelbaum PS. Assessment of patients' competence to consent to treatment. *N Engl J Med* 2007; **357**: 1834–40.

28. Jeste DV, Palmer BW, Appelbaum PS. A new brief instrument for assessing decisional capacity for clinical research. *Arch Gen Psychiatry* 2007; **64**: 966.

29. Dunn LB, Nowrangi MA, Palmer BW, Jeste DV, Saks ER. Assessing decisional capacity for clinical research or treatment: a review of instruments. *Am J Psychiatry* 2006; **163**: 1323–34.

30. Keyserlingk EW, Glass K, Kogan S, Gauthier S. Proposed guidelines for the participation of persons with dementia as research subjects. *Perspect Biol Med* 1995; **38**: 319–61.

31. Black BS, Rabins PV, Sugarman J, Karlawish JH. Seeking assent and respecting dissent in dementia research. *Am J Geriatr Psychiatry* 2010; **18**: 77–85.

32. Karlawish J. Research involving cognitively impaired adults. *N Engl J Med* 2003; **348**: 1389–92.

33. Morain SR, Joffe S, Largent EA. When is it ethical for physician-investigators to seek consent from their own patients? *Am J Bioeth* 2019; **19**: 11–18.

34. Cho MK, Magnus D, Constantine M, et al. Attitudes toward risk and informed consent for research on medical practices: a cross-sectional survey. *Ann Intern Med* 2015; **162**: 690.

35. Kelley M, James C, Kraft SA, et al. Patient perspectives on the learning health system: the importance of trust and shared decision making. *Am J Bioeth* 2015; **15**: 4–17.

36. Largent EA, Karlawish J. Rescuing research participants after Alzheimer trials stop early: sending out an SOS. *JAMA Neurol* 2020; **77**: 413–14.

37. Pierce AL, Cox CG, Nguyen HT, et al. Participant satisfaction with learning Alzheimer disease clinical trial results. *Alzheimer Dis Assoc Disord* 2018; **32**: 366–8.

Chapter 38

SPARKing Drug Development for Alzheimer's Disease in Academia

Daria Mochly-Rosen and Kevin V. Grimes

38.1 Introduction

Translating academic discoveries into novel therapeutics that address unmet patient needs can be a daunting task. Even the most promising research findings generally fail to progress beyond publication in an academic journal. Biopharmaceutical companies and healthcare investors consider the majority of academic discoveries to be too risky to commit the substantial resources required for a drug-development campaign. Further de-risking requires skills and expertise that are typically beyond the scope of academic institutions. The resultant gap between academic discovery and biopharmaceutical investment has been termed the "valley of death." The Stanford SPARK program was established to help academic laboratories cross this chasm by providing education in the product development process, project-specific mentorship by seasoned volunteer advisors, and modest funding. SPARK has helped over 50% of participating faculty to advance their discoveries to commercial partnerships and/or clinical trials.

38.2 Scope of the Problem

Drug discovery and development is a time-consuming, expensive, and risky endeavor. The average time from discovery to US Food and Drug Administration (FDA) approval is approximately 10 years [1]. Depending on which methodology is applied, the cost has been estimated to range from $985 million to $2.6 billion, when the expenditures on failed programs are included [2, 3]. Perhaps most alarming, the rate of success in receiving FDA approval after human studies has been initiated is only 14% [4]. This high risk of failure is unsurprising. Preclinical research is typically conducted in relatively homogeneous cell lines, induced pluripotent stem cells, or animal models. Shifting to clinical studies in a heterogeneous patient population with a disease that is often incompletely understood is a large leap indeed. It is small wonder that the biopharmaceutical industry is risk averse.

Drug development is extremely complex, requiring the mastery of multiple "applied science" disciplines to succeed. To achieve the desired efficacy and safety profile, a new drug must engage its intended target with the required concentration and time of occupancy, while avoiding off-target effects. An oral drug for Alzheimer's disease (AD) must undergo intestinal absorption and first-pass hepatic metabolism, travel through the bloodstream with a reasonable protein binding profile, cross the blood–brain barrier, perhaps cross the target cell's plasma membrane, bind to its target, and exert the desired effect – all while avoiding any untoward effects. A small-molecule drug will typically have to go through an iterative process of optimization to achieve the desired specificity, potency, solubility, bioavailability, ability to cross the blood–brain barrier, pharmacokinetics, and safety profile. The academic team must also ensure that strategies for protecting intellectual property and regulatory filings are given appropriate consideration early in the process. Clearly, successfully traversing this level of complexity requires a team approach and the expertise of many individuals.

Obtaining funding for this applied science stage of academic research can also be challenging, as most reviewers for granting agencies prefer to support discovery research or, occasionally, later-stage clinical trials. Academic reviewers may consider drug discovery more pedantic and plodding and therefore less exciting and intellectually challenging. This cultural disconnect can carry over into opinions that academics may have regarding industry scientists and vice versa. While academics may incorrectly characterize industry scientists as doing more mundane and tedious work, industry scientists may regard academics as undisciplined and sloppy. The lack of reproducibility of academic research is a serious problem [5] that has caught

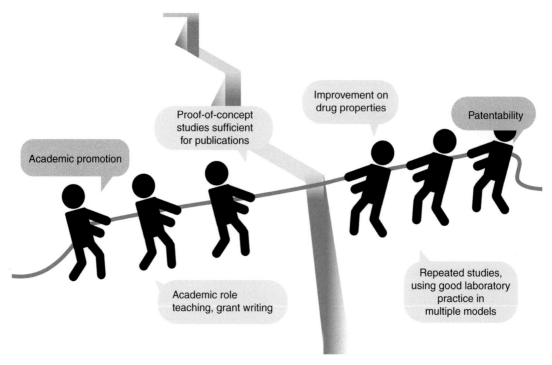

Figure 38.1 The disconnect between academic incentives and translational research in academia.

the attention of federal funding agencies and is yet another barrier to licensing academic inventions to biopharmaceutical partners.

Complicating matters further, there is a misalignment in incentives for academics to engage in drug development (Figure 38.1). Success in an academic career is generally tied to the publication of novel basic research discoveries in high-impact journals and obtaining large research grants. This leaves little time or incentive for academics to engage in the complex iterative process of drug development. It may be especially risky for a non-tenured faculty to devote substantial time to therapeutic development.

38.3   Social Responsibility

The vast majority of academic research in the United States is funded by taxpayers through federal grants, and our citizens appropriately expect these expenditures will result in clinical advances that will reduce morbidity and mortality, improve quality of life, and reduce costs to the healthcare system. Academic researchers have an ethical obligation to ensure that their discoveries benefit not only their careers, but the society that makes their research possible. Translation of their discoveries should become second nature in academia.

Academic researchers must also consider their responsibility to trainees. The majority of graduate students and postdoctoral fellows in science and engineering programs will choose careers in industry. There are seven times as many PhD graduates as there are new faculty positions each year. In the biomedical sciences, it is estimated that only 25% of PhD graduates are in tenure-track positions 5 years after graduation [6]. If faculty are to succeed in our educational mission, academic programs must provide the requisite knowledge and resources to better prepare students and trainees for success in careers beyond academia.

38.4   SPARK Program

The Stanford SPARK Program was established 14 years ago with the overarching goal of advancing promising academic discoveries to medical advances that address important unmet patient needs. The program is a partnership between university scientists and volunteer advisors from the local biopharmaceutical ecosystem. SPARK closes the translational gap by convening basic researchers, clinician scientists, and industry scientists in the same room to share ideas on how to advance early-stage research into a novel therapeutic. An illustration that summarizes the SPARK approach is provided in Figure 38.2.

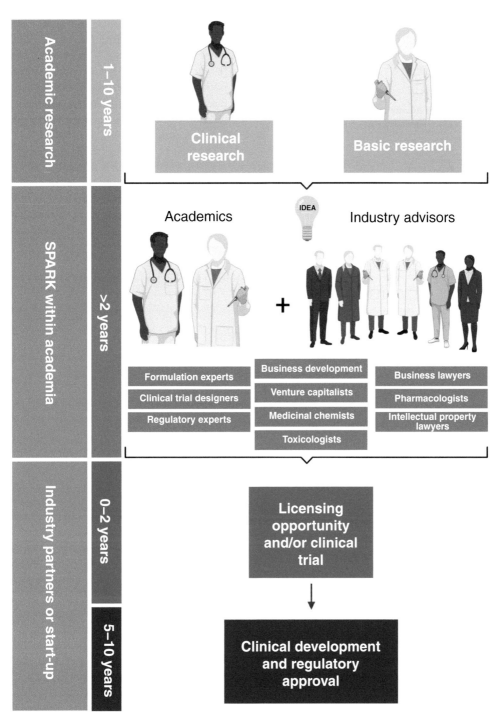

Figure 38.2 Translation of academic ideas to licensing and/or clinical trials by SPARK. The scheme emphasizes that the ideas for translational research stem from years of academic work by bench scientists and academic clinicians who are experts in their field but lack the know-how to bring their ideas to fruition. Once a project team is selected to join SPARK, they receive advice from many industry experts in the various disciplines of drug discovery, development, and commercialization. Importantly, all the discussions in SPARK meetings are confidential, allowing budding ideas to mature without impeding them from being patented, an essential feature to enable the subsequent high cost development steps. After 2 years of training in the many aspects of drug development, the project may be licensed and/or move to clinical trial in academia. In some cases, licensing occurs while the project is still within SPARK; often, however, licensing requires an additional 1–2 years. An additional 5-10 years are then required for licensed projects to complete clinical development and receive regulatory approval. There are many reasons for a project failure during development, including business decisions. It is therefore essential that the success of an academic translational research program is measured by what is under the control of the program. In SPARK's case, we measure our success by the impact of the educational program, and by the number of projects that are licensed and/or entered clinical studies.

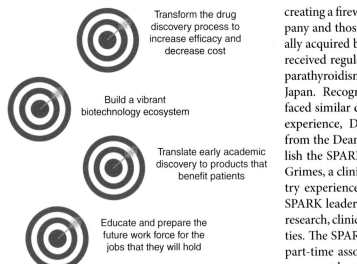

Transform the drug discovery process to increase efficacy and decrease cost

Build a vibrant biotechnology ecosystem

Translate early academic discovery to products that benefit patients

Educate and prepare the future work force for the jobs that they will hold

Figure 38.3 SPARK's goals.

SPARK has four primary missions (Figure 38.3):

(1) to educate faculty, postdoctoral fellows, and graduate students on the translational research process so that development of therapeutics based on promising discoveries becomes second nature at our institution;

(2) to help advance novel therapeutics and diagnostics to clinical study or the commercial sector;

(3) to build a vibrant biotechnology industry locally; and

(4) to promote more efficient, cost-effective, and innovative approaches to drug discovery and development.

Daria Mochly-Rosen founded the SPARK Program in 2006 in response to the challenges that she faced in advancing her peptide therapeutics to a commercial partnership for further development. After failing to garner interest from existing biopharmaceutical companies, she and her graduate student decided to start their own company. They pitched to scores of biotechnology venture capital funds before a syndicate of venture investors recognized the value of her research and agreed to provide Series A funding to launch KAI Pharmaceuticals. Dr. Mochly-Rosen took a 1-year leave of absence from the university to serve as the Chief Scientific Officer of the company. In about 1 year, KAI began clinical studies. After returning to Stanford, she continued to serve on the board of directors and the scientific advisory board, which necessitated

creating a firewall between the activities at the company and those of her laboratory. KAI was eventually acquired by Amgen and its drug, etelcalcetide, received regulatory approval for secondary hyperparathyroidism in the United States, Europe, and Japan. Recognizing that all Stanford academics faced similar difficulties and armed with her prior experience, Dr. Mochly-Rosen received support from the Dean of the School of Medicine to establish the SPARK Program. She recruited Dr. Kevin Grimes, a clinician scientist with 15 years of industry experience to serve as her co-director, so the SPARK leadership team had close ties to the basic research, clinical medicine, and industry communities. The SPARK team has now grown to include a part-time associate director, three project managers, a postdoctoral fellow, and an executive assistant.

38.5 Components of a Successful Program

A critical step for any university-based translational accelerator is to develop a close working relationship with the technology transfer office. Ideally, both parties recognize that they are working in parallel to advance university research to benefit society. Fortunately, from its inception, SPARK received the support of Stanford's Office of Technology Licensing (OTL). OTL assisted SPARK in identifying the most promising faculty inventions while continuing to lead discussions with potential industry partners and negotiate licensing deals.

Another critical step in establishing a translational research program in academia is to obtain support of faculty colleagues. At SPARK's beginning, a number of prominent faculty members were very much opposed to the idea of filing patents on the inventions of academic researchers. After all, these discoveries were funded by taxpayers and should be freely available. They were also concerned that engaging with industry partners might co-opt the university's research agenda away from discovery research. While these are reasonable concerns, there are compelling counter arguments. First, without patents to allow a period for return on the substantial investment required to obtain regulatory approval, commercial partners will not develop our discoveries. In fact, failing to file a patent will virtually ensure that our discoveries will not benefit patients. Second, SPARK's aim is to advance discoveries to improve patient outcomes regardless of financial return. Third, SPARK forms partnerships with individual scientists that represent multiple biopharmaceutical sectors and not with individual companies. Lastly, we select approximately a dozen faculty-led projects from the many hundreds that are ongoing. The university's basic research enterprise continues to thrive.

A third essential step is to identify a pool of senior industry advisors to support the program. SPARK started with only five industry advisors and we grew our advisor panel in accordance with the needs of the program. By our fifth year, we had enlisted the help of over 100 advisors. Our advisors include individuals with a broad strategic view including healthcare investors and senior officers of biopharmaceutical companies. We also have advisors with very deep expertise in the core areas of drug development in such varied disciplines as medicinal chemistry, antibody development, pharmacokinetics, biomarker development, regulatory science, clinical trial design, formulation, manufacturing, and many others. Serving in an advisory capacity can be particularly appealing to retired members of the biopharmaceutical workforce. To facilitate advisor participation, we hold our weekly meetings after working hours from 5:30 to 7:30 p.m., and we provide a light dinner. Advisors sign a confidential disclosure agreement and agree to assign any inventions around the SPARK project to the university. Most of our advisors have PhDs and MDs and have been mentored during their training and careers. As an expression of "scientific altruism," they are now mentoring individuals who will benefit from their knowledge and expertise. Our advisors truly seem to enjoy hearing about cutting-edge science and helping to advance the research to benefit patients. A common comment after our sessions is, "That was fun!" SPARK has become a biotech community of very talented individuals.

Of course, funding is another essential element for advancing our projects. Over the years, SPARK has provided an average of $50,000 per project per year. Project teams submit funding requests tied to concrete milestones in the development process. For example, a team might request $25,000 to develop an assay appropriate for the high-throughput screening facility, $50,000 to perform iterative structure–activity relationship studies while optimizing a small-molecule lead, or $30,000 to perform in vivo proof-of-concept studies. The Stanford SPARK Program has received funding from the Dean of the School of Medicine, the Maternal Child Health Research Institute (which is supported by the Lucile Packard Children's Hospital), clinical departments, various National Institutes of Health (NIH) grants, company foundations, and family foundations. However, as the program is not endowed, each year is a new challenge in raising sufficient funds to support the SPARK projects.

38.6   Selection Process

Each July, SPARK sends out a request for proposals via email across the campus, including the School of Medicine, Bioengineering, Chemistry and Chemical Engineering, Biology, Neuroscience, and other life-science programs and institutes. The application is not onerous – only two pages including: (a) a description of the intended product, (b) a brief discussion of the underlying science, (c) the clinical indication/need and why the proposed therapeutic will be a major advance beyond the current standard of care, (d) what the team hopes to accomplish with 2 years of SPARK support, (e) long-term plans – license to existing company vs. start-up company vs. conducting the clinical trial at Stanford, and (f) a brief description of the team members. SPARK defines therapeutic broadly and we support small-molecule development, monoclonal antibody and protein therapies, nucleic acid and gene therapies, and genomically engineered cell therapies. Proposals are due in late September. We receive 40–50 proposals and convene a panel of senior advisors to review and select the most promising proposals as finalists. Twenty project teams are invited to present as finalists over four evenings in early December and approximately 12 will be selected for SPARK participation.

Our selection criteria are as follows (Figure 38.4):

(1)   the product addresses a serious unmet medical need;

(2)   novelty of approach – the focus is on first-in-class therapeutics; and

(3)   feasibility of development – this is a broad category and includes that the science is ready for translation; the team is open to mentorship and advice; there is a clear and achievable path for preclinical and clinical development; the product will be embraced by patients, providers, and payers; and that the competition will not make the product irrelevant by the time it achieves regulatory approval.

441

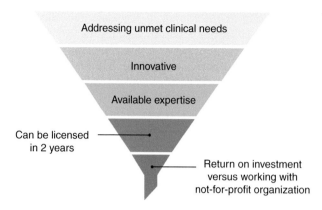

Figure 38.4 Criteria for SPARK project selection.

Of note, financial return is not a criterion. In fact, SPARK gives special consideration to projects that address global health needs, maternal and child health projects that are less likely to attract industry support, and repurposing of generic drugs for new serious clinical indications.

38.7 Educational Program

SPARK seminars are held each Wednesday evening from 5:30 to 7:30 p.m. with a brief hiatus during the summer and winter holidays. Weekly participation is mandatory for at least one member from each SPARK team. The attendance has grown from approximately 10 faculty and trainees in the first year to well over 100 attendees each week currently. The audience includes approximately 50 members of active SPARK projects, 30 industry mentors, and another 20 graduate students and postdoctoral fellows who attend to learn about the process of therapeutic development. We hold seminars on various topics in drug and diagnostic discovery and development every other week, which are often given by our SPARK advisors or invited speakers (Table 38.1).

On the intervening weeks, four SPARK project teams will present their progress and challenges from the prior several months. We emphasize that presenters should not give talks about their science, but rather discuss their project's trajectory and indicate where they need help. Our advisors and audience members ask clarifying questions and offer advice regarding next steps for the project. Hierarchy and ego are left at the door; a first-year graduate student may question or offer advice to a senior faculty member. Of course, the advisors, who have the requisite knowledge, generally have the strongest positions. On occasion, two or more experts in a given discipline may offer varying opinions. These opinions may be further discussed, but we do not attempt to arrive at a consensus. Ultimately, it is up to the SPARK project team to choose their path forward.

Not aiming for a consensus is an important distinction from industry's practice, where consensus-building is an essential part of the culture. To build on the out-of-the-box thinking and the reward for being-the-first culture of academia, SPARK encourages the project teams to take risks. And if they fail, we all learn and share the knowledge. This is another distinction from industry, where taking the time to summarize and publish a failed approach is not a priority, in contrast to the publish or perish culture in academia. Since there can be considerable benefit in learning from failure, such reports by academic translational research programs support the industry as well.

When we first initiated the program, we expected that the attendees would be primarily limited to the postdoctoral fellows and graduate students with active projects. To our surprise, the majority of faculty members also faithfully attend the seminars and updates. SPARK has been successfully educating the educators, which is essential to creating a culture of translation.

38.8 Start with the End in Mind

Unlike our basic research, where we can pivot to follow the most interesting direction of our science, therapeutic development requires a single-mindedness and a firm commitment to reaching the endpoint. Our mantra at SPARK is: "Start with the end in mind." This means defining the specific clinical problem that we are addressing and tailoring our project to provide the optimal solution. We must consider the type of therapeutic (small molecule, monoclonal antibody, etc.), risk–benefit ratio, route of delivery and dosing frequency, acceptability of on-target side effects, intellectual property status, regulatory path, preclinical and clinical development, potential commercial upside, and alternative not-for-profit development paths. It is essential to have a firm understanding of the clinical need and how the proposed product compares to the standard of care and the competition that is currently in the pipeline.

The first exercise that our SPARK teams are assigned is to create their target product profile (TPP). The TPP describes the essential characteristics of the intended drug product (Table 38.2).

Table 38.1 SPARK seminar topics

Case history of a recently approved therapeutic

Overview of drug discovery and development

Starting with the end in mind – feasibility and target product profile

Project management

Intellectual property

Working with the OTL

Assessing unmet medical needs and clinical indications

Robustness and reproducibility of academic research

Design thinking and team science

Target identification and validation

High-throughput screening and evaluating hits

Small-molecule optimization: from lead to development candidate

Repurposing drugs for new indications

Machine learning in drug discovery

Therapeutic antibody and protein development

Preclinical pharmacology and in vivo models

Pharmacokinetics, absorption, distribution, metabolism, and excretion

Preclinical safety and toxicology evaluation

Formulation

Pharmacogenomics

Drug–drug interactions and special populations

Development of biomarkers and diagnostics

Nucleic acid and gene therapies

Genomically modified cell therapies

Chimeric antigen receptor T-cell therapy

Regulatory science, incentives, and strategies

Clinical trial design and conduct

Understanding your market and commercial potential

Creating value in biotechnology

Commercialization panel – what investors are looking for

How to pitch your project

Value-based pricing of novel therapeutics

Non-profit drug development

Legal aspects of starting a company

Table 38.2 SPARK target product profile

Product description	Type of agent (small molecule, antibody, cell therapy, etc.) Proposed target (agonist or antagonist) Other distinguishing features
Indications and usage	Clinical indication(s) – lead indication Intended patient population Any co-administered therapies Improvement over current standard of care
Development and preclinical	Target selectivity Planned efficacy assays (in vitro) In vivo models of disease
Preclinical safety	Known safety concerns (on- or off-target) Desired/achievable therapeutic window Planned safety assays (in vitro, in vivo)
Clinical pharmacology	Pharmacokinetics Absorption, distribution, metabolism, excretion Drug interactions Pharmacodynamics Duration of effect
Dosing and administration	Route of administration Frequency of administration Dosage
How supplied/ storage	Formulation (excipients) Estimated shelf-life Required storage conditions (temperature, light, etc.)
Financial considerations	Cost of goods Cost of development Projected pricing/cost to patient Benefits/acceptability to third-party payers/insurers Potential partners
Regulatory considerations	Orphan designation Expedited review Precedents regarding trial population/endpoints
Intellectual property	Patentability Freedom to operate Desired licensing outcome
Competition	Same clinical indication Same target or mechanism

443

The document can be used as a road map or blueprint for guiding development. The TPP is a living document and can be revised and more detailed as the project advances, but if at any point it becomes clear that an essential attribute cannot be met, the project should be discontinued or at least a substantial pivot in approach is required.

We also emphasize the need for a team member to assume the role as project manager. Therapeutic development is an extremely complex multidisciplinary process with many interdependent tasks. The team may have multiple advisors as well as relationships with other labs, university discovery and technology service centers, and contract research organizations. These collaborations require active management. Time is perhaps our most precious resource and delays to achieving regulatory approval may literally result in increased patient suffering and mortality.

38.9   Project Mentorship

Perhaps the most important component of the SPARK Program is direct mentorship to specific projects provided by the SPARK advisors. Often these relationships arise organically when an advisor offers to help after a team presents their progress report. The program leadership also introduces advisors to project teams when it becomes clear that the team will benefit from their particular expertise. The extent of support may range from an hour-long meeting with a regulatory science expert to discuss high-level strategy with the FDA, to multiple meetings with a clinical trialist over several months to design an investigator-sponsored clinical trial, to weekly meetings with a medicinal chemist over 2 years to iteratively optimize a small-molecule lead candidate. When a project becomes ready for commercialization, SPARK mentors may make introductions to potential investors or chief executive officer candidates.

38.10   Commercialization

Approximately 70% of SPARK projects may be attractive to the commercial sector and SPARK leadership maintains relationships with various biotechnology venture firms and academic liaisons from biopharmaceutical companies. In addition, SPARK holds pitch sessions at the annual Biotechnology Innovation Organization (BIO) International Convention and the BIO Investor Forum. Once a SPARK project generates traction with a potential investor or commercial partner, SPARK depends on Stanford's OTL to take over and negotiate potential licenses.

38.11   SPARK Outcomes

SPARK has defined success as advancing a project either to commercial partnership or directly to a clinical trial in the university healthcare system. By these metrics, SPARK has achieved a success rate of over 60% (Figure 38.5). SPARK start-up companies have raised on average $20 million. Two SPARK start-ups have gone public and a third has a pharma deal worth nearly $900 million dollars.

Success rate

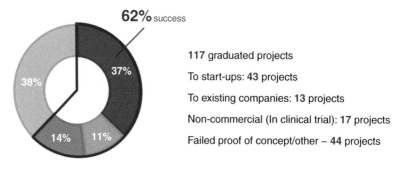

62% success

117 graduated projects

To start-ups: **43** projects

To existing companies: **13** projects

Non-commercial (In clinical trial): **17** projects

Failed proof of concept/other – **44** projects

Figure 38.5 Summary of SPARK projects and their outcomes, as of 2019. The shaded segments represent the following: 37%, licensed to start-up company; 11%, licensed to existing biopharmaceutical company; 14%, advanced to clinical study without a commercial partner; 38%, failed to advance to a desired outcome (typically because of failed proof-of-concept experiment, loss of key personnel, or other team performance factors).

SPARK has created other successes that are important within the context of academia. It has educated many hundreds of faculty, postdoctoral fellows, and graduate students on translational research. These individuals represent both the current and future educators and innovators in academic research and the future leaders in the biopharmaceutical industry. Another unexpected SPARK success has been the follow-on research funding that SPARK projects have received. According to our faculty surveys, they have received 6–8 dollars in federal or foundation research grants for each dollar that they have received from SPARK.

38.12 SPARK Projects for AD and Neurodegeneration

While the pathophysiology of AD is incompletely understood, academics have tenaciously pursued novel approaches to better understand the disease mechanisms and identify new therapeutics targets (Figure 38.6), many of which have been the focus of researchers at Stanford University. Over SPARK's 14 years in operation, 11 projects that promised to modify disease progression in neurodegenerative

diseases were selected for participation. Each of these projects focused on a novel molecular target and their therapeutic approaches included the development of three repositioned drugs, one monoclonal antibody, and a number of novel small molecules. A particular obstacle for drugs targeting the central nervous system (CNS) is crossing the blood–brain barrier, and several of our advisors have particular expertise in overcoming this challenge. These SPARK projects have led to five start-up companies and one license to an existing company; only one of the start-ups has since folded. The remaining five unlicensed projects are still under development within SPARK.

One successful SPARK project led to the founding of CuraSen Therapeutics, Inc., a start-up company that is developing novel treatments for AD, Parkinson's disease, and other neurodegenerative diseases. CuraSen was based on the science of Dr. Mehrdad Shamloo, a professor in neurosurgery at Stanford, who joined SPARK in 2015 to advance his research to find drugs that would restore or replace damaged noradrenergic signaling pathways originating in the locus coeruleus (LC). The LC nucleus transmits norepinephrine to activate the limbic system and cerebral cortex. Early loss of

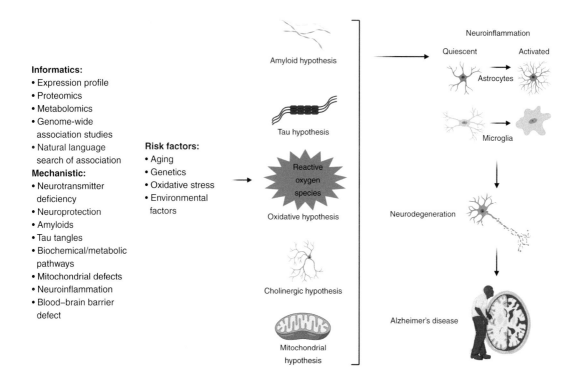

Figure 38.6 Approaches to identify the molecular mechanisms causing AD and to identify new therapeutic targets.

neurons in the LC is a hallmark of AD and related diseases. This loss results in increased inflammation, dysregulated metabolism, and progressive neurodegeneration.

The first insight into the role of the LC in neurodegeneration came from a study using a mouse model of trisomy (Down syndrome), which is also associated with accelerated neurodegeneration and an AD-like phenotype. Using xamoterol, a beta-1-adrenergic receptor partial agonist, the researchers showed that restoring norepinephrine-mediated neurotransmission could reverse cognitive dysfunction in this mouse model [7]. Subsequent studies showed that xamoterol enhances memory in the Thy1-hAPPLond/Swe + (amyloid precursor protein) mouse model of Alzheimer's [8], and suppresses neuroinflammation and pathology in the 5×FAD mouse model of AD [9].

Since beta-1-adrenergic receptor activation causes worsening of heart failure, a common co-morbidity in elderly AD patients, the ideal drug would achieve high levels in the brain while minimizing systemic exposure. During his participation in SPARK, Dr. Shamloo obtained substantial advice and support in medicinal chemistry to generate a superior CNS-penetrable analog of their original compound [10]. He also obtained considerable advice regarding formulation, patent strategy, and company building. In 2016, with the help of SPARK advisor Dr. Robert Booth, Dr. Shamloo founded CuraSen. In October 2017, CuraSen raised $54.5 million in Series A financing. In 2019, CuraSen began clinical trials using existing beta-1-adrenergic receptor activators, which helped inform their subsequent clinical programs. In September of 2020, the company initiated Phase 1 clinical studies of their proprietary beta-1-adrenergic receptor agonist, the drug developed while Dr. Shamloo's project was mentored in SPARK. According to the company's press release, 70 healthy volunteers and patients with a variety of neurodegenerative diseases including mild cognitive impairment and Parkinson's disease will be treated. A Phase 2 study began recruiting patients in July of 2021.

This example illustrates (i) how compelling basic research suggested the use of an existing drug (repositioning) to provide a rapid proof of concept in multiple animal models of AD; (ii) how limitations of the existing compound helped focus the medicinal chemistry efforts to overcome these pharmacological challenges; and (iii) how working persistently and iteratively through structure–activity relationships led to a proprietary new chemical entity that has entered clinical studies.

38.13 The Formula for Effective Translation of Academic Discoveries to Benefit Patients

As should be apparent from the above, the principles of our program are simple (Figure 38.7) but distinct from academic incubators: a single inventor or a small team is taken out of their academic environment, mentored by experts (often one expert in each field), and then moves out to their start-up. An incubator structure is efficient in company building, but misses out on building on key opportunities, including the following:

1. Building mutual respect between scientists in academia and in industry by simply spending extended times together to learn the strengths

---

The formula for effective translation of academic discoveries to benefit patients

Overcoming cultural divide by

o Mixing many volunteer industry advisors with many academicians

o Meeting in one room, year round

o Meeting on university campus, to integrate the industry knowledge with academic thinking

Building on the risk-taking innovative culture of academia

o No hierarchy; multiple opinions are encouraged

o *Not* aiming to reach a consensus

o Learning from successes AND failures

Figure 38.7 Key elements that help in SPARK's success.

of basic and applied research. This experience is transformative to SPARK participants and the industry experts alike; it makes future partnerships seamless.

2. Holding the translational research meetings on campus and making them available not only to those who are actively working on a project, but also to trainees who plan industry careers. This fulfills the educational priority of universities to prepare students for the careers that they will pursue.

3. Exposing SPARK participants to the whole process of drug development, regardless of the stage of their project. A holistic understanding of the entire enterprise improves efficiency. Drug discovery and development is full of interdependent activities. Focusing only on the expertise needed for the next step, rather than the whole chain of expertise, limits the possibilities for innovating the process.

4. Exposing trainees to contacts and role models for the many possible career opportunities outside academia.

5. Educating the educators, so that translational research becomes second nature. This prepares our faculty for future opportunities to translate their research to benefit patients.

6. By holding discussions with many advisors at the same time, and allowing many opinions to be heard, breakthroughs in the translational research process are more likely to occur and may increase the efficiency and decrease the cost of drug development.

We believe that the SPARK model provides essential elements that are congruent with the academic mission to develop novel therapeutic approaches that will help patients and improve societal health. Such efforts may also give rise to innovative and less costly approaches to drug discovery and development in both academia and industry.

38.14 Why Should We Translate Our Discoveries?

The recent COVID-19 pandemic has made it increasingly clear that there is immense value in educating our faculty and trainees in the translational process to ensure that their cutting-edge research advances into novel therapeutics for unmet patient needs. Indeed, it is our social responsibility to deliver better health to our society, train the next generation of basic and translational scientists, and to stimulate the biotechnology industry to provide high-quality employment to our graduates. Translating our discoveries will facilitate the development of cures and disease-modifying therapies for the diseases that still plague our society, including AD and other neurodegenerative diseases, refractory cancers, and the next unexpected pandemic. If successful, we can reduce suffering and death while also reducing the untenably escalating costs of our healthcare system.

Acknowledgments

The authors wish to thank the funders of the SPARK program including the Dean of the Stanford University School of Medicine, the Maternal and Child Health Research Institute, the NIH Clinical and Translational Science Award, and the Weston Havens Foundation; the many faculty members, students, and postdoctoral fellows that have participated in the program; and especially to the many industry advisors that volunteer to support the program and share their much-valued knowledge. We thank Lucia Lee for the figure preparations and illustrations and Dr. Kate Samardzic for help in preparing the manuscript for submission.

The authors declare no conflicts of interest.

References

1. PhRMA Foundation. Biopharmaceutical research and development: the process behind new medicines. 2015. Available at: www.phrma.org/-/media/Project/PhRMA/PhRMA-Org/PhRMA-Org/PDF/P-R/rd_brochure.pdf (accessed December 4, 2020).

2. Wouters OJ, McKee M, Luyten J. Estimated research and development investment needed to bring a new medicine to market, 2009–2018. *JAMA* 2020; **323**: 844–53.

3. DiMasi JA, Grabowski HG, Hansen RW. Innovation in the pharmaceutical industry: new estimates of R&D costs. *J Health Econ* 2016; **47**: 20–33.

4. Wong CH, Siah KW, Lo AW. Estimation of clinical trial success rates and related parameters. *Biostatistics* 2019; **20**: 273–86.

5. Begley CG, Ellis LM. Raise standards for preclinical cancer research. *Nature* 2012; **483**: 531–3.

6. Schillebeeckx M, Maricque B, Lewis C. The missing piece to changing the university culture. *Nat Biotechnol* 2013; **31**: 938–41.

7. Salehi A, Faizi M, Colas D, et al. Restoration of norepinephrine-modulated contextual memory in a mouse model of Down syndrome. *Sci Transl Med* 2009; **1**: 7ra17.

8. Coutellier L, Ardestani PM, Shamloo M. B1-adrenergic receptor activation enhances memory in Alzheimer's disease model. *Ann Clin Transl Neurol* 2014; **1**: 348–60.

9. Ardestani PM, Evans AK, Yi B, et al. Modulation of neuroinflammation and pathology in the 5×FAD mouse model of Alzheimer's disease using a biased and selective beta-1 adrenergic receptor partial agonist. *Neuropharmacology* 2017; **116**: 371–86.

10. Yi B, Jahangir A, Evans AK, et al. Discovery of novel brain permeable and G protein-biased beta-1 adrenergic receptor partial agonists for the treatment of neurocognitive disorders. *PloS One* 2017; **12**: e0180319.

The Role of Professional Associations and Patient Advocacy in Advancing Alzheimer's Drug Development

Amir Kalali and Gil Bashe

39.1 Introduction

First described in 1906, Alzheimer's disease (AD) remains among the most burdensome non-communicable – emotionally and economically – neurological illnesses, robbing people of memories and cognitive ability. Alzheimer's Disease International's (ADI) annual World Alzheimer Report estimates that there are more than 50 million people living with dementia globally. Advocacy groups, working with professional associates, estimate that this patient community will increase to 152 million by 2050. In 2019, ADI reported that someone develops dementia every 3 seconds, and the current annual economic burden of this neurological illness is estimated at almost $1 trillion, a staggering figure, expected to double by 2030.

No longer willing to be kept at arm's length, patient and professional associations demand, and have secured, a voice at innovation and policy tables. Clinical researchers and drug developers must take this new advocacy voice into account in planning their programs. Once focused on study design and company priorities, lead investors and drug-development teams must now expand their efforts to include the professional, patient, and policy advocacy landscape. These groups are essential to setting research and policy priorities and are influential voices in securing funding at the federal, state, and private investment levels.

In 2011, Senator Susan Collins (R–ME) and then-Representative (now Senator) Edward Markey (D–MA), co-founder of the 1999 Congressional Task Force on Alzheimer's Disease, co-sponsored the National Alzheimer's Project Act (NAPA). NAPA directed the US Department of Health and Human Services (HHS) Secretary to "be responsible for the creation and maintenance of an integrated national plan to overcome Alzheimer's [disease]." These efforts were driven by professional and patient associations seeking to emphasize that AD, like cancer, was epidemic and could engulf and impoverish both the developed and developing world.

Several major goals were articulated in the NAPA legislative language including to "prevent and effectively treat AD by 2025." President Obama noted the importance of this goal during his State of the Union address that same year. The bill outlined five priorities, relevant to drug development effort elements, to be considered in developing study designs and outreach to professional associations:

(1) prevent and effectively treat AD by 2025;
(2) optimize care quality and efficiency;
(3) expand supports for people with AD and their families;
(4) enhance public awareness and engagement; and
(5) track progress and drive improvement.

Subsequently, the NAPA Advisory Council established three working groups to accomplish these lofty goals: Research, Long-Term Care and Supports, and Clinical Services. Each year, the subcommittees report on their progress and make recommendations for plan updates to the HHS Secretary and Congress, as required by law. This has continued throughout following administrations.

39.2 Expanding Roles of Advocacy Organizations

Advocacy organizations have expanded their efforts from caregiver support and policy making and are now driving new research possibilities. Long considered awareness-building allies in the drug-development process, patient and professional associations have taken on a new role to accelerate clinical trial recruitment, fund research efforts, and advocate with regulatory authorities for approval to market new therapies.

In other non-communicable disease categories, such as cancer, cardiovascular disease, and diabetes, patient and professional associations have been sought out as a second clinical home for scientists eager to share and present new data around approaches to manage these life-threatening illnesses. However, the slow pace of success in moving discovery and development approach ideas from laboratory bench to people's home medicine chests in order to better manage cognitive disorders and dementia has these groups reevaluating their participatory approach in the drug-development process.

Scientists would be well served in dedicating efforts to brief staff and volunteer medical advisory boards on their study efforts. Additionally, lay advocates – driven by mission and experience – have become immersed in the science of their categories. Along with MD, PhD, and MBA, the title of patient advocate has an influential sway in the rooms of biopharmaceutical companies and state and federal representatives' offices.

In many cases, companies dedicated to exploring possible therapies for AD have dedicated senior staff focusing on advocacy relations. These corporate leaders are not determining whether third-party groups should receive funding for charitable events; rather, how to strengthen ties to advance clinical trial recruitment and support during open-microphone sessions at US Food and Drug Administration Patient Advisory meetings.

No longer expected to play a secondary "supporting role," more and more associations are entering the research funding process, seeking to advance promising new approaches. Once viewing each other as competitors for donations and grants, professional and patient organizations are looking to each other to co-fund promising research ideas, much like private equity groups invite other funds to mutually support a start-up enterprise. This has placed these groups in a new role from their founding. While fund-raising efforts such as walks, galas, golf outings, and conference sponsorships still occupy their workflow, the focus on these monies in the digital era has shifted from awareness building to being leading sources for research funds.

These associations are now neutral meeting grounds for advocates, clinicians, drug-development sponsors, regulatory leaders, and scientists to share approaches, data, and ideas. There are routes that have been explored and failed. Study designs that need new eyes. Diagnostics and imaging technologies that may alert physicians and their patients to earlier diagnoses and the possibilities of better management through clinical trial participation. Patient and professional associations can be both scientific and keen funders. The territory is vast: the National Institutes of Health (NIH) ClinicalTrials.gov site now lists more than 2,500 ongoing studies for AD. With the pool for patient and family participation limited, association involvement in these trials is a "Good Housekeeping" seal of approval and signals independent eyes on these studies.

39.3 Important AD and Related Dementia Organizations

The following three organizations are important:

- **Alzheimer's Association**: The Alzheimer's Association is the largest and oldest non-profit organization dedicated to dementia and cognition decline. Launched in 1980, it formed as the Alzheimer's Disease and Related Disorders Association, Inc., with chapters across the United States. It started as a patient advocacy organization working with the then-nascent National Institute on Aging (NIA) and pharmaceutical companies, then initiating clinical development programs. The Alzheimer's Association continues to provide education, research funding, advocacy, local support, and resources for families and professionals.

- **Alzheimer's Drug Discovery Foundation (ADDF)**: Founded in 1998 by Leonard A. Lauder and Ronald S. Lauder, the ADDF is the only philanthropy solely focused on accelerating the development of drugs to prevent and treat AD.

- **Cure Alzheimer's Fund (CureAlz)**: Also known as the Alzheimer's Disease Research Foundation, CureAlz is focused on supporting research on AD treatment and prevention. The organization was founded by three families who were frustrated by the slow pace of research for the condition. Since its founding in 2004, CureAlz has contributed over $110 million to research, and its funded initiatives have been responsible for several key breakthroughs, including the groundbreaking "Alzheimer's in a Dish."

Today, both academic and industry researchers should be aware of and seek to establish ties to a number of leading groups in the AD community. Along with their work to raise awareness of the disease and offer emotional support to caregivers, these groups are in the frontlines of setting US and global priorities on research and patient and caregiver support. In fact, the Congressional Task Force on Alzheimer's Disease was launched with support from the Alzheimer's Association. This advocacy and Beltway policy effort worked successfully to unanimously pass the National Alzheimer's Project Act (PL-111–375). This bipartisan task force has also been instrumental in securing funding for research at the NIH and raising awareness of this disease by way of congressional briefings. Professional and patient advocacy groups in this sector are must-have allies.

The three groups mentioned above are noted for their funding support for research. However, there are many other associations that are key to mobilizing awareness around clinical trials – from diagnostic modalities, to new diet and memory support approaches, to drug discovery. These groups should be on the radar screens for all those engaged in bringing promising management techniques and therapies – scientists from academic medical centers, contract research organizations, and biopharmaceutical companies – from whiteboard to patient bedside:

- The American Brain Foundation was established in 1992 by its research partner, the American Academy of Neurology (AAN), and connects clinical researchers with funding possibilities in order to increase awareness of brain disease. This is a noted meeting ground for some 32,000 neurologists and other AAN members. In 2019, it reported that it had provided more than $24 million for research on several types of brain disease, including AD and other types of dementia.
- Alzheimer's Disease International (ADI) was founded in 1984 to overcome AD and is the umbrella organization that draws on the data, voices, and input of more than 100 global AD associations. ADI's annual reports are considered the most comprehensive source for dementia-related programs, economic analysis, and worldwide approaches.
- The Alzheimer's Family Center (AFC) comprises two organizations and has a

local focus versus a national mandate. Its geographic importance and numbers served make it quite important in the care and advocacy conversation. Located in Orange County, CA, AFC is tasked with serving area residents living with dementia through day-care support critical to caregiver well-being. Its funds are directed to its own programming.

- Alzheimer's Foundation of America (AFA) was founded in 2002 by a caregiver whose mother lived with AD for more than a decade. AFA seeks to provide resources to caregivers, including family education, free memory-screening services, dementia care training for professionals, and support groups nationwide.
- Alzheimer's Research and Prevention Foundation (ARPF) focuses on preventing AD through research, education, and memory screenings. The ARPF was established in 1993 and its efforts include holistic and integrative medicine. At a time when therapies are limited, ARPF informs professionals around brain health as well as dementia prevention strategies.
- BrightFocus Foundation, launched in 1973 as the American Health Assistance Foundation, targets AD and other research areas. It has funded more than $100 million in research grants for AD.
- Fisher Center for Alzheimer's Research Foundation (FCARF) was founded by philanthropists Zachary Fisher and David Rockefeller in 1995. Their goal was to build a top-of-the-line research center to seek a cure for AD. Along with funding research, FCARF provides educational resources through their website, publishes a quarterly magazine called *Preserving Your Memory*, and uses the majority of their donations to partner with many other national and international researchers who share similar goals.
- Lewy Body Dementia Association (LBDA) is committed to advocating for, educating, and supporting those affected by Lewy body dementia (LBD). LBD is the second most common form of dementia. Its progression is similar, albeit much less known than AD.
- The Long Island Alzheimer's and Dementia (LIAD) Center is a local AD charity formed to serve those in this New York suburban

451

community who live with dementia. The LIAD Center offers several different programs targeting a different stage or challenge of AD and provides social work services to family members to help maintain their well-being.

39.4 Other Relevant Professional Organizations

In addition to AD-focused organizations there are several organizations whose work has an impact on advancing new treatments for AD. These include:

- The International Society for CNS Drug Development (ISCDD): Founded in 2002, this was the first independent non-profit organization to bring together scientists from industry, regulators, and academia involved in central nervous system (CNS) drug development to collaborate on initiatives to accelerate the development of new treatments.

- The International Society for CNS Clinical Trials and Methodology (ISCTM): Founded in 2004, this is an independent non-profit organization, focused on methodological issues in CNS drug development.

- International Psychogeriatric Association (IPA): Founded in 1980, this is an independent non-profit organization dedicated to advancing geriatric mental health.

- The Decentralized Trials and Research Alliance (DTRA): Founded in 2020, this is an independent non-profit organization focused on accelerating research participation, made accessible to everyone, which is enabled by the consistent, widespread adoption of appropriate decentralized research methods (previously also described as remote or virtual). DTRA has a particularly wide stakeholder base that allows the whole ecosystem to collaborate on initiatives advancing its mission.

39.5 The Common Role of Professional Organizations

These forums all have in common the principle that research entities, including biopharmaceutical companies, should not be working in silos. They should be sharing learnings and best practices and maximizing the value of finite funding for research and development.

An example of where these organizations are very useful is the ability to allow multiple organizations to collaborate to achieve consensus in areas such as definitions, outcome measures, best practices, etc., which allows the acceptance and adoption of new approaches by the field and the regulatory authorities. Conditions such as AD cannot be addressed by single entities no matter how large or well funded. It will take a network of collaborative organizations to ensure success.

Under President Obama, the share of NIH money being directed toward AD research increased by 56% to $986 million, including $57 million for research dedicated to vascular and other related dementias. Subsequent funding increases have transformed the NIA from a mid-size NIH institute to the fifth largest among 27 NIH institutes. While 2020 saw a decrease in funding, the NIA still maintains a $2.6 billion overall budget. For researchers seeking to tap these funds, a strong and broad connection to the leading professional and patient groups is essential, and securing support from third-party groups eager to pursue innovative approaches is necessary to overcome a disease that less than two decades ago could only be diagnosed at death. The professional association connection is vital to advancing discoveries that will improve the human condition.

Drivers of innovation should assess their connection to groups using this priority checklist:

(1) ensure the trial design considers the needs and abilities of the caregiver and patient;

(2) determine whether trial information is readily understood and addresses questions;

(3) assess what information would encourage accelerated patient trial enrollment;

(4) evaluate the frequency of face-to-face or remote connection;

(5) prepare advocates to address their families', third-party, and medical stakeholders' questions;

(6) look toward external messaging priorities with regulators or media outlets;

(7) know the progress of trial enrollment and scientific publications or presentations;

(8) keep current in regulatory milestones; and

(9) participate in ambassador programs that help peer-to-peer communication.

The shift away from paternal, arms-length connection to patients and their caregivers has taken place. Now, the AD community, with a myriad of groups to amplify their voice in a decision-making forum, expects to be engaged as partners in science. Researchers at all points of the diagnostic and drug-development continuum should be asking the key question: "If this study impacted my family, what would I need or want to know?" The best approach to secure strong professional and patient connections is to filter efforts through the powerful lens of empathy and mutual respect.

Alzheimer's Disease Neuroimaging Initiative

Charles Bernick

40.1 Introduction

As we ventured into the twenty-first century, therapeutic pharmaceutical options for Alzheimer's disease (AD) were limited to a handful of medications having modest symptomatic effects. However, even at that time, there was tremendous interest in developing disease-modifying therapies, spurred on by accumulating knowledge regarding the underlying disease mechanisms. Success in animal models led to testing of various strategies (anti-inflammatories, statins, antioxidants, immunotherapies, etc.) in cohorts with AD dementia. These initial efforts, unfortunately, did not result in any positive results [1].

At the same time, it was becoming increasingly recognized that the pathological processes leading to the clinical manifestations of AD began years before symptoms occurred. Moreover, the concept that there was a period of time between the onset of mild cognitive symptoms with independent function and dementia, termed mild cognitive impairment (MCI), gained traction. It was found that the "amnestic" subtype of MCI, characterized by the presence of subjective memory complaints, objective memory impairment, and otherwise normal daily function, was associated with a relatively high annual conversion rate to AD dementia (12%/year compared to 1–2%/year for age-matched individuals without MCI) [2]. Thus, it became attractive to think that MCI represented a stage at which potential disease-modifying therapies might be more effective, and that previous studies were doomed to failure because they initiated therapy at the point of dementia, where the disease process had progressed too far.

There were other factors, though, that had hindered AD drug development. Early AD clinical trials utilized psychometric test batteries such as the Alzheimer's Disease Assessment Scale – cognitive subscale (ADAS-cog) as primary outcome measures. These measures had several limitations including poor test–retest reliability, reducing their statistical power and necessitating larger sample sizes and longer study duration to detect a significant difference in the rate of change between treatment groups [3]. The issue of increased duration of clinical trials is magnified when utilizing an MCI cohort, as rates of cognitive and functional decline are not linear in the progression of AD; the slope of decline in MCI cohorts tends to be less steep than in those with AD dementia, thus requiring longer study periods to see a disease-modifying treatment effect. Furthermore, cognitive and functional outcomes are usually unable to separate a symptomatic (improved cognitive performance) from a disease-modifying (interfering with neurodegeneration) effect. Conversely, an effective disease-modifying therapy could fail to show a cognitive-enhancing effect, at least initially, and thus be considered ineffective if only clinical measures are used.

Given these limitations to clinical trial conduct, there was a need in the field to seek out biomarkers that could be employed as a means to identify individuals with AD pathology at the earliest stages in the disease course, to be used as direct measures of neuronal health and disease progression, have some clinical relevance, and that could potentially be used as outcome measures in clinical trials. Theoretically, these biomarkers would allow trials to be conducted with smaller sample sizes and shorter observation time [4].

In response to this imperative for improved biomarkers in clinical trials of AD therapies, the Alzheimer's Disease Neuroimaging Initiative (ADNI) was launched in 2004, as a research project to study the rate of change of cognition, function, brain structure and function, and biomarkers in a cohort of elderly controls, subjects with MCI, and subjects with AD dementia.

40.2 ADNI Origins and Development

ADNI was initially funded in 2003 as a 6-year, $67 million public–private collaboration by the National Institute on Aging (NIA) and the National Institute of Biomedical Imaging and Bioengineering of the National Institutes of Health (NIH), several pharmaceutical companies (Pfizer, Wyeth, Eli Lilly, Merck, GlaxoSmithKline, AstraZeneca, Novartis, Eisai, Elan, Forest Laboratories, Bristal Meyers Squibb), foundations (Alzheimer's Association, Institute for Study of Aging), and the NIH Foundation. Fifty-six sites across North America were recruited to participate with the target enrollment of 200 elderly controls, 400 subjects with MCI, and 200 with AD dementia [5].

The overall goals of the study were [5]:

(1) the development of methods leading to uniform standards for acquiring longitudinal, multi-center MRI and fluorodeoxyglucose (FDG) positron emission tomography (PET) data on healthy elderly controls, MCI, and AD dementia patients;

(2) the use of these optimized methods for acquisition of imaging data in the ADNI cohort and validation of these imaging surrogates with concurrently acquired biomarkers and cognitive and functional measures;

(3) the identification of clinical measures and biomarkers (imaging and fluid) that provide maximum power for the diagnosis of MCI and AD and assessment of treatment effects in clinical trials; and

(4) the creation of an accessible imaging and clinical data repository with information on longitudinal changes in imaging and fluid biomarkers and cognitive function in healthy controls and subjects with MCI and AD dementia.

ADNI was extended in 2009 during the ADNI GO phase, which assessed the existing ADNI 1 cohort along with 200 new participants with "early" MCI. The objective of this phase was to examine biomarkers at an earlier stage of the disease, as it had become clear that the MCI patients enrolled in the original ADNI cohort were so far advanced in the disease process that the data were not capturing early MCI changes. MRI protocols were also adjusted in the ADNI GO phase [6].

In 2011, ADNI 2 began and was designed to expand ADNI 1 and make the data more relevant for drug discovery by enrolling more early MCI participants. Assessment continued of participants from the ADNI 1/ADNI GO phases in addition to adding new participant groups including 150 elderly controls, 100 early MCI subjects and 150 "late" MCI, and 150 mild AD dementia patients. A new cohort, significant memory concern (SMC), was also added in ADNI 2 to address the gap between healthy controls and MCI. A major addition to ADNI 2 was the addition of amyloid PET with florbetapir at all ADNI 2 sites and on all ADNI 2 and ADNI GO subjects. MRI moved to 3-T rather than the 1.5-T instruments used in ADNI 1 [7].

ADNI 3 began in 2016 [8], with an expanded goal of determining the relationships between the clinical, cognitive, imaging, genetic, and biochemical biomarker characteristics across the entire spectrum of AD. ADNI 3 added tau PET imaging with the ligand flortaucipir, for potential use in clinical trials for subject selection, as a baseline covariate and as an outcome measure. In addition, the amyloid-beta tracer, florbetaben, was incorporated for all new subjects enrolled in ADNI 3, with the aim to compare amyloid tracers by a common scale (Centiloid scale). MRI sequences were expanded, with advanced diffusion MRI and task-free functional MRI sequences implemented on systems that are capable and that resemble the Human Connectome Project. During ADNI 3, the cohort was replenished and expanded.

40.3 ADNI Structure

ADNI is governed by a steering committee that includes representatives from all funding sources as well as principal investigators of the ADNI sites, and is organized as eight cores, each with different responsibilities, under the direction of an Administrative Core, led by Dr. Michael Weiner, as well as a Data and Publications Committee (DPC). The eight cores comprise (1) the Clinical Core, responsible for subject recruitment, collection and quality control of clinical and neuropsychological data, testing clinical hypotheses, and maintaining databases; (2) the MRI and (3) PET cores, responsible for developing imaging methods, ensuring quality control between neuroimaging centers, and testing imaging hypotheses; (4) the Biomarker Core, responsible for the receipt, storage, and analysis of biological samples and development of immortalized cell lines for genetic analysis; the distribution of samples for further analyses is under the control of a resource allocation committee which is completely independent from all ADNI investigators; (5) the Genetics Core, responsible for genetic characterization and analysis of participants as well as banking DNA, RNA, and immortalized cell lines at the National Cell Repository for Alzheimer's Disease; (6) the Neuropathology Core, responsible for analyzing brain pathology obtained at autopsies of ADNI participants; (7) the Biostatistics Core, responsible for statistical analyses of ADNI data; and (8) the Informatics Core, responsible for managing data-sharing functions [6].

40.4 Public–Private Partnership

The immense value to biomedical research that comes from collaborative efforts has been well documented and can result in higher research productivity, reduced research risk, and increased innovation through the sharing of knowledge and resources [9]. ADNI stands as one of the first and largest AD research collaborations between government, pharmaceutical companies, and foundations.

Much of ADNI's success is due to the establishment of research standards among the partners. Prior to the funding of ADNI, the NIA held a series of workgroups that included both academic and industry scientists to discuss the development of common protocols for the various measures (i.e., clinical, neuropsychological, neuropsychiatric, neuroimaging, and fluid biomarker) included in the study with the aim of implementing the best methods for data collection and standard operating procedures.

One of the major ways that ADNI distinguishes itself is in the ongoing involvement of its private partners. Participating not only financially, but also in a guidance capacity from before the inception of the study, the industry partners joined together to form the Private Partner Scientific Board (PPSB). Managed by the Foundation for the NIH, the PPSB is an independent forum for all ADNI private-sector partners (pharmaceutical companies, biotechnology companies, and non-profit organizations). The role of the PPSB is to share information, as well as to provide private-sector views and expertise regarding ADNI. Over the course of ADNI this group has not only contributed industry expertise to the project but has also undertaken and funded add-on projects that were not originally included in the original grant [10].

A schematic of ADNI structure is given in Figure 40.1.

40.5 Data

A diverse array of clinical, radiological, and fluid biomarker data have been collected throughout the course of ADNI. The choice of measures has been focused on identifying methods for earlier diagnosis of AD and more precise tools to track disease

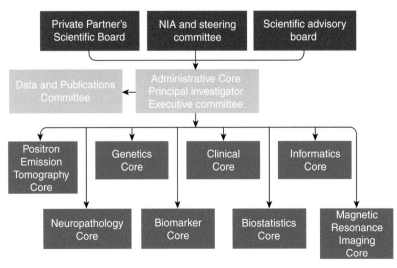

Figure 40.1 Administrative structure of ADNI.

course and response to therapies in clinical trials. As new knowledge and technologies accrued during the study, additional clinical and biomarker measures were introduced into the protocol.

The types of data collected can be categorized into the following groups:

- **Clinical**: The clinical data are comprised of information about each subject including recruitment, demographics, physical examinations, cognitive assessment data, and diagnosis. The cognitive assessments include measures such as the Alzheimer's Disease Assessment Scale – cognitive subscale (ADAS-cog), Cog State Battery, Clinical Dementia Rating, Montreal Cognitive Assessment, Neuropsychiatric Inventory, and Geriatric Depression Scale [11].

- **Imaging**: Both MRI and PET imaging have been fundamental to ADNI and have evolved throughout the study period.

    MRI sequences that are available include: structural, fluid-attenuated inversion recovery (FLAIR), T2 gradient recalled echo, diffusion tensor imaging (DTI), task-free functional MRI (fMRI), arterial spin labeling, and T2 hippocampus. However, there has been changes in the MRI protocol through the study. DTI and fMRI scans were added in ADNI GO and ADNI 2, whereas participants from ADNI 1 only received structural MRIs (add processing protocol) [12].

    PET imaging also varied during the different phases of ADNI. Patients in ADNI 1 initially received ^{11}C Pittsburgh compound B (PiB) scans. However, the protocol was amended before the conclusion of the study to include the adoption of florbetapir scans over PiB scans due to processing time limits. Therefore, PiB was only used on a small set of participants (approximately 100) in ADNI 1. In ADNI 1, only a subset of participants received FDG PET imaging. Tau and amyloid PET imaging were performed on all participants at their initial ADNI 3 visit. The subsequent tau imaging schedule depended on amyloid status: 80% of amyloid-positive and 20% of amyloid-negative participants were scheduled to have three additional tau scans, whereas the remaining 80% of amyloid-negative and 20% amyloid-positive participants would have one additional tau scan. Amyloid PET imaging is performed on every 2-year schedule, either

with florbetapir (participants continuing from ADNI 2) or florbetaben (newly enrolled participants). FDG PET imaging was performed on MCI and AD participants at baseline only [8].

- **Biospecimens**: A variety of fluid biospecimens are collected in ADNI including urine, blood serum and plasma, buffy coat, apolipoprotein-E (*APOE*)/genome-wide association studies (GWAS), cell immortalization, RNA, and cerebrospinal fluid (CSF). Investigators can request samples from the Biofluid Biobank; also available are highly standardized amyloid beta 42 ($A\beta_{42}$), total tau (t-tau), and hyperphosphorylated tau 181 (p-tau$_{181}$) measurements on CSF samples [13].

- **Genetics**: Genotyping and sequencing data have been generated for ADNI 1, ADNI GO, and ADNI 2 subjects and can be requested by ADNI investigators. Available data include *APOE* genotyping, translocase of outer mitochondrial membrane 40 (TOMM40) poly-T variant, and GWAS [14].

40.6 Data Capture and Distribution

The potential of advancing scientific collaboration with the goal of improving knowledge and treatment of disease through the practice of open data sharing had been recognized for decades. However, the willingness of scientific communities to accept a sharing model built upon contributions across institutions, laboratories, and investigators has been more recent and exemplified by ADNI.

Before the project began, the NIA realized that the amount of data that ADNI could generate would exceed what the ADNI investigators were able to analyze on their own. It was decided that data would be stored in a database hosted by the Laboratory of Neuroimaging (LONI), currently housed at the University of Southern California, and that the data would be available nearly immediately after acquisition, following quality-control analysis. Unlike customary policies of prior studies, there was no embargo on the availability of the resources generated by ADNI – no special access or period of exclusive use with respect to either the data or the biofluid and DNA samples from the participants – for either the ADNI investigators or the private partners. In addition, there are no preemptive intellectual-property rights associated with the data in the database. The data and the samples are open to the entire scientific research community, establishing a precedent for policies that facilitate federally funded research. All data generated from the use of ADNI samples are also made immediately available on the ADNI LONI website [15].

As a result, ADNI data have been queried millions of times by investigators around the world, mostly from university researchers, followed by pharmaceutical/biotechnology companies, scanner manufacturers, government scientists, and other members of the public, including high-school teachers.

The longitudinal collection of data in ADNI has been challenging to arrange in a useful form given the complex, heterogeneous, and extensive nature of the data. As outlined above, in the earliest ADNI phase (ADNI 1), different study cohorts (healthy control, MCI, and AD subjects) followed different protocols. In subsequent ADNI phases (ADNI GO and ADNI 2), additional cohorts were added for early MCI, late MCI, and SMC subjects and new clinical assessments were added, florbetapir PET scans replaced PiB PET scans [8] and additional vendor-specific MRI scanning sequences were added. Throughout the study, image and biospecimen analysts have returned results at different times and for different subsets of subjects. All of these study changes and additions have contributed toward an increasingly valuable but disparate data set. However, a stringent set of methods have been established to allow transfer of data from clinical examinations and fluid and imaging biomarkers, application of quality-control measures, synchronization of data, and assurance of data safety.

ADNI data are widely shared but remain restricted to investigators who agree to the terms of the ADNI data-use agreement and receive the approval of the DPC. The ADNI repository provides online, web-based interfaces for managing the full range of data-access and control activities. These include (1) an online data-use application; (2) an online application review system that enables rapid evaluation and an approve/disapprove application; (3) automated user-account creation and notification for approved applicants; (4) online progress-report notifications that notify investigators when a progress report is due and to automatically terminate accounts of non-responsive investigators; and (5) an online manuscript submission system whereby investigators may submit

manuscripts to the DPC for review as required under the ADNI data-use agreement.

40.7 Worldwide ADNI

One of the major goals of the original ADNI project was to standardize methods for measuring a variety of biomarkers. Standardization of protocols has enabled ADNI to collect comparable data from multiple sites and has spread globally to Europe, Asia, Australia, and South America. Data sharing without embargo has expanded to the Worldwide ADNI (WW-ADNI) initiatives as well.

WW-ADNI is an umbrella organization created and managed by the Alzheimer's Association. The goal in creating WW-ADNI was to harmonize protocols and results across different geographical ADNI sites so that researchers will have access to comparable worldwide data [16].

Among the worldwide initiatives, the ADNI platform was first introduced into Europe in the form of a small cross-sectional pilot study, E-ADNI, which aimed to assess the feasibility of utilizing ADNI procedures to multiple European countries. A number of other data collection programs in Europe include (1) AddNeuroMed, a public–private initiative with a cohort of 700 control, MCI, and AD subjects across Europe that used ADNI protocols for structural MRI; (2) Pharmacog, which overlaps the most with ADNI and which aims to predict cognitive properties of new drug candidates for neurodegenerative diseases; (3) Swedish ADNI, a small-scale initiative that used ADNI protocol and subsequently has merged into the larger Swedish BrainPower initiative; and (4) Italian ADNI, a larger project with 480 patients enrolled. These studies have in common the use of standardized ADNI protocols for at least some of their data collection. Several data-repository projects have been implemented in Europe. NeuGRID is the European equivalent of LONI, and out-GRID aims to synergize neuGRID, LONI, and the Canadian repository, CBRAIN, and to develop full interoperability. CATI (Centre pour l'Acquisition et le Traitement de l'Image) is the French repository for data sets within that country.

The Australian version of ADNI, termed AIBL, has similar goals to ADNI and uses ADNI protocols for its imaging studies. AIBL, however, is taking a specific focus on investigating lifestyle factors involved in AD. By collecting extensive neuropsychological and lifestyle data, the study aims to understand which health and lifestyle factors protect or contribute to AD. Like ADNI, however, all data are made available through LONI and are funded by the Alzheimer's Association.

The Japanese ADNI (J-ADNI) was conceived in 2006 when ADNI was beginning in North America and at the end of the Japanese study J-COSMIC (Japan Cooperative SPECT Study on Assessment of Mild Impairment of Cognitive Function). J-ADNI further advanced the development of an infrastructure to conduct global clinical trials of AD drugs in Japan and was important to Japanese researchers in fostering international collaboration.

40.8 ADNI, Biomarkers, and Clinical Trials

Despite the successful development and approval of several cholinesterase inhibitors, along with the N-methyl-D-aspartate receptor modulator, memantine, it was close to 20 years before another drug for AD received approval. There are many reasons offered for this disappointing record including drug selection, dosing, and decisions about moving certain agents along the clinical trial pathway; subject selection; choice (and variability) of outcome measures; and trial duration.

ADNI was created to collect and integrate knowledge of AD pathophysiology, imaging and fluid biomarkers, and various clinical and neuropsychological measures with the goal of identifying the best biomarker or combination of biomarkers that reflect disease progression and are most likely to predict response to therapy. ADNI investigators have advanced the design of pre-dementia trials, influencing regulators in the United States and abroad. These advances have included the move from time-to-endpoint designs to continuous outcome measures as primaries, the use of biomarker-based subject selection, single primary outcomes in prodromal trials, and cognitive endpoints in pre-dementia clinical trials [17–19].

With an increasing focus on the development of disease-modifying therapies, ADNI biomarker work is specifically aimed at this aspect of AD drug development. Some of the more immediate applications that have come out of ADNI involve cohort selection, outcome measures, and other issues related to trial design.

40.8.1 Cohort Selection

In selecting an appropriate cohort for clinical trials, one barrier in the past has been the use of clinical AD and MCI criteria. It is known that clinical criteria used in the past have lacked specificity, with some patients diagnosed with MCI or dementia due to AD not having AD pathology. Moreover, as AD "prevention" studies were launched, clinical criteria had insufficient sensitivity (it is not possibly to reliably identify cognitively normal subjects who have amyloid pathology using clinical measurements). In the past, subjects who fulfilled clinical criteria for AD but without AD pathology were likely enrolled in trials due to a lack of amyloid measures. One of the major accomplishments of ADNI has been to validate amyloid phenotyping via CSF or amyloid PET imaging. ADNI has shown that a CSF profile of low $A\beta_{42}$ and elevated t-tau and p-tau$_{181}$ characterizes AD [20]. Similarly, a positive amyloid PET scan identifies the presence of fibrillar amyloid plaques and demonstrates the presence of plaques in nearly all AD, 60% of MCI, and 20–30% of cognitively normal elderly [21]. Furthermore, a novel staging approach used florbetapir PET data from across the full ADNI cohort to define a four-stage model of amyloid progression similar to that reported in neuropathological studies. Successive stages were associated with progressively lower CSF $A\beta_{42}$ levels and with more severe diagnostic stages. Unlike dichotomous systems of defining amyloid positivity, stage I captured the earliest signs of amyloid deposition, suggesting that the system may aid the selection of participants for clinical trials of amyloid-modifying therapies [22]. If amyloid measures to ensure the presence of the AD process is used in studies submitted as part of a new drug application (NDA), then the labeling for the drug will need to include this in the indication.

Because detecting a disease-modifying effect in AD depends on demonstrating a difference in slope of trajectory between treated and placebo groups, it is necessary that the placebo group shows notable decline over the study period. The cognitively normal group of ADNI showed almost no change in a 12-month period. Moreover, placebo participants in seven randomized controlled trials over the past decade were found to have highly variable trajectories of cognitive change in a recent study [23]. These findings may be due to differences in entry criteria, distribution of APOE ε4 (APOE-4) status, co-morbidities and resilience factors, and outcome measures. Thus, particularly for MCI and prevention studies, identifying a biomarker profile that can predict the likelihood of decline within the study period and outcome measures that are sensitive to change in these groups would enhance the chance of recognizing an effective therapy. ADNI is well positioned to characterize this biomarker profile.

40.8.2 Outcome Measures

Due to requirements for drug approval, AD clinical trials used measures of memory, cognition, and/or function as outcomes. These are imperfect measures as they are subject to high test–retest variability and are influenced by factors other than changes due to AD. A "biological marker" that represents progression of AD pathology, correlates with symptomatology (especially memory and cognitive decline), and is not affected by non-AD pathology could be used as a surrogate outcome measure, overcoming the problems associated with the current clinical measures. Biomarkers studied in ADNI can be used in all phases of drug development. Amyloid measured in the CSF could provide evidence of target engagement and provide insight into the mechanistic impact of agents on amyloid metabolism which would be appropriate for Phase 1 studies.

In Phase 2 studies, sponsors must decide on whether to do long, large studies to demonstrate proof of concept or smaller, shorter trials utilizing biomarkers not proven to predict success. The first approach has a lower risk but increased cost; the latter strategy is faster and less expensive but carries a greater risk of ending up with a negative outcome in Phase 3 trials. Biomarkers are helpful in this setting because they can enrich the cohort and detect drug effects with few patients exposed for shorter periods of time than simply using clinical measures.

In regard to potential biomarker outcome measures, despite some early hopes, brain amyloid burden, measured with amyloid PET or in CSF, does not correlate well with disease severity and has not yet been proven an effective surrogate outcome. Several counterintuitive results in which increased brain atrophy was reported in response to anti-amyloid therapy have also ruled out volumetric MRI measures as satisfactory surrogate markers for therapeutic amyloid reduction. However, other MRI measures being explored in ADNI may still be a highly useful outcome measure for neuroprotective interventions. On the other hand, pathological studies have indicated that AD symptomatology is more closely associated with tau tangles than amyloid deposits [24], and that brain tau correlates with cognition [25], suggesting a cause–effect relationship between tau tangles, synaptic dysfunction/synapse loss/neurodegeneration, and cognitive function. With the introduction of PET tau ligands, the possibility that tau PET could ultimately be used as a surrogate marker for AD clinical trials has emerged. However, synaptic loss correlates most closely with cognitive impairment in AD, so it is possible that CSF synaptic protein biomarkers such as neurogranin could play a significant role as a surrogate marker in concert with biomarkers of AD pathology.

Phase 3 trials require clinical outcomes for the NDA, and sample sizes cannot be reduced using biomarkers. Moreover, larger samples are needed to provide the necessary exposures to detect safety or tolerability issues associated with the trial agent. Biomarkers, however, are required to support a disease-modifying type claim unless randomized start or randomized withdrawal trial designs are utilized to demonstrate disease modification. Several ADNI biomarkers could serve as outcomes in prevention trials including CSF t-tau or p-tau, p-tau/$A\beta_{42}$ ratio, or tau PET imaging. None are validated surrogates but might act as unvalidated surrogates or could serve as key secondary outcomes in trials using clinical measures as primary outcomes.

Until a validated biomarker that is linked with clinical meaningfulness becomes available there remains a need for a clinical outcome measure that is sensitive to change in preclinical and MCI stages of AD. Using data from ADNI, among other cohorts, a composite clinic outcome measure termed ADCOMS was developed that included elements from several commonly used cognitive and functional scales [26]. The ADCOMS had better sensitivity over individual tests to detect clinical decline in MCI and mild AD, thus reducing the sample sizes required in various simulations.

40.8.3 Sample Size

Data from ADNI studies have been used to determine sample sizes for clinical trials required to show a 20–25% reduction in disease progression [22]. Biomarkers provide a numerical advantage over clinical measures in enriching the cohort and demonstrating a disease-modifying effect. For example, based on modeling from ADNI, an MCI trial using a combination of hippocampal volume and amyloid positivity, defined by explicit cut points, reduced the required sample sizes by 45–60% depending on the outcome measure used. Enrichment with hippocampal volume followed by amyloid positivity, combined with the use of ADAS-cog13 as an outcome measure, reduced the sample size required to detect a 30% treatment effect with 80% power from 908 to 363, the estimated trial cost from $83 million to $45 million, and the estimated trial time from 5.2 years to 4.3 years [27].

However, caution must be exercised in extrapolating these calculations directly to clinical trials. The ADNI calculations are based on studying the rate or amount of change occurring in a structure in a given time (e.g., hippocampal change in 12 months) and calculating how many patients would be required to show a drug–placebo difference if the drug had a 20–25% effect. An agent, however, that decreased amyloid production by 25% might not have a 25% effect on MRI volumetrics since these are measures of neurodegeneration and the relationships between amyloid production and neurodegeneration are unknown. Power calculations for trials should allow for these uncertainties.

40.9 ADNI Caveats

There are some characteristics of ADNI that may influence how the data are applied to clinical trial design. Notably, the sample is very well educated, with educational levels of 14.7–16 years indicating that most subjects had completed several years of college. Patients with higher education levels tend to have later onset of AD and faster progression after onset. This high level of education may complicate extrapolating some results to other trials, particularly international trials which tend to include more persons with low educational levels. Similarly, most trials have more women than men, while the ADNI cohort has the reverse (percentage of females ranging from 35.4 to 48). This might affect the generalization of some aspects of ADNI.

The ADNI cohort provides data on more mild AD patients and anticipates the likely inclusion of more mild patients in clinical trials. Extrapolating biomarker data from ADNI to typical protocols including mild-to-moderate AD (typically a Mini-Mental State Examination [MMSE] score range of 16–26) is difficult; patients with more severe disease tend to progress more rapidly and may have different biomarker–clinical relationships.

The clinical definition of MCI also bears on the likelihood of evolution to AD dementia. The definition of MCI used to define the ADNI cohort differs from the definition of MCI developed by Petersen et al. [2]. The definition employed in the ADNI MCI population is more defined operationally with MMSE score ranges and thresholds for neuropsychological assessments. Patients with more than mild depression or more than minimal vascular symptoms are excluded. These differences will affect the composition of the trial population and the ADNI biomarker findings will apply most readily to MCI populations using the same MCI definition. Minor differences in MCI definitions have substantial effects in clinical trials as evidenced by the markedly different percentages of APOE-4 carriers across MCI trials [28]. Results must be extrapolated from trial to trial with caution; and ADNI results also must be generalized with careful consideration of the sample selection criteria.

40.10 Conclusion

Beginning over 15 years ago, ADNI continues to provide the global scientific community with high-quality data to address critical questions about the development and progression of AD. From the demonstration that biomarkers can detect AD disease changes years prior to the onset of symptoms, to revealing the complexities of AD disease progression, ADNI has helped guide a shift in focus toward designing clinical trial interventions earlier in the disease process. Furthermore, through development of novel biomarkers and measures that can be applied to subject selection and outcome measures, ADNI has provided tools that may be incorporated to complete clinical trials and determine therapeutic effectiveness much faster and at a lower cost.

References

1. Schneider LS, Mangialasche F, Andreasen N, et al. Clinical trials and late-stage drug development for Alzheimer's disease: an appraisal from 1984 to 2014. *J Intern Med* 2014; **275**: 251–83.

2. Petersen RC, Doody R, Kurz A, et al. Current concepts in mild cognitive impairment. *Arch Neurol* 2001; **58**: 1985–92.

3. Becker RE, Greig NH. Alzheimer's disease drug development in 2008 and beyond: problems and opportunities. *Curr Alzheimer Res* 2008; **5**: 346–57.

4. Cummings JL. Integrating ADNI results into Alzheimer's disease drug development programs. *Neurobiol Aging* 2010; **31**: 1481–92.

5. Mueller SG, Weiner MW, Thal LJ, et al. The Alzheimer's Disease Neuroimaging Initiative. *Neuroimaging Clin N Am* 2005; **15**: 869-xii.

6. Weiner MW, Aisen PS, Jack CR, et al. The Alzheimer's Disease Neuroimaging Initiative: progress report and future plans. *Alzheimers Dement* 2010; **6**: 202–11.e7.

7. Weiner MW, Veitch DP, Aisen PS, et al. 2014 Update of the Alzheimer's Disease Neuroimaging Initiative: a review of papers published since its inception. *Alzheimers Dement* 2015; **11**: e1–120.

8. Weiner MW, Veitch DP, Aisen PS, et al. The Alzheimer's Disease Neuroimaging Initiative 3: continued innovation for clinical trial improvement. *Alzheimers Dement* 2017; **13**: 561–71.

9. Lee S, Bozeman B. The impact of research collaboration on scientific productivity. *Soc Stud Sci* 2005; **35**: 673–702.

10. Jones-Davis DM, Buckholtz N. The impact of ADNI: what role do public–private partnerships have in pushing the boundaries of clinical and basic science research on Alzheimer's disease. *Alzheimers Dement* 2015; **11**: 860–4.

11. Aisen PS, Petersen RC, Donohue MC, et al. Clinical Core of the Alzheimer's Disease Neuroimaging Initiative: progress and plans. *Alzheimers Dement* 2010; **6**: 239–46.

12. Jack CR, Bernstein MA, Borowski BJ, et al. Update on the MRI core of the Alzheimer's Disease Neuroimaging Initiative. *Alzheimers Dement* 2010; 6: 212–20.

13. Kang J, Korecka M, Figurski MJ, et al. The Alzheimer's Disease Neuroimaging Initiative 2 Biomarker Core: a review of progress and plans. *Alzheimers Dement* 2015; **11**: 772–91.

14. Saykin AJ, Shen L, Yao X, et al. Genetic studies of quantitative MCI and AD phenotypes in ADNI: progress, opportunities, and plans. *Alzheimers Dement* 2015; **11**: 792–814.

15. Toga AW, Crawford KL. The Alzheimer's Disease Neuroimaging Initiative Informatics Core: a decade in review. *Alzheimers Dement* 2015; **11**: 832–9.

16. Carillo MC, Bain LJ, Frisoni GB, Weiner MW. Worldwide Alzheimer's Disease Neuroimaging Initiative. *Alzheimers Dement* 2012; **8**: 337–42.

17. Donohue MC, Gamst AC, Thomas RG, et al. The relative efficiency of time-to-threshold and rate of change in longitudinal data. *Contemp Clin Trials* 2011; **32**: 685–93.

18. Aisen PS, Andrieu S, Sampaio C, et al. Report of the task force on designing clinical trials in early (predementia) AD. *Neurology* 2011; **76**: 280–6.

19. Aisen PS, Vellas B, Hampel H. Moving towards early clinical trials for amyloid-targeted therapy in Alzheimer's disease. *Nat Rev Drug Discov* 2013; **12**: 324.

20. Shaw LM, Vanderstichele H, Knapik-Czajka M, et al. Cerebrospinal fluid biomarker signature in Alzheimer's Disease Neuroimaging Initiative subjects. *Ann Neurol* 2009; **65**: 403–13.

21. Jack CR Jr., Lowe VJ, Weigand SD, et al. Serial PIB and MRI in normal, mild cognitive impairment and Alzheimer's disease: implications for sequence of pathological events in Alzheimer's disease. *Brain* 2009; **132**: 1355–65.

22. Veitch DP, Weiner MW, Aisen PS, et al. Understanding disease progression and improving Alzheimer's disease clinical trials: recent highlights from the Alzheimer's Disease Neuroimaging Initiative. *Alzheimers Dement* 2019; **15**: 106–52.

23. Petersen RC, Thomas RG, Aisen PS, et al. Randomized controlled trials in mild cognitive impairment: sources of variability. *Neurology* 2017; **88**: 1751–8.

24. Nelson PT, Alafuzoff I, Bigio EH, et al. Correlation of Alzheimer disease neuropathologic changes with cognitive status: a review of the literature. *J Neuropathol Exp Neurol* 2012; **71**: 362–8.

25. Braak H, Braak E. Staging of Alzheimer's disease-related neurofibrillary changes. *Neurobiol Aging* 1995; **16**: 271–8.

26. Wang J, Logovinsky V, Hendrix SB, et al. ADCOMS: a composite clinical outcome for prodromal Alzheimer's disease trials. *J Neurol Neurosurg Psychiatry* 2016; **87**: 993–9.

27. Wolz R, Schwarz AJ, Gray KR, Yu P, Hill DL, Alzheimer's Disease Neuroimaging Initiative. Enrichment of clinical trials in MCI due to AD using markers of amyloid and neurodegeneration. *Neurology* 2016; **87**: 1235–41.

28. Jelic V, Kivipelto M, Winblad B. Clinical trials in mild cognitive impairment: lessons for the future. *J Neurol Neurosurg Psychiatry* 2006; **77**: 429–38.

Financing Alzheimer's Disease Drug Development

Jayna Cummings, Amanda Hu, Angela Su, and Andrew W. Lo

41.1 Introduction

Alzheimer's disease (AD), the most common cause of dementia, is arguably one of the largest unmet medical needs of our time, affecting the daily life of an estimated 6.2 million Americans aged 65 or older, and millions more across the globe. AD ranks sixth among the top 10 leading causes of death in the United States and, until June 7, 2021, when the controversial aducanumab (Aduhelm™) received US Food and Drug Administration (FDA) approval using the accelerated approval pathway, it was the only condition for which there were no treatments available to prevent, cure, or slow it. Without the development of a significant medical breakthrough, the number of people aged 65 or older with AD in the United States is projected to more than double to 12.7 million by 2050, and its related costs to the US healthcare system are expected to more than triple, from $355 billion in 2021 to more than $1.1 trillion by 2050. In addition, the estimated 15.3 billion hours of unpaid assistance provided by informal caregivers (often family members and friends) are valued at $256.7 billion, imposed by a lack of other treatment options [1]. Whether the FDA's approval of aducanumab can help to stem this tide remains to be seen.

Despite these staggering numbers, and the large market they represent, drug development in this critical field has been slow. Between 1998 and 2017, there were an estimated 146 medicines for AD unsuccessfully developed, and only four approvals [2]. Until 2021, not one single novel medication had been approved to treat AD in the US since 2003, and the five FDA-approved AD drugs available during that time treated only the symptoms of the disease. The focus in AD research has shifted to disease-modifying therapeutics, but the failure of several costly Phase 3 trials in recent years has hastened the withdrawal from this field by several big pharmaceutical companies, as well

as many private-sector investors. The recent aducanumab approval may change this trend.

These dynamics imply that the risks associated with developing drugs for AD are higher than for other diseases, often outweighing the allure of the substantial revenues of an effective disease-modifying AD therapy. A new AD drug could be worth tens of billions of dollars upon approval. Indeed, upon the approval of aducanumab, it was estimated that Biogen could stand to make $112 billion in the United States alone if it could reach one-third of the estimated 6 million Americans living with AD [3]. However, this is highly speculative and must be weighed against the very high probability of failure and the risk of total loss – the high cost of AD drug development poses an enormous financial risk to investors. Across the entire pharmaceutical industry and all diseases, the overall success rate of drug-development programs is 13.8% [4], and the median and average costs to bring a new therapy to market are estimated to be $985.3 million and $1.3 billion, respectively, with a cost of capital of 10.5% [5]. An AD drug-development program costs an estimated $5.7 billion (with an 11% cost of capital) and lasts about 13 years [6], with an overall failure rate of 99% [7]. In contrast, cancer drug-development programs have a median cost of $793.6 million (with a 9% cost of capital) and a median development time of 7.3 years [8], with an estimated success rate of 3.4% [4].

The higher cost of AD drug development stems from our current understanding of AD, or lack thereof. Despite recent scientific breakthroughs, many of AD's biological causes and underlying mechanisms remain unknown. For instance, it is still unclear whether the biomolecular hallmarks of AD, amyloid plaques and tau tangles, are causes or symptoms of the disease. Further confounding the drug-development process are the limitations of preclinical models in translating AD findings to humans, the lack of surrogate AD biomarkers, and the difficulty of diagnosing and monitoring the progression of AD. While Congress allocated more funding to the National Institutes of Health (NIH) to study AD, greater private-sector investment will be required to bring this new knowledge forward. Ironically, greater financial resources are required in order to reduce the costs and risks of AD drug development, which will be necessary to attract greater private-sector investment and address these challenges.

41.2 The Funding Landscape for AD Drug Discovery and Development

Every stage of the drug discovery and development process, from basic preclinical research to marketing approval, requires financial resources. Each stage also carries with it a level of risk, uncertainty, and complexity driven by our current biological understanding of a given disease, target, or mechanism (Figure 41.1). Familiarity with the available range of funders, investors, and financing methods within the biopharmaceutical ecosystem and their corresponding appetites for risk are critical to advancing AD drug development.

In this section, we consider the general progression of such an advance in chronological format,

according to the typical timeline of therapeutic development. However, some funding bodies and investors will finance research and development at multiple stages in the drug discovery and development process as a result of increasing collaboration across stakeholder groups.

41.2.1 Government Funding

In the United States, the NIH invests tens of billions of dollars annually in medical research, making it the largest single public funder of biomedical research in the world. With more than 80% of the NIH's funding awarded for extramural research (outside of the federal government) through its competitive grants process, the NIH is the principal supporter of investigator-initiated research leading to new targets and potential new interventions. Studies suggest that this pursuit has been largely successful. For example, one study found that NIH funding contributed to every new molecular entity (NME) approved between 2010 and 2016, focusing primarily on drug targets versus the NMEs themselves [9]. Within the NIH, the National Institute on Aging (NIA) is the primary agency supporting and conducting AD research, working closely with the National Institute of Neurological Disorders and Stroke (NINDS) to establish research priorities and fund projects.

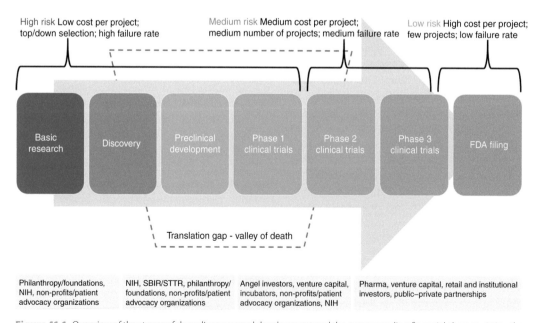

Figure 41.1 Overview of the stages of drug discovery and development and the corresponding financial characteristics, the natural funders and investors for each stage, and the most appropriate financing method.

Through a number of collaborations with industry and non-profit partners, the NIA and NINDS have established several initiatives to support and accelerate the discovery process.

With the passage of the National Alzheimer's Plan Act (NAPA) in 2011, the United States metaphorically declared a "war on Alzheimer's." In 2012, the National Plan to Address Alzheimer's Disease was released, establishing five goals to prevent future cases of AD and its related dementias, and to better meet the needs of American families currently confronting the disease [10]. Prompted by the growing burden of AD in the aging US population, and following the first goal of the National Plan to "prevent and effectively treat AD by 2025," NIA funding increased substantially between 2011 and 2020, from $448 million to $2.8 billion [11]. NAPA was also followed by the launch of the Brain Research through Advancing Innovative Neurotechnologies (BRAIN) initiative in 2013, a public–private research initiative inspired by the Human Genome Project, one aimed at revolutionizing our understanding of the brain and new ways to treat, cure, and prevent brain disorders such as AD.

Nevertheless, considering the outsized socioeconomic burden of AD, the NIH budget allocated to AD is comparatively small. For instance, medical care costs associated with cancer survivorship in 2015 were an estimated $183 billion (in 2019 US dollars) and projected to increase to $246 billion by 2030 [12], significantly smaller than the projected costs of AD to the United States, yet the National Cancer Institute's budget in 2020 was over $7 billion, more than twice as large as the funding to AD (see Figure 41.2 for a comparison of NIH budget allocations for cancer vs. AD).

Given the socioeconomic burden of AD, governments should have a strong incentive to invest heavily in translational research. Less risk-averse than individual and institutional investors, the government is uniquely positioned to invest in the long-term interests of its citizens and engage key stakeholders from across the biomedical ecosystem in developing new treatments and technologies.

The NIH is one of the few sources of funding that spans across the entire drug-development process, albeit to a smaller extent as it moves into later-stage development. For example, the Small Business Innovation Research (SBIR) and Small Business Technology Transfer (STTR) programs exist to help bridge the gap between early-stage research and clinical development by encouraging small domestic businesses to engage in research and development (R&D) with potential for commercialization. Federal agencies with extramural R&D budgets exceeding $100 million are required to allocate 3.2% to fund small businesses through

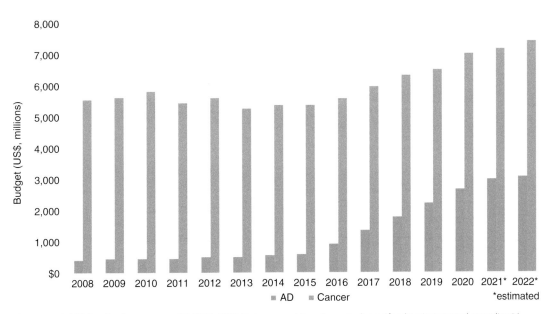

Figure 41.2 NIH funding for cancer vs. AD, 2008–2022. Data source: https://report.nih.gov/funding/categorical-spending#/.

the SBIR program. Similarly, federal agencies with extramural R&D budgets greater than $1 billion are required to reserve 0.45% to fund the STTR program. Currently, 11 federal agencies participate in the SBIR program, and five of them also participate in the STTR program. The NIA's SBIR and STTR grants and contracts went from approximately $26.5 million in 2011 to $87.7 million in 2018.

41.2.2 Philanthropy and Foundations

Philanthropists are individuals who give their time, money, experience, or reputation, whether directly or through a foundation, to serve a greater good and help create a better world. They are not typically interested in financial returns, but rather the measurable impact of their donation in addressing a chosen cause. As a result, philanthropic capital can fill in the gaps where commercial and government funding cannot, providing seed funding for high-risk, high-reward projects that may otherwise be too undeveloped to receive funding from other sources.

Although philanthropy represents only a small portion of overall scientific funding – an estimated 2–4% [13] – it is a powerful resource that can help demonstrate a proof of concept and attract additional funding from government or other sources to build infrastructure for drug discovery and development [14].

In some cases, philanthropists and foundations have collaborated to leverage their investments and enable more serious drug discovery efforts. For example, in July 2018, several major philanthropists, including Leonard Lauder, Bill Gates, the Dolby family, and the Charles and Helen Schwab Foundation, jointly created the Diagnostics Accelerator program, an initiative of the Alzheimer's Drug Discovery Foundation (ADDF), with an initial funding commitment totaling almost $35 million. The Diagnostics Accelerator serves as a "call to action" to the research community, encouraging and advancing the development of new diagnostics and biomarkers, which will improve our understanding of the disease and the design of clinical trials.

41.2.3 Non-Profit and Advocacy Organizations

Advocacy and other non-profit organizations typically play an important role in funding basic and early-stage research through research grants. Equally as important, however, is the expertise and access to patients these organizations can bring to the drug discovery and development process. Like foundations and philanthropy, non-profit and advocacy organizations are well suited to fund exploratory and early-stage research since they prioritize the impact of research over financial returns. The key difference between foundations and philanthropy versus non-profit and advocacy organizations is their source of funding – for the former, it is typically a single donation from an individual or family, while for the latter, it is gifts and donations from the general public, philanthropists, and other grant opportunities.

The Alzheimer's Association is the largest non-profit funder of AD research in the world, currently investing more than $208 million in 590 projects across 31 countries. It funds projects across the research spectrum, aimed at increasing the scientific understanding of AD, brain health, and disease prevention, identifying new treatment strategies, and improving care for people suffering from AD and their families.

Non-profit and advocacy organizations also undertake other important initiatives aimed at improving the lives of patients, including raising disease awareness, lobbying for regulatory changes and increased funding, referring patients to clinical trials, and providing resources and support to families.

41.2.4 Angel Investors

Angel investors are a growing sector of funding, investing an estimated $4.3 billion in 2019 [15]. Usually one of the first groups of investors in early-stage clinical development, angel investors are typically high-net-worth individuals who invest smaller amounts of money in a specific product, service, or industry in exchange for equity or convertible debt in a start-up company. In 2019, an estimated 21% of transactions involving an angel investor were in the healthcare and biotechnology sectors; the largest percentage of transactions (28.7%) were in the technology and software sector [15].

In addition to injecting capital into an early-stage company, angel investors may also provide valuable contacts and advice for the entrepreneur. Also known as seed investors, angel funders, or private investors, angel investors typically invest in the initial stage of an endeavor. This means that their investments are risky, and they are subject to high dilution rates as the company issues more equity. As a result, angel investors look for companies with potentially very high returns on investment (ROI). Due to its risky nature, angel investors typically look for an ROI of 10-fold or more, in addition to using risk-management measures such as exit strategies and future growth and acquisition plans. Many early-stage companies need smaller initial investments, on the order of $5 million, while venture capital firms typically prefer to make investments of at least $25 million. Angel investors help to bridge that capital gap [16].

For an entrepreneur, angel investors are able to offer a much-needed boost in cash on terms less strict than those of traditional lenders. Contracts with angel investors usually carry fewer stipulations, partly due to the fact that angel investors frequently invest in the entrepreneur, rather than the business. While banks may not be willing to lend to an entrepreneur, angel investors offer an opportunity for entrepreneurs to keep building their company while keeping a solid bank balance. Most entrepreneurs find their angel investors through personal contacts, although a growing number of angel investors are shifting to online crowdfunding sites. Securing an angel investor may be difficult, as most investors specialize in certain sectors of their own choosing.

41.2.5 Venture Capital

Historically, venture capital (VC) has been the primary funding source for start-ups, financing the work needed to translate new knowledge into effective therapies. However, after the downturns of 2008 and 2011, investors began to withdraw capital, particularly in the early-stage life-science space, when their returns no longer sufficiently compensated them for their high risk and long lock-up periods, resulting in a contraction of VC funds and greater focus on later-stage companies [17]. Between 2009 and 2014, the total VC invested in all industry sectors increased significantly from $20.3 billion to $39.6 billion, while the investment in life-science companies shrank as a percentage of total investments, from 35.7% to 19.9%. Over the same time period, there were significant shifts from early- to later-stage investments in healthcare. The percentage of early-stage investments dedicated to healthcare decreased

from 62% to 45%, while the amount invested in later-stage life-science companies increased from 38% to 55% [18].

These trends in VC funding are driven by the increasing risk and uncertainty of the drug-development process [19]. Today, while some VC firms are willing to invest in early-stage biotechnology companies with strong data to support their technology, the vast majority continue to hold off until a program is sufficiently de-risked. Large pharmaceutical companies have become the main customers for VCs, which has a direct impact on the disease indications these companies are willing to pursue [14]. Their typical investment time horizons are 3–7 years. VC investing primarily involves milestones and exit opportunities such as licensing agreements, co-development agreements, and stock sales or initial public offerings (IPOs).

Given these considerations, it is no surprise that VC investment in AD has been low. According to a 2019 BIO report, between 2008 and 2017, the amount of venture investment in US companies with lead-stage programs in AD totaled only $741 million, compared to $12.2 billion over the same period for novel oncology drugs [20].

41.2.6 Biotechnology Initial Public Offerings

The year 2020 was a banner year for biotechnology IPOs despite – or perhaps because of – the COVID-19 pandemic. Eighty-two biotechnology companies debuted on the Nasdaq stock exchange, raising a total of $15 billion. To put this in perspective, 2019 saw 55 biotechnology IPOs that raised $5.6 billion. This trend may seem to bode well for AD therapeutics, but the unfortunate reality is that very few of those IPOs were of companies focused on AD. Using a slightly different sample of biotechnology IPOs raising more than $50 million, BioPharma Dive classified the IPOs according to therapeutic area, and Table 41.1 shows the same trend away from AD – which is part of the central nervous system (CNS) category – that Big Pharma has exhibited. Therefore, as friendly as the IPO market may seem to the life sciences in general, it is unlikely to imply greater levels of financing for AD biotechnology companies unless something dramatic changes.

With the rise in funding levels for AD research from the NIA starting in 2016, a number of

Table 41.1 All biotechnology IPOs on US exchanges that raised more than $50 million, stratified by therapeutic area

Therapeutic focus	2020	2019	2018
Cancer	34	15	17
Rare disease	12	3	8
Immune	6	4	5
CNS	4	6	1
Infections	6	0	5
Other*	8	10	8

*"Other" includes liver, eye, heart, gastrointestinal, metabolic, ear, skin, and kidney.

Source: BioPharma Dive (www.biopharmadive.com/news/biotech-ipo-performance-tracker/587604/).

translational opportunities in AD should start appearing within the next few years (assuming a 10-year gestation lag between fundamental science and therapeutic application). It is imperative to prepare for that moment by creating the business ecosystem needed to fund this translational effort, and it must begin soon, given the time lags involved in launching such endeavors.

41.2.7 Pharmaceutical Companies

As our understanding of biology and human disease has grown over the last two decades, new approaches to therapeutic interventions have caused seismic shifts in the respective roles of biotechnology and pharmaceutical companies. Prior to the 1980s, pharmaceutical companies were typically fully integrated enterprises, taking projects from preclinical drug discovery through clinical development to marketing and commercialization. This was the era of chemistry, in which small molecules were the dominant therapeutic class.

However, the use of microbes for producing chemical feedstocks and the development of recombinant DNA technology ushered in the era of biology, in which large-molecule therapeutics have begun to take the market share away from more traditional medicines. This trend away from chemistry toward biology has greatly increased the complexity of drug development because many of today's therapeutics are the product of living organisms such as engineered T-cells or viral vectors, and these are often more difficult to incorporate into scalable manufacturing processes than large arrays of precisely controlled chemical reactors.

With the entrance of thousands of smaller biotechnology companies, the role of pharmaceutical companies in drug discovery and early-stage clinical development has declined and companies have come to rely on smaller biotechnology firms to fill their pipelines with later-stage assets through licensing and partnership agreements and mergers and acquisitions. In 2019, big pharmaceutical companies spent nearly $83 billion on R&D, with larger shares going toward pre-human/preclinical research (15.7%) and Phase 3 clinical trials (28.9%), and smaller shares going toward Phase 1 and Phase 2 clinical development (8.8% and 9.7%, respectively) [21].

In this new context, it is unsurprising that AD drug development among big pharmaceutical companies has stalled despite a lucrative market for AD therapeutics, estimated at $30 billion in the United States alone. Based on the current state of the field, the late-stage pipeline for AD lacks a diversity of targets and the cost and duration of AD trials simply make it too risky for companies, given their fiduciary responsibility to maximize shareholder value. The string of high-profile Phase 3 failures focused on amyloid beta in recent years has only raised more red flags (see Figure 41.3), leading several prominent big pharmaceutical companies – including AstraZeneca, Bristol-Myers, GSK, and, most recently, Pfizer and Amgen – to reduce or eliminate entirely their focus on CNS disorders. The controversy surrounding aducanumab, an experimental drug to treat AD with questionable efficacy founded on the amyloid hypothesis, has compounded these concerns, a topic we will turn to in Section 41.5.

However, the setbacks have also helped to illuminate several of the key issues in AD drug development, and the recent approval of aducanumab has inspired greater attention to the field. It has been estimated that the value of the global pipeline of late-stage disease-modifying AD therapeutics would increase from $338 billion to $788 billion with the development of diagnostics and biomarkers that improve our ability to identify and treat individuals likely to develop AD [22].

Once the science has progressed and the fruits of increased government spending on basic and early-stage research have come to bear, Big Pharma will be ready and waiting to do its part in bringing new products to patients.

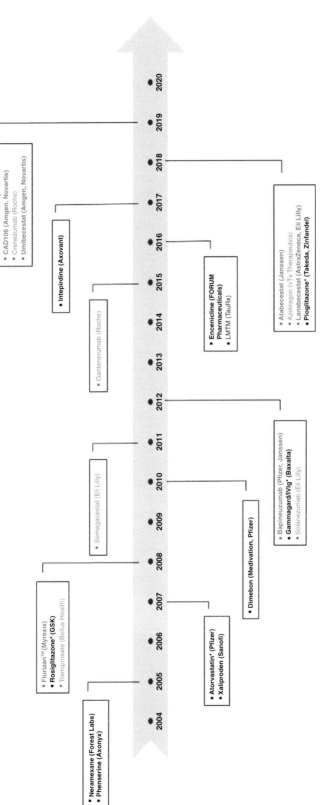

Figure 41.3 Timeline of Phase 2/3 and Phase 3 trials for disease-modifying candidates sponsored by industry that failed to meet their primary endpoints since 2003. Bolded text indicates discontinued development program and blue text indicates an amyloid-related target. *, Repurposed drug for AD; **, approved by FDA via Accelerated Approval pathway in 2021.

41.3 Alternative Business Models and Financing Structures

The risk and uncertainty of AD drug discovery and development require new business models and financing structures to successfully traverse the "valley of death," the wide funding gap between early-stage research and clinical development. As we have seen, there is great future potential for AD investment and research, yet the past and present AD landscape has been quite bleak.

Despite failed trial after failed trial, however, and few successful targets, there has been a recent surge to revitalize AD drug development. New financing models are a substantial contributor to this new outlook, which could accelerate the development of a more diverse set of AD drugs. These models are normally supplemental to the general drug financing structure outlined in Section 41.2, but they may have significant benefits, especially in the case of AD. We review some of these new financing models below.

41.3.1 A Portfolio Approach

To reduce the risk and uncertainty inherent to the drug-development process, financial engineering techniques may be used to create large private-sector funds ("megafunds") to support a portfolio of biomedical research projects simultaneously, techniques that were originally proposed for the oncology space [23]. By spreading the risk of translational medicine across a much larger pool of investors, and increasing the number of "shots on goal" in drug development, the risk to all investors will be lowered, and the chances of one or two successes are much higher.

Although such a megafund would require a large upfront investment, the profits from even one or two successes of a portfolio of oncology projects would be more than enough to cover the cost of the failures. In taking a portfolio approach, the overall risk would be lowered to a point where both debt and equity could be issued by the megafund, which would allow it to gain access to the much larger capacity and more patient capital of debt markets. Employing financial techniques such as portfolio theory and securitization, the oncology portfolio entity can be shown to generate returns that the more conservative and larger institutional funds, which have typically avoided investment in the biopharmaceutical industry, would now find

attractive, e.g., pension funds, insurance companies, endowments, foundations and trusts, and money market and mutual funds.

However, when applying the same model to AD, Lo et al. found that with the current scientific understanding of AD, the simulated investment performance of a megafund containing 64 projects was mixed at best, with mediocre expected returns for higher probabilities of success and lower correlations between prospective AD projects, and highly negative expected returns for lower probabilities of success and higher correlations [24]. The most sobering results involved the parameters closest to our current-day understanding of AD, yielding an expected return of −14.3% and a 13% probability that no project would reach fruition. These risk–reward profiles imply that debt financing an AD megafund would be virtually impossible under current conditions, and a private-sector megafund would not be economically viable. This finding may help to explain the 18-year drought in novel drug approvals for AD prior to 2021: given our current understanding of AD translational research, there is an insufficient number of shots on goal.

Despite an improved outlook for AD drug development, the current pipeline of AD drugs in clinical development – 121 agents across nine disease-modifying targets [25] – does not reflect the level of diversity required to improve the performance of an AD megafund. This suggests that government investment in AD drug discovery and development remains vital in building a strong pipeline of research. Indeed, in addition to funding basic and early-stage research, the government could help to attract greater private-sector investment by providing a guarantee to megafund investors to help reduce their risk of default. Such a government guarantee could also improve the megafund's credit rating and lower its cost of capital which, in turn, should attract more investors [26].

41.3.2 Public–Private Partnerships

The current challenges in AD drug development require collaboration across the stakeholder communities to mobilize resources and better facilitate the development process, from early-stage research to clinical practice. A public–private partnership, involving at least one public entity and one private entity, allows partners to share certain risks that otherwise might deter them from investment in the first place, while increasing scale, focusing their priorities, and optimizing the use of available knowledge and resources.

An illustrative example of such a partnership is the Dementia Discovery Fund, a VC fund established in coordination with the UK government under the leadership of former Prime Minster David Cameron. Launched in 2015 with a $100 million commitment from six global pharmaceutical companies, the UK government, and the non-profit Alzheimer's Research UK under the management of SV Health Investors, the Dementia Discovery Fund's goal is to deliver new drug approaches for the diagnosis and treatment of dementia by 2025. Since its launch, the Dementia Discovery Fund has raised an additional $250 million from investors, including the US-based AARP interest group, the National Football League Players Association, and Bill Gates. The fund is targeting early interventions and disease-modifying treatments that go beyond the amyloid hypothesis [27].

Similar to a public–private partnership, a non-profit/for-profit hybrid organization combines the unique capabilities of each organizational structure and provides a continuous development path between early-stage research and discovery to commercialization. The non-profit part of the organization, driven by a social mission, is responsible for funding research at the earliest stages of the drug discovery and development process using philanthropic and donor contributions. Its goal is to identify promising research with potential for commercialization, and guide it through the discovery process and valley of death, so that once a target or compound is sufficiently validated by its research, the for-profit part of the organization can then take the lead in shepherding the project through clinical development toward revenue generation. Part of the income from licensing, royalties, or sale of an asset can then be donated back to the non-profit part of the organization to create a self-sustaining funding model.

Examples of this model include the CZ Biohub and the Parker Institute for Cancer Immunotherapy. Both are non-profit entities that fund innovative early-stage research with an eye toward developing intellectual property. Each partners with academic institutions, but maintains its own portfolio of diverse technologies that are available for licensing. These organizations serve as a bridge between academia and industry, helping

to navigate the cultural differences and translate scientific discoveries into new diagnostics and therapies.

41.3.3 Venture Philanthropy

Venture philanthropy refers to a funding model in which a non-profit or "mission-driven" organization makes investments that have the potential to generate financial returns to advance its philanthropic mission. Investments are not made with a profit motive, and instead any returns are reinvested to support the non-profit organization's mission. With the success of the Cystic Fibrosis Foundation (CFF)'s investment in the development of Kalydeco in 2012 and the subsequent sale of its rights to future royalties to Royalty Pharma in 2014 for $3.3 billion, interest in the venture philanthropy model has exploded.

Motivated by its mission to reduce the burden of disease in people with cystic fibrosis, the CFF invested $150 million over a period of 12 years to fund cystic fibrosis programs in development at Vertex Pharmaceuticals. As a rare disease, cystic fibrosis was not originally a key market for drug developers, requiring the CFF's active role to advance the development of a treatment. For Vertex, financing from the foundation provided two key advantages: significant clinical expertise in the disease, and a low cost of generally non-dilutive capital [28].

In the case of AD, the ADDF is one of the most prominent organizations employing a venture philanthropy model to accelerate the speed of drug development. Investing in early-stage clinical trials and preclinical drug discovery research, the ADDF serves to bridge the valley of death and reinvests any financial rewards to continue working toward its mission to conquer AD.

41.3.4 Royalty Investments and Adaptive Financing

New investment companies have emerged in response to the challenges facing biotechnology and pharmaceutical companies – including the so-called "patent cliff," the changing investor landscape, and the increasing complexity of translational medicine – to bridge the biopharmaceutical funding gap by purchasing economic interests in royalty streams. This type of funding mechanism allows the patent-holders, typically universities, hospitals, and medical research centers, to monetize their intellectual property, providing them with much-needed cash to fund new research. The largest of these royalty investment companies in the biopharmaceutical industry is Royalty Pharma, with more than $10 billion in assets. Royalty Pharma invests in late-stage clinical trials and approved therapeutics, and their current portfolio contains rights to 42 approved and marketed products and several more in the pipeline.

Although Royalty Pharma focuses on late-stage products, making them unlikely investors in AD at this stage, some of their investments have employed unique financing structures that could be applied to AD therapeutic development. In particular, "adaptive financing," a creative synthetic royalty structure used to finance Sunesis Pharmaceuticals' Phase 3 adaptive clinical trial of vosaroxin for acute myeloid leukemia. As an adaptive trial, changes in design or analyses were possible based on the examination of data by an independent data safety monitoring board (DSMB) at an interim point in the trial. In this case, the DSMB could determine whether to stop the study early, continue as planned, or increase the sample size. While Sunesis had sufficient capital to fund the original trial, they were seeking an additional $25 million to fund the potential expansion of the study, pending the DSMB's interim analysis. Royalty Pharma conditionally agreed to invest the $25 million in exchange for payments tied to the outcomes of the trial and the DSMB's decisions. This adaptive structure created a win–win situation for both parties – Sunesis received a funding commitment, allowing them to focus on preparing regulatory filings and commercial launch, and Royalty Pharma was able to limit its exposure to the risk of a negative outcome while also positioning itself to receive a sizable royalty if vosaroxin were approved [29].

Chaudhuri and Lo have proposed modeling this type of financially adaptive clinical trial as a sequence of real options to improve decision making throughout the course of a clinical trial and maximize economic value to the sponsor [30]. They find that when a potential therapy is ineffective, an adaptive financing structure can decrease the expected cost to the sponsor by up to 46% in terms of total expenditures, number of patients, and trial duration. Mitigating the downside risk – achieved by amortizing the large fixed costs associated with clinical trials over time – will lead to an increase in value for sponsors and investors in the form of lower costs of capital and larger valuations when a therapy is effective [30].

41.4 Lessons Learned

The challenges of AD drug development reflect the broader shift in the development process from a linear course of development to a complex ecosystem in which finance plays an outsized role. The increased risk and complexity of the drug-development process has led to an outflow of capital for the riskiest ideas – but the potentially most transformative ones – as investors and other stakeholders seek other more attractive opportunities. At the same time, biotechnology and pharmaceutical companies have determined that their R&D dollars are better spent on later-stage assets that have already been sufficiently de-risked. The result is the valley of death between early-stage research and clinical development, where many promising discoveries are left to languish due to insufficient capital.

There is a need for alternative funding models to support AD research and innovation, since there is currently little investment in this space, and those investments are considered high risk. The new models described in Section 41.3 have great potential to lower investor risk and increase funding to early-stage AD companies and research, in the hopes of creating a more robust and diversified drug landscape. There have been multiple instances of collaborative success with these new funding models, which involve effective communication between the private and public sectors, as well as between company and investor.

At the same time, biomedical experts play a critical role in promoting the use of these new funding models. They can communicate to potential investors the excitement in the scientific community regarding new discoveries about the biological basis of AD and new potential methods for modifying the course of the disease. Investors respond not only to risk, but also to reward, and so far the only message they have received is that developing a drug for AD is futile.

However, there is reason for hope. As this volume goes to press, Eli Lilly released the stunning announcement that its Phase 2 clinical trial of donanemab, an investigational antibody targeting the N3pG form of beta amyloid, "showed significant slowing of decline in a composite measure of cognition and daily function in patients with early symptomatic Alzheimer's disease compared to placebo" [31]. But wary investors recall the many positive Phase 2 trials of Figure 41.3 that ultimately failed in much more costly Phase 3 trials. Why should this time be any different?

Unless scientists, clinicians, and biopharmaceutical executives can change this narrative, no new business models or funding opportunities will be forthcoming. Articulating a broader strategy for dealing with AD – perhaps through the chapters in this volume and with better scientific underpinnings – may be the catalyst needed to re-engage the private sector in this critically underserved area.

41.5 Aducanumab, Financing Drug Development, and Regulatory Practices

With the approval of aducanumab on June 7, 2021, the entire AD landscape has shifted dramatically. Given that this approval occurred just as this volume was going to press, much of the information contained in these pages do not reflect the full import of this momentous decision by the FDA. Therefore, we conclude with a few observations on what such an approval might mean for the path forward.

Perhaps the most obvious implication is that this event has greatly increased the uncertainty surrounding AD therapeutics in several respects. First, the FDA's decision to ignore a near-unanimous negative recommendation by its own advisory committee of experts creates uncertainty about the underlying drivers of the approval process. Second, Biogen's decision to price aducanumab at $56,000 per year of treatment – which is much higher than even the most optimistic cost-effectiveness estimates – creates uncertainty about the potential backlash from payors and politicians. Third, the decision to await further data before deciding whether or not to add aducanumab to the formulary by several prominent hospitals and health insurers due to lack of demonstrated efficacy – including the Cleveland Clinic, Mount Sinai, and six affiliates of Blue Cross Blue Shield, all as of July 17, 2021 – creates uncertainty for Biogen shareholders and other investors of AD therapeutics, as well as for independently insured employers considering the impact of this treatment on their budgets. And finally, the fact that the first approved

AD drug in 18 years targets amyloid beta creates uncertainty for the entire AD biopharmaceutical ecosystem that has invested in other mechanisms such as the presenilin, calcium (Ca^{2+}) dysregulation, lysosome, and tau hypotheses [32].

Increased uncertainty is usually viewed by economists as a disincentive for investors, hence the current environment is likely to delay current and pending AD investment initiatives. Why invest now in an atmosphere of high uncertainty when waiting a year or two can lead to lower-risk opportunities? The highly controversial and confusing approval of aducanumab may also contribute to the general impression among investors that the AD therapeutics space is risky and should be deprioritized from an investment perspective. This could be one of the most unfortunate and long-lasting consequence of the aducanumab approval.

Although several official investigations and reviews have now been launched by various entities, it will take months, if not years, to fully understand the motivation underlying this landmark decision. However, public statements made by FDA officials and records obtained by journalists support the view that regulators were persuaded by compelling scientific evidence confirming aducanumab's ability to clear amyloid plaques in most trial participants [33]. Critics have countered with the observation that clearance of Aβ by itself has, to date, demonstrated little to no clinical benefits for AD patients, hence it should not have served as the basis for approval. This debate highlights an important aspect of the FDA approval process, and a potential path forward.

At the heart of this controversy is the use of human judgment and discretion in overriding statistical evidence. One possible interpretation of the FDA's decision is that, in weighing the burden of disease, the lack of progress to date, and the waning interest in AD among biopharmaceutical companies against the potential benefits of a therapy that, for the first time in history, successfully demonstrated efficacy in counteracting a specific biochemical property of the disease itself, the regulators decided the potential benefit to AD patients of approval outweighed the uncertainties. Even if direct clinical benefits were not observed, it is not unreasonable to conclude that the reduction in amyloid is potentially worth backing, especially in the absence of any other more compelling alternatives. And with no approved drugs in 18 years for a disease affecting more than 6 million Americans at a cost of $355 billion in 2021, it is easy to see how a case could be made to employ human judgment and discretion to approve a drug that some believe has not met traditional statistical thresholds of efficacy. Desperate times call for desperate measures.

41.6   The Path Forward

If the utilitarian logic described above was the basis of the aducanumab approval, the concern with such a narrative is its lack of transparency and the confusion and uncertainty it creates. There is, however, a middle ground in which human judgment can be applied while still preserving transparency and incorporating statistical evidence in a completely rigorous fashion. That middle ground is Bayesian decision analysis (BDA), and it has been proposed precisely for the drug and device approval process so as to allow regulators to weigh various factors in rendering decisions that will affect many stakeholders [34–39].

The basic idea of BDA is to render a decision – approval or no approval – that minimizes the expected loss from the two possible types of incorrect decisions: a type I error or false positive (approving an ineffective treatment), and a type II error or false negative (not approving an effective treatment). The benefits of such an approach are most easily seen by comparing BDA with the traditional hypothesis-testing approach: choose a desired type I error rate, say 5%, and evaluate the statistical significance of the clinical evidence against this threshold. If results are inconsistent with the null hypothesis of no efficacy at a significance level, or p-value, of less than 5%, then we reject the null hypothesis and, in our context, approve the therapeutic.

The question asked and answered by BDA is "why 5%?" For fatal diseases that have no existing treatments, patients may be willing to accept a higher false positive rate, especially if it yields a lower false negative rate, as is often the case. In the BDA framework, the regulatory approval threshold is determined by explicitly minimizing the expected loss to patients due to *both* type I and II errors, where the expected loss is the sum of the measured impact of false positives and false negatives, each weighted by their respective probabilities.

Of course, a prerequisite for applying BDA is estimating the costs of false positives and negatives, which can be a challenge since some of those costs are in the form of patient preferences, the impact of side effects, and the opportunity cost of missing out on potentially effective treatments, all of which have to be measured. However, these considerations are presumably already being weighed by regulators, hence BDA provides a more systematic framework in which to make these measurements. For example, in the application of BDA to clinical trial data for a device to treat Parkinson's disease [39], researchers collaborated with the FDA and the Michael J. Fox Foundation to survey patients regarding their risk–reward preferences of the device, and these measured preferences were incorporated in computing the optimal false positive and negative rates for the clinical trial.

One important concern with this approach is that it could lead to a larger number of false positives, especially for diseases like AD that impose huge burdens and where there are no effective treatments. And once a drug is approved, it is often very difficult to withdraw from the market even if its efficacy is less than expected. Such an outcome is not altogether bad – after all, the whole point of BDA is to be more aggressive in developing therapeutics for the most burdensome diseases.

Nevertheless, to address the potential of more false positives, we propose creating a new category of regulatory approval that consists of a temporary license to market "speculative" therapies for treating high-impact diseases for which there are no existing effective therapeutics, such as pancreatic cancer, glioblastoma, and AD. Such a "spec-license" would not allow off-label use, and would expire after a period of 2 or 3 years, during which the licensee is required to collect and share data on the performance of its therapeutic. If the accumulated data on efficacy are positive, the license converts to a standard approval at the end of the trial period, otherwise the therapy is withdrawn upon expiration. Regulators should have the right to terminate the spec-license at any time in response to adverse events or significantly negative efficacy data.

This new type of license may seem similar to the FDA's "accelerated approval" program through which aducanumab was approved. The key difference is that, under a spec-license, the approval is only temporary for a set period of time, but provides a clear pathway through which more evidence can be collected – during which time the drug manufacturer can charge for the drug – and the drug can be more easily withdrawn if that evidence does not warrant full approval. It would greatly accelerate the pace of therapeutic development for a number of underserved medical needs, including AD, without limiting regulatory flexibility in any way, or imposing large and potentially irreversible costs on the healthcare system for therapeutics that have yet to fully establish their clinical value.

BDA offers a systematic, rational, transparent, reproducible, and practical framework in which regulators' decisions can be clearly understood by and communicated to all stakeholders while explicitly incorporating their feedback. If we have learned any lessons from the aducanumab controversy, it is the fact that all parties would benefit from greater transparency and predictability in the regulatory approval process.

Acknowledgments

We thank Zoe Lewin for helpful comments and editorial assistance. Research funding for this project was provided by the MIT Laboratory for Financial Engineering and its sponsors (listed at https://lfe.mit.edu/about/sponsors/). No funding bodies had any role in study design, data collection and analysis, decision to publish, or preparation of this manuscript. No direct funding was received for this study. The authors were personally salaried by their institutions during the period of writing (though no specific salary was set aside or given for the writing of this manuscript).

DISCLAIMER: The view and opinions expressed in this article are those of the authors only, and do not necessarily represent the views and opinions of any institution or agency, any of their affiliates or employees, or any of the individuals acknowledged above.

Disclosures

Dr. Lo reports personal investments in private biotechnology companies, biotechnology venture capital funds, and mutual funds. Dr. Lo is a co-founder and principal of QLS Advisors LLC, a healthcare investment advisor, and QLS Technologies Inc., a healthcare analytics and consulting company; an advisor to AlphaSimplex Group, Apricity Health, Aracari Bio, BrightEdge Impact Fund, Enable Medicine, FINRA, Lazard, Quantile Health, SalioGen Therapeutics the Swiss Finance Institute, and Thalēs; and a member of the Board of Overseers at Beth Israel Deaconess Medical Center and the NIH's National Center for Advancing Translational Sciences Advisory Council and Cures Acceleration Network Review Board. During the most recent 6-year period, Dr. Lo has received speaking/consulting fees, honoraria, or other forms of compensation from: AlphaSimplex Group, Annual Reviews, Bernstein Fabozzi Jacobs Levy Award, BIS, BridgeBio Pharma, Cambridge Associates, CME, Financial Times, Harvard Kennedy School, IMF, JOIM, National Bank of Belgium, New Frontiers Advisors (for the 2020 Harry M. Markowitz Prize), Q Group, Research Affiliates, Roivant Sciences, and the Swiss Finance Institute.

References

1. Alzheimer's Association. 2021 Alzheimer's disease facts and figures. *Alzheimers Dement* 2021; **17**: 327–406.

2. PhRMA. Alzheimer's medicines: setbacks and stepping stones. Available at: www.phrma.org/en/Alzheimer-s-Medicines-Setbacks-and-Stepping-Stones (accessed November 30, 2020).

3. Garde D, Feuerstein A. Why Biogen may be sitting on the most lucrative product in pharmaceutical history. Available at: www.statnews.com/2021/06/07/why-biogen-may-be-sitting-on-the-most-lucrative-product-in-pharmaceutical-history/ (accessed July 23, 2021).

4. Wong CH, Siah KW, Lo AW. Estimation of clinical trial success rates and related parameters. *Biostatistics* 2019; **20**: 273–86.

5. Wouters OJ, McKee M, Luyten J. Estimated research and development investment needed to bring a new medicine to market, 2009–2018. *JAMA* 2020; **323**: 844–53.

6. Scott TJ, O'Connor AC, Link AN, Beaulieu TJ. Economic analysis of opportunities to accelerate Alzheimer's disease research and development. *Ann N Y Acad Sci* 2014; **1313**: 17–34.

7. Cummings JL, Morstorf T, Zhong K. Alzheimer's disease drug-development pipeline: few candidates, frequent failures. *Alzheimers Res Ther* 2014; **6**: 37.

8. Prasad V, Mailankody S. Research and development spending to bring a single cancer drug to market and revenues after approval. *JAMA Intern Med* 2017; **177**: 1569–75.

9. Cleary EG, Beierlein JM, Khanuja NS, McNamee LM, Ledley FD. Contribution of NIH funding to new drug approvals 2010–2016. *Proc Natl Acad Sci USA* 2018; **115**: 2329–34.

10. US Department of Health and Human Services. National Plan to Address Alzheimer's Disease. 2012. Available at: https://aspe.hhs.gov/national-plan-address-alzheimers-disease (accessed December 23, 2020).

11. National Institutes of Health. Estimates of funding for various research, condition, and disease categories (RCDC). 2020. Available at: https://report.nih.gov/funding/categorical-spending#/ (accessed July 19, 2021).

12. Mariotto AB, Enewold L, Zhao J, Zeruto CA, Yabroff KR. Medical care costs associated with cancer survivorship in the United States. *Cancer Epidemiol Biomarkers Prev* 2020; **29**: 1304–12.

13. Keller K, Briggs L, Riley E. Alzheimer's disease: a center for strategic philanthropy giving smarter guide. Available at: https://milkeninstitute.org/sites/default/files/reports-pdf/FINAL-Alz-GSG2_2.pdf (accessed December 23, 2020).

14. Finkbeiner S. Bridging the valley of death of therapeutics for neurodegeneration. *Nat Med* 2010; **16**: 1227–32.

15. Angel Resource Institute. Halo report: annual report on angel investments. 2020. Available at: https://angelresourceinstitute.org/ (accessed December 30, 2020).

16. Castiglia O. Biotech angels bedeviled by dilution. Available at: www.forbes.com/sites/mergermarket/2020/01/06/biotech-angels-bedeviled-by-dilution/?sh=512e619c6486 (accessed July 19, 2021).

17. Ford D, Nelsen B. The view beyond venture capital. *Nat Biotechnol* 2014; **32**: 15–23.

18. Fleming JJ. The decline of venture capital investment in early-stage life sciences poses a challenge to continued innovation. *Health Aff* 2015; **34**: 271–6.

19. National Venture Capital Association. NVCA and MedIC Coalition release patient capital 3.0: confronting the crisis and achieving the promise of venture-backed medical innovation. Available at: www.prweb.com/releases/2013/4/prweb10670100.htm (accessed December 30, 2020).

20. Thomas D, Wessel C. The state of innovation in highly prevalent chronic diseases. Volume IV: Alzheimer's disease therapeutics. Available at: http://go.bio.org/rs/490-EHZ-999/images/BIO_HPCD4_ALZHEIMERS.pdf (accessed November 20, 2020).

21. PhRMA. 2020 PhRMA annual membership survey. Available at: https://phrma.org/Report/2020-PhRMA-Annual-Membership-Survey (accessed December 30, 2020).

22. Cole MA, Seabrook GR. On the horizon: the value and promise of the global pipeline of Alzheimer's disease therapeutics. *Alzheimers Dement (N Y)* 2020; **6**: e12009.

23. Fernandez J-M, Stein RM, Lo AW. Commercializing biomedical research through securitization techniques. *Nat Biotechnol* 2012; **30**: 964–75.

24. Lo AW, Ho C, Cummings J, Kosik KS. Parallel discovery of Alzheimer's therapeutics. *Sci Transl Med* 2014; **6**: 241cm5.

25. Cummings J, Lee G, Ritter A, Sabbagh M, Zhong K. Alzheimer's disease drug development pipeline: 2020. *Alzheimers Dement (N Y)* 2020; **6**: e12050.

26. Fagnan DE, Fernandez J-M, Lo AW, Stein RM. Can financial engineering cure cancer? *Am Econ Rev* 2013; **103**: 406–11.

27. Al Idrus A. Dementia Discovery Fund reels in $350 M for disease-modifying drugs. Available at: www.fiercebiotech.com/dementia-discovery-fund-reels-350m-for-disease-modifying-drugs (accessed January 1, 2021).

28. Kim E, Lo AW. Venture philanthropy: a case study of the Cystic Fibrosis Foundation. Available at: https://ssrn.com/abstract=3376673 (accessed January 1, 2021).

29. Lo AW, Naraharisetti SV. New financing methods in the biopharma industry: a case study of Royalty Pharma, Inc. *J Invest Manag* 2014; **12**: 4–19.

30. Chaudhuri SE, Lo AW. Financially adaptive clinical trials via option pricing analysis. *J Econom* 2020; DOI: 10.1016/j.jeconom.2020.08.012.

31. Eli Lilly. Lilly's donanemab slows clinical decline of Alzheimer's disease in positive Phase 2 trial. Jan 11, 2021. Available at: https://investor.lilly.com/news-releases/news-release-details/lillys-donanemab-slows-clinical-decline-alzheimers-disease (accessed January 18, 2021).

32. Kocahan S, Zumrut D. Mechanisms of Alzheimer's disease pathogenesis and prevention: the brain, neural pathology, *N*-methyl-D-aspartate receptors, tau protein and other risk factors. *Clin Psychopharmacol Neurosci* 2017; **15**: 1–8.

33. Sevigny J, Chiao P, Bussière T, et al. The antibody aducanumab reduces Aβ plaques in Alzheimer's disease. *Nature* 2016; **537**: 50–6.

34. Montazerhodjat V, Chaudhuri SE, Sargent DJ, Lo AW. Use of Bayesian decision analysis to minimize harm in patient-centered randomized clinical trials in oncology. *JAMA Oncol* 2017; **3**: e170123.

35. Chaudhuri SE, Ho MP, Irony T, Sheldon M, Lo AW. Patient-centered clinical trials. *Drug Discov Today* 2018; **23**: 395–401.

36. Isakov L, Lo AW, Montazerhodjat V. Is the FDA too conservative or too aggressive? A Bayesian decision analysis of clinical trial design. *J Econom* 2019; **211**: 117–36.

37. Chaudhuri S, Lo AW, Xiao D, Xu Q. Bayesian adaptive clinical trials for anti-infective therapeutics during epidemic outbreaks. *Harvard Data Sci Rev* 2020;DOI: https://doi.org/10.1162/99608f92.7656c213.

38. Chaudhuri SE, Lo AW. Incorporating patient preferences via Bayesian decision analysis. *Clin J Am Soc Nephrol* 2021; **16**: 639–41.

39. Hauber B, Mange B, Zhou M, et al. Parkinson's patients' tolerance for risk and willingness to wait for potential benefits of novel neurostimulation devices: a patient-centered threshold technique study. *MDM Policy Pract* 2021; **6**: 2381468320978407.

Chapter 42

Valley of Death and the Role of Venture Philanthropy in Alzheimer's Disease Drug Development

Lauren G. Friedman, Meriel Owen, Alessio Travaglia, and Howard Fillit

42.1 Introduction

With a growing aging population, the number of individuals with Alzheimer's disease (AD) worldwide is projected to reach 131.5 million by 2050 [1]; however, with the exception of the approval of aducanumab (Aduhelm™) in 2021, there are limited therapies that can slow or halt progression in patients at all stages of the disease or prevent the onset of symptoms. Despite the critical need for new disease-modifying therapies, there are significant barriers to translational research that transforms fundamental research discoveries into therapeutic products for clinical practice [2]. The estimated cost of developing a drug for AD is more than double the average cost of developing drugs for other indications [3]. These exorbitant costs are primarily driven by expensive late-phase clinical trials that require large numbers of patients and long treatment durations to detect differences in cognitive and behavioral endpoints.

Over 99% of drugs in development for AD have failed to advance to regulatory submission [4]. These failures can be attributed to multiple factors including complex underlying pathophysiology, limited translatable preclinical animal models, biological heterogeneity amongst patients, and a historical lack of sensitive and reliable biomarkers that can detect changes in pathology and accurately predict clinical outcomes such as cognition. Despite the huge potential market size and compelling societal benefit, the high cost of AD drug development combined with historically high attrition rates for AD and other neurodegenerative diseases has led some large pharmaceutical companies to exit from neuroscience research and development (R&D) [5]. All these factors can slow progress and decrease the number of opportunities to advance new therapies for patients. Expanding and supporting a wider range of novel therapies for AD requires innovation, ample funding, and resources that employ creative approaches to tackle this incredible challenge.

42.2 Diverse Funding Ecosystem

While the pharmaceutical industry is the main driver of drug development, many of the disease-modifying drugs currently in clinical development for AD are sponsored by or were originally developed in academic laboratories and small biotechnology companies. Before reaching the clinical development stage, early-stage biotechnology and academic drug discovery programs may face significant challenges that are associated with the arduous and expensive process of developing drugs, often succumbing to what is known as the "valley of death," the gap in translating laboratory discoveries into human clinical trials [6]. Many drug programs stall at this stage due to a lack of funding, failure to generate promising data, or lack of experienced management and multidisciplinary expertise required to develop and commercialize drugs. In order to address the valley of death, a diverse and robust financial ecosystem involving government, industry, venture capital (VC), and philanthropy is required [7].

In the United States, the National Institutes of Health (NIH) serve as the primary non-dilutive funding source (meaning no equity is required in exchange for funding) for AD research. Much of this funding is dedicated to exploratory research grants that help expand our understanding of the biological mechanisms driving disease, identifying new targets, and, increasingly, supporting drug discovery and development campaigns. The NIH also supports start-up companies with non-dilutive funding through its Small Business Technology

Transfer and Small Business Innovation Research grants, which serve as a key channel through which drug programs can spin out of academic labs into for-profit entities. Although the funding committed by the NIH has recently increased and continues to bolster the research pipeline, these types of grants can be competitive and take up to a year or more from grant submission to receipt of funding.

VC funders partner with companies to make investments with the expectation of generating financial returns. In general, investors seek clear exit strategies (typically through licensing deals, acquisitions, or initial public offerings) and returns on investment within several years of the initial financing [8]. Given the perceived risk, high attrition rates, long development timelines, and costly clinical trials, investors have traditionally prioritized other disease indications, resulting in fewer deals in the AD space per year. However, in recent years, venture firms such as Dolby Family Ventures and specialized funds like the Dementia Discovery Fund have established dedicated AD therapeutics portfolios, where companies can leverage drug-development and business expertise from internal investment teams and external networks for guidance and potential strategic partnerships.

The pharmaceutical industry is the largest funder of drug discovery and development worldwide and serves as the primary source of funding for late-phase clinical trials [9]. Between 1995 and 2002, pharmaceutical investment in neuroscience research doubled from $2.5 billion to $5.3 billion; however, dwindling numbers of regulatory approvals coupled with longer clinical trial durations and lengthier US Food and Drug Administration (FDA) review timelines changed the risk–reward calculus, causing many companies to move away from neuroscience R&D investment in the following years [5]. Withdrawal from the central nervous system (CNS) space by large companies detracts from the pipeline in academia and industry, and across the spectrum from target discovery to clinical trials and biomarker development. Despite recent exits from neuroscience by several large pharmaceutical companies, industry continues to look toward academia and early-stage biotechnology companies as sources of innovation; however, they often lack critical data (i.e., demonstration of in vivo CNS exposure, favorable drug-like properties, or acceptable safety profiles) needed to de-risk

programs to attract investors or strategic pharmaceutical partners.

Pharmaceutical partners and other investors often only consider programs that have reached certain inflection points, such as drug candidate selection or clinical proof of concept, but funding at these stages is still limited. In the past decade, multiple disease foundations have started to fill this funding gap. The Alzheimer's Association is the largest non-profit funder of AD research, and supports studies that enhances our understanding of the disease pathophysiology, dementia risk, patient care, and health disparities. In recent years, the Alzheimer's Association has increased funding toward translational research and early-phase clinical trials. Other foundations including BrightFocus Foundation, the Tau Consortium, Alzheimer's Research UK, the Alzheimer's Drug Discovery Foundation (ADDF), and the Weston Brain Institute contribute to the funding landscape that supports translational research and early-stage clinical development. Foundations offer deep disease-focused expertise and can have close ties with stakeholders associated with the disease, including patients, caregivers, and thought leaders from academia and industry.

Together, the NIH, VC investors, large pharmaceutical companies, and disease foundations drive the development of innovative and novel drugs for AD. Research funded by these groups has greatly improved our understanding of the disease and advanced multiple drugs into human clinical trials.

42.3 Venture Philanthropy: A Hybrid Funding Model

Despite this diverse ecosystem of funding sources for AD drug development, the valley of death persists where many programs in academia and early-stage biotechnology stagnate or fail. Crossing the valley of death requires more than strong science. It necessitates a seasoned team with drug-development expertise, project management, and negotiation skills. Companies also need a strong intellectual-property protection strategy, the ability to raise and manage funds, and a demonstrable competitive advantage over other approaches to the disease [2]. These skill sets are highly multidisciplinary and often require many years to acquire.

To help address the challenges faced by programs in the valley of death, the venture

481

philanthropy model has emerged as one of the drivers of translational research to provide funding, as well as access to resources and drug-development expertise. Venture philanthropy combines principles from VC investing with mission-related funding to support the development of high-risk/high-reward therapies [10]. Depending on the organization, funding is provided to academic centers in addition to for-profit companies but is structured to enable returns on investment. Funding can take various forms, including royalty-bearing grants to academic institutions and convertible promissory notes, equity purchases, or other instruments to companies. If programs yield financial returns, they are funneled directly into supporting more research in furtherance of the venture philanthropy's charitable mission [11].

The most notable example is the Cystic Fibrosis Foundation (CFF) [12]. After the discovery of the mutations in the cystic fibrosis transmembrane conductance regulator (*CFTR*) gene that render CFTR protein defective in cystic fibrosis [13–15], the CFF recognized that substantial investment was needed to accelerate the research and development of drugs that could restore CFTF function, to treat the root cause of the disease. In response, the CFF adopted a venture philanthropy model that would enable investment in for-profit companies and attract interest from industry for an underfunded rare disease like cystic fibrosis. The CFF invested a total of $150 million over 12 years in Aurora Bioscience and its successor, Vertex Pharmaceuticals. In addition to capital, the CFF contributed extensive clinical expertise to guide study design, access to patient registry data, and an established network of clinical and care centers. The funding and resources were crucial in developing ivacaftor (Kalydeco®), a CFTR potentiator that became the first FDA-approved disease-modifying therapy for cystic fibrosis patients [16]. The CFF sold their royalty rights for cystic fibrosis therapies developed by Vertex for a record-breaking $3.3 billion return on investment, providing capital to reinvest into expanding the therapeutic pipeline for cystic fibrosis [17].

Following the CFF's example, increasing numbers of disease foundations are creating venture philanthropy arms to accelerate therapeutic development. The Juvenile Diabetes Research Foundation (JDRF) and the Multiple Myeloma Research Foundation have both launched investment funds as self-sustaining vehicles to drive more capital,

knowledge, and talent into their respective disease areas. These funds also leverage internal expertise and tools from the foundations, including access to biobanks and genomics data to guide strategies for drug discovery, clinical networks to speed trial start-up, and guidance on clinical trial designs [18, 19].

While venture philanthropies can fund earlier-stage or more novel approaches that may be viewed as too risky for traditional investors, their investment decisions are rooted in assessing scientific rigor, the potential commercialization path, and the eventual impact on patients. Similar to VC firms, venture philanthropies apply rigorous scientific and business due diligence to evaluate investment opportunities. Many employ internal teams of MD and PhD-trained scientists and consult with external leaders from academia, industry, and VC to guide investment decision making. The extensive due diligence and guidance from disease, drug, and business development experts can serve as third-party validation for academic and biotechnology programs that can attract additional investors and industry partnerships.

Through their extensive networks, foundations with venture philanthropy models can partner with other disease foundations or early-stage investors to augment funding and, in some cases, provide mechanisms to help academic programs cross the valley of death. For example, JDRF partnered with PureTech Ventures to form a venture-creating vehicle that identified licensing opportunities from academia, formed new companies around the technologies, and provided expertise, resources, and capital [20]. Venture philanthropies have also established collaborations with industry partners to leverage pharmaceutical investment and internal drug-development expertise. For example, Fast Forward, the National Multiple Sclerosis Society's wholly owned commercial development subsidiary, partnered with EMD Serono (a US division of Merck KGaA), to advance early-stage drug development for multiple sclerosis [21].

42.4 A Role for Venture Philanthropy in AD Drug Development

Venture philanthropies are well positioned to tackle some of the major challenges associated with AD drug development and have been increasingly making an impact in accelerating the development of treatments for AD. The ADDF was among the first life-science venture philanthropies and was founded in 1998 with the sole mission of developing therapies to treat and prevent AD and related dementias. The ADDF has invested over $150 million to advance hundreds of AD drug candidates developed in academia and early-stage ventures through the drug-development pipeline. As of 2018, the ADDF had provided funding to support nearly 20% of all disease-modifying AD drugs in clinical development [22].

Over the last two decades, the pharmaceutical industry invested heavily in candidate therapies that target key pathologies involved in AD – namely amyloid-beta deposits and hyperphosphorylated tau. We now know that AD has multiple underlying causes, from misfolded proteins to inflammation, vascular dysfunction, and other mechanisms that are affected by aging, with each representing novel drug targets [23]. Given the complexity of the underlying biology, the heterogeneity in pathological and clinical presentations, and the greater risk associated with developing therapies for AD, industry prioritized validated targets like amyloid that have genetic links and are associated with disease hallmark pathology.

As the field has expanded beyond amyloid-targeted drugs, public and private funders have invested in programs with diverse mechanisms or modes of action in order treat the numerous underlying causes related to aging biology. Venture philanthropies like the ADDF have used a "multiple shots on goal" portfolio strategy by making smaller-sized investments in distinct and diverse programs to increase the odds that one or more will be effective [24]. Since venture philanthropies are focused on accelerating drug development instead of driving profits, they can also support the investigation of repurposed drugs – approved drugs tested for new indications. Clinical trials that test repurposed drugs can generate human proof-of-mechanism data to validate AD drug targets. Due to the limited patent protection around repurposed agents, there are fewer commercial incentives for traditional investors to support this type of research [25]. However, venture philanthropies can collaborate with academic groups to identify paths for commercialization that may include novel formulation development or medicinal chemistry campaigns to generate new chemical matter.

In addition to providing capital for preclinical and clinical research, venture philanthropies can address other critically unmet needs that are required to support drug development. One of the biggest barriers to AD clinical development has been the lack of sensitive and reliable biomarkers that can identify and stratify patients for trials, demonstrate target engagement, and monitor disease progression and treatment response. As more drug targets are pursued, the toolbox of biomarkers that complement clinical development must expand. The ADDF has been supporting biomarker studies since its founding. In the early 2000s, ADDF seed-funded research at the University of Pennsylvania to support the development of Amyvid™ (^{18}F-labeled florbetapir), a positron emission tomography agent that binds amyloid aggregates and measures brain amyloid load. The radioligand was eventually licensed by Avid Radiopharmaceuticals and developed by Eli Lilly and Company, becoming the first FDA-approved diagnostic test for AD [26]. Since then, Amyvid™ has been used in multiple clinical trials to enroll patients with evidence of brain amyloid accumulation and to measure brain amyloid reduction [27, 28]. While neuroimaging and cerebrospinal fluid biomarkers are currently used in clinical trials with high diagnostic accuracy, they involve expensive and/or invasive procedures that limit their widespread use. To increase the number of reliable, affordable, and accessible biomarkers available for clinical trials, and ultimately clinical practice, the ADDF partnered with Bill Gates and other funders to launch the Diagnostics Accelerator (www.alzdiscovery.org/research-and-grants/diagnostics-accelerator), a $50 million fund to fast-track the development of blood biomarkers, eye scans, digital tests, and other biomarkers. Initiatives like these have enabled venture philanthropies to help advance AD biomarker development that will dramatically reduce the cost of clinical trials. In 2020, the ADDF provided funding to clinically validate C_2N Diagnostics' mass-spectrometry-based amyloid-beta blood test, which predicts brain amyloid pathology and will ultimately be used to screen patients for clinical trials at lower cost.

In order to bridge the gap between academic drug discovery and early-phase clinical development, resources and guidance beyond funding are needed to help lower the barriers for AD drug development. Initiatives like the ADDF–Harrington Scholar program, in collaboration with the Harrington Discovery Institute, aim to advance academic discoveries into medicines for AD and related dementias. The ADDF–Harrington award provides funding for preclinical programs and committed support from a team of pharmaceutical industry veterans with expertise tailored to the needs of selected projects. For example, a program at Vanderbilt University was the recipient of the ADDF–Harrington Scholar award, which provided funding and guidance on formulation and interpretation of safety pharmacology and toxicology data to advance a novel M1 muscarinic receptor positive allosteric modulator into first-in-human clinical trials [29]. Acadia Pharmaceuticals and Vanderbilt entered into an exclusive licensing agreement to further develop and commercialize the drug [30]. Past collaborations, like the ADDF's partnership with Pfizer's Center for Therapeutic Innovation, provided other avenues for co-funding and access to pharmaceutical resources for drug discovery programs.

While partnerships between pharmaceutical companies and foundations have been instrumental in helping researchers cross the valley of death, few educational opportunities outside of industry are available to train the next generation of academic researchers in therapeutic development, particularly for chronic CNS diseases which present unique challenges. To help bridge the knowledge gap, the ADDF sponsors an annual Drug Discovery for Neurodegeneration workshop. This interactive meeting is co-funded by the National Institute on Aging and is designed as an introductory course that covers all aspects of therapeutic development for neurodegenerative diseases. The ADDF also organizes advisory panel meetings that bring together leaders from academia, biotechnology organizations, pharmaceutical companies, and other foundations to provide guidance on relevant AD drug discovery topics and results in peer-reviewed publications. Recommendations on a range of topics have included best practices for AD preclinical animal-study design and conduct [31] and evaluating and interacting with contract research organizations in academia and early-stage biotechnology companies [32].

42.5 Conclusions and Future Directions

Over the past 20 years, the venture philanthropy model has been building momentum among disease-focused foundations. In recent years, the size of non-profit investments in AD programs has grown as more candidate therapies enter clinical trials and reach later-stage milestones. Venture philanthropies like the ADDF have helped academic groups reach critical inflection points and have increased funding in early-stage biotechnology companies. As a result, the ADDF's investments are starting to pay off. For example, the ADDF invested in Tetra Therapeutics in 2016 to support the development of a novel phosphodiesterase-4D inhibitor for AD and fragile X syndrome with neuroprotective properties. Shinogi recently acquired Tetra in a deal valued at $500 million and, as a result, the ADDF received returns that tripled the original investment. Reaching these milestones means more critical funds can be deployed to advance AD therapeutics, providing capital to fund more discovery programs to feed the therapeutic pipeline, expand the size of investments that can support clinical trials, and continue to fund the development of biomarker tools to bolster these programs. Moving forward, venture philanthropy can continue to serve as an important funding model that can support the pipeline of AD drugs in development to deliver much-needed treatments to patients.

References

1. Prince MJ, Wimo A, Guerchet MM, et al. World Alzheimer Report 2015: the global impact of dementia: an analysis of prevalence, incidence, cost and trends. Available at: https://kclpure.kcl.ac.uk/portal/en/publications/world-alzheimer-report-2015--the-global-impact-of-dementia(ae525fda-1938-4892-8daa-a2222a672254)/export.html (accessed November 23, 2020).

2. Seyhan AA. Lost in translation: the valley of death across preclinical and clinical divide – identification of problems and overcoming obstacles. *Transl Med Commun* 2019; **4**: 18.

3. DiMasi JA, Grabowski HG, Hansen RW. Innovation in the pharmaceutical industry: new estimates of R&D costs. *J Health Econ* 2016; **47**: 20–33.

4. Cummings JL, Morstorf T, Zhong K. Alzheimer's disease drug-development pipeline: few candidates, frequent failures. *Alzheimers Res Ther* 2014; **6**: 37.

5. Choi DW, Armitage R, Brady LS, et al. Medicines for the mind: policy-based "pull" incentives for creating breakthrough CNS drugs. *Neuron* 2014; **84**: 554–63.

6. Finkbeiner S. Bridging the valley of death of therapeutics for neurodegeneration. *Nat Med* 2010; **16**: 1227–32.

7. Cummings J, Reiber C, Kumar P. The price of progress: funding and financing Alzheimer's disease drug development. *Alzheimers Dement (N Y)* 2018; **4**: 330–43.

8. Thomas D, Wessel C. The state of innovation in highly prevalent chronic diseases. Volume IV: Alzheimer's disease therapeutics. Available at: http://go.bio.org/rs/490-EHZ-999/images/BIO_HPCD4_ALZHEIMERS.pdf (accessed November 23, 2020).

9. Cummings J, Lee G, Mortsdorf T, Ritter A, Zhong K. Alzheimer's disease drug development pipeline: 2017. *Alzheimers Dement (N Y)* 2017; **3**: 367–84.

10. Hanson SL, Nadig L, Altevogt BM, et al. Workshop on venture philanthropy strategies to support translational Research Planning Committee. In *Venture Philanthropy Strategies to Support Translational Research: Workshop Summary*. Washington, DC: National Academies Press; 2009: 59–68.

11. Lopez JC, Suojanen C. Harnessing venture philanthropy to accelerate medical progress. *Nat Rev Drug Discov* 2019; **18**: 809–10.

12. Esther Kim AWL. Venture philanthropy: a case study of the Cystic Fibrosis Foundation, April 2019. Available at: https://ssrn.com/abstract=3376673 (accessed November 23, 2020).

13. Kerem B, Rommens JM, Buchanan JA, et al. Identification of the cystic fibrosis gene: genetic analysis. *Science* 1989; **245**: 1073–80.

14. Riordan JR, Rommens JM, Kerem B, et al. Identification of the cystic fibrosis gene: cloning and characterization of complementary DNA. *Science* 1989; **245**: 1066–73.

15. Rommens JM, Iannuzzi MC, Kerem B, et al. Identification of the cystic fibrosis gene: chromosome walking and jumping. *Science* 1989; **245**: 1059–65.

16. Sloane PA, Rowe SM. Cystic fibrosis transmembrane conductance regulator protein repair as a therapeutic strategy in cystic fibrosis. *Curr Opin Pulm Med* 2010; **16**: 591–7.

17. Senior M. Foundation receives $3.3-billion windfall for Kalydeco. *Nat Biotechnol* 2015; **33**: 8–9.

18. Perkins LM, Young AQ, Giusti K. One foundation's strategy to accelerate drug discovery through genomics. *Sci Transl Med* 2011; **3**: 78cm11.

19. Ramsey BW, Nepom GT, Lonial S. Academic, foundation, and industry collaboration in finding new therapies. *N Engl J Med* 2017; **376**: 1762–9.

20. Orelli B. JDRF teams with VC PureTech to promote startups. *Nat Biotechnol* 2013; **31**: 1065.

21. Osherovich L. Fast forward in MS. *Science-Business eXchange* 2009; **2**: 858.

22. Alzheimer's Drug Discovery Foundation. 2018 Alzheimer's clinical trials report. Available at: www.alzdiscovery.org/research-and-grants/clinical-trials-report/2018-report (accessed November 23, 2020).

23. Hara Y, McKeehan N, Fillit HM. Translating the biology of aging into novel therapeutics for Alzheimer disease. *Neurology* 2019; **92**: 84–93.

24. Lo AW, Ho C, Cummings J, Kosik KS. Parallel discovery of Alzheimer's therapeutics. *Sci Transl Med* 2014; **6**: 241cm245.

25. Shineman DW, Alam J, Anderson M, et al. Overcoming obstacles to repurposing for neurodegenerative disease. *Ann Clin Transl Neurol* 2014; **1**: 512–18.

26. Yang L, Rieves D, Ganley C. Brain amyloid imaging: FDA approval of florbetapir F18 injection. *N Engl J Med* 2012; **367**: 885–7.

27. Honig LS, Vellas B, Woodward M, et al. Trial of solanezumab for mild dementia due to Alzheimer's disease. *N Engl J Med* 2018; **378**: 321–30.

28. Sevigny J, Chiao P, Bussiere T, et al. The antibody aducanumab reduces Abeta plaques in Alzheimer's disease. *Nature* 2016; **537**: 50–6.

29. Conley AK, Blackford J, Rook J, et al. Functional activity of the muscarinic positive allosteric modulator VU319 during a Phase 1 single ascending dose study. *Am J Geriatr Psychiatry* 2020; **28**: S114–15.

30. Acadia Pharmaceuticals and Vanderbilt University. Acadia Pharmaceuticals and Vanderbilt University announce exclusive license agreement and research collaboration [press release]. Available at: www.businesswire.com/news/home/20200507005980/en/ACADIA-Pharmaceuticals-and-Vanderbilt-University-Announce-Exclusive-License-Agreement-and-Research-Collaboration (accessed November 23, 2020).

31. Shineman DW, Basi GS, Bizon JL, et al. Accelerating drug discovery for Alzheimer's disease: best practices for preclinical animal studies. *Alzheimers Res Ther* 2011; **3**: 28.

32. Lane RF, Friedman LG, Keith C, et al. Optimizing the use of CROs by academia and small companies. *Nat Rev Drug Discov* 2013; **12**: 487–8.

Chapter 43

Alzheimer's Association Funding and Policy for Alzheimer's Disease Drug Development

Maria C. Carrillo, Emily A. S. Meyers, and Heather M. Snyder

43.1 Introduction

Alzheimer's disease (AD) is a public health challenge that grows in urgency every year. Aging is one of the main risk factors for AD and AD-related dementia (AD/ADRD), and as the population of Americans over the age of 65 increases, the prevalence of AD continues to grow. According to the annual report published by the Alzheimer's Association [1], in 2020 the population of individuals over the age of 65 in the United States was 56 million, with 1 in 10 individuals living with AD dementia. This population is projected to grow to 88 million by 2050.

The impact of AD/ADRD does not rest solely on the individual with the disease. Caregivers – professional or unpaid individuals providing care for a family member, friend, or another person in their community – provide support for individuals with AD/ADRD not only in activities of daily living, but also financially and emotionally. For the more than 6 million Americans living with AD today, more than 16 million family members, friends, or other unpaid caregivers are providing care for them. It was estimated that the cost of care for someone with dementia was $357,297 in 2019, with 70% of this cost borne by family caregivers in the form of unpaid caregiving and out-of-pocket expenses. Caregivers for individuals with AD face special challenges including anxiety, depression, and impact on their physical health. Recently, research in this area has expanded, including means to address and support the challenges experienced by caregivers [1].

As a nation, in 2021, the cost of caring for people with AD and other dementias was estimated at $355 billion. Of this amount, the total cost to Medicare and Medicaid was estimated at $239 billion, and an estimated $76 billion is paid out-of-pocket by families and individuals living with AD.

On a global scale, the World Alzheimer Report 2015 [2] estimates that 46.8 million people worldwide were living with dementia in 2015, a number that was projected to double every 20 years. In 2015, 58% of individuals with dementia lived in low- or middle-income countries, as classified by the World Bank, a number that is expected to increase to 68% by 2050. Further, the global cost of dementia was $818 billion in 2015 and, at the time of their report, was estimated to be a trillion dollar disease by 2018.

These data stress the need and urgency of action to address not only the clinical need for drug development to delay or prevent symptoms of AD, but also methods of supporting individuals with AD and their families financially and emotionally.

43.2 Mission and Vision of the Alzheimer's Association

The Alzheimer's Association is the leading voluntary health organization in AD care, support, and research. The Alzheimer's Association leads the way to end AD and all other dementia – by accelerating global research, driving risk reduction and early detection, and maximizing quality care and support. Since its formation in 1980, the Alzheimer's Association works on a national and local level to provide care and support for all those affected by AD/ADRD.

The Alzheimer's Association is the largest AD/ADRD advocacy organization in the world, fighting for critical AD/ADRD research and care initiatives at the state and federal level. Working with and through the Alzheimer's Impact Movement (AIM), a separately incorporated advocacy affiliate, the Alzheimer's Association has developed and grown bipartisan support for critical policy priorities. AIM is a separately incorporated advocacy affiliate of the Alzheimer's Association. Further, the Alzheimer's Association has helped to drive bipartisan support in the US Congress for historic research funding for AD/ADRD at the National Institutes of Health (NIH). In 2021, annual funding for AD/ADRD research reached $3.2 billion.

As the largest non-profit funder of AD/ADRD research in the world, the Alzheimer's Association is committed to advancing vital research toward methods of treatment, prevention, and, ultimately, a cure. It provides direct funding to researchers, including supporting and expanding the AD drug-development pipeline. This support is not only financial, but includes the promotion of sharing of knowledge and data, gathering key individuals from academia and industry to advance research and drug development. It also accelerates clinical trial research through the Alzheimer's Association TrialMatch™, a clinical trials matching service for people living with the disease, caregivers, and cognitively unimpaired volunteers.

43.3 Complexity and Continuum of AD

AD is a complex disease. Despite the role for processes downstream of amyloid-beta and tau accumulations as neuropathological events in AD, the precise mechanisms for neuronal dysfunction, synapse loss, dendrite pruning, and/or cell death that occur in AD remain uncertain. There is an urgent and pressing need to identify therapeutic strategies capable of preventing neuronal damage, targeting the pre-existing damage, or a combination of the two. There is growing evidence that dysfunction – and even death – of other types of cells may contribute to disease pathology. Thus, as an example (in addition to neuronal targets or other cellular types), it is essential to understand this biology and potentially develop therapeutics that target these cellular mechanisms of astrocytes, oligodendrocytes, microglia, and even endothelial cells on blood vessels in order to halt, diminish, and/or reverse the brain cell degeneration seen in AD/ADRD.

In 1984, the criteria for the clinical diagnosis of AD were established by the National Institute of Neurological and Communicative Disorders and Stroke (NINCDS) and the Alzheimer's Disease and Related Disorders Association (ADRDA) workgroup. Many important advances have been made since that time, including the ability to map the biological processes of AD and the elucidation of the clinical spectrum of the disease. In 2011, the Alzheimer's Association, in collaboration with the National Institute on Aging (NIA) at the NIH, published an expert consensus on redefined diagnostic guidelines for clinical and research use [3]. These guidelines – known as the 2011 NIA–AA guidelines (see Box 43.1 and Figure 43.1) – set the stage of AD as a disease continuum including preclinical, mild cognitive impairment (MCI) due to AD, and dementia due to AD phases, with

Box 43.1 2011 NIA–AA guidelines

The AD Continuum

The progression of AD, from brain changes that are unnoticeable to the person affected to brain changes that cause problems with memory and, eventually, physical disability, is called the AD continuum.

On this continuum, there are three broad phases: preclinical AD, MCI due to AD, and dementia due to AD (see Figure 43.1). The AD dementia phase is further broken down into the stages of mild, moderate, and severe, which reflect the degree to which

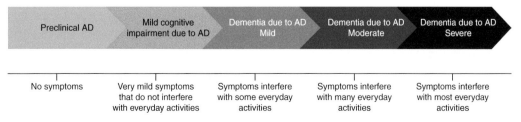

Figure 43.1 Alzheimer's disease AD continuum. Note, although the arrows are of equal size, the components of the AD continuum are not equal in duration.

Box 43.1 (cont.)

symptoms interfere with one's ability to carry out everyday activities.

While we know the continuum starts with preclinical AD and ends with severe AD dementia, how long individuals spend in each part of the continuum varies. The length of each phase of the continuum is influenced by age, genetics, gender, and other factors.

Preclinical AD

In this phase, individuals have measurable brain changes that indicate the earliest signs of AD (biomarkers), but they have not yet developed symptoms such as memory loss. Examples of measurable brain changes include abnormal levels of amyloid beta as shown on positron emission tomography (PET) scans and in analysis of cerebrospinal fluid (CSF), and decreased metabolism of glucose as shown on PET scans. When the early changes of AD occur, the brain compensates for them, enabling individuals to continue to function normally.

While research settings have the tools and expertise to identify some of the early brain changes of AD, additional research is needed to fine-tune the tools' accuracies before they become available for widespread use in hospitals, doctors' offices, and other clinical settings. It is important to note that not all individuals with evidence of AD-related brain changes go on to develop symptoms of MCI or AD dementia. For example, some individuals have amyloid-beta plaques at death but did not have memory or cognitive problems in life.

Mild Cognitive Impairment Due to AD

People with MCI due to AD have biomarker evidence of AD brain changes (for example, abnormal levels of amyloid beta) plus subtle problems with memory and thinking. These cognitive problems may be noticeable to family members and friends, but not to others, and they do not interfere completely with the individual's ability to carry out everyday activities. The mild changes in cognitive abilities occur when the brain can no longer compensate for the damage and death of nerve cells caused by AD.

Among those with MCI, one analysis found that after 2 years' follow-up, 15% of individuals older than 65 had developed dementia. Another study found that 32% of individuals with MCI developed AD within 5 years' follow-up [4–6]. A third study found that among individuals with MCI who were tracked for 5 years or longer, 38% developed dementia. However, in some individuals, MCI reverts to normal cognition or remains stable. In other cases, such as

when a medication inadvertently causes cognitive changes, MCI is mistakenly diagnosed and cognitive changes can be reversed with medication changes. Identifying which individuals with MCI are more likely to develop AD/ADRD is a major goal of current research.

Dementia Due to AD

Dementia due to AD is characterized by noticeable memory, cognitive, or behavioral symptoms that impair a person's ability to function in daily life, along with evidence of AD's-related brain changes. Individuals with AD dementia experience multiple symptoms that change over a period of years. These symptoms reflect the degree of damage to nerve cells in different parts of the brain. The pace at which symptoms of dementia advance from mild to moderate to severe differs from person to person.

Mild AD Dementia

In the mild stage of AD dementia, most people are able to function independently in many areas but are likely to require assistance with some activities to maximize independence and remain safe. They may still be able to drive, work, and participate in favorite activities.

Moderate AD Dementia

In the moderate stage of AD, which is often the longest stage, individuals may have difficulties communicating and performing routine tasks, including activities of daily living (such as bathing and dressing); become incontinent at times; and start having personality and behavioral changes, including suspiciousness and agitation.

Severe AD Dementia

In the severe stage of AD dementia, individuals need help with activities of daily living and are likely to require around-the-clock care. The effects of AD on individuals' physical health become especially apparent in this stage. Because of damage to areas of the brain involved in movement, individuals become bedbound. Being bed-bound makes them vulnerable to conditions including blood clots, skin infections, and sepsis, which triggers body-wide inflammation that can result in organ failure. Damage to areas of the brain that control swallowing makes it difficult to eat and drink. This can result in individuals swallowing food into the trachea (windpipe) instead of the esophagus (food pipe). Because of this, food particles may deposit in the lungs and cause lung infection. This type of infection is called aspiration pneumonia, and it is a contributing cause of death among many individuals with AD.

specific guidelines based on the scientific knowledge at the time. The preclinical stage is proposed for research use and encompasses the pathophysiological process of AD that is thought to begin years before clinical symptoms are present [7]. Growing evidence of this can be seen through the use of biomarkers in brain imaging, CSF, and, in more recent work, blood/plasma. MCI due to AD defines the phase where an individual transitions from asymptomatic to symptomatic [8]. The utilization of biomarkers – such as brain imaging, CSF, and others – can increase the certainty of the diagnosis of MCI due to AD. The dementia phase of the disease defines the point that cognitive impairment interferes with daily living, and suggests the need for pathological confirmation of related brain changes, such as amyloid plaques, tau tangles, and neurodegeneration [9]. This paradigm of the disease as a continuum sets the stage for therapeutic interventions across the entire disease continuum, including possible prevention. Estimates for a hypothetical intervention delaying disease onset 5 years could potentially result in a 57% reduction in the number of individuals living with AD dementia by 2050 [10].

To assist in the diagnosis of AD, Jack and colleagues outlined a research framework to classify certain biomarkers that are indicators of deposition of amyloid beta (A), pathological tau (T), and neurodegeneration (N) (A/T/N) [11]. This system proposes to focus on a diagnosis using biological factors, rather than clinical symptoms of cognitive impairment. The system for staging severity of the disease was determined by evaluating pathological changes. In 2018, the Alzheimer's Association, in collaboration with the NIA, convened experts to develop a research framework to enable enhanced efforts for diagnosing and identifying clinical trial participants across the entire AD continuum, which may contribute to therapeutic development [12]. The NIA–AA Research Framework is to enable innovation and further discovery; it is premature and inappropriate to use this framework currently in a clinical setting.

In addition to the complex continuum of the disease progression, the prevalence of the disease is not the same between men and women and between race and ethnicities, adding an additional layer of complexity. Further AD research continues to identify many diverse biological targets of AD, beyond the hallmark presentations of amyloid-beta plaques, tau tangles, and cell death. Taken together, these characteristics of the disease identify many challenges to drug development in AD therapy.

43.4 Alzheimer's Association Funding to Accelerate Drug Development

43.4.1 Philosophy

There is a significant gap in funding opportunities to advance potential target identification to pre-investigation drug discovery programs, which includes the identification and development of potential drugs before they are tested in humans. There is a need for funding to bridge this gap, departing from traditional funding mechanisms, which combines both expertise and the necessary know-how with the needed resources to translate more potential therapies to human studies. Such funding and programs should focus on high-risk/high-reward endeavors that advance multiple drug strategies for further testing and to advance such studies to human trials.

The Alzheimer's Association believes that all potential treatment avenues must be advanced, and all methods must be explored for advancing combination therapies. No stone can be left unturned in the vigorous search for better treatments and prevention of AD/ADRD.

The Alzheimer's Association International Research Grant Program lies at the heart of its commitment to advance AD/ADRD research. Since awarding the first grants in 1982, the Alzheimer's Association has grown into the largest private, non-profit funder of AD/ADRD research. As of July 2021, it is investing over $250 million in more than 750 active best-of-field projects in 39 countries.

The driving force behind the Alzheimer's Association International Research Grant Program is its desire to improve the quality of life for people affected by AD/ADRD. Key goals include:

- achieving new insights into the discovery science of AD/ADRD;
- using these insights to identify and advance novel approaches to risk assessment, diagnosis, treatment, and prevention;
- improving care and support for those living with the disease; and
- furthering the understanding of risk, risk reduction strategies, and prevention.

489

It seeks to:

- foster a diverse, inclusive scientific community that meets the needs of researchers at every career stage, with an emphasis on engaging and supporting early career investigators and those new to AD/ADRD research;
- design a nimble program offering grant programs that evolve to reflect a rapidly accelerating field;
- ensure the quality of its funded research through rigorous peer review, with input from the Alzheimer's Association's International Research Grant Program Council and Medical and Scientific Advisory Group; and
- support all scientifically legitimate avenues of investigation to nurture a robust pipeline of fresh ideas including the molecular pathophysiology of the biological underpinnings.

43.4.2 Funding Initiatives to Accelerate Drug Discovery

Launched in 2010 as a joint collaboration between the NIA and the Alzheimer's Association, the International Alzheimer's and Related Dementias Research Portfolio (IADRP) collates and categorizes the portfolios of major organizations for areas of shared priorities as well as areas of opportunities to inform coordination and collective efforts that seek to advance AD/ADRD research. Such coordination requires continued assessment of the funding landscape in the United States and internationally.

As reflected in IADRP, in 2019, new funding by the Alzheimer's Association spanned a diverse number of potential therapeutic targets, including metabolism, neurogenesis, oxidative stress, tau, apolipoprotein-E (ApoE), and other lipid-related mechanisms, amyloid beta, and inflammation-related biology. IADRP is reflective of the Alzheimer's Association's portfolio for the last 10 years of funding (https://iadrp.nia.nih.gov/).

Specific funding programs to stimulate the drug discovery and development activities in the field are necessary. To that end, in partnership with the Tau Consortium of the Rainwater Charitable Foundation, the Alzheimer's Association has funded 13 projects (as of January 2021) through a program aimed to stimulate the drug discovery and development pipeline. This program, the Tau

Pipeline Enabling Program, leverages the field's advances in knowledge on the mechanisms of tau and related biological pathways (e.g., microtubule stability, inflammation, axonal transport). The potential to target tau and tau-related biological pathways is emerging as a promising therapeutic strategy and the program seeks to accelerate the discovery of potential new therapies for tauopathies. The intent of this program is to enrich the pipeline for therapy development by facilitating the translation of academia-derived ideas into practical application [13]. In short, it bridges the gap between innovative but resource-constrained researchers and the larger pharmaceutical companies that are looking for drug candidates to be taken into human trials.

The strategic goal of the Alzheimer's Association funding of early-stage clinical trials, through its robust Part the Cloud Translational Research program, is to increase the options for potential interventions in early stages of neurodegeneration and to encourage the discovery and development of a wide range of interventions that target biology with strong scientific rationale for AD/ADRD.

The Alzheimer's Association believes that there are urgent unmet needs for discovering and developing novel therapeutic targets, as well as addressing new paradigms for testing potential interventions that target the complex biological underpinnings of AD/ADRD. Given the uncertainty regarding the precise mechanisms of neurodegeneration, Part the Cloud, in partnership with Bill Gates, has funded nearly 30 potential therapeutic trials (on experimental or repurposed drugs). Identifying therapies that target mitochondrial/bioenergetics and inflammation may have the potential to treat complex underlying biology of AD/ADRD, while also gaining a deeper understanding of multiple diseases that affect the brain. As of the time of writing, Part the Cloud – including this partnership – has funded in total over $60 million in innovative Phase 1 and Phase 2 clinical trials.

43.5 Importance of Biomarkers in Research and Clinical Discovery

The use of biomarkers in AD and ADRD has been a turning point in both our understanding of disease progression and the design and implementation of clinical trials. With the advancement of the 2011

NIA–AA guidelines, significant attention to both the development and validation of biomarkers in larger and diverse populations continues to be a key research priority. The Alzheimer's Association has both funded efforts and advocated for efforts to ensure these advancements continue. Just as important as developing tools that accurately detect the biological changes associated with AD/ADRD is the need to ensure accuracy and standardization measures that can be applied globally. Today, advances in brain imaging, fluid (CSF and blood), and other emerging biomarkers such as retinal imaging, skin biopsies, and saliva measures are continuing to emerge and advance.

43.5.1 PET Brain Imaging as a Biomarker

Imaging techniques can detect hallmark characteristics of AD, including deposition of amyloid beta and tau, as well as others, in living individuals using PET. In 2001, funding from the Alzheimer's Association to Dr. William Klunk and Dr. Chet Mathis at the University of Pittsburgh enabled the development of the first and still widely used PET imaging agent to detect amyloid beta in living persons (Pittsburgh Compound B [PiB]). Further funding from the Alzheimer's Association in 2006 enabled the addition of amyloid PET to the initiation of the longitudinal study, Alzheimer's Disease Neuroimaging Initiative (ADNI) – laying the essential foundation to develop PET imaging as a tool in AD research and clinical trials.

Because amyloid-beta plaques are one of the hallmark pathological features of AD, the clinical utility of imaging biomarkers is momentous. Proper use of these tools is critical to fully capture their benefits, and this led the Alzheimer's Association, together with the Society of Nuclear Medicine and Molecular Imaging, to develop appropriate-use criteria for amyloid PET [14]. The Alzheimer's Association is in the process of updating these criteria reflecting progress in the field, as well as the expansion to other PET imaging targets such as tau.

To further standardize the use of amyloid PET imaging, the Alzheimer's Association supported the sharing of the Centiloid project through the Global Alzheimer's Association Interactive Network. The Centiloid project aimed to develop a common quantitative output value across tracers and methods for amyloid PET imaging. These efforts laid the groundwork for both the development of and the standardization of AD imaging biomarkers.

43.5.2 Fluid Markers for AD

As techniques and technologies continue to evolve, global standardization efforts by the Alzheimer's Association are essential in considering the use of CSF and blood biomarkers.

The Alzheimer's Association established the Global Biomarker Standardization Consortium (GBSC) in 2010 to gather key researchers and clinicians from academia, industry, regulatory agencies, and government leaders in AD/ADRD, to achieve internationally accepted reference materials and reference methods for use in global clinical practice. Such standards are essential to ensure that analytical measurements are reproducible and consistent across multiple laboratories and across multiple kit manufacturers.

The quality control (QC) work group was one of the first initiatives of the GBSC, and it had the goal of standardizing the measurement of potential AD biomarkers in CSF [15, 16]. In addition, the program has assisted in the development of international reference materials and methods. Today, more than 90 laboratories participate in the program in over 20 countries, with the long-term goal of improving the quality of biofluid biomarker measurements, in both CSF and blood. In addition to the standardization of CSF analysis by the QC program, the Alzheimer's Association also convened a multidisciplinary workgroup to develop appropriate-use criteria for the safe and optimal use of CSF procedures and testing for AD [17].

The QC program has led to the creation of additional work groups focused on pre-analytical factors for handling and processing of both CSF and blood. These consortia, the CSF Pre-Analytics Consortium and the Standardization of Alzheimer's Blood Biomarkers (SABB), are pre-competitive collaborations that include experts from industry and academia. The CSF Pre-Analytics Consortium recently published a protocol for use in clinical practices to minimize the systemic differences in the biomarker measurements. The SABB work group formed in 2019 and the analysis is ongoing.

The GBSC continues to evaluate the use of emerging biomarkers in the field of AD. Recent advances in the detection of amyloid beta, neurofilament light chain, and hyperphosphorylated tau in blood/plasma have led the GBSC to support round-robin studies to evaluate current techniques. Outcomes from these studies will improve knowledge on how assays compare to each other and whether there are candidate reference materials to standardize measurement.

43.6 The Alzheimer's Association as a Global Convener to Accelerate Drug Discovery

Convening the research community is a pivotal aspect in the philosophy of the Alzheimer's Association and is essential for accelerating knowledge and research. To that end, it hosts a number of conferences annually in order to facilitate communication.

The Alzheimer's Association International Conference (AAIC®) is the largest and most influential international meeting dedicated to advancing dementia science. These annual meetings gather scientists from all over the world to share research discoveries that may lead to methods of prevention and treatment, and to improvements in the diagnosis of AD.

The AAIC serves as an annual compendium of activities and advances. Each year there are often updates on the clinical trial pathway and activities. For instance, the AAIC 2020 included presentations from more than 18 Part the Cloud awardees, who shared updates on their trials. The AAIC also serves as a platform to announce impactful research outcomes, specifically the advancement in blood tests that may be able to detect AD more easily and accurately, and with greater certainty.

The AAIC Satellite Symposium (SS) was an important development by the Alzheimer's Association and international partners to provide accessibility to researchers from all corners of the world and to provide these opportunities year round. Often held in areas around the world that may be less accessible or may not have the necessary infrastructure required for the AAIC, the satellite symposia allow for exciting scientific discussions, receive local media coverage to further raise awareness, and recognize local individuals as key resources in their community. By holding the AAIC SS throughout the year, the meetings make a difference globally by being instrumental in convening researchers worldwide, enabling collaborations and breakthroughs in AD research.

The AAIC Neuroscience Next (NN) is the most recent addition to the AAIC portfolio, with the inaugural meeting in November 2020. AAIC NN was developed as a means to engage early-career researchers from cognitive, computational, behavioral, and other areas of neuroscience research to stimulate research in AD and ADRD. A goal of the conference is to take a broad look at the neuroscience field in order to uncover cross-functional discoveries that can be applied to a number of brain disorders, including AD.

In addition to the AAIC-related meetings, the Alzheimer's Association, in partnership with the Tau Consortium of the Rainwater Charitable Foundation and Cure PSP, convened the Tau 2020 Global Conference. The first-of-its-kind meeting focused on a single protein – spanning the tauopathy brain diseases – and assembled leading tau experts from academia, industry, government, and the philanthropic sector. Key issues included expanding awareness of recent advances, increasing support for research, and fostering global partnerships. Discussions highlighted potential advancements and aspects that bring the field closer to drug-target and -therapy development.

For the past 15 years, the Alzheimer's Association has led the Alzheimer's Association Research Roundtable (AARR) to convene discussion and focused meetings to address challenges and barriers in the clinical development of AD and ADRD, including trials and drug development. The AARR is a consortium of senior scientists from the pharmaceutical, biotechnology, diagnostics, imaging, and cognitive-testing industries, and senior staff and advisors of the Alzheimer's Association with the mission of advancing the research, development, and management of new treatments for AD. The AARR benefits from the contribution of state-of-the-field scientific discourse, debate, and information sharing, aimed at advancing the field of AD research and development.

Discussions of the AARR have led to the development of specific work groups, including the ARIA Workgroup. Amyloid-related imaging abnormalities (ARIA) are based on reports of vasogenic edema in clinical trials of anti-amyloid therapies. The US Food and Drug Administration (FDA) set specific safety guidance for participants to enroll and be retained in these trials in 2010. The ARIA Workgroup convened a group of experts from industry and academia to review the available data and clinical trial experience, in order to develop expert guidance on these safety recommendations. The workgroup developed recommendations based on the data, and then presented these recommendations to the FDA while also publishing them in *Alzheimer's & Dementia: The Journal of the Alzheimer's Association*. The FDA later revised their safety guidance and criteria for subject inclusion and monitoring ARIA in these clinical trials.

Building off the AARR model, the association convenes the Alzheimer's Association Business Consortium (AABC). The AABC was organized with the mission to advance AD/ADRD research and innovation in small- and medium-size biotechnology, diagnostics, medical device, and contract research organizations. Currently, over 60 companies are part of the AABC and work in areas of common interest pre-competitively to advance both the field of AD/ADRD research and the goals of its member organizations. They provide leadership and direction to the group's areas of focus, which include, but are not limited to, collaborations, recognition and visibility, and knowledge and information sharing.

43.7 Alzheimer's Association National Strategy

43.7.1 Clinical Trial Recruitment Efforts

The Alzheimer's Association is committed to accelerating the global research community and knowledge.

There are varying levels of risk for developing AD, including differences in biological sex, race, and ethnicity. It is essential that clinical trial participants are a reflection of all communities, in order to fully understand the impact of risk and potential benefit of interventions to all. In 2018, the NIA published a national strategy that highlights practical and proactive approaches to help study sites engage a wider and more diverse number of participants [18]. The Alzheimer's Association assisted in facilitating the development of this document that focuses on four main themes: increase awareness and engagement at a broad, national level; build and improve capacity and infrastructure at the study-site level; engage local communities and support participants; and develop an applied science of recruitment.

To facilitate trial identification, the Alzheimer's Association offers TrialMatch™, which is a free matching program that connects individuals living with AD, caregivers, and healthy volunteers with current research studies. TrialMatch features a continuously updated database of both pharmacological and non-pharmacological trials, all over the country and online. Individuals provide certain information and are matched to studies based on their personal background, diagnosis, and treatment history. Though TrialMatch is not directly involved in AD research, it is a catalyst to accelerate clinical trial recruitment and results, and serve as a pivotal step toward development of AD therapy.

The Alzheimer's Association US Study to Protect Brain Health Through Lifestyle Intervention to Reduce Risk (US POINTER) is a 2-year clinical trial to evaluate whether lifestyle interventions that simultaneously target many risk factors protect cognitive function in older adults who are at increased risk for cognitive decline. US POINTER consists of five active sites across the country, with the goal of recruiting participants representative of the population. Add-on studies further investigate the biology behind the main study, including a neuroimaging study, sleep study, microbiome study, and neurovascular study.

The Alzheimer's Association also leads and co-funds the Imaging Dementia – Evidence for Amyloid Scanning (IDEAS) and New IDEAS studies. In 2013, after the Centers for Medicare & Medicaid Services announced that they would not provide coverage for PET imaging scans due to insufficient evidence, the IDEAS study aimed to determine the clinical usefulness and value of incorporating amyloid PET imaging in diagnosing AD/ADRD. More than 18,000 individuals have participated in the study and early results indicate that this imaging significantly influenced the clinical management of patients with mild cognitive impairment and dementia. The New IDEAS study follows in the footsteps of the original study, but with a focus on increasing diversity in participants. In addition, to adding participants, the New IDEAS study also includes a biorepository to store saliva and blood samples from the participants, which are matched to the brain scan data. This will allow accessibility for researchers to test and validate new genetic and blood biomarkers for dementia in a diverse population.

Together, these research initiatives aim to advance the knowledge and accuracy of risk and diagnosis of AD.

43.7.2 Alzheimer's Association Network and Community Engagement

As a science-led, advocacy-based organization, a core aspect of the Alzheimer's Association's mission is to provide support, care, and education to all stakeholders, keeping them informed and engaged. There are over 70 local Alzheimer's Association chapters across the United States, and these chapters are a vital part of the organization. The Alzheimer's Association is in communities nationwide, extending its reach. In addition to support options, it has both an international, national, and local relationship with the community's scientific researchers, including Alzheimer's Association grant recipients.

Through this nationwide network, the Alzheimer's Association provides essential education to lay and scientific audiences in the community, which includes sharing the importance of clinical trials. Many of the clinical trial efforts led by the Alzheimer's Association have sites that are spread across the country, and local chapters in those areas are encouraged to promote awareness of ongoing trials and the importance of participation in studies. The chapters also advocate for participation in the TrialMatch program.

43.8 The Alzheimer's Association and the Drug-Development Ecosystem

While there are many challenges to the development of therapies for AD and ADRD, the Alzheimer's Association has never been more optimistic than it is today. This stems from recent advancements in understanding and measuring the emerging pathology of disease, in thinking about the disease as a continuum, developing tools to actively monitor disease-related changes in a living person, and new strategies for identifying and enrolling participants in clinical trials, as well as confirmation of drug–target engagement.

The Alzheimer's Association has been involved in every major advancement in AD/ADRD research since the 1980s, and is the world's largest non-profit funder of AD/ADRD research. The

Alzheimer's Association directly funds science and unites the scientific academic, government, and industry leaders worldwide to accelerate research. A few examples highlighted in this chapter include:

- the AAIC, the world's largest and most influential international meeting dedicated to advancing dementia science;
- the Part the Cloud program, which has invested over \$60 million to advance nearly 60 clinical trials (as of July 2021) – these studies are targeting a wide variety of known and potential new aspects of the disease, such as inflammation and other promising new targets for therapy; and
- leadership of the US POINTER, the first study of multi-component lifestyle interventions to protect cognitive function in a large-scale US-based population.

We must expand all potential treatment avenues and also explore methods for combining these approaches. AD and ADRD are complex, and their effective treatment and prevention will likely also be a complex – but achievable – task. All currently pursued treatments that are considered safe should be continued to determine their efficacy.

References

1. Alzheimer's Association. 2020 Alzheimer's disease facts and figures. *Alzheimers Dement* 2020; **16:** 391–460.

2. Alzheimer's Disease International. *World Alzheimer Report 2015: The Global Impact of Dementia.* London: Alzheimer's Disease International; 2015.

3. Jack CR, Jr., Albert MS, Knopman DS, et al. Introduction to the recommendations from the National Institute on Aging–Alzheimer's Association workgroups on diagnostic guidelines for Alzheimer's disease. *Alzheimers Dement* 2011; 7: 257–62.

4. Petersen RC, Lopez O, Armstrong MJ, et al. Practice guideline update summary: mild cognitive impairment. *Neurology* 2018; **90:** 126–35.

5. Ward A, Tardiff S, Dye C, Arrighi HM. Rate of conversion from prodromal Alzheimer's disease to Alzheimer's dementia: a systematic review of the literature. *Dement Geriatr Cogn Disord Extra* 2013; 3: 320–32.

6. Mitchell AJ, Shiri-Feshki M. Rate of progression of mild cognitive impairment to dementia: meta-analysis of 41 robust inception cohort studies. *Acta Psychiatr Scand* 2009; **119:** 252–65.

7. Sperling RA, Aisen PS, Beckett LA, et al. Toward defining the preclinical stages of Alzheimer's disease: recommendations from the National Institute on Aging–Alzheimer's Association workgroups on diagnostic guidelines for Alzheimer's disease. *Alzheimers Dement* 2011; **7**: 280–92.

8. Albert MS, DeKosky ST, Dickson D, et al. The diagnosis of mild cognitive impairment due to Alzheimer's disease: recommendations from the National Institute on Aging–Alzheimer's Association workgroups on diagnostic guidelines for Alzheimer's disease. *Alzheimers Dement* 2011; **7**: 270–9.

9. McKhann GM, Knopman DS, Chertkow H, et al. The diagnosis of dementia due to Alzheimer's disease: recommendations from the National Institute on Aging–Alzheimer's Association workgroups on diagnostic guidelines for Alzheimer's disease. *Alzheimers Dement* 2011; **7**: 263–9.

10. Karlawish J, Jack CR, Jr., Rocca WA, Snyder HM, Carrillo MC. Alzheimer's disease: the next frontier – special report 2017. *Alzheimers Dement* 2017; **13**: 374–80.

11. Jack CR, Jr., Bennett DA, Blennow K, et al. A/T/N: an unbiased descriptive classification scheme for Alzheimer disease biomarkers. *Neurology* 2016; **87**: 539–47.

12. Jack CR, Jr., Bennett DA, Blennow K, et al. NIA–AA Research Framework: toward a biological definition of Alzheimer's disease. *Alzheimers Dement* 2018; **14**: 535–62.

13. Alzheimer's Association. The Tau Pipeline Enabling Program (T-PEP). Available at: www.alz.org/research/for_researchers/grants/types-of-grants/partnership_funding_programs/the_tau_pipeline_enabling_program_(t-pep)_(2) (accessed July 24, 2021).

14. Johnson KA, Minoshima S, Bohnen NI, et al. Appropriate use criteria for amyloid PET: a report of the Amyloid Imaging Task Force, the Society of Nuclear Medicine and Molecular Imaging, and the Alzheimer's Association. *J Nucl Med* 2013; **54**: 476–90.

15. Mattsson N, Andreasson U, Persson S, et al. CSF biomarker variability in the Alzheimer's Association quality control program. *Alzheimers Dement* 2013; **9**: 251–61.

16. Carrillo MC, Blennow K, Soares H, et al. Global standardization measurement of cerebral spinal fluid for Alzheimer's disease: an update from the Alzheimer's Association Global Biomarkers Consortium. *Alzheimers Dement* 2013; **9**: 137–40.

17. Shaw LM, Arias J, Blennow K, et al. Appropriate use criteria for lumbar puncture and cerebrospinal fluid testing in the diagnosis of Alzheimer's disease. *Alzheimers Dement* 2018; **14**: 1505–21.

18. National Institute on Aging. Together we make the difference: national strategy for recruitment and participation in Alzheimer's and related dementias clinical research. Available at: www.nia.nih.gov/research/recruitment-strategy (accessed July 20, 2021).

The Role of Philanthropy in Alzheimer's Disease Therapeutic Development

Cara Altimus

44.1 Introduction

Following a series of major clinical trial failures and pharmaceutical company exits from the space, Alzheimer's disease (AD) and related dementias have risen in the public consciousness. However, the healthcare crisis precipitated by AD is growing in magnitude. Today 7.2 million Americans live with AD and other dementias, and this number is expected to nearly double to 13 million in just 20 years [1]. While priorities for biomedical funding are often justified by how much life is lost or the cost to a healthcare system, the cost of AD and related dementias is far greater. Consider that 10% of people over age 65 currently suffer from AD and related dementias – and that for every one of them, their personal histories and identities are lost forever [2].

Despite 146 candidate therapies trialed between 1998 and 2017, the stark reality remains that only one therapeutic that impacts the underlying pathophysiology of AD – aducanmab – has been approved [3]. Scientists believe that there are multiple factors causing slow scientific progress: the disease develops gradually, going undetected for years; the cell biology of AD is complex, and has proven difficult to model; and the task of identifying clinical trial participants can only be described as Herculean.

These clinical failures have precipitated multiple large pharmaceutical companies to divest from neuroscience research, abandoning portfolios that might lead to a cure. High-profile pharma exits from AD research have left a gap that philanthropy can step in to fill, playing a leading role in providing funding and driving major innovation. While philanthropy is a relatively small player in the medical research ecosystem, making up approximately 3% of all of US funding for research and development [4], it remains a unique and less constrained source of biomedical research capital, and it is one that is poised to grow. Michael Milken, medical philanthropist and Chairman of the Milken Institute, said "Philanthropy is far more than just writing checks. It takes an entrepreneurial approach that seeks out best practices and empowers people to change the world" [5]. When philanthropists and foundations fully embrace the unique attributes of their capital and use it strategically to fill key funding gaps, incentivize new behaviors, and innovate the medical research system, the results could have major, positive impacts for science and for patients.

44.2 AD Research Funding Landscape

Following notable clinical trial failures in AD research, researcher and funder communities are redoubling efforts to develop new hypotheses explaining the underlying disease mechanisms so that new therapeutic targets might be identified and developed. Congress has dramatically increased AD funding to support this growth, with dedicated funding rising from approximately $600 million in 2015 to $2.8 billion in 2020 [6]. And the community has seen significant private investments as well. For example, in 2018, the Alzheimer's Drug Discovery Fund partnered with a coalition of philanthropists to launch the Diagnostics Accelerator to develop novel biomarkers for the early detection of AD [7]. In a rapidly changing landscape with several major public and private investments, it is ever more important to identify the specific challenges that philanthropy is uniquely positioned to tackle and encourage these engagements. At the Center for Strategic Philanthropy (CSP) we work on the principle that if philanthropists are able to identify the specific gaps where the larger funds are missing and either higher risk tolerance is needed, or nimbleness is valued, then philanthropic dollars can leverage the existing and growing federal funds to be truly catalytic.

44.3 Targeted Philanthropic Investment for AD

While biomedical philanthropy represents a critical area for investment, it is also a complex system that requires understanding current scientific trends, industry stakeholders and incentives, as well as the health policy landscape that regulates how therapeutic agents reach patient communities. Trends show year-on-year growth in biomedical philanthropy, and it is poised to grow. Among the 190 billionaires who have promised to donate at least half of their wealth, health is noted as the highest priority [8].

Our team at CSP works with philanthropists and foundations to identify specific routes for scientific investment. Over the last 3 years, we have worked with several partners to build programs and initiatives focused on AD and related dementias. Across our work, we have spoken with more than 100 researchers, interviewed more than 50 non-profit organizations, and convened funders, resulting in four identified areas for targeted philanthropic investment:

1. **Filling in the valley of death:** Broadly, philanthropists can play a pivotal role in navigating the early stages of translational research. This is the stage where a scientific discovery shows therapeutic potential but still needs to be developed prior to any in-human testing. This is a common spot for good science to get stuck. The National Institutes of Health (NIH) is a strong funder of discovery-focused research, but that funding is typically insufficient to develop a treatment sufficiently for an investor or pharmaceutical company to have confidence that they will be able to get the therapeutic to market.

2. **Investing in people:** Despite leaps in AD research funding, there is a critical need to focus on the workforce to ensure that young scientists – including women and people of color – are able to achieve sufficient opportunity to secure stable research positions. It is also crucial to foster cross-disciplinary collaboration so that experts from other disciplines are able to apply hypotheses or approaches from other disciplines to AD research.

3. **Elevating patient and carer perspectives:** Many philanthropists invest in medical research following personal experiences with the medical community. These perspectives bring major value-add to the scientific process and can be leveraged to drive progress, bring real-life experience, and create priorities that align with community need.

4. **Changing the conversation:** Finally, philanthropy might be a minority investor in the research community; however, its impact can be transformative for changing the culture. Funding policies can promote (or even require) data sharing, and create open-access publications to facilitate faster exchange of ideas. They can also drive gender and equity in the sciences. Further, as philanthropists select grant recipients or advisors, they are tilting the field of future funding, making these decisions critical for field success.

44.4 Bridging the Valley of Death

One of the most prominent gaps that philanthropy has filled in biomedical research over the past two decades is the translational "valley of death." Many foundations have adopted a venture philanthropy strategy, funding not only translational academic research programs but also commercial entities. Venture philanthropy treats funding as an investment rather than a gift, with expectations of social return, efficiency, and oversight. There is growing evidence that these programs are efficient in moving early-stage assets into the clinic and setting them up for longer-term development and regulatory approval.

The most well-known success story is the Cystic Fibrosis Foundation (CFF), which has deployed a successful venture philanthropy model for the last 20 years. To date, it has invested nearly $500 million in medical products, the most well-known being Kalydeco®, the first disease-modifying therapy for cystic fibrosis by Vertex Pharmaceuticals. The CFF negotiated a term that allowed Vertex to receive a royalty stream from the sales of the product. Kalydeco was approved in 2012, and the CFF sold its royalty stream for $3.3 billion to Royalty Pharma in 2014. The CFF also developed a network of more than 120 care centers that allowed for swift enrollment of patients with a particular kind of genetic mutation for clinical trials. This is a model for how philanthropic capital can unlock a path to systems change.

Many other disease research organizations have crafted programs that direct funding toward research in academic laboratories or early-stage biotechnology companies to bridge the valley of death. Take, for example, the Leukemia and Lymphoma Society, which funds over $45 million in blood cancer research annually. Their Therapy Acceleration Program (TAP), with 19 projects in the portfolio, is a venture philanthropy started in 2007 that partners with biotechnology companies to accelerate the development of novel therapies. During the past decade, TAP has helped to move dozens of preclinical efforts into clinical trials and, in 2017, two of their partnerships yielded US Food and Drug Administration (FDA) approvals: Celator's Vyxeos (acquired by Jazz Pharmaceuticals) for treating high-risk acute myeloid leukemia and Kite Pharma's (acquired by Gilead) chimeric antigen receptor T-cell therapy for lymphoma patients.

44.4.1 Applying Venture Philanthropy to AD Research

The various models of venture philanthropy highlight that the goal of accelerating therapeutic development is common – and that the mechanisms are as varied as the players and disease spaces. This diversity of venture philanthropy approaches is necessary. Each disease space is unique with specific scientific challenges, funding landscape, and in some cases existing treatments. In AD, the scientific challenges are great, funding has recently increased, and the therapeutics that modify the disease trajectory do not yet exist. This unique combination of circumstances necessitates a highly engaged strategy with informed investments.

Where can philanthropic investments lead to better therapeutics? Here we outline key facets of a translational investment program for AD.

44.4.1.1 Increase Access to Critical Translational Steps

While the process of drug development is often described at great length in scientific literature, several key steps require specialized expertise and access to resources that are not equally available to all researchers and institutions. These resources include compound libraries, high-throughput screening techniques, computational modeling, and access to medicinal chemists.

As major public investments provide new capital for basic science, new targets are being identified. Philanthropists can empower individual research teams to move these findings closer to testable hypotheses by providing access to early steps in translational development. This approach has been successful in other research communities through facilitating access to contract research organizations (CROs). CROs are private organizations that provide specialized research support to investigators or pharmaceutical companies on a contractual (outsourced) basis. They have the internal expertise and resources to conduct critical translational experiments in an unbiased and highly replicable manner, thereby producing data required to de-risk investment for a potential industry or funding partner.

An example of this type of program can be found within the Chordoma Foundation, which operates the Drug Screening Program. This program provides a mechanism for the research community to rapidly evaluate promising therapies in preclinical models of disease through a centralized hub where multiple screenings can occur in parallel. The program is operated through a partnership with a cancer-specific CRO, South Texas Accelerated Research Therapeutics (START) that specializes in cancer drug development. The Chordoma Foundation contracts with START to evaluate up to 10 therapeutic concepts per year, but others can use the same program on a fee-for-service basis. Additionally, the program provides each funded investigator study-design support, including dosing and model selection, which gives the grantees an additional leg up when moving to late-stage development.

If translated to AD and related dementias, it will be critical to ensure that partnership programs are able to navigate neurological drug development, which is an especially complex field of study. Neurotherapeutics holds unique challenges, including high rates of off-target activity, the blood–brain barrier, and in vivo models for secondary screening.

44.4.1.2 Create a Start-Up Culture

Recently, philanthropists and non-profit organizations have started to experiment with assisting academic investigators in the transition to a start-up company. This support mechanism is most relevant in the later stages of translational development, such as when data are being prepared for regulatory review to allow clinical trial.

Some non-profit organizations work with academic investigators who are taking the first steps to launch a start-up company. This typically includes raising initial (also known as seed) funds, licensing the technology from the academic institution, and developing contracts with support organizations. Non-profit organizations working in this space may play the role of an angel investor, providing early funding to the start-up and a stamp of confidence for the company's work. In these situations, non-profit organizations often offer more favorable terms than are available through traditional funder networks, because they operate with different objectives.

Importantly, this mechanism of promoting a greater number of start-up companies drives a shift in incentives from those typical in an academic setting (publication and NIH grants) to those more common in business (increase in value). These differences can drive accelerated therapeutic development because the incentive structure driving "increased value" is more aligned with creating a patient-ready asset.

There are a number of successful models for how to invest in new companies. For example, Multiple Myeloma Research Foundation supports this stage of development through the Biotech Investment Awards program. This proposal-based grant program aims to accelerate the development of innovative treatments for myeloma through the support of rapid testing of therapeutics in multiple myeloma. Grants are milestone driven, and payments are awarded after successful completion of milestones as outlined in each applicant's proposal.

44.4.1.3   Teach the Off-Topic Skills

Many biomedical researchers have neither the requisite experience in drug development, nor the necessary network to identify resources and funding to perform early translational steps. These scientists need more than funding – they need a support system. Private funders can fill these critical gaps in a number of ways:

- **Educate**: Philanthropically funded programs can provide academic investigators with opportunities to build their skills, providing training on topics including business development, legal agreements, guidance on requirements for FDA submission relevant to the disease space, and medicinal chemistry.

- **Mediate**: Communication between academic laboratories and industry is difficult because there are often competing priorities. Academics are focused on novel science, while industry is focused on making drugs. Some non-profit programs serve as the arbitrator or mediator in collaborative efforts, acting as a neutral third party in the arrangements. They assist in streamlining the processes and ensure that each side understands the milestones and terms of the agreement.

- **Match**: Finding the right partners is critical to the drug-development process. Private funders have unique networks and can facilitate interactions between investigators, partners, and funders at various stages of the development process. Additionally, philanthropic organizations may take an active role in developing the team required to move a therapeutic forward.

The Harrington Discovery Institute, which runs the Innovation Support Center, provides support to scientists through mentorship by a panel of experts who have demonstrated success in drug development. This panel of mentors advises on elements of development and the assessment of commercial potential. The Harrington Discovery Institute also takes an active role in identifying and securing funding, which bridges projects from academic settings to the final teams that will be able to commercialize the therapeutic. During this process, the Harrington Discovery Institute identifies the most efficient vehicles for the particular project, which include company creation, sponsored research agreements, and intellectual property augmentation. Ultimately, this program does not provide direct funds to investigators, but it provides access to experts and funding streams enhancing the potential for commercial success.

If applied to AD, this type of program could be highly impactful as most universities do not have sufficient expertise in neurotherapeutic drug development.

44.5   People-First Strategies

The NIH prioritizes the development of the biomedical workforce in numerous ways, ranging from creating and funding training programs at universities to developing funding mechanisms to support research independence. However, the professional growth of a scientist is long and challenging. Notably, between 1980 and 2016, the average age for securing an investigator's first NIH grant rose steadily from age 35 to 43. Even more worrisome is the pipeline for grant funding: there remain few opportunities for independent research funding prior to the attainment of a faculty position, and funding rates for mid-career investigators (age 41–55) are declining, while funding rates for established career investigators (>56) are climbing [9]. This threatens the pipeline of scientific talent, delays scientific independence, and stunts research. More concerning, these patterns threaten to entrench old ideas in biomedical research. Further evidence for this phenomenon is the growing trend showing that proposals that already had some scientific data score more favorably. An important way to break these patterns is to ensure that a new generation of researchers has sufficient support to pursue new ideas and bring new technologies to tough problems.

As the influx of federal funds attracts researchers to pursue AD research, philanthropists can play a key role in keeping talent focused, and providing support to accelerate cross-discipline science.

44.5.1 Fellowships

Research fellowships are typically short-term, lasting from several months to a few years, and focused on professional development and training. Programs generally align with a career phase and are an opportune mechanism for young scientists to transition and integrate into a new field. An AD-focused fellowship would likely be most impactful in late trainee career stages such as postdoctoral training, late graduate studies, or early-stage faculty. Additionally, in these career-stage-oriented awards, there is benefit to targeting researchers with prior experience in AD and new researchers because the goal is to increase the diversity of ideas in the discipline.

Further, receiving a fellowship is considered an honor and can increase the probability of receiving future federal funding. The National Bureau of Economic Research reported that fellowships promote the retention of scientists in the workforce pipeline. NIH fellowship recipients go on to be awarded a larger percent of NIH grants and also represent an increasing fraction of faculty positions in academic research institutions. Research

fellowships can be an effective strategy to encourage scientists to join a field and build a career pipeline to help grow specific disciplines.

44.5.2 Cross-Field Integration

A related but distinct avenue of workforce development is the intentional integration of technologies, ideas, and approaches from other disciplines. For example, genetic studies have implicated a growing number of targets with known activity in the human immune response. However, pursuing these targets will require integration of immunologists in AD research. Similarly, we are seeing a large influx of health data that could be leveraged to understand risk and potential treatments; however, these data sets are complex and require specialized expertise to navigate. As such, data scientists, computer scientists, and statisticians must be brought into the research community. A final example stems from the types of biological targets being identified. While a majority of therapeutic approaches have been predicated on individual proteins, there is a growing literature on the neural circuits underlying AD. A few researchers are exploring the application of neural-device technologies to the development of new treatment modalities; however, neural-device development and application requires a complex array of researchers ranging from engineers, neurosurgeons, and material scientists.

While scientists generally acknowledge the importance of interdisciplinary research, the peer review process has been routinely criticized for favoring dominant research and entrenched hypotheses over interdisciplinary work. This may happen if reviewers feel that funds are limited, pushing individuals to favor the "safe bet" over an "out of box" idea. However, in AD, this strategy led to *only* five FDA approvals for treatments targeting AD symptoms and a majority of funding rewarded to ideas and scientists who have had a long history in the field.

Philanthropy can play a transformative role in getting ideas from other disciplines to the forefront by taking a seed-funding approach. This way, researchers can generate preliminary data that can be included in an application for NIH funding, and give new entrants the leg up needed to be competitive. Additionally, this approach leverages likely follow-on funding from the NIH, which is possible because of the recent influx of funding.

44.6 Patient Perspective

Across our tenure-advising philanthropists, we have noted that individuals do not stumble upon biomedical philanthropy, rather it finds them. Many passionate philanthropists have engaged in biomedical research because they are directly impacted by a disease. However, it is the direct experience, and in many cases frustration, with current medical care that motivates their engagement. Unfortunately, the prevalence of AD is growing around the world and, as such, our likelihood of experiencing it through caring for a loved one, or directly suffering from neurodegeneration ourselves is also increasing.

Both scenarios have been major drivers of philanthropic investment and innovation in AD over the last several years. For example, the Alzheimer's Society UK, a philanthropically funded organization, supported the development of Jelly Drops, which combat dehydration in dementia patients. Moving closer to therapeutic development, the BG3, the Gates investment team, has made major investment in developing quantitative biomarkers, which is needed to create tools to definitively diagnose AD. In other research communities, philanthropists have funded patient-preference surveys that are used to drive the direction of innovation so that it is better able to target the aspects of disease that are most impactful to patients' lives. If done in AD, this kind of initiative could help funders and researchers prioritize the greatest needs of those living with AD, including those with early symptoms and caregivers.

44.7 Focus on Culture

Many scientists share that the cultural currents of scientific research are shifting. Periods of low NIH funding rates (lower than 20%) have driven a sense of scarcity of funding and led to fierce competition between research groups. However, there is a growing realization that biomedical research should ultimately benefit patients, and the more these timelines can be accelerated, the greater the benefit to patients is possible. This shift has led to more data and resource sharing, greater adoption of open-access publications, and increased effort for workforce and scientific diversity.

One potential driver of the seed change is the start of a generational shift in the scientific workforce. Analysis of the scientific workforce has shown an aging population beyond that seen in the broader US workforce; however, a deep dive into these demographic shifts shows that the large cohort of baby boomers, paired with the elimination of mandatory retirement in universities, has driven this change such that the share of scientists over the age of 55 increased from 18% to 33% between 1993 and 2010 [10]. Ten years later, it is expected that the turnover of the baby-boomer cohort has begun, creating space for a new generation of investigators, And greater turnover brings the opportunity for new practices.

Philanthropic funders can lead this change by promoting actions and behaviors that have outsized impact on the research community, but may be perceived as out of alignment with traditional academic research incentives. Examples include: requiring open-access publication of findings, supporting the publication of data in databases that are available to other researchers, inclusion of diverse samples/subjects (gender, ethnicity, etc.), supporting research to replicate key studies, promoting meaningful collaboration, and publishing negative results so that others might incorporate the findings in their experimental plans. All of these changes require intention and support. As philanthropists partner with researchers, these community-bolstering mechanisms should be included in funding agreements and, where needed, additional funding provided to allow the research teams to successfully incorporate them within the studies.

Aligning Science Across Parkinson's, a recently launched program seeking to drive basic science discovery for Parkinson's disease, created strong grant terms focused on open-science priorities. Open-access publication, use of pre-print servers, and data sharing are required for funding and evaluated in all rounds of follow-up funding.

44.7.1 Diversity in Leadership

Many philanthropists rely on the established research community to provide program guidance, grant-application review, and/or mentoring for grant recipients through participation on advisory boards. These positions can be highly impactful for an investigator's career; however, we have noted that a vast majority of these roles are held by luminaries in the field. Greater diversity of career stage, gender, race, country of origin, and perspective can have an outsized impact on the field and individuals' careers. From the perspective of philanthropic impact, any program working in AD needs a robust breadth of topical knowledge. However, expansion of those who are advising philanthropists will give more individual researchers a greater understanding of the field priorities and landscape, and set more individuals up for success in future grant competition.

44.8 Conclusion

In our tenure as philanthropy advisors and as biomedical research experts, our team at CSP can see that the spectrum across which philanthropic investment is needed is vast, and that it can feel overwhelming. However, this is where the opportunity lies – philanthropists are uniquely positioned to look across the landscape and engage in the spaces that other sources of capital are less able.

The funding landscapes supporting drug development in AD have shifted dramatically over the last 5 years, and philanthropy can infuse needed energy, expertise, and connections in ways that will accelerate development. While I have outlined specific ways that philanthropy can support translational development, the research teams, and the business case for follow-on investment, there are other important mechanisms not specifically outlined here. In any philanthropic endeavor, we encourage donors to be an agent of needed change, driving increased collaboration, inclusive science, and ultimately a focus on the patient communities that might benefit from the advance.

References

1. Super N, Ahuja R, Proff K. Reducing the cost and risk of dementia. Available at: https:// milkeninstitute.org/sites/default/files/reports-pdf/ Reducing%20the%20Cost%20and%20Risk%20 of%20Dementia%20Full%20Report-FINAL-for-posting_0.pdf (accessed November 25, 2020).

2. Alzheimer's Association. 2020 Alzheimer's disease facts and figures. *Alzheimers Dement* 2020; **16**: 391–460.

3. PhRMA. Research. Alzheimer's medicines: setbacks and stepping stones. Available at: www .phrma.org/en/Alzheimer-s-Medicines-Setbacks-and-Stepping-Stones (accessed November 25, 2020).

4. Research!America. U.S. Investments in Medical and Health Reserach and Development, 2013–2017. Available at: www.researchamerica .org/sites/default/files/Policy_Advocacy/2013-2017InvestmentReportFall2018.pdf (accessed November 25, 2020).

5. Milken M. Giving pledge letter 2010. Available at: https://givingpledge.org/Pledger.aspx?id=245 (accessed November 25, 2020).

6. Alzheimer's Impact Movement. Alzheimer's and dementia research. Available at: https://alzimpact .org/issues/research#:~:text=Today%2C%20 funding%20for%20Alzheimer's%20 and,increase%20for%20fiscal%20year%202020 (accessed November 25, 2020).

7. Losak A. New coalition of philanthropists including Bill Gates, Leonard Lauder commit more than $30 million. Available at: www.alzdiscovery .org/news-room/announcements/new-coalition-of-philanthropists-including-bill-gates-and-leonard-lauder-co (accessed November 25, 2020).

8. The Giving Pledge. Giving pledge. 2020. Available at: https://givingpledge.org/PledgerList.aspx (accessed November 25, 2020).

9. Charette MF, Oh YS, Maric-Bilkan C, et al. Shifting demographics among research project grant awardees at the National Heart, Lung, and Blood Institute (NHLBI). *PloS One* 2016; **11**: e0168511.

10. Blau DM, Weinberg BA. Why the US science and engineering workforce is aging rapidly. *PNAS* 2017; **114**: 3879–84.

Chapter 45

National Institute on Aging's Alzheimer's Disease Translational Research Program: Diversifying the Drug-Development Pipeline for the Treatment and Prevention of Alzheimer's Disease and Related Dementias

Laurie Ryan, Suzana Petanceska, and Lorenzo Refolo

45.1 Introduction

It is estimated that as many as 5.8 million Americans aged 65 and older currently have Alzheimer's disease (AD) dementia, with the prevalence in the United States projected to increase to 13.8 million by 2050. AD is the most common dementia diagnosis and the sixth leading cause of death for Americans. In addition, many others have related forms of dementia, such as Lewy body disease, frontotemporal degeneration, and vascular cognitive impairment, either alone or more commonly mixed with AD pathology. The social and economic costs of these disorders are enormous. One analysis of healthcare spending found that total costs for a person with probable dementia in the last 5 years of life was an estimated $287,000, compared with $175,000 for an individual with heart disease and $173,000 for someone with cancer [1, 2]. The recent advances in understanding the neurobiology of AD offer unprecedented opportunities to discover new treatments for AD. However, despite these scientific advances, the development of effective AD therapies has been challenging. Drug discovery and development for the treatment of AD and AD-related dementias (AD/ADRD) is extremely expensive and time-consuming, and the possibility of disappointment looms at every phase of discovery. It has been estimated that half the candidate therapies fail during preclinical research – the phase when important information on feasibility, testing, and drug safety is collected. And, if a promising therapy does advance to the clinic, there's an extremely high failure rate during Phase

2 and Phase 3, primarily due to lack of efficacy and/or toxicity [3].

The National Institutes of Health (NIH) is the largest funder of AD and ADRD research in the world. The National Institute on Aging (NIA), part of the NIH, leads the federal effort on AD/ADRD research. On January 4, 2011, the National Alzheimer's Project Act (NAPA) became law. It declared prevention, treatment, and care to be a priority for the United States and ordered the creation of a National Plan to Address Alzheimer's Disease. The National Plan was initially released in 2012. The first goal of the plan is to find effective ways to treat or prevent dementia by 2025. As part of the strategic planning process for the implementation of the goals of the National Plan, the NIH holds a series of AD/ADRD Research Summits held in alternate years. Two focus on treatment and prevention of AD/ADRD while the third focuses on better approaches to care, services, and support. The NIH AD Research Summits [1] bring together a multi-stakeholder community including government, industry, academia, private foundations, and patient advocates to formulate an integrated, translational research agenda to enable the development of effective therapies (disease-modifying and palliative) across the disease continuum for the cognitive as well as neuropsychiatric symptoms of AD/ADRD. Recommendations from the summits in turn inform the development of Research Implementation Milestones (www.nia.nih.gov/research/milestones), which show concrete steps that the NIH and other stakeholders in the AD/

ADRD research and development (R&D) ecosystem need to take to meet the goals of the National Plan. The recommendations and subsequent milestones are then translated into new NIA–NIH programs and funding initiatives. Since the first NIH AD Research Summit in 2012, the NIA's funding for AD/ADRD research has steadily increased, allowing continued expansion and diversification of the drug-development portfolio and the development of translational infrastructure programs to accelerate the discovery of effective therapies.

45.2   Bridging the Valley of Death with a Pipeline of Funding Opportunities

Since 2005, the NIA has been developing a robust translational research program for the treatment and prevention of AD dementia [4, 5]. The program has two major components: the first is a series of funding initiatives that span target discovery and early validation through late-stage clinical drug development (Figure 45.1). The goal of this component is to deliver new investigational new drugs (INDs) and new drug applications (NDAs) for a diverse portfolio of therapeutic targets. The second component is a suite of translational research infrastructure programs; the goal of this component is to help the community of researchers in academia, biotechnology, and pharmaceutical industry more effectively execute each step of the critical path. The pipeline of funding opportunities for drug discovery, preclinical, and clinical drug development utilizes a variety of grant mechanisms from small exploratory grants (R21) to large cooperative agreements (U01). The NIA's small business grants program provides support for all steps of drug discovery and preclinical drug development through early clinical development (for details see Chapter 48).

45.2.1   AD Drug Development Program

The most robust funding initiative for preclinical drug development is the NIA's Alzheimer's Drug Development Program (ADDP) – this funding vehicle provides seamless support for the development of small molecules and biologics, from mid-stage preclinical drug development through Phase 1 trials. This is a milestone-driven program that utilizes the cooperative grant mechanism. The program offers two entry points: (i) hits optimization through INDs and (ii) preclinical lead selection through Phase 1 trials. Since its inception in 2006 the ADDP has supported 38 preclinical drug-development projects. Of these, nine have secured an IND and entered clinical development and are currently supported by a combination of the NIA's clinical drug development funding opportunities and Small Business Innovation Research (SBIR) grants program and/or by multiple non-profit or for-profit funders. These clinical drug candidates target nine different molecular targets that underlie

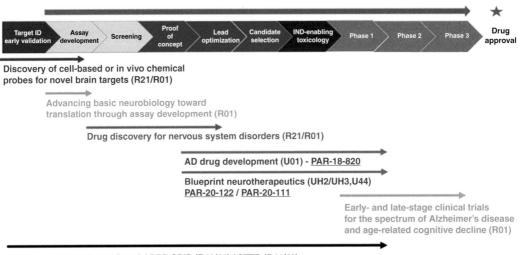

Figure 45.1 A pipeline of NIA and Trans-NIH translational research funding opportunities.

multiple aspects of the disease process such as neuroinflammation, proteostasis, synaptic plasticity, neurogenesis, amyloid-beta oligomer aggregation, and signaling.

45.2.2 Blueprint Neurotherapeutics Program

The NIA's ADDP is complemented by the Trans-NIH Blueprint Neurotherapeutics (BPN) funding initiatives. The BPN program supports preclinical drug development for small molecules through Phase 1 trials and utilizes a virtual model; researchers receiving support through the program receive access to NIH-funded consultants and contract research organizations that specialize in medicinal chemistry, pharmacokinetics, toxicology, formulations development, chemical synthesis under good manufacturing practices, and Phase 1 clinical testing. Since the launch of the BPN program, the NIA has supported five preclinical drug-development projects for five first-in-class small molecules – one of these, BPN-14770 (a selective allosteric inhibitor of phosphodiesterase 4D) by Tetra Therapeutics, secured IND status and additional NIA funding through the SBIR program, and recently completed a Phase 2 trial. In 2020, Tetra was acquired by the pharmaceutical company Shionogi; Shionogi will advance the late-stage clinical development of BPN-14770 in AD and other central nervous system disorders such as fragile X syndrome.

45.2.3 Drug Repurposing and Combination-Therapy Development

The promise and current limitations to successful drug repurposing and combination-therapy development for AD were one of the major topics of discussion at the three NIH AD Research Summits; the summit participants called for establishing new research programs that combine computational and experimental approaches to advance data-driven drug repurposing and combination-therapy development. In 2017, the NIA launched the funding initiative, Translational Bioinformatics Approaches to Advance Drug Repositioning and Combination Therapy Development for Alzheimer's Disease, and encouraged the use of existing, and development of new, computational methods to identify drugs already in use for other conditions, which are predicted to be efficacious in AD/ADRD as individual compounds or as

drug combinations. To date, this NIA program has supported over 20 projects which bring together experts in data science (network biology, systems pharmacology, machine learning, and artificial intelligence) with experts in disease biology and clinical research. The teams are leveraging the universe of publicly available big data on AD and other conditions (genomic, multi-omic, drug data, and electronic health records) to generate better predictions regarding repurposable drugs and drug combinations, and to create the knowledge, tools, and resources needed for successful drug repositioning and combination-therapy development for AD/ADRD. The new phase of this funding initiative is encouraging academic partnerships focused on integration of clinical and phenotypic data with molecular data generated in biosamples from failed trials for AD/ADRD, for the purpose of identifying the molecular determinants of responder phenotypes to enable precision drug repositioning and combination-therapy development. Another research area of high interest is projects aimed at developing methods that can assess the synergy or additivity between candidate therapeutics, including synergy between candidate drugs and non-pharmacological perturbations (i.e., diet, sleep, cognitive training).

45.2.4 Clinical Development Programs: Embedding Biomarkers and Data-Sharing Requirements

The NIA supports early-stage AD/ADRD trials (Phase 1 and Phase 2) and late-stage AD/ADRD trials (Phase 2/3 and Phase 3) via two R01 funding initiatives. Early-stage clinical development is also supported though the NIA's SBIR (see Chapter 48). In addition, trials conducted through the NIA's clinical trials infrastructure, the Alzheimer's Clinical Trials Consortium (ACTC), are supported via a separate funding opportunity (see below for more details). These three funding opportunities support clinical trials, testing promising pharmacological (small molecules and biologics, novel, and repurposed drugs) and non-pharmacological interventions in individuals with age-related cognitive decline and across the AD/ADRD spectrum, from presymptomatic to more severe stages of disease. Applications are welcome from academic investigators as well as investigators from biotechnology and pharmaceutical companies.

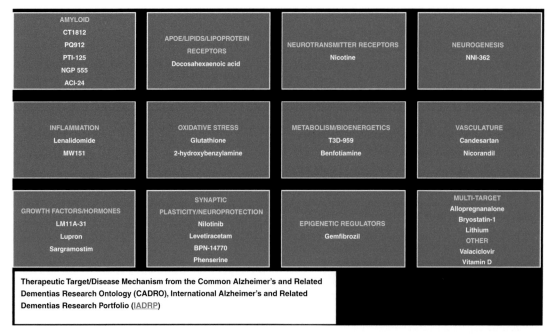

Figure 45.2 NIA-supported early-stage clinical drug development (Phase 1 and Phase 2) 2013–2019.

Some of the salient features of these three funding initiatives are expectations for the inclusion of biomarkers and biosamples collection. For early-stage trials, investigators are expected to incorporate pharmacodynamic biomarkers as well as to collect and store blood and other biosamples for future genomic and other "omic" analyses aimed at interrogating treatment responsiveness and examining predictors of decline and progression. Late-stage trials are expected to include a combination of biomarkers (fluid, imaging), cognitive, and functional measures as outcomes and to collect DNA and other biosamples to enable subsequent interrogation of treatment responsiveness, as well as examination of predictors of decline in the groups receiving placebo. Moreover, all these initiatives include requirements for data and biosamples sharing. Registration trials are expected to share resources according to the Collaboration for Alzheimer's Prevention (CAP) principles [6], which entails making screening/pre-randomization data and biosamples available within 12 months of completing enrollment and making placebo- and treatment-arm data and samples available after regulatory approval or within 18 months after the completion or early termination of a trial. For earlier-stage trials, resources must be shared upon acceptance of primary publication or within 9 months of trial completion, whichever comes first [7].

Between 2013 and 2019, the NIA supported 40 early-stage drug trials via the early-stage and SBIR initiatives, involving 29 compounds against 14 different disease mechanisms (Figure 45.2).

45.3 Translational Infrastructure Programs for Data-Driven and Predictive Drug Development: Laying the Foundation for a Precision-Medicine Approach to AD Therapy Development Using Systems-Based Approaches

Over the last 7 years, the NIA's funding for AD and ADRD research has steadily increased, allowing continued expansion and diversification of our drug-development portfolio and translational infrastructure programs to help advance future therapeutics (Figure 45.3). The translational infrastructure programs were developed in response to a series of recommendations from the NIH AD Research Summits (2012, 2015, 2018); they support cutting-edge research built around open-science and open-source principles. Collectively they are designed to rapidly deliver critical data resources, knowledge, and research tools to help the R&D community in academia

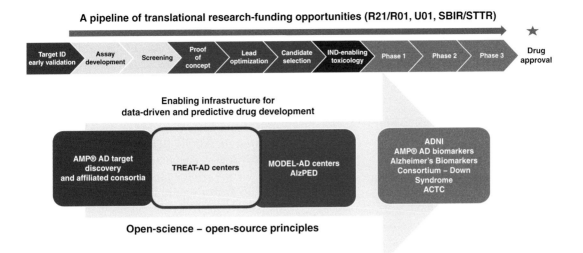

Figure 45.3 The NIA AD Translational Research Program: diversifying the therapeutic pipeline.

and industry more effectively execute each step of the critical path and enable a true precision-medicine approach to AD/ADRD therapy development [8].

45.3.1 Accelerating Medicines Partnership® Program for Alzheimer's Disease

Accelerating Medicines Partnership® Program for Alzheimer's Disease (AMP® AD) is an innovative pre-competitive public–private partnership among the NIH, pharmaceutical industry, and non-profit organizations aimed at increasing the likelihood of success for new candidate drugs by validating existing, and identifying new, disease-relevant targets by harnessing the power of big data and enabling rapid and broad data sharing. Led by the NIA and managed by the Foundation for the NIH (FNIH), the AMP® AD program has two components: Target Discovery and Preclinical Validation and Biomarkers in Clinical Trials. The Target Discovery and Preclinical Validation Project is implementing a systems-biology approach to discover and validate the next generation of therapeutic targets using an open-science research model; the program supports a consortium of six multi-institutional, multidisciplinary academic teams and a data coordinating center at Sage Bionetworks. It leverages decades-old public investment in epidemiological research, genetics, and brain-tissue banking by generating high-quality multi-omic data and deploying cutting-edge computational and experimental

methods to deliver deeper understanding of the complex biology of AD/ADRD, identify the next generation of therapeutic targets, and make all data, methods, and insights rapidly available, without embargo, to researchers around the world. Since its launch in 2014, the program has delivered an unparalleled amount of high-quality molecular and biological data and enabled many new mechanistic disease insights, significantly expanding the AD target landscape (www.nia.nih.gov/research/amp-ad).

The data, methods and candidate targets delivered by the AMP® AD research teams are made available through the NIA-supported big-data infrastructure: AD Knowledge Portal [9, 10], a FAIR data repository (www.go-fair.org), and the portal-linked, open-source platform, Agora (www.agora.io/en). Agora is an interactive, web-based tool designed to allow researchers to access detailed information on more than 500 candidate targets (including druggability assessment contributed by the AMP® AD industry partners) nominated by AMP® AD teams and to evaluate any gene of interest against a series of AMP® AD-verified genomic analyses delivered. More than 500 unique candidate drug targets along with a wealth of supporting evidence and data have been made publicly available to date.

To date over 3,000 researchers from around the world (~60% from academic and ~40% from industry) have accessed these data resources.

In February 2021, the NIH launched the second phase of the AMP® AD program (AMP® AD 2.0) by expanding the scope of the initial Target Discovery component to enable a true precision-medicine approach to target and biomarker discovery.

45.3.2 AMP® AD-Affiliated Systems-Biology Consortia

The AMP® AD-affiliated systems-biology consortia are summarized in Figure 45.4, and described in the subsections below.

45.3.2.1 M²OVE-AD

Molecular Mechanisms of the Vascular Etiology of Alzheimer's Disease (M²OVE-AD) focuses on deconstructing the metabolic and vascular etiology of AD. The program established by the NIA in collaboration with the National Institute of Neurological Disorders and Stroke (funding initiative RFA-AG-15–010) aims to understand how the various vascular and metabolic factors influence the emergence of cerebrovascular disease and AD clinical–pathological features. It generates high-quality multi-omic data from brain and blood samples collected across several natural history and population studies where occurrence of both neurodegeneration and vascular disease have been characterized, and the program has used network-biology approaches to integrate these data with data on neuroimaging, vascular physiology, and cognitive measures.

45.3.2.2 Resilience-AD

The NIA's Resilience-AD program aims to understand the molecular determinants of cognitive resilience in individuals at high risk for AD. Specifically, it aims to generate deeper understanding of the mechanisms by which

gene–environment interactions lead to cognitively resilient phenotypes in the presence of high risk for disease, and identify new therapeutic targets amenable to prevention strategies, using both pharmacological and non-pharmacological approaches. The Resilience-AD research teams are generating high-quality multi-omic data using biosamples collected in individuals who resist/escape AD/ADRD despite having high AD risk (such as centenarians, individuals homozygous for the apolipoprotein ε4 allele, individuals with Down syndrome, and individuals who remained cognitively normal despite the presence of disease biomarkers established by neuroimaging or by postmortem neuropathological assessment). They apply a variety of network-biology approaches to derive molecular drivers of resilience and examine the mechanisms by which these genes/proteins operate across multiple cell-based and animal models.

45.3.2.3 Psych-AD

The Neuropsychiatric Symptoms in AD (Psych-AD) program is focused on understanding the molecular mechanisms underlying the neuropsychiatric symptoms in AD/ADRD. The projects integrate epidemiological research, multi-omic profiling (bulk-tissue and single-cell/single-nucleus profiling) and mechanistic studies via systems- and network-biology approaches, with a goal to discover the molecular ties between various neuropsychiatric symptoms and AD/ADRD and to identify and characterize new therapeutic targets and biomarkers for the treatment of neuropsychiatric symptoms in AD/ADRD. The program is a result of a series of funding-opportunity announcements launched between 2018 and 2020, developed as a collaboration between the NIA and the National Institute for Mental Health.

45.4 A Precision-Medicine Approach to the Development of Mouse Models of Late-Onset AD and Preclinical Efficacy Testing: MODEL-AD

The Model Organism Development and Evaluation for Late-Onset Alzheimer's Disease (MODEL-AD) consortium was launched in 2016; it brings together multiple institutions supported by two U54 center grants: one at the University of California at Irvine

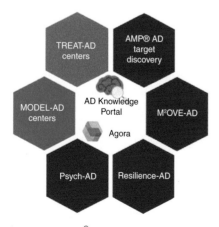

Figure 45.4 AMP® AD-affiliated systems-biology consortia.

and the other at Indiana University in collaboration with Jackson Labs, Sage Bionetworks, and the University of Pittsburgh. The MODEL-AD mission is to ameliorate several major factors contributing to the poor predictive power of animal-model preclinical studies. To this end, during their first 5-year funding cycle, the MODEL-AD goals are to:

- create 50 new mouse models using CRISPR (clustered regularly interspaced short palindromic repeats) and knock-in models;
- carry out high-capacity screening of all models and deep phenotyping of the most promising models to align mouse and human phenotypes across multiple outcomes (molecular omics, neuropathology, imaging);
- establish a preclinical efficacy testing pipeline to enable rigorous preclinical efficacy testing of promising candidate therapeutics; and
- provide broad, unrestricted distribution of all data and models for use in research and therapy development.

To date, the MODEL-AD teams have made available over 40 new genetically modified (knock-in) mouse models to researchers in academia and industry without costly licensing fees or intellectual property barriers. The data generated as part of the process of initial characterization and deep phenotyping are made available on a continuous basis via the AD Knowledge Portal. A key component of MODEL-AD is the Preclinical Efficacy Testing Core (PTC). The PTC is responsible for establishing a pipeline for rigorous preclinical testing of promising candidate treatments. In 2020, the PTC launched the Screening the Optimal Pharmaceutical for Alzheimer's Disease (STOPAD) portal, enabling drug developers from academia and industry to nominate candidate compounds. Compounds that are selected for preclinical efficacy testing will be paired with a genetically modified mouse model appropriate for the molecular process that is being targeted [11, 12].

45.5 Enabling Reproducible and Translatable Preclinical Efficacy Testing: AlzPED

As discussed earlier, it is difficult to translate positive preclinical study results into similar positive clinical outcomes. One of the chief culprits is poor rigor in design, methodology, and evaluation of preclinical studies. To help improve the rigor,

reproducibility, and translatability of preclinical investigations, the NIA and the NIH Library along with the Alzheimer's Drug Discovery Foundation and the Alzheimer's Association joined forces to create the Alzheimer's Disease Preclinical Efficacy Database (AlzPED). AlzPED, launched in 2016, is a publicly available, searchable, knowledge base that hosts more than 1,000 published studies regarding the preclinical testing of candidate therapeutics in animal models of AD/ADRD. It aims to illuminate the experimental design and reporting practices of preclinical efficacy testing studies for researchers, funding agencies, and the public. It also houses data on 188 animal models, 890 therapeutic agents, 173 therapeutic targets, and more than 1,500 AD-related outcome measures. In 2018, AlzPED became a platform for creating citable reports and preprints of unpublished studies, including studies with negative findings to reduce publication bias in favor of studies reporting positive findings [3].

45.6 Accelerating Therapy Development for Novel Targets: TREAT-AD

The TaRget Enablement to Accelerate Therapy Development for Alzheimer's Disease (TREAT-AD) consortium is the newest addition to the NIA's translational infrastructure established through the Alzheimer's Centers for Discovery of New Medicines funding initiative. It consists of two translational centers (TREAT-AD Center at Emory University, Sage Bionetworks, and Structural Genomic Consortium and TREAT-AD Center at Indiana University School of Medicine and Purdue University) with a common mission: to diversify and accelerate therapy development for AD/ADRD through the development of open-source tools, reagents, and methods for robust validation of candidate targets delivered by AMP® AD and other target discovery programs and by integrating a set of novel targets into drug discovery campaigns. Each TREAT-AD center brings together expertise in data science, computational biology, disease biology, structural biology, assay development, medicinal chemistry, pharmacology, and clinical research. The consortium will deliver high-quality target-enabling tools, including crystal structures, antibodies, chemical probes, and cell-based assays, for an array of novel targets; initiate drug discovery for a diverse portfolio of novel targets; and make all data, tools, and methods available to researchers in academia and the biotechnology and pharmaceutical industry, for laboratory research and drug discovery.

45.7 Clinical Trials Infrastructure

45.7.1 Alzheimer's Disease Neuroimaging Initiative

The Alzheimer's Disease Neuroimaging Initiative (ADNI) is a longitudinal multi-center study designed to develop clinical, imaging, genetic, and biochemical biomarkers for the early detection and tracking of AD. The overall goal of ADNI is to validate biomarkers for use in AD clinical treatment trials. It was first launched in 2004 as a landmark pre-competitive public–private partnership that enabled broad sharing of all data. It is a structured partnership overseen by the Private Partner Scientific Board (representatives from private, for-profit, and non-profit entities). ADNI has had a significant impact on both clinical and basic science research. It has helped optimize biomarkers for use in trials through validation studies, reproducibility studies, and statistical analysis. It has also generated new knowledge about underlying physiopathology and genetic contributions to the disease and has inspired similar consortia around the world [13].

45.7.2 Alzheimer Clinical Trials Consortium

Launched in late 2017, the Alzheimer Clinical Trials Consortium (ACTC) is a next-generation clinical trials infrastructure designed to harness best practices and latest methods for AD/ADRD trials. The ACTC is a cooperative agreement (U24) between the NIA and ACTC investigators. It includes 35 member sites across the United States along with numerous participating sites in the United States and other countries. ACTC trials are supported by a funding opportunity for Phase 1b to Phase 3 trials of pharmacological and non-pharmacological interventions in individuals across the AD/ADRD spectrum from presymptomatic to more severe stages of disease. A key area of focus for the ACTC is improving diversity in recruitment and in the clinical trial workforce. The Minority Outreach and Recruitment Team is developing central and local partnerships with diverse communities to enhance representation of these under-represented groups in AD/ADRD trials. The ACTC Inclusion and Diversity Committee has been conducting mentorship activities for

ACTC junior investigators and trial study staff. Additionally, the ACTC Patient Advisory Board has been constituted with a focus on inclusion of individuals from under-represented populations as well as from across the disease spectrum. Sharing (data and biosamples) is another key element of the ACTC, and it is part of the NIA's enabling infrastructure for data-driven and predictive therapy development. All design, methods, procedures, etc. developed will be shared with the larger research community as will trial data and biosamples per the NIA requirements noted earlier.

The ACTC successfully launched its first trial in 2020 in collaboration with Eisai and Biogen, the AHEAD 3–45 study evaluating efficacy and safety of lecanemab (BAN2401) in participants with preclinical AD and elevated amyloid, and also in participants with early preclinical AD and intermediate amyloid. Two other trial grants were funded in fiscal year 2020. One is a Phase 2 trial of CT1812 in mild-to-moderate AD. The development of CT1812, a small-molecule antagonist of the sigma-2 receptor, has long been supported by the NIA through its preclinical and clinical therapy development programs. The other trial is a Phase 2 study testing the efficacy of an oral combination of two cannabinoids, tetrahydrocannabinol and cannabidiol, for the treatment of agitation in participants with severe dementia. In addition to these trials, the ACTC supports several other NIA-funded studies including the Trial Ready Cohort for the Prevention of Alzheimer's Dementia (TRC-PAD) and the Trial-Ready Cohort – Down Syndrome (TRC-DS), both of which develop trial-ready cohorts of AD biomarker-positive individuals for enrollment in future trials. TRC-DS is part of the larger ACTC-DS, which is a component network of the ACTC established for conducting AD clinical trials in the Down syndrome population.

45.7.3 AMP® AD Biomarkers in Clinical Trials Project

AMP® AD, as noted above, is an NIH-led pre-competitive public–private partnership to identify and validate the most promising biological targets of AD to advance diagnostic and drug development. The first phase, AMP® AD 1.0, consisted of two components: the Biomarkers Project and the Target Discovery and Preclinical Validation Project. The Biomarkers Project incorporated tau positron emission tomography imaging into two NIH-funded prevention trials (A4 trial and DIAN-TU). Data sharing under AMP® AD includes making the screening data and biosamples available after enrollment completion and making post-randomization data and biosamples available as soon as possible after completion without compromising trial integrity. The Anti-Amyloid Treatment in Asymptomatic Alzheimer's Disease (A4) trial has achieved the first milestone by making the screening data and biosamples available (via the Laboratory of Neuroimaging, LONI). This is the first registration trial to ever do so and the first paper using the screening data from A4 was published in 2020 [14]. The trial is currently ongoing with anticipated completion in 2022.

45.8 Training a Diverse and Cross-Disciplinary Translational Workforce

Complementing the NIA's translational infrastructure is support for cross-disciplinary training programs funded through the NIA's Institutional Training Programs to Advance Translational Research funding initiative on AD/ADRD. Through several funded programs across the United States, the NIA is supporting a new generation of translational scientists, with expertise in biology, data science, engineering, and drug development, who are able to participate and lead team-science programs from target discovery to clinical trials.

The Institute on Methods and Protocols for Advancement of Clinical Trials in Alzheimer's and Related Dementias (IMPACT-AD) is an AD/ADRD clinical trials training course to build and diversify the next generation of AD clinical trialists. It was developed by ACTC investigators and funded via a U13 in fiscal year 2020. Members of the first class came from a variety of demographic backgrounds (age, race, ethnicity, etc.), specialties (physicians, psychologists, statisticians, etc.), environmental backgrounds (rural, urban, etc.), and career stage/current position.

Funding opportunities for new fellowship and career development programs aimed at promoting diversity in translational research for AD/ADRD were recently released (PAR-21-217, 21-218, and 21-220) as was an AD/ADRD clinical trial short courses funding opportunity announcement (PAR-21-141) to increase diversity and provide education in state-of-the-art clinical research skills in AD/ADRD [15].

45.9 Toward an Open-Science Research Ecosystem for Therapy Development

Open science is an inclusive, participatory approach to research in which learning is accelerated by making data, research methods, and research tools available to all qualified researchers. Rapid and broad sharing of data and tools is particularly important in the new era of biomedical research, marked by the rise of big data and novel analytical approaches to better understand human wellness and disease in a person-specific manner. Over the last two decades, the NIA has led and contributed to the development of transformative open-science research programs and open-science collaborations and partnerships.

One of the key recommendations from a large multi-stakeholder community participating in the NIH AD Research Summits was a call to enable and propagate open-science practices across the R&D continuum. The collective input was the impetus for the NIA to develop the array of translational infrastructure programs described above, AMP® AD and affiliated target discovery consortia and the MODEL-AD and TREAT-AD centers. All operate under open-science principles to rapidly deliver data, knowledge, and research tools necessary to overcome key barriers to developing effective therapies. These calls for open science extended to clinical trials. Sharing data, both summary and participant levels, and biosamples from clinical trials, is critical for helping us understand factors that impact the success or failure of therapeutic agents, including differences in how AD/ADRD unfolds in individual participants and how different people respond to treatment. This helps avoid duplicating trials unnecessarily and increases the speed and efficiency of the clinical trial enterprise. Yet, this has rarely been done in the clinical trial space. In 2015, the Institute of Medicine published the first set of guidelines outlining responsible clinical trial data sharing for the entire biomedical community [16]. At the same time, a coalition of stakeholders including the FDA, NIA, Alzheimer's Association, clinical trialists, and trial sponsors developed the Collaboration for Alzheimer's Prevention [6] described earlier. Similarly, the NIA began raising the bar for data and resource sharing from AD/ADRD clinical trials with the AMP® AD Biomarkers Project. As mentioned above, the A4 study, part of AMP® AD, became the very first trial to make its screening data and biosamples available. Starting in 2018, the NIA codified these data-sharing expectations across the NIA AD/ADRD clinical trial funding initiatives as described above.

The NIA continues to expand the use of open-science practices across the NIA-supported research enterprise and engage with AD/ADRD private-sector stakeholders to develop an open-science research ecosystem capable of meeting the needs of all patients and individuals at risk of the disease.

References

1. National Institutes of Health. NIH professional judgment budget for Alzheimer's disease and related dementias for fiscal year 2022. Available at: www.nia.nih.gov/sites/default/files/2020-07/bypass-budget-report-FY-2022.pdf (accessed January 18, 2021).

2. Kelley AS, McGarry K, Gorges R, Skinner JS. The burden of health care costs for patients with dementia in the last 5 years of life. *Ann Intern Med* 2015; **163**: 729–36.

3. Refolo L. From mouse to medicine: improving preclinical research in Alzheimer's disease. Available at: www.nia.nih.gov/research/blog/2017/02/mouse-medicine-improving-preclinical-research-alzheimers-disease (accessed January 18, 2021).

4. Petanceska S, Ryan L, Silverberg N, Buckholtzet N. Commentary on "A roadmap for the prevention of dementia II. Leon Thal Symposium 2008." Alzheimer's disease translational research programs at the National Institute on Aging. *Alzheimers Dement* 2009; **5**: 130–2.

5. Buckholtz NS, Ryan LM, Petanceska S, Refolo LM. NIA commentary: translational issues in Alzheimer's disease drug development. *Neuropsychopharmacol Rev* 2012; **37**: 284–6.

6. Weninger S, Carrillo MC, Dunn B, et al. Collaboration for Alzheimer's prevention: principles to guide data and sample sharing in preclinical Alzheimer's disease trials. *Alzheimers Dement* 2016; **12**: 631–2.

7. Ryan L, Petanceska S. Raising the bar on data and biosample sharing from AD/ADRD clinical trials. Available at: www.nia.nih.gov/research/blog/2020/12/raising-bar-data-and-biosample-sharing-ad-adrd-clinical-trials (accessed January 18, 2021).

8. Sperling RA, Jack CR, Jr., Aisen PS. Testing the right target and right drug at the right stage. *Sci Transl Med* 2011; **3**: 111cm33.

9. Petanceska S, Refolo L. Open science delivers a wealth of AD/ADRD research data to a portal near you. Available at: www.nia.nih.gov/research/blog/2020/11/open-science-delivers-wealth-ad-adrd-research-data-portal-near-you (accessed January 18, 2021).

10. Greenwood AK, Montgomery KS, Kauret N, et al. The AD knowledge portal: a repository for multi-omic data on Alzheimer's disease and aging. *Curr Protoc Hum Genet* 2020; **108**: e105.

11. Oblak AL, Forner S, Territo PR, et al. Model Organism Development and Evaluation for Late-Onset Alzheimer's Disease: MODEL-AD. *Alzheimers Dement* 2020; **6**: e12110.

12. Sukoff Rizzo SJ, Masters A, Onoset KD, et al. Improving preclinical to clinical translation in Alzheimer's disease research. *Alzheimers Dement* 2020; **6**: e12038.

13. Weiner MW, Veitch DP, Aisen PS, et al. Recent publications from the Alzheimer's Disease Neuroimaging Initiative: reviewing progress toward improved AD clinical trials. *Alzheimers Dement* 2017; **13**: e1–85.

14. Sperling RA, Donohue MC, Raman R, et al. Association of factors with elevated amyloid burden in clinically normal older individuals. *JAMA Neurol* 2020; **77**: 735–45.

15. Bernard M. Announcing NIA's new crop of research concepts! Available at: www.nia.nih.gov/research/blog/2020/09/announcing-nias-new-crop-research-concepts (accessed January 18, 2021).

16. Institute of Medicine. *Sharing Clinical Trial Data: Maximizing Benefits, Minimizing Risk.* Washington, DC: The National Academies Press; 2015.

Chapter 46

Alzheimer's Disease Drug Discovery and the Evolution of Start-Up Biotechnology Companies: Cognition Therapeutics, Inc. as a Case Study

Susan Catalano

46.1   Introduction

Alzheimer's disease (AD) afflicts about 6 million people in the United States and 50 million worldwide, and the number of patients is expected to more than double by 2050. Disease-modifying therapies for AD continue to be a huge unmet medical need. With the exception of the recently approved drug aducanumab, only symptomatic treatments are currently available which briefly slow cognitive decline for an average of 6 months by regulating neurotransmitter levels.

Large biopharmaceutical company and investor interest in particular disease areas are linked. Investors build companies that develop medicines which are licensed to large biopharmaceutical companies who take them the final mile through expensive late-stage clinical trials, approval, and marketing. Rarely are they successful enough with a new medicine to grow sufficiently quickly to take on those challenges themselves. Nowhere is this less likely to happen than in diseases of the central nervous system (CNS), where the sheer complexity of the biology results in an industry-leading ~90% failure rate. Large biopharmaceutical company interest in discovering and developing therapeutics for diseases of the central and peripheral nervous system has waxed and waned over the years, and industry scientists have faced increases or reductions in staffing levels in parallel, with consequent disruptions or discontinuation of therapeutic discovery research that often takes years to complete in such complicated diseases.

Since I began working in AD therapeutic discovery and development in 2003 there have been many changes in the landscape. Several large pharmaceutical companies have consolidated through mergers and acquisitions, the number of large and mid-sized companies focused on neurodegeneration has dwindled, and big pharmaceutical companies have largely discontinued drug discovery and development of AD-modifying therapeutics due to several large, expensive late-stage clinical trial failures.

Yet the need for novel approaches to slow or stop AD progression has never been greater; dementia care worldwide was estimated to cost more than $1 trillion annually in 2018 [1] and $280 billion in the United States in 2019. AD is the only leading cause of death that is still on the rise [2]. Over 75% of AD patients live at home, where more than 10 million Americans provide 8.5 billion hours of unpaid care at a cost of more than $94 billion. However, no dollar amount can possibly describe the real cost of AD: the loss of loved ones and an entire generation of wisdom when families need it most. In recent years, the task of stopping this disease has fallen to smaller biopharmaceutical start-up companies, who nevertheless face significant hurdles to field novel therapeutics in this space against the backdrop of investor and large pharmaceutical company pessimism.

Those hurdles are both financial and scientific. When the National Alzheimer's Project Act (NAPA) was passed by the US government in 2011, the Leaders Engaged on Alzheimer's Disease (LEAD) Coalition was begun in response and continues to this day. Associated with the LEAD Coalition's initial organization, one of the scientific leaders from the biopharmaceutical industry approached me to ask what I thought the field required to achieve NAPA's number 1 goal: Prevent and effectively treat Alzheimer's by 2025. My response was that the field would need at least 10 new investigational new drugs (INDs) per year (each with a different, novel mechanism of action) for the next 10 years to have a chance at achieving that goal. This prediction has been borne out; attempts to repurpose existing medicines to slow or halt the disease have been tried but have not met with success.

This chapter presents a case study of how one small company discovered and developed CT1812, a disease-modifying AD small-molecule experimental therapeutic that works by a novel mechanism of action, with the support of its investors and the National Institutes of Health (NIH). As the co-founder of this company, Cognition Therapeutics, Inc., this account is necessarily personal and hopefully serves as an inspiration to other entrepreneurs considering a similar undertaking. It's been an amazing journey, and as you'll see several times throughout this story, it was only possible because of many major sources of support: (1) our investors and the National Institute on Aging (NIA), who continue to support the company financially; (2) the extraordinary dedication of the finest, most productive scientists I've ever had the pleasure to work with; (3) colleagues in the field who have been quite generous with their advice and help; and (4) the patients and their families and caregivers who volunteer for clinical trials. It has been a privilege to work with all of these folks.

The views expressed here are my own and not necessarily those of the company or its shareholders or advisors, regulatory authorities, or the NIH. CT1812 is an investigational therapeutic that has not been approved for any use by the FDA. The relative benefit of the drug compared to its risks is still being evaluated and has not been determined. The risk–benefit profile will be evaluated after adequate placebo-controlled clinical trials of CT1812 have been completed.

46.2 History of Scientific Accomplishments and Fundraising

Figure 46.1 summarizes Cognition's history of scientific accomplishments to date. Cognition was incorporated on August 21, 2007, by me and my pharmaceutical industry veteran co-founders Gilbert Rishton, Anthony Giordano, and Franz Hefti. At the time, the company was just an idea of how to find disease-modifying therapeutics (i.e., those capable of slowing or stopping AD). We believed that by using a unique method for constructing novel brain-penetrant CNS-drug-like small-molecule libraries (the process of "conditioned extraction," pioneered by co-founder Gilbert Rishton) and novel screening assays using mature primary neurons in vitro, we could discover drug candidates capable of blocking the toxic effects of the amyloid-beta (Aβ) oligomers thought to cause AD.

This collective approach to drug discovery (commonly referred to as "platform technology") was unique, and we first approached state economic development corporations (EDCs) for financial support to begin operations. Such state agencies distribute small amounts of seed capital to start businesses under very favorable terms for the company, and typically require the businesses to stay in that geographic area for some period of time to contribute to economic growth in the region. Based on our co-founder's prior experience with agencies in the state of Pennsylvania, we approached EDCs in the city of Pittsburgh, and were successful in receiving start-up capital from Innovation Works and the Pittsburgh Life Sciences Greenhouse (PLSG). I relocated to Pittsburgh and began to build our laboratory facilities in incubator space secured by the PLSG in November of 2007, putting together laboratory benches we still use with a borrowed

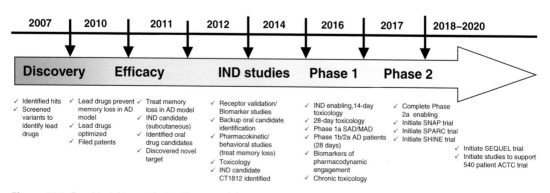

Figure 46.1 Cognition's history of scientific accomplishments to date. MAD, multiple ascending dose; SAD, single ascending dose.

manual screwdriver. We attracted an Executive in Residence from the PLSG, Dr. Hank Safferstein, to step into the chief executive officer (CEO) role and help develop and execute on a unique and powerful public–private financing and operating plan for the company. Pittsburgh has a high concentration of neuroscience faculty and students in its universities, and the ease of staffing the company with experienced neuroscientists has been a noteworthy advantage in the company's history. Combined with the low cost of operations (i.e., rent, etc.), the environment in Pittsburgh allowed us to pioneer the discovery and development of medicines that work by novel mechanisms of action in a way that would not have been likely elsewhere.

In order to model a disease that takes place in the aging brain, I knew we would need to model the mature brain in our in vitro screening system. It would be critical to use primary neurons and glia instead of surrogate cells because the process of synaptic plasticity is not fully replicated in any surrogate system used to this day, despite considerable technical advances. In addition, it was important that these primary neurons and glia were from brain areas affected in AD (we use hippocampal and neocortical cells) and allowed to mature in the dish before use in screening assays. This is because it requires at least 3 weeks of growth in vitro for primary neurons to achieve peak numbers of synapses [3, 4], exhibit spontaneous oscillatory activity [5, 6], and express the full complement of synaptic proteins found in the adult [7]. Cognition is one of the only places in the world that routinely produces such mature cultures in the 384-well microtiter plate format suitable for screening large numbers of small molecules, and this process is described in a recent paper [8].

Prior evidence suggested that low, sub-lethal concentrations of Aβ oligomers trigger a rapid reduction in the amount of neurotransmitter receptors at the synaptic plasma membrane of neurons; this loss of receptors at the cell surface appeared to be the basis for the Aβ-oligomer-mediated inhibition of electrophysiological measures of synaptic plasticity, and thus learning and memory. This reduction was accompanied by a retraction of the spines where synapses are located. Importantly, both neurotransmitter receptor expression, spines, and learning and memory function would recover after Aβ oligomers were washed out, suggesting their negative effects were reversible [9–12]. An assay that modeled these early, reversible disease-related changes might

discover effective AD drugs. We chose to adapt the previously published 3-(4,5-dimethylthiazol-2-yl)-2,5-diphenyltetrazolium bromide (MTT) assay that uses cargo dye to measure the rate of endocytosis and exocytosis in neurons and glia for use with these cultures [13–15]. By measuring the trafficking rate of endosomal/lysosomal lipid vesicles and associated transmembrane receptors in neurons and glia, we could measure a process important for normal synaptic plasticity, learning, and memory that was impacted by the AD toxin, Aβ oligomers. Small molecules that dose-dependently blocked Aβ-oligomer-induced deficits in trafficking rate (whether added before or after oligomers) but did not affect trafficking rate when dosed in the absence of oligomers were forwarded on to further testing. The disease relevance of this assay was borne out by its ability to predictably identify compounds that restored learning and memory to normal in transgenic AD mice [8, 16–19].

This culture system and assay were challenging to field, so I knew we would need very high-quality starting material. It would be pointless to begin by screening commercially available CNS-drug-like small-molecule libraries; such compound collections are typically rich in scaffolds that are based on existing CNS drugs, and modulating neurotransmission was unlikely to result in successful disease-modifying AD therapeutics (as I'll get to below). I reached out to Dr. Gilbert Rishton, whom I had seen speak about a new process he pioneered for generating small-molecule libraries called conditioned extraction. This process involved starting with low-molecular-weight oils like ginger oil (available in kilogram quantities from the flavors and fragrances industry), removing chemically reactive groups (that typically create assay artifact via covalent reactions) through simple chemical modification, and separating the resulting mixtures via flash chromatography [20–23]. This resulted in mixtures of 5–10 compounds suitable for screening that had ideal CNS-drug-like physicochemical properties: they were low-molecular-weight, lipophilic, and contained the fundamental elements of what was once a biologically active scaffold, but, most importantly, they were novel. I asked Gil to join our new company as a co-founder and bring this process with him, and to my delight he agreed. We have never had to engineer blood–brain-barrier penetration into our leads or drug candidates and have patents on multiple series issued or pending. Because of this

515

excellent library, we easily identified the high-affinity receptor targets of active molecules with secondary counterscreens available at contract research organizations (CROs) and found novel drug candidates in record time.

At one point we briefly considered using acronyms for these platform systems. The library generation technology was christened NICE (for Novel Improved Conditioned Extraction) and the cultures and screening assays were called EASSY (for Early Alzheimer's Screening System). We abandoned it after our lab folks strongly expressed their displeasure, since the screening systems were anything but nice and easy.

The following year while we worked to screen libraries and identify our first hit molecules, the United States was hit by an economic disaster precipitated by the subprime mortgage crisis (the Great Recession). The NIH moved swiftly to mobilize funding to support the nation's research infrastructure through the Small Business Catalyst Awards for Accelerating Innovative Research, with funds made available in the American Recovery and Reinvestment Act. With the help of our CEO Dr. Hank Safferstein, we applied for and received our first NIH grant in 2009. Also in this year we secured our first angel investor, Ogden CAP Associates, who have supported us ever since. In 2010, we received our first patent for our library-generation technology, demonstrated that our lead compounds prevented memory loss in an AD mouse model, and applied for and received funding from the Alzheimer's Drug Discovery Foundation, a unique venture philanthropy organization supported entirely by the Lauder family (an act of generosity with few equals). Around this time, we secured our second major investor, Golden Seeds, a network of angel investors who support women-led companies. It's hard to overstate the personal and professional support they've given us and me personally over the years. We also received funding early on from Tech Coast Angels, an inspiring and well-connected California-based network of investors. I've enjoyed personal relationships with many of these investors, most of whom have a personal connection to the disease, and I draw significant inspiration from these truly wonderful people.

Over the ensuing years as I frequently traveled to visit academic collaborators or interview and audit CROs, I would also give an update to one of our angel investor groups in that city or pitch to a new angel group that our existing investors

introduced us to. Through this activity we widened our network of investors to include groups such as Cowtown Angels, Ariel Savannah Angel Partners, Bangor Angels, Bluetree Allied Angels, Sofia Angels, Central Texas Angel Network, Houston Angel Network, Maine Angels, and BIOS Partners. Their support has been critical to the company's survival.

We continued to improve the potency of our small molecules through the iterative process of medicinal chemical engineering known as structure–activity relationship (SAR) optimization, culminating in the nomination of CT1812 as an IND candidate in 2013. Our phenotypic screens had led us to understand that it was binding affinity at sigma-2 receptors that was responsible for CT1812's potent anti-Aβ-oligomer activity, but we also knew that high affinity at sigma-2 receptors was not enough (i.e., we had high-affinity sigma-2 receptor ligands that were inactive). This means that CT1812 and its active relatives occupy a unique binding pocket on the receptor associated with this activity, known as a pharmacophore, and this uniqueness was borne out by the many issued patents on the drug candidate and its analogs. CT1812 is the world's first selective sigma-2 allosteric antagonist taken to the clinic for any disease or condition whatsoever; this is referred to as a first-in-class medicine. It means there is no roadmap for how to develop it and this required us to find out how to quantitatively measure whether the drug engaged its target in patients, i.e., what proteins or lipids in a patient's clinical biofluid sample (blood or cerebrospinal fluid [CSF]) would change with dose when the drug bound to sigma-2 receptors. Without target-engagement biomarkers detectable in patients, it is impossible to predict if the drug is getting where it needs to go and affecting function, so it is impossible to predict its likelihood of success. These proteins or lipids whose changing concentrations signal the drug's dose-dependent impact on the receptor's function and disease biology are referred to as biomarkers. The necessity for discovering these biomarkers adds to the cost and time of developing drug candidates, one of the hallmark features of first-in-class drug development.

The fact that we would need to drug a new target to stop AD came as no surprise. Aβ oligomers cause a range of negative impacts on brain cells, which vary by concentration; at low concentrations the oligomers subtly perturb the process of synaptic plasticity (the molecular basis for learning and memory) and at high concentrations they can rapidly kill cells. Cell death is a complicated process, and by the time a cell has committed to dying, there are so many molecular signaling pathways gone wrong that a drug acting at a single receptor is unlikely to stop it. The only tractable intervention point is "upstream," where the perturbations are subtle and relatively simple. The first symptom in AD is an anterograde amnesia – a failure to encode new memories – which is a perturbation of the molecular process of synaptic plasticity. For this reason, at the outset of the company, I chose to focus our efforts on finding drug candidates to stop the actions caused by low concentrations of Aβ oligomers. I knew it was likely that we'd find neurotransmitter receptor targets that appeared to be involved, yet I knew this would be a "red herring": the two classes of drugs currently on the market for AD modulate neurotransmission, but provide brief symptomatic relief that does not last; neither stops the disease process. Many other existing drugs modulate the process of neurotransmission, yet there was no epidemiological evidence suggesting that any of these stopped the progression of AD. Moreover, many initiatives to systematically examine the impact of existing drugs on AD (a term referred to as "repurposing") had been attempted over the years and have not yielded success. I remember one conversation with a large biopharmaceutical company executive in which he was speculating about potential neurotransmitter receptor targets, and I said "You know you're not going to stop Alzheimer's disease by modulating neurotransmission." That stopped the conversation dead in its tracks. Clearly we would have to choose a different class of target, and do the hard work of understanding the disease itself at the same time we were attempting to drug it.

Of all the possible intervention points and compound mechanisms of action we could have discovered that would block the toxic effects of Aβ oligomers in a phenotypic screen, it was not surprising that what we discovered was one that was far upstream: ligand displacement. Aβ oligomers behave like a ligand binding to a receptor: several laboratories had demonstrated that oligomers bind specifically and saturably to a single receptor site on synapses at neurons, and they only become toxic when they bind to this receptor site. This pharmacological (or "lock and key") receptor–ligand mechanism can be targeted very effectively with brain-penetrant small molecules.

Other mechanistic goals (disruption of oligomer structure or prevention of their formation) do not have a successful track record of being achieved with brain-penetrant small molecules, and blocking individual pathways downstream of the toxicity caused by oligomers with small molecules has not met with clinical success to date.

As we conducted formal good laboratory practice toxicology studies of CT1812, we began discussions with the US Food and Drug Administration (FDA) in a pre-IND meeting in 2014, in which the agency provides feedback on plans for development and early clinical testing of a drug candidate. As we prepared to interview clinical trial sites and contractors for our first-in-human clinical trials, I traveled to Australia to visit the Nucleus Network site and, while there, met with Scale Investors. We gained the support of Scale Investors and chose Nucleus Network for our first clinical trial site and began the study in 2015. I was there for the first human dose, a very fulfilling experience that few scientists ever get to witness. The experience was so positive that we continued with our first patient study and expanded to six sites within Australia, overseen by Neuroscience Trials Australia. The US FDA granted CT1812 Fast Track status in 2016.

While this happened, many folks in our small group of scientists volunteered to assist with fielding the Phase 1 and Phase 1b/2a clinical trials, further straining the resources of the laboratory in Pittsburgh who were responsible for continuing to discover and develop backup drug candidates. We benefitted from the expert advice of PharmaDirections and worked side by side with them, doing whatever it took to manage the process. In a large organization, experts with prior experience are typically hired to advance the drug through development. Insufficient funding precluded us from this path, but fortunately our dedicated laboratory staff rose to the challenge, listened carefully to expert advisors, and executed flawlessly, while never growing above the original six members. It provided me with a valuable lesson: never underestimate the capabilities of dedicated scientists who share the vision of impacting the disease and are willing to do whatever it takes to make that happen.

Scientifically, having no prior disease-modifying AD therapeutics presents a challenge; rather than engineer a faster-onset antidepressant that works by the same mechanism of action as existing drugs, which can be evaluated side by side in clinical trials, there is no comparator, no "gold-standard" therapeutic to guide discovery or development. Added to this was the extra challenge of the nature of the previous attempts to slow or stop AD; while many demonstrated excellent target engagement, others did not, and their failure could not be explained biologically. Added to this was the scientific challenge and added cost of developing a first-in-class mechanism. We therefore faced a formidable risk that is unacceptable to larger biopharmaceutical companies, and therefore most large institutional investors. Without the support of competitive peer-reviewed grants from the NIA, enabled by congressionally mandated increases to its budget (itself enabled by many effective advocacy organizations), we would not have survived.

We designed a series of clinical trials to examine the biology that our first-in-class drug impacted. We were enabled to do this by the inspiring group of clinical scientists and expert AD trialists on our Medical Advisory Board. Dr. Lon Schneider was unstinting in his generosity and patience; without his help to understand the NIH system for clinical trial support, and write grants to obtain it, CT1812 may never have reached the clinic. Our development strategy was to discover biomarkers of target engagement and disease modification in small clinical pharmacology trials conducted in parallel with a large, simple, fully powered Phase 2 study to determine if the drug worked to slow or stop disease in mild-to-moderate patients. For the latter study, there was some guidance; many prior clinical studies of the symptom-modifying anticholinesterase drugs had shown that a significant change from placebo-treated patients (a 3-point change on the Alzheimer's Disease Assessment Scale – cognitive subscale test) could be detected with 6 months of daily treatment with about 40 patients per group. Our biology told us that CT1812 could be capable of slowing or stopping disease (a term referred to as disease modification), but as part of this process should also impact cognitive test scores with 6 months of treatment like the existing symptom-modifying drugs. We knew that the odds were high that the expensive later stage of development would be handled by a larger company that had licensed our drug candidate; our task was to demonstrate that it worked to change cognitive abilities in patients AND provide objective biomarker evidence that demonstrated target engagement and an impact on relevant biology. With the help of our advisors and experts, we submitted seven clinical

grants. These were favorably reviewed by our peers and the grants have supported all of CT1812's clinical development. Program officers at the NIA were patient and helpful during this process and were a key element of our first major source of support.

This was incredibly hard work, and I drew personal support and inspiration for it from family, friends, and the patients themselves. Many companies receive requests from patients or their caregivers for access to experimental medicine. I remember a correspondence I received from one patient, over the years watching the handwriting in the signature of the neatly typed letters gradually deteriorate. On one occasion I took the lab folks on a tour of the Carnegie Art Museum run by volunteers for patients suffering from AD. Watching the interactions of these generous volunteers with the patients was a very moving experience for all of us.

My advice to young entrepreneurs who sincerely desire to impact patients suffering from diseases with no available treatments is: never hold back, never give up, and don't leave anything on the table. It is harrowing to contemplate dedicating decades of your life to something that, after all, might not work, but that's what it takes, and every day thousands of my scientific colleagues do exactly that. Working side by side with them all these years has been the greatest honor of my life. This work continues to this day by a dedicated team of scientists and industry professionals.

46.3 CT1812's Mechanism of Action

Available evidence points to accumulation of the $A\beta_{42}$ protein, and its self-association into toxic oligomers that cause synaptic dysfunction and loss, as a central pathogenic feature of AD. CT1812 is the first highly brain-penetrant small molecule that selectively displaces Aβ oligomers bound to neuronal receptors at synapses (Figure 46.2) and facilitates their clearance from the brain into the CSF. CT1812 thus lowers the Aβ-oligomer binding affinity to their receptors. By displacing Aβ oligomers from the site where they cause toxic changes (i.e., when they are bound to receptors at synapses), CT1812 acts like a shield to protect synapses from toxic oligomer effects. As long as it remains above threshold concentrations (brain concentrations corresponding to 80% receptor occupancy, which is achieved with once-daily oral dosing), CT1812 prevents these displaced oligomers from rebinding

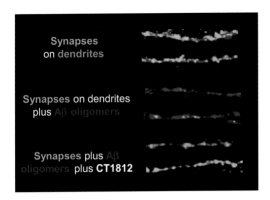

Figure 46.2 CT1812 displacement of synaptotoxic Aβ oligomers from their receptors restores synapse number to normal.

to their synaptic receptors. And because its brain concentrations are in vast excess compared to the concentration of oligomers in the brain, CT1812 will continue to shield synapses as concentrations of Aβ oligomers rise throughout the disease. Early clinical studies indicated that CT1812 is well tolerated at these doses [18, 24]. CT1812's mechanism of action is genetically validated: the Icelandic mutation (A673 T) confers a four-fold lower risk of AD on carriers, and oligomers formed from this mutation-containing protein bind with four-fold lower affinity to receptors than wild-type protein [25]. CT1812 is the only drug candidate that mimics the effect of this AD-protective mutation.

Initial clinical studies of CT1812 in AD patients provided preliminary evidence of target engagement, reduction of synaptic damage, and disease modification. When administered once daily for 28 days to mild-to-moderate AD patients, CT1812

significantly increases Aβ oligomers, reduces synaptic degeneration markers (synaptotagmin, neurogranin, and hyperphosphorylated tau at specific amino acid residues), and normalizes protein, lipid, and metabolite levels (that are dysregulated in AD patients compared to age-match normal controls) in patient CSF compared to placebo [18]. In AD, cognitive impairment correlates most closely with synapse number [26–29]. CT1812's synaptoprotective mechanism of action (Figure 46.3) has the potential to halt or slow cognitive decline with long-term administration, which will significantly alleviate the suffering of AD patients. This hypothesis is being tested in four ongoing Phase 2 clinical trials at sites in the United States, Australia, and the European Union, all supported by NIH grants.

One possible molecular basis for these observations is the direct role that sigma-2 receptor complex component proteins, namely progesterone receptor membrane component 1 (PGRMC1) [30–32] and transmembrane protein 97 (TMEM97) [33], have in both intracellular lipid vesicle trafficking, cholesterol synthesis, and autophagy. PGRMC1 contains several immunoreceptor tyrosine-based activation motif (ITAM) consensus sequences and binds directly to several vesicle-trafficking regulatory proteins including N-ethylmaleimide-sensitive factor (NSF), microtubule-associated proteins 1A/1B light chain 3B (MAP1LC3B), ultraviolet radiation resistance-associated gene (UVRAG), unc-51-like autophagy activating kinase 2 (ULK2), autophagy related 5 (Atg5), and RB1-inducible coiled-coil protein 1 (RB1CC1) [34, 35]. PGRMC1 regulates trafficking of a wide variety

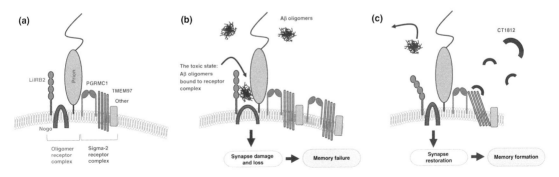

Figure 46.3 Hypothesized mechanism of CT1812 action. (a) The sigma-2 receptor complex includes the proteins PGRMC1 and TMEM97. The sigma-2 receptor complex binds directly to and tightly regulates the oligomer receptor complex which includes the proteins LilRB2, neurite outgrowth inhibitor (Nogo) receptor, and cellular prion protein. (b) In AD, Aβ builds up and forms oligomers. When oligomers bind to oligomer receptors, abnormal signaling leads to synapse damage and loss, and memory failure. The sigma-2 receptor complex upregulates to compensate, but cannot overcome the toxic signaling. (c) CT1812 binds to the sigma-2 receptor complex and changes its shape (allosteric antagonist), which in turn changes the oligomer receptor's shape. This destabilizes the oligomer binding site and displaces oligomers from synapses without affecting normal synapse protein function. Synapse number and memory are restored to normal levels.

of transmembrane receptors between subcellular compartments and the plasma membrane and is required to stabilize these receptors in the plasma membrane (including epidermal growth factor receptor [EGFR] [36], membrane progesterone receptor alpha [mPRα] [37], glucagon-like peptide receptor type 1 [GLP-1 R] [38], netrin receptor [UNC-40/deleted in colorectal cancer; UNC-40/DCC] [39], and insulin receptors [40]); reduction of PGRMC1 levels observed in human mutation carriers results in internalization of these receptors and elimination of PGRMC1's ability to bind cytochrome P450 family 7 subfamily A member 1 (CYP7A1) [41].

Direct binding of PGRMC1 to MAP1LC3B and UVRAG is required for normal autophagy [35]. Both lipid vesicle formation/trafficking and autophagy place large demands on cellular lipid membrane synthesis and degradation, and both PGRMC1 and TMEM97 directly regulate cholesterol synthesis. Most of TMEM97's sequence (aa 10–158) is an expanded emopamil binding protein superfamily (EXPERA) domain, likely to possess direct sterol isomerase catalytic activity [42]. Human mutations in EXPERA domain proteins lead to several disease syndromes, including those with a neurological phenotype [43]. TMEM97 itself binds directly to NPC1 (the protein that is mutated in the sphingolipid storage disorder Nieman–Pick's disease); reduction of TMEM97 upregulates NPC1 and restores cholesterol synthesis and trafficking in Nieman–Pick patients' cells [44]. PGRMC1 interacts with *Nr4a1* (an immediate early gene required for the induction of several genes encoding steroidogenic enzymes) to regulate neurosteroid synthesis or signaling in neuronal cell lines [45], a possible protective mechanism in response to neuroinflammatory signaling. In non-neuronal cells, PGRMC1 regulates cholesterol synthesis via two direct binding interactions; to cytochrome P450 proteins [46] and to insulin-induced gene protein (Insig) and sterol regulatory element binding protein (SREBP) cleavage-activating protein (SCAP) [47, 48]; under low cholesterol conditions, Insig/SCAP dissociates from PGRMC1 and translocates to the nucleus where they trigger sterol-regulatory-element-related gene transcription. Finally, both PGRMC1 and TMEM97 bind directly to the low-density lipoprotein (LDL) receptor; this complex binds LDL, apolipoprotein-E, and monomeric and oligomeric Aβ and contributes to their internalization into neurons, one potential

mechanism for oligomer clearance from the brain [30]. Sigma-2 receptor ligands block alpha-synuclein oligomer-induced impairment of autophagy in neurons, and so may be effective therapeutics in Parkinson's disease and the related alpha-synucleinopathies, multiple system atrophy, and dementia with Lewy bodies [49].

The linkage of this receptor's biology (which is still coming into focus) with AD was made possible by the discovery of CT1812. In order to learn more about this receptor's function, we brought together the scientific community of researchers who studied this receptor (many of whom had never met each other) for the first time in an annual meeting: International Symposium on Sigma-2 Receptors: Role in Health and Disease, now in its fifth year [50].

AD is a complex disease that we believe will ultimately be treated via polypharmacology – combinations of medications directed at different targets [51]. Many therapeutic strategies (such as anti-inflammatories and anti-tau agents) will undoubtedly provide relief to AD patients; however, these approaches will not be effective unless the negative effects of increasing concentrations of toxic Aβ oligomers that underlie disease progression are effectively addressed.

Together, these results provide encouraging evidence of the impact of CT1812 on multiple aspects of disease in AD patients and support further development of this drug candidate so that the relative benefit and risks of CT1812 can be more thoroughly evaluated. CT1812 is currently being studied in four randomized, double-blind, placebo-controlled Phase 2 studies (6 months to 1 year in treatment duration) in patients with mild-to-moderate AD: SNAP (NCT03522129), SPARC (NCT03493282), SHINE (NCT03507790), and SEQUEL. An additional 18-month study in 540 early-stage AD patients (Mini-Mental State Examination [MMSE] 20–30) is being planned in collaboration with the Alzheimer's Clinical Trial Consortium (ACTC) clinical trial network. The safety and tolerability of CT1812 will continue to be explored in all clinical trials.

CT1812 is still being evaluated in the clinic, and the risks versus the benefits are still coming into focus. The relative benefit of these effects to the risks of the drug have not been determined. Additional studies will be required to determine if there is a health benefit, and if this benefit outweighs the risks of the drug.

Acknowledgments

This chapter is dedicated to a long list of folks who made this achievement possible, and my deepest gratitude goes out to all of them: first and foremost, to my family for putting up with my absence all these years and supporting me through the many tough times. My co-founders Drs. Gilbert Rishton, Anthony Giordano, and Franz Hefti believed in the idea and launched us on our way. Our CEO Dr. Harold T. Safferstein shared the vision and the journey and was instrumental in growing the company from an idea through multiple Phase 2 trials. The founding scientists at CogRx did all the hard work to discover and develop CT1812 and its analogs, going "once more into the breach" again and again: Dr. Nicholas J. Izzo, Dr. Gary Look, Kelsie Mozzoni LaBarbera, Courtney Rehak, Raymond Yurko, Jessica Ravenscroft, Colleen Silky Limegrover, Nicole Knezovich, Lora Waybright, Emily Watto, Kelsey Sadlek, and Mikalya Wilson. They give me faith in humanity, and are all awesome, as were the interns we had early on: Elizabeth Brough, Zanobia Syed, John Hong, Thomas Walko III, Harrison Wostein, Megan Wardius, Brianna Layman, Colleen Bodnar, and Erika Pack. Our Scientific Advisory Board – Drs. Cindy Lemere, John Cirrito, Rob Malenka, Rolf Craven, Harry LeVine, Dominic Walsh, Michael Cahill, Tara Spires-Jones, and Bob Mach – provided wisdom and guidance and connection to a larger world of expertise for our studies. Our dedicated Medical Advisory Board Steering Committee – Drs. Lon Schneider, Steve DeKosky, and Michael Grundman – designed the trials with me and charted a rapid course to determine if our drug worked; Dr. Roger Morgan oversaw the safety of our trials, and Drs. Kaj Blennow, Henrik Zetterberg, Mary Sano, Larry Ereshevsky, Alison Goate, and Michael Woodward provided expert advice on trial conduct and endpoints measures. My colleagues within the AD basic research and therapeutics discovery and development field have supported our innovative new science and drug candidate through the publication and grant peer-review process, and I'm very grateful for their support. The founding Clinical Operations team at Cognition Celine Houser and Alyssa Galley did an amazing job of managing the complexity of multiple trials with graceful diplomacy, and we couldn't have done it without Michelle Higgin, Julie Pribyl, and Chris Viau of PharmaDirections. Cameron Hughes and the staff at Nucleus Networks did a great job with our first-in-human trials, as did Tina Soulis and the staff at Neuroscience Trials Australia with our first-in-patient trial. The people of Australia are very warm and welcoming, and I'd like to thank the patients and their caregivers there who participated in our early clinical trials. I'd like to thank the founding Board of Directors of Cognition Therapeutics, Inc., including Mr. Robert Gailus of Ogden CAP, Dr. Franz Hefti, Dr. Irwin Sher, Dr. Aaron Fletcher of BIOS Partners, Dr. Nada Jain and Ms. Peggy Wallace of Golden Seeds, and Mr. Mark Breedlove, who believed in that vision and whose vote of confidence was summarized by something Franz Hefti once said to me in a board meeting "You've delivered everything you said you would deliver, and that's rare." We could not have done this without the support of Cognition's investors: John Manzetti at the Pittsburgh Life Sciences Greenhouse PLSG and Accelerator Fund, Rich Lunak and Larry Miller at Innovation Works, Jo Ann Corkran and Loretta McCarthy and the investors at Golden Seeds, Cowtown Angels, BIOS Partners, Ariel Savannah Angel Partners, Bangor Angels, Bluetree Allied Angels, Sofia Angels, Central Texas Angel Network, Houston Angel Network, Maine Angels, Scale Investors, Tech Coast Angels, and individual angel investors, who wanted a therapeutic that could stop AD, and supported us despite the odds. I'm very proud to say that I think there is a good chance that that is exactly what we've delivered. The National Institute on Aging program officers Neil Buckholtz, Laurie Ryan, Suzana Petanceska, and Larry Refolo were very supportive; we could not have discovered CT1812 and conducted its clinical development without the support of our peers and National Institutes of Health (NIH). We also received support from the National Institute of Neurological Diseases and Stroke, the Michael J. Fox Foundation, and the Alzheimer's Drug Discovery Foundation (ADDF). Howard Fillit at the ADDF has always been very supportive. The NIH infrastructure is supported by congress and the US taxpayers; I am very fortunate to be able to work in a democracy that values research and supports therapeutic discovery and development. I ask forgiveness from the other folks who were so generous with their time and resources, whose names are too numerous to mention. Finally, to the patients and their caregivers and family members all over the world who volunteered for our trials; you never left our thoughts for a minute, and you should rest assured we did everything humanly possible to get this therapy to you as fast as our resources allowed.

References

1. Patterson C. World Alzheimer Report 2018. The state of the art of dementia research: new frontiers. Available at: www.alz.co.uk/research/WorldAlzheimerReport2018.pdf (accessed January 29, 2021).

2. Heron M. Deaths: leading causes for 2016. Available at: www.cdc.gov/nchs/data/nvsr/nvsr67/nvsr67_06.pdf (accessed January 29, 2021).

3. Grabrucker A, Vaida B, Bockmann J, Boeckers TM. Synaptogenesis of hippocampal neurons in primary cell culture. *Cell Tissue Res* 2009; **338**: 333–41.

4. Ramakers GJA, Kloosterman F, van Hulten P, van Pelt J, Corner MA. Activity-dependent regulation of neuronal network excitability. In *Neural Circuits and Networks*, Torre V, Nicholls J (eds.). Berlin: Springer; 1998: 141–51.

5. Banker G, Goslin K. Types of nerve cell cultures, their advantages, and limitations. In *Culturing Nerve Cells*, Banker G, Goslin K (eds.). Cambridge, MA: MIT Press; 1998: 11–36.

6. Opitz T, De Lima AD, Voigt T. Spontaneous development of synchronous oscillatory activity during maturation of cortical networks in vitro. *J Neurophysiol* 2002; **88**: 2196–206.

7. Torre V, Nicholls J (eds.). *Neural Circuits and Networks*. Heidelberg: Springer; 1998.

8. LaBarbera KM, Limegrover CM, Rehak C, et al. Modeling the mature CNS: a predictive screening platform for neurodegenerative disease drug discovery. *J Neurosci Methods* 2021; **358**: 109180.

9. Kamenetz F, Tomita T, Hsieh H, et al. APP processing and synaptic function. *Neuron* 2003; **37**: 925–37.

10. Lacor PN, Buniel MC, Chang L, et al. Synaptic targeting by Alzheimer's-related amyloid β oligomers. *J Neurosci* 2004; **24**: 10191–200.

11. Reed MN, Hofmeister JJ, Jungbauer L, et al. Cognitive effects of cell-derived and synthetically derived Aβ oligomers. *Neurobiol Aging* 2011; **32**: 1784–94.

12. Hsieh H, Boehm J, Sato C, et al. AMPAR removal underlies Abeta-induced synaptic depression and dendritic spine loss. *Neuron* 2006; **52**: 831–43.

13. Hong H-S, Maezawa I, Yao N, et al. Combining the rapid MTT formazan exocytosis assay and the MC65 protection assay led to the discovery of carbazole analogs as small molecule inhibitors of Abeta oligomer-induced cytotoxicity. *Brain Res* 2007; **1130**: 223–34.

14. Kreutzmann P, Wolf G, Kupsch K. Minocycline recovers MTT-formazan exocytosis impaired by amyloid beta peptide. *Cell Mol Neurobiol* 2010; **30**: 979–84.

15. Liu Y, Schubert D. Cytotoxic amyloid peptides inhibit cellular 3-(4,5-dimethylthiazol-2-yl)-2,5-diphenyltetrazolium bromide (MTT) reduction by enhancing MTT formazan exocytosis. *J Neurochem* 1997; **69**: 2285–93.

16. Izzo NJ, Staniszewski A, To L, et al. Alzheimer's therapeutics targeting amyloid beta 1–42 oligomers I: Abeta 42 oligomer binding to specific neuronal receptors is displaced by drug candidates that improve cognitive deficits. *PLoS One* 2014; **9**: e111898.

17. Izzo NNJ, Xu J, Zeng C, et al. Alzheimer's therapeutics targeting amyloid beta 1–42 oligomers II: sigma-2/PGRMC1 receptors mediate Abeta 42 oligomer binding and synaptotoxicity. *PLoS One* 2014; **9**: e111899.

18. Izzo NJ, Yuede CM, LaBarbera KM, et al. Preclinical and clinical biomarker studies of CT1812: a novel approach to Alzheimer's disease modification. *Alzheimers Dement* 2021;DOI: https://doi.org/10.1002/alz.12302.

19. Rishton GM, Look G, Ni Z-J, et al. Negative allosteric modulators of the sigma-2 receptor: discovery of investigational drug CT1812 for Alzheimer's Disease. *ACS Med Chem Lett*; DOI: https://doi.org/10.1021/acsmedchemlett.1c00048.

20. Rishton GM. Reactive compounds and in vitro false positives in HTS. *Drug Discov Today* 1997; **2**: 382–4.

21. Rishton GM. Nonleadlikeness and leadlikeness in biochemical screening. *Drug Discov Today* 2003; **8**: 86–96.

22. Rishton GM. Aggregator compounds confound amyloid fibrillization assay. *Nat Chem Biol* 2008; **4**: 159–60.

23. Arai H, Beierle K, Fullenwider C, Kaj Z. Chemically conditioned extracts of ginger oil: leadlike "alkaloidal" compounds derived from natural extracts via reductive amination. American Chemical Society Western Regional Meeting, Anaheim, CA, Jan 22, 2006. Available at: http://acs.confex.com/acs/werm05/techprogram/S2455.HTM.

24. Grundman M, Morgan R, Lickliter JD, et al. A Phase 1 clinical trial of the sigma-2 receptor complex allosteric antagonist CT1812, a novel therapeutic candidate for Alzheimer's disease. *Alzheimers Dement (N Y)* 2019; **5**: 20–6.

25. Limegrover CS, LeVine H, Izzo NJ, et al. Alzheimer's protection effect of A673 T mutation may be driven by lower Aβ oligomer binding affinity. *J Neurochem* 2021; **157**: 1316–30.

26. Masliah E, Terry RD, Alford M, DeTeresa R, Hansen L. Cortical and subcortical patterns

of synaptophysinlike immunoreactivity in Alzheimer's disease. *Am J Pathol* 1991; **138**: 235–46.

27. DeKosky ST, Scheff SW. Synapse loss in frontal cortex biopsies in Alzheimer's disease: correlation with cognitive severity. *Ann Neurol* 1990; **27**: 457–64.

28. Scheff SW, Price DA. Synaptic pathology in Alzheimer's disease: a review of ultrastructural studies. *Neurobiol Aging* 2003; **24**: 1029–46.

29. Colom-Cadena M, Spires-Jones T, Zetterberg H, et al. The clinical promise of biomarkers of synapse damage or loss in Alzheimer's disease. *Alzheimers Res Ther* 2020; **12**: 21.

30. Riad A, Zeng C, Weng C-CC, et al. Sigma-2 receptor/TMEM97 and PGRMC-1 increase the rate of internalization of LDL by LDL receptor through the formation of a ternary complex. *Sci Rep* 2018; **8**: 16845.

31. Riad A, Lengyel-Zhand Z, Zeng C, et al. The sigma-2 receptor/TMEM97, PGRMC1, and LDL receptor complex are responsible for the cellular uptake of $A\beta_{42}$ and its protein aggregates. *Mol Neurobiol* 2020; **57**: 3803–13.

32. Xu J, Zeng C, Chu W, et al. Identification of the PGRMC1 protein complex as the putative sigma-2 receptor binding site. *Nat Commun* 2011; **2**: 380.

33. Alon A, Schmidt HR, Wood MD, et al. Identification of the gene that codes for the σ 2 receptor. *Proc Natl Acad Sci USA* 2017; **114**: 7160–5.

34. Behrends C, Sowa ME, Gygi SP, Harper JW. Network organization of the human autophagy system. *Nature* 2010; **466**: 68–76.

35. Mir SU, Schwarze SR, Jin L, et al. Progesterone receptor membrane component 1/sigma-2 receptor associates with MAP1LC3B and promotes autophagy. *Autophagy* 2013; **9**: 1566–78.

36. Ahmed IS, Rohe HJ, Twist KE, Craven RJ. PGRMC1 (progesterone receptor membrane component 1) associates with epidermal growth factor receptor and regulates erlotinib sensitivity. *J Biol Chem* 2010; **285**: 24775–82.

37. Thomas P, Pang Y, Dong J. Enhancement of cell surface expression and receptor functions of membrane progestin receptor α (mPRα) by progesterone receptor membrane component 1 (PGRMC1): evidence for a role of PGRMC1 as an adaptor protein for steroid receptors. *Endocrinology* 2014; **155**: 1107–19.

38. Zhang M, Robitaille M, Showalter AD, et al. Progesterone receptor membrane component 1 is a functional part of the GLP-1 receptor complex in pancreatic beta cells. *Mol Cell Proteomics* 2014; **1**: 3049–62.

39. Runko E, Kaprielian Z. *Caenorhabditis elegans* VEM-1, a novel membrane protein, regulates the guidance of ventral nerve cord-associated axons. *J Neurosci* 2004; **24**: 9015–26.

40. Hampton KK, Anderson K, Frazier H, Thibault O, Craven RJ. Insulin receptor plasma membrane levels increased by the progesterone receptor membrane component 1. *Mol Pharmacol* 2018; **94**: 665–73.

41. Mansouri MR, Schuster J, Badhai J, et al. Alterations in the expression, structure and function of progesterone receptor membrane component-1 (PGRMC1) in premature ovarian failure. *Hum Mol Genet* 2008; **17**: 3776–83.

42. Sanchez-Pulido L, Ponting CP. TM6SF2 and MAC30, new enzyme homologs in sterol metabolism and common metabolic disease. *Front Genet* 2014; **5**: 1–9.

43. Online Mendelian Inheritance in Man, OMIM®. Johns Hopkins University, Baltimore, MD. MIM Number: 300205:11/20/2019. Available at: https://omim.org/.

44. Ebrahimi-Fakhari D, Wahlster L, Bartz F, et al. Reduction of TMEM97 increases NPC1 protein levels and restores cholesterol trafficking in Niemann–Pick type C1 disease cells. *Hum Mol Genet* 2015; **25**: 3588–99.

45. Intlekofer KA, Clements K, Woods H, et al. Progesterone receptor membrane component 1 inhibits tumor necrosis factor alpha induction of gene expression in neural cells. *PLoS One* 2019; **14**: e0215389.

46. Rohe HJ, Ahmed IS, Twist KE, Craven RJ. PGRMC1 (progesterone receptor membrane component 1): a targetable protein with multiple functions in steroid signaling, P450 activation and drug binding. *Pharmacol Ther* 2009; **121**: 14–19.

47. Suchanek M, Radzikowska A, Thiele C. Photoleucine and photo-methionine allow identification of protein–protein interactions in living cells. *Nat Methods* 2005; **2**: 261–7.

48. Hughes AL, Powell DW, Bard M, et al. Dap1/PGRMC1 binds and regulates cytochrome P450 enzymes. *Cell Metab* 2007; **5**: 143–9.

49. Limegrover CS, Yurko R, Izzo NJ, et al. Sigma-2 receptor antagonists rescue neuronal dysfunction induced by Parkinson's patient brain-derived α-synuclein. *J Neurosci Res* 2021; **99**: 1161–76.

50. Izzo NJ, Colom-Cadena M, Riad AA, et al. Proceedings from the Fourth International Symposium on Sigma-2 Receptors: Role in Health and Disease. *eNeuro* 2020; **7**: 1–7. Available at: http://eneuro.org/lookup/doi/10.1523/ENEURO.0317-20.2020.

51. Frautschy SA, Cole GM. Why pleiotropic interventions are needed for Alzheimer's disease. *Mol Neurobiol* 2010; **41**: 392–409.

Introduction to Venture Capital in Alzheimer's Disease Drug Development

Laurence Barker, Jonathan Behr, and Christian Jung

47.1 Introduction

Venture capital plays a pivotal role in providing funding for emerging technologies. This is as important for biotechnology as it is for developing software and social media platforms. Often research scientists discover potential disease treatments then struggle to find the support to transform these ideas into an approved medicine. This requires partners not only able to provide the necessary capital but also the commercial and industry expertise.

Providing this form of private equity is a vital first step in developing treatments for diseases like Alzheimer's disease (AD). Without this source of capital many of these ideas would languish in the laboratory as larger biotechnology and pharmaceutical firms are often unwilling to take on the risk of such early-stage projects. But once proof of concept has been demonstrated and initial clinical trials have been undertaken, it is often these larger companies that will purchase smaller biotechnology firms from their venture capital funders. Venture capital often provides the vital bridge between a laboratory experiment and a promising therapeutic.

Venture capitalists frequently deploy capital where others fear to tread and, like every other investor, they need to make a profit. Without the potential for a return, no investor will ever assign capital to a potential therapeutic.

The medical need for therapies to treat AD is undeniable. Current drugs provide some symptomatic relief at best. Despite the approval of aducanumab (Aduhelm™) for AD, which was only approved in 2021, no drug has been definitively shown to modify the course of AD. In other words, there is tremendous profit potential for an effective therapy. Yet despite this commercial advantage, few venture capital firms had previously invested in this disease area. That's because AD has proved a particularly difficult disease to treat.

The primary challenge has been a lack of understanding about both the underlying biology and pathology of AD. This lack of knowledge led the industry to focus on only one or two targets – namely amyloid beta and tau – rather than exploring other potential mechanisms. In addition, it has been tricky to identify the right patients for specific drugs due to the heterogeneity of the disease. Clinical trials are also difficult to undertake because they need to be large and long lasting, which makes them expensive to conduct.

These factors have all contributed to a high failure rate for potential treatments. During a period of 10 years, 413 AD trials were performed with an overall success rate of just 0.4% [1]. As a result, several pharmaceutical companies decided to no longer progress research and development (R&D) in this field. In the face of so many challenges, it might seem just too risky an area even for a venture capitalist. But there are ways to improve the odds of succeeding in this difficult disease area. Of note, the timing and manner of approval of aducanumab has reenergized interest in the space.

47.2 The Dementia Discovery Fund

47.2.1 A New Way to Fund Neurodegenerative Therapies

The Dementia Discovery Fund (DDF) was established to bridge a gap in funding early-stage AD drug discovery and was designed to help to improve the odds of success. David Cameron, then Prime Minster of the UK, played a pivotal role in the DDF's formation. He recognized funding was insufficient to help innovative ideas for treating AD to become marketable products. As the UK was hosting the G8 council meeting in 2013, he made dementia its focus.

In 2014, the UK government's Department of Health and Social Care was asked to devise a framework to tackle this condition more effectively. The result was a partnership between this department, some of the world's largest pharmaceutical companies, and the charity Alzheimer's Research UK. The mission of the DDF was then formed with initial investors; it needed leadership and management, so a bidding process ensued. SV Health Investors, championed by Kate Bingham, won the bid to become the fund manager in a competitive selection process held in 2015. This life-sciences venture capital firm has over 25 years of experience and has invested in more than 200 companies, helping bring many important new medicines to patients (see Figure 47.1).

The original investors – biotechnology and pharmaceutical companies, government agencies, and charities – were then joined by venture philanthropists, advocacy groups, and health investors in creating a £250 million fund, with a mandate to invest in novel dementia therapeutics.

The DDF represents the first time charities, government, and pharmaceutical companies, together with public and private investors, have had this level of collaboration with venture capitalists. If successful, the DDF will have a positive global impact for society and individuals while generating long-term returns for investors.

47.2.2 Improving the Odds

Establishing the DDF was a good first step toward the goal of developing viable treatments for AD and the fund needed to maximize approaches that were able to improve the odds of its success in a challenging area. The DDF is unique. Most venture capital healthcare funds do not have such a focus on a particular disease area. The DDF has deepened its knowledge by building a team with in-depth expertise of neuroscience drug discovery and development in this area. This expertise complements other team members' venture investment experience.

In addition, the DDF has established an influential and knowledgeable scientific advisory board, which has representatives from seven pharmaceutical companies. These individuals provide advice and guidance about how to discover and develop drugs for dementia. They also point out the obvious pitfalls to avoid. Often, this advice represents not only the individuals' expertise but also that of others in the organization. If one of the DDF's investments shows promise, they may well inform their business development groups. There is, however, no compunction to do deals with these firms.

From its inception, the DDF, with advice from its scientific advisory board, moved away from the industry's tendency to repeatedly double down on only a few potential pathways and instead looked at a broad range of mechanisms which potentially contribute to the development of AD. To this end, the DDF identified four areas of focus – neuroinflammation, mitochondrial dynamics, synaptic physiology and function, and trafficking and membrane biology. These areas have evolved as the DDF learns from its investments, its network, and new scientific research findings.

While the investors drive the decision-making process, access to deep scientific expertise makes the DDF able to make better investments and to continue to support companies actively. This combination improves the odds of success. By

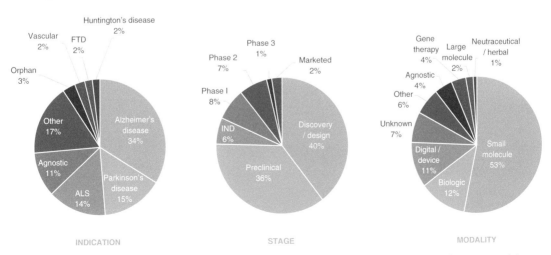

INDICATION   STAGE   MODALITY

Figure 47.1 DDF deal flow in 2019: a rich pipeline of opportunities. ALS, amyotrophic lateral sclerosis; FTD, frontotemporal dementia; IND, investigational new drug.

combining a focus on dementia with the rigor of for-profit venture capital investing, the DDF has been able to build the expertise required to make sound investment decisions in dementia disease. This includes an evolving understanding of the biology of AD, identifying the right biomarkers, designing effective clinical trials, creating connections with leaders in their scientific field, and the ability to implement the most productive management team.

The DDF is a science-first fund which takes a proactive approach to investing. It investigates areas where the science is mature enough to support drug discovery and – with suitably informed and structured investment – has the potential to generate new therapies.

47.2.3 Investment Process

For the DDF, a therapeutic investment opportunity must be based on credible, innovative science in the dementia space, with the potential to be translated into life-changing therapeutics for patients. The DDF has established itself in the dementia disease ecosystem over the 6 years since its inception. Strong relationships with researchers and clinicians specializing in this field as well as close ties to institutional investors and partnership with pharmaceutical companies give it a proprietary pipeline of greater than 300 investment opportunities a year (see Figure 47.2).

47.2.3.1 Selecting Investment Candidates

The DDF allocates capital to a range of propositions. While not funding academic research, it will invest in early-stage opportunities, which may subsequently grow into larger companies with more funding as they achieve key development milestones. The DDF can also use its expertise to guide these early-stage companies through milestones if helpful. It can also allocate capital to later-stage

companies, further along the R&D path, which also benefit both from the DDF's capital and expertise.

For the DDF to decide to invest in a particular project or company, it must meet certain criteria. The first criteria being whether an investment will fit the DDF's strategy. Does the project or company have the potential to deliver a drug which would transform a dementia indication?

The DDF also assesses the strength of the project's science. In particular, it looks for strong evidence to support the pathway or mechanism's role in disease. That may include human genetic and molecular evidence, in vitro studies, and cellular or animal models. Given the poor predictive nature of preclinical models to date, the DDF assigns a greater weight to human data [2, 3]. There is a balance to be struck between innovation and requiring evidence up front to support the hypothesis that a given approach will work. If a project is a good strategic fit and the science is interesting and compelling but not definitive, then the DDF will, if needed, make an initial investment to test a hypothesis or to confirm a particular result.

There is a second tier of criteria which are required for any successful venture. These criteria include aspects such as the team, the market opportunity, the competitive landscape, and intellectual property. For example, a company requires a strong team in order to succeed. This will require the combination of both scientific and managerial expertise. Where this is lacking, the venture investors can build the team needed for success.

A potential product also needs a market opportunity of sufficient size to enable the DDF to more than earn back the initial investments. The DDF will also scope out the market opportunity for a particular technology, as well as the competitive landscape, to ensure the potential therapeutic could be the first or best in class. There also needs to be the potential to secure intellectual property

Figure 47.2 DDF limited partners (not exhaustive).

such as patents to protect the proprietary product when it gets to market.

A strong development plan is another critical component for a DDF investment. For an investment to progress beyond the initial payment, the DDF needs clear milestones to determine whether or not it should continue to invest. There is intense collaboration between the DDF and its potential investments to map out a clear plan.

The DDF will use its expertise and knowledge to build an overall investment thesis for a company that relies on all of these criteria. Sometimes, however, there are investments of special interest which may not yet meet these criteria. The DDF can then use its own financing and scientific expertise to supplement any missing business strengths. When considering whether or not to invest, the DDF is not just thinking about its own requirements but also those of other future co-investors. The DDF syndicates to provide a company with sufficient funding to take a product through to clinical proof of principle, which is an established hand-off point to pharmaceutical partners. Occasionally, the DDF makes small investments in technologies which will make a major improvement in the ability of many companies to develop drugs to treat AD. Past investments include a compound library and a technology to increase the transmission of a drug across the blood–brain barrier.

47.2.4 How Does the DDF Structure Its Investments?

A venture capital fund structures its investments to ensure its capital is used to most effectively advance a company through milestones which build shareholder value and eventual returns. In the case of the DDF, these returns are derived from the successful development of dementia therapeutics.

Investments need to match the closed-end structure of the DDF, which has a finite amount of capital, and therefore individual investments cannot require too significant a proportion of the capital. Their life cycles also need to complement that of the venture capital fund (meaning the company needs to return capital to investors within the fund lifetime). To reflect the early nature of many of the DDF's investments, the fund has been structured to last 15 years, rather than the typical decade of most venture funds, to help enable the DDF to support its investments through to key value inflection points.

As outlined previously, the DDF has a number of criteria it uses to determine whether a company represents a good investment opportunity. If an opportunity is a good match, the DDF will then look at how best to structure this investment.

47.2.4.1 Creating Companies

As the development of dementia drugs is still challenging, there are a limited number of investable companies. The DDF uses its team of scientific experts to evaluate companies needing investment and also scientific discoveries which are not currently being developed by companies. If there is a promising technology – which matches the DDF's criteria but has no corporate structure – the DDF will use its venture partners and wider network to develop this into a company. In these scenarios, the DDF helps shape and form these companies by building the executive team. The venture partners often act as interim chief executive or chief scientific officers. These executives will help build the initial team, pull the company's proposition together, and will often lead the company through the first few financing rounds.

The DDF will work in close collaboration with academic founders whose role is often differentiated from that of the venture capitalists and management. The founders will often become scientific advisers to the company and its internal team and receive equity as a company founder. In contrast to work carried out by the academic founders, the venture capitalists will determine the amount of investment needed to drive the company to its first proof of concept. They will look for other investors to build a syndicate to fund this first phase.

47.2.4.2 Investing in More Mature Companies

Not every investment made by the DDF involves building a company from the foundations up. Sometimes these first steps have already been taken by the founder, an independent entrepreneur, or another investor, such as another venture capital firm.

The DDF will evaluate the company to decide whether it wants to become the lead investor. The role of the lead investor is to structure a financing round and propose the investment terms, which requires valuing the company. The DDF will also help recruit other investors; a process known as syndication. This is necessary to find sufficient capital for both the immediate and future financing rounds. The DDF will also join syndicates formed by other lead investors.

The lead investor is responsible for the majority of the due diligence – whether it is scientific, commercial, or corporate. Even when the DDF is not the lead investor, however, it will still conduct its own independent due diligence on, at a minimum, the scientific aspects of the investment. Whether the DDF is leading the syndicate or only a member, it is still an active investor, meaning it will play a role in governance and oversight of the investment, and support the company's team in key decision making, to ensure the highest likelihood of success. Venture capital firms help to shape the company by providing input on strategy, development plans, proposed hires, and the structure of the investment round.

The structure of investments made by venture capital firms will usually provide particular rights and controls. A diligent fund will use these rights in combination with their expertise to increase the likelihood of the company's success.

47.3 Financing Structures Used in Venture Capital Investments

47.3.1 Common and Preferred Equity

When a private company is created, the equity it issues is common stock. When additional investment is added – whether from the original investor or another venture capital fund – preferred equity is used.

These two forms of equity have different purposes. The common equity, often referred to as "sweat equity," most often goes to founders and represents the work done in creating a company. In contrast, preferred equity is created when the company is growing its capital base. It has additional rights over the common stock, which usually include economic rights, such as the ability to earn dividends and liquidation preferences, and can include anti-dilution rights. These protect the value of an investor's holdings through the issuance of additional shares if a future investment comes in at a lower price. Preferred equity also has non-economic rights such as voting rights and protective provisions. These non-economic rights can vary but usually include approval or veto rights over certain corporate decisions, as well as a preemptive right which guarantees the ability to make future investments, and the right for certain shareholders or classes of shareholders to appoint board members.

Importantly, there are often votes that require a certain threshold of the preferred shares to pass. For example, the triggering of subsequent investment tranches needs to pass a certain threshold of preferred shares. This prevents the common shareholders from forcing the preferred holders to stump up additional capital.

This level of control is a way venture capital firms ensure that companies consider and apply the guidance of their investors and one reason why the selection of its investors is an important decision for a company.

47.3.2 Convertible Debt

Venture capital companies will sometimes choose to make their investments using a special type of mid-term debt, which can later be converted into equity. There are non-debt instruments that serve the same purpose, such as Simple Agreements for Future Equity (known as "SAFEs"). Convertible debt is often used when the value of a company cannot be agreed either because the company is at a very early stage or because it is facing short-term challenges.

This instrument can be converted into equity once a particular trigger has been reached. Its activation tends to be when a subsequent financing round of a particular size has been completed and/or when the debt term is reached. It is important that this subsequent financing has been led by another investor, to provide an independent valuation. The debt is also often structured so, when converted into shares, these are priced at a discount to the value of the company. This discount – plus interest – compensates the venture firm for investing at a time of greater risk.

47.3.3 Milestones

Venture capitalists often release a total investment in a series of tranches. Financing is structured this way to protect investors from sinking too much capital into a company before knowing whether it is making progress toward its long-term goals. Milestones – which are an objective measure of a development that creates value for the company – are trigger points to release additional tranches of capital. For instance, for early drug discovery, developing a molecule with a particular chemical profile that demonstrates activity in initial in vitro laboratory assays relevant to AD treatment could be a good point at which to release additional funding. Drug-development milestones could also include the achievement of certain data sets. For example, demonstrating that a drug candidate has a particular type of effect in an animal model. And for an advanced project, the acceptance of a drug application by a regulator to start clinical studies would be an important breakthrough followed by clinical development.

Milestones will happen more frequently for early-stage projects, making it easy to turn off the capital as soon as one is missed. This enables a venture capital firm to invest in riskier projects without overcommitting to an unsuccessful investment. However, once the drug makes it to clinical trials, the financing rounds become larger and the time between milestones becomes much longer.

47.3.3.1 Using Milestones to Realize Profits

As outlined, the purpose of venture capital financing is to bridge the gap between early-stage innovation and creating a high-value drug candidate which is of interest to investors other than venture capital firms. This could be large pharmaceutical companies or public markets.

When others are willing to buy, this allows venture capital funds to exit their investments and realize their returns. Typical exits include the sale of the company, licensing or partnering of a particular compound, or the flotation of a company on a stock exchange. The triggers for these exits are usually milestones in drug development such as a compound entering a clinical trial or some demonstration of benefit to a patient in early-stage clinical studies.

Venture capital investors hope to realize value before incurring the expense of long clinical studies necessary to show the impact of a drug candidate on disease. But given the high risk of dementia research, it is challenging to convince other investors there is sufficient risk-adjusted value in these projects without carrying out human drug trials.

47.4 Case Studies

The following case studies illustrate how the DDF uses its investment process in real life, including how it builds companies and works with others to raise financing.

47.4.1 Therini Bio

Therini Bio is a company created out of academia due to the actions of venture capitalists. Professor Katerina Akassoglou, Professor of Neurology at the University of California San Francisco, discovered that fibrin, a blood-clotting factor, is implicated in the toxic inflammation which damages neurons in neurological diseases including AD. Professor Akassoglou discovered molecules which reduce this inflammation and the subsequent damage to neurons.

The DDF led a seed-round $9.5 million financing with Dolby Family Ventures, an AD-focused family office, and the Alzheimer's Drug Discovery Foundation (ADDF) to develop these molecules into therapeutics that target fibrin. The initial focus of the company will be on AD and multiple sclerosis.

A key component of the company creation is to bring in management. In this case, one of the DDF's venture partners joined as the chief executive officer to structure the development and seed-financing plan, recruit a small team, and get the company up and running. This included the transition of key R&D work from the academic laboratory to the company. The DDF has board representation and is the principal driver behind the company at this early stage. It has subsequently built a broader syndicate through an additional financing round to advance the fibrin-targeted therapies.

47.4.2 Cerevance

Cerevance was built around a technology with the potential to develop treatments for multiple diseases. The DDF chose to invest because it wanted to apply this platform to dementia, including AD. The DDF co-led Cerevance's initial $29 million financing round alongside Lightstone Ventures, to harness a technology platform, invented in the Howard Hughes Medical Institute laboratory of Nathaniel Heintz, PhD, at Rockefeller University. Rather than relying on animal models to reveal critical pathways and receptors present in vulnerable cell populations as well as their molecular responses, the technology enables the molecular analysis of specific cell types in human brain tissue. The DDF played an active role on the board and as neurodegenerative science advisory to the company to drive a focus and utilization of the platform for dementia. Alongside the platform technology, the company licensed in some more advanced central nervous system (CNS) programs, which enabled Cerevance to hit significant milestones sooner and increased the value of the company. This helps to balance the inherent risk associated with the early stage of the platform-derived programs and for future financing to take place at a more attractive valuation.

In 2020, Cerevance closed an oversubscribed $65 million Series B financing round to advance several therapies into clinical development, including those for AD.

47.5   The Role of DDF in Drug Development

When the DDF was started in 2015, there was an investment gap for early-stage companies developing therapeutics for dementia, including AD. Many pharmaceutical companies had deemed the disease too high risk and did not fund therapeutic development. As previously explained, the purpose of the DDF was to bridge this gap and to help innovations receive the level of funding needed.

Numerous organizations have recognized the need for high-quality dementia research and supported development through large research grants. These studies have improved the understanding of dementia and the progress toward tackling AD. While grants deepen scientific understanding, they do not provide the risk capital needed to translate this knowledge into a drug. Turning a laboratory innovation into a drug-development candidate can cost at least 10 times as much as a typical National Institutes of Health (NIH) grant. Although there is an increase in grants to demonstrate preclinical activity of drug candidates, formal development is beyond the mandate of grant-funding bodies.

Life-science venture capital bridges this translation gap and is designed to provide funding to high-risk early-stage investments. By using milestones and finance tranches, just enough can be invested to get a company to the next development stage. This process also limits loss when investments fail – which is to be expected with venture capital.

This is "hands-on" investing: venture capital firms can provide the necessary skills and executives to help build a company which would be attractive to other investors – particularly those which do not specialize in AD.

The DDF investments have created a pipeline of companies and programs with which biotechnology and pharmaceutical companies can partner or could be taken onto an initial public offering. Not only does this pipeline offer the possibility of new drugs but it will hopefully catalyze additional industry interest in AD. Now the science is better understood and programs are more advanced, there is a greater chance of investment success.

47.5.1   Evolution

Neurodegenerative research has evolved since 2015, with the launch of the DDF leading the vanguard of initiatives. More non-profit initiatives and investors are now active in this area of research and development. This has improved the pipeline of available investments as well as providing more venture capital available for syndication (see Figure 47.3).

While the amount of capital invested over the last two decades in researching dementia is much less than in more established fields such as oncology and inflammation, this has had an indirect benefit for neurodegenerative disease researchers. As the capital invested in neurodegenerative disease increases, advances in other areas can be applied to this field, which should accelerate drug development there accordingly.

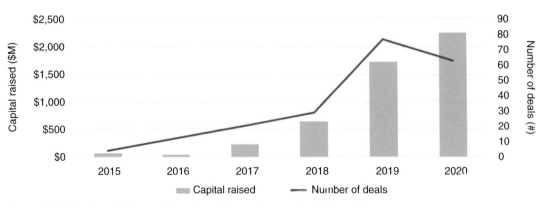

Figure 47.3 Early-stage venture capital investment in neurodegenerative therapeutics.

47.5.2   Reducing Development Risk

As more capital has been attracted to neurodegenerative disease, it is easier to form syndicates with other investors at earlier stages of a company's life cycle and its drug-development program. Forming syndicates has a direct benefit to the companies as it allows venture capital firms to build stronger financing strategies earlier in the life span of a company, which will give the drug-development program a greater chance of success. Not only does the company get better access to capital but also to greater expertise.

Early syndication helps an investor better mitigate its risks. Working with co-investors reduces the amount of time one fund acts as a solo investor, which is a high-risk strategy. For a company looking for investment, receiving funding becomes more likely when the burden of risk can be shared. Sharing the investment burden with others allows a fund to also retain more of its finite capital so it can continue to participate through to a particular company's later financing rounds. This ensures funding can be continued throughout the drug-development process as well as allowing the venture capital funds to contribute their expertise to later-stage companies. Both of these increase the company's likelihood of success.

As modeling suggests that it will take an estimated $38.4 billion over a decade to deliver a robust pipeline of AD therapeutics, attracting capital through syndication gives the DDF the greatest chance of providing the seed financing to build that development pipeline [4]. But while venture capitalists like to use this mechanism to minimize the risk of capital investment, there is an active debate about whether this is the right way forward.

47.6   Changes in Disease Treatment

Traditional treatment of a large number of diseases has relied on small-molecule drugs. While this is no longer the case in other areas of disease, it has taken longer for newer approaches to transfer across to the treatment of neurodegenerative disease. But there are other methods of disease treatment being developed such as monoclonal antibodies, nucleic acid-based therapies, and antisense oligonucleotides, as well as the use of gene therapies. These therapies are matched to the targeted pathology to modulate, which helps researchers more effectively target a particular mechanism or pathway affecting disease.

The risk profile of these drugs is very different to those of small molecules, and for some applications they can reduce the overall risk, time, and cost of getting a medicine into a patient and having an effect. Both this risk profile and the particular pathology being targeted are considerations which will motivate the choice of particular approach to disease treatment.

Companies are now developing new therapeutics which could be used across a range of different diseases. For example, one of DDF's investments is developing small molecules which can be used to interact with certain RNA structures. This technology can be applied to a number of different diseases from CNS to oncology, which attracts a broader range of investors who might have greater interest in diseases other than AD.

47.6.1   Precision Medicine

We are seeing a shift toward a precision approach to treating disease, including AD. This stratifies patients into specific subgroups based on various factors, including genetics and specific pathophysiologies. This reflects the recognition that disease symptoms may be caused by different mechanisms depending on these different features and should therefore be treated differently.

Precision medicine can reduce risk by using certain drug-development paths. Venture capitalists like to use indications that necessitate shorter clinical trials and have clearer endpoints to test the mechanism of a drug. This allows investors to determine more quickly whether this is a mechanism which will impact disease in the clinic. This will reduce the risk of taking the drug into an AD trial where it is much harder and more costly to ascertain efficacy.

The mechanism tested must, however, be one which can have a direct read-across to AD or another form of dementia. For example, there is tau pathology in both progressive supranuclear palsy and AD, or synuclein pathology in both Parkinson's disease and dementia with Lewy bodies. Many of the companies that DDF has invested in are using this approach – testing the mechanism of their compound in another indication, such as another neurodegenerative disease, and, when they have greater confidence, trying it in AD.

As the understanding of the disease increases and researchers separate out the different strands of AD into different pathologies, treatment will become more bespoke. This will make it easier to develop therapies to treat AD as there will be greater insights of which biomarkers are affected, allowing companies to develop more detailed plans for clinical trials and improve the chances of clinical success.

47.7   Conclusion

The purpose of the DDF was to provide a source of funding which would bridge the investment gap between grant funding innovative dementia research and large pharmaceutical companies. The lack of disease understanding and number of high profile failures meant the pipeline of dementia drugs had dried up.

Five years later the formation of DDF has led to a vanguard of other initiatives, which has both increased the understanding of this disease as well as attracting more venture capital to this area of high unmet medical demand. This is the key to success because venture capital is the most effective form of private investment capital in high-risk areas like dementia drug discovery, which will increase the likelihood of a treatment for AD.

This increase in capital invested in dementia research has not only increased the pipeline of available drugs but also broadened the number of mechanisms and pathologies being pursued. Applying the lessons from other disease areas is helping to accelerate and reduce the risk of drug development for AD.

References

1. Cummings JL, Morstorf T, Zhong K. Alzheimer's disease drug-development pipeline: few candidates, frequent failures. *Alzheimers Res Ther* 2014; **6**: 37.

2. Sabbagh JJ, Kinney JW, Cummings J. Animal systems in the development of treatments for Alzheimer's disease: challenges, methods, and implications. *Neurobiol Aging* 2013; **34**: 169–83.

3. Windisch M. We can treat Alzheimer's disease successfully in mice but not in men: failure in translation? A perspective. *Neurodegen Dis* 2014; **13**: 147–50.

4. Lo AW, Ho C, Cummings J, Kosik KS. Parallel discovery of Alzheimer's therapeutics. *Sci Transl Med* 2014; **6**: 241cm245.

Chapter 48

Federal Small Business Support for Small Businesses Pursuing Alzheimer's Disease Drug Development

Pragati Katiyar, Armineh L. Ghazarian, Zane Martin, and Todd Haim

48.1 Introduction

Developing effective Alzheimer's disease (AD) therapeutics requires significant total investment as well as funding at all stages and within all sectors of the drug-development industry. Start-up companies and small biotechnology companies, critical elements of that industry, play an outsize role in the pivotal early stages of drug development. Because of the public health need to address AD and the exorbitant cost of AD care [1, 2], new therapeutics that enhance treatment of AD are crucial. In 2011, Congress acted on the need for new therapeutics by passing the National Alzheimer's Project Act (NAPA), with an ambitious goal to both prevent and effectively treat AD and AD-related dementia (AD/ADRD) by 2025 [3, 4].

AD drug development does not come without challenges. In 2013, a G8 summit titled "Tackling gaps in developing life-changing treatments for dementia" identified six innovation gaps that require advances [5]:

(1) understanding the biological processes affected by newly identified genetic risk factors;

(2) understanding neuronal resilience for novel drug development;

(3) drug-target validation;

(4) selection of appropriate subjects for proof-of-concept clinical trials;

(5) improving drug–target engagement in humans; and

(6) innovative approaches for clinical trials for the early detection of the disease.

The immense cost and time required for developing therapeutics is another challenge. The average therapeutic takes approximately 13 years and $5.6 billion to progress from the laboratory to final US Food and Drug Administration (FDA) approval [4]. Private investors typically consider this cost high risk and are reluctant to invest in AD therapeutic development upfront, making federal funding critical [6].

48.2 Role of Small Business in AD Drug Development

The development of an AD therapeutic is a long, multi-stage journey. Each stage involves efforts from various players, and this robust development landscape includes efforts from different corners of the research and development (R&D) enterprise that is critical to ultimate success. Large pharmaceutical companies and investors are vital players in this journey, providing much-needed capital for downstream development and commercialization. But small businesses are uniquely positioned to take advantage of federal funding mechanisms that big pharmaceutical companies cannot access, fostering crucial development in early research stages. Each stage of the drug-development process depends on certain sources of funding (Figure 48.1). Advancing innovations from academic medical centers to pharmaceutical companies often involves an intermediate step of moving the innovations to start-ups. Upon reaching value inflection points, the start-ups may be able to transition the innovations to pharmaceutical companies through partnership, co-development, mergers, and acquisitions [7]. Early-stage development activities conducted by start-up companies often rely on the National Institutes of Health (NIH) and its small business funding programs.

48.3 NIH SBIR/STTR Programs

The Small Business Innovation Research (SBIR) and Small Business Technology Transfer (STTR) programs are two small business funding programs available at the NIH. They support US small

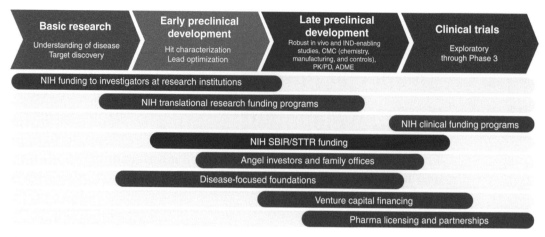

Figure 48.1 The four overall stages of drug development rely on various private and public funding sources.

businesses' scientific and technological innovations with potential for commercialization using set-aside federal funding. Although the terms SBIR and STTR represent separate programs, this chapter will refer to those programs collectively as the *small business programs*.

The first SBIR program was established in 1977 at the National Science Foundation (NSF) to address concerns about the potential loss of US competitiveness with increasing globalization [8]. Senator Edward Kennedy and the NSF Senior Program Officer, Roland Tibbetts, understood the important role small businesses play in driving innovations and boosting the economy by creating jobs. They also recognized that, due to lack of funding, many small businesses fail without materializing the full potential of their innovations. The first SBIR program at the NSF became the precursor of the current federal agency-wide SBIR program.

The US Congress started the federal agency-wide SBIR program in 1982 to help small businesses reach key value inflection points, not only to encourage innovation but also to prevent failures [9]. A key value inflection point is a point at which specific milestones in one phase must be achieved to create value that enables entrance to the next phase of development. The path toward commercialization involves several key value inflection points.

The STTR program, started in 1992, requires collaboration between the small business awardee and a major US research institution. Both the SBIR and STTR programs use congressionally mandated set-aside funds to provide US small businesses with early-stage capital to stimulate R&D with the goal of moving innovative technologies closer to commercialization [10, 11].

Although the SBIR and STTR programs share the same objective, they have a few critical differences (Table 48.1).

Table 48.1 Comparison of SBIR and STTR programs

	SBIR	STTR
Percentage set-aside of the federal agency's extramural R&D budget	3.2%	0.45%
Non-profit research partner (university or federal agency)	Permits and encourages research partnership	Requires a formal collaboration with a non-profit research institution
Principal investigator	Must be primarily employed with the small business at the time and for the duration of the award	Can be employed with either the small business or the non-profit research partner
Percentage of the award budget that must go to small business (not a subcontractor)	At least 67%	At least 30% must go to the small business and at least 40% must go to a single partnering US research institution
Number of participating federal agencies	11	5

48.4 SBIR/STTR Funding at the NIH

By statute, any federal agency with an annual extramural R&D budget of at least $100 million must set aside 3.2% of that budget for the SBIR program. Agencies whose extramural R&D budgets exceed $1 billion are required to set aside an additional 0.45% for the STTR program. During fiscal year (FY) 2020, the NIH invested an estimated $1.187 billion in promoting innovations from small businesses across the United States. Because the NIH is the largest public funder of biomedical research, the set-aside results in an extremely significant source of funding for small businesses and the largest source of seed funding for small businesses working on biomedical research [4, 12, 13].

The NIH small business funding has steadily increased since 1998 (Figure 48.2), and a sample funding analysis for 2018 small business awards across the NIH's institutes and centers shows funding opportunities in various biomedical fields as each NIH institute and center focuses on a specific biomedical field or disease area (Figure 48.3) [14].

Securing small business funding provides many benefits that are essential for emerging small businesses. For example, the NIH SBIR/STTR funds are non-dilutive, which means they do not affect the small company's stock or shares, and because the funding is not a loan, no repayment is required. Non-dilutive funding reduces innovators' and potential partners' risk of giving up any equity or ownership while supporting data generation for the initial proof of concept.

With funding from the NIH, small businesses retain their intellectual property (IP) rights [15] and can access additional federal resources, such as early market intelligence, entrepreneurial training, business development resources, and a seal of approval for their product from a panel of expert peer reviewers, all of which can facilitate further fundraising efforts [16]. The Bayh–Dole Act deals with IP arising from federally funded research and allows investigators the first right to patent their inventions.

48.5 Role of Small Business in the AD Drug-Development Ecosystem

In the United States, attention to AD and ADRD increased with the 2011 passage of NAPA, which calls for a coordinated national plan to accelerate research and care. Under the national plan, the National Institute on Aging (NIA) and National Institute of Neurological Disorders and Stroke (NINDS) at the NIH lead the research effort by

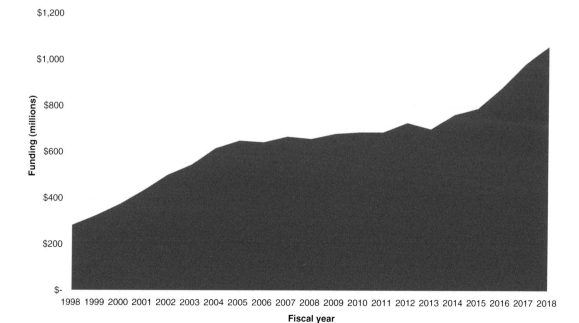

Figure 48.2 NIH SBIR/STTR funding from 1998 to 2018, showing a steady increase.
Source: https://report.nih.gov/nihdatabook/category/8.

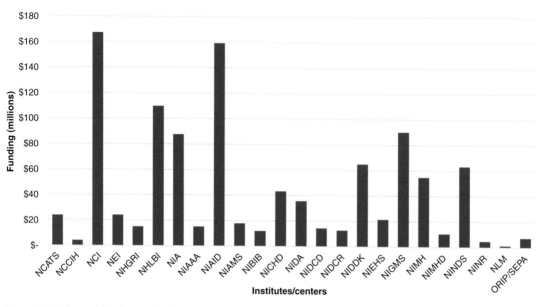

Figure 48.3 A sample funding analysis for 2018 SBIR/STTR awards across the NIH's institutes and centers. Source: https://report.nih.gov/nihdatabook/category/8.

hosting research summits with experts from academia, industry, and advocacy groups to highlight the most promising lines of research, including therapeutic development. In 2015, the NIA received a dramatic increase in congressionally directed appropriations for AD/ADRD research. The funding also increased the NIA's ability to award not only small businesses but also academic investigators who partner with small businesses to develop their research into a marketable product. Through this early-stage seed funding, small businesses can leverage their unique position and take advantage of these funding opportunities to further develop their research ideas to attract downstream investments, translating their innovative research into viable commercial products.

Based on AD Research Summits in 2012 and 2015, the NIA Small Business Committee, which comprises representatives from each of the four NIA extramural research program divisions and evaluates gaps in the research ecosystem to be filled by small business funding, announced new small business funding opportunity announcements (FOAs) in 2017. These small business FOAs encourage research on and commercialization of novel therapies, devices, and other

healthcare programs and services to prevent the onset of AD/ADRD, and to reduce their burden on individuals, their families, and society at large (Advancing Research on Alzheimer's Disease and Alzheimer's-Disease-Related Dementias: PAS-17-064; PAS-17-065 [17, 18]). Through this recently reissued FOA, PAS-19-316, current budget caps for SBIRs are $500,000 for Phase I SBIR awards and $2.5 million for Phase II SBIR awards (SBIR project phases have no correlation to clinical trial phase nomenclature). Phase I SBIR/STTR awards support proof-of-concept studies, while Phase II SBIR/STTR awards support continued R&D. To date, these funding initiatives have resulted in 115 AD/ADRD small business grants to 94 institutions for projects across the drug pipeline, from drug discovery to early-stage clinical trials, and across a broad range of therapeutic target categories that represent the promise of the broad global pipeline of AD therapeutics, including beta-amyloid, tau, inflammation, growth factors and hormones, metabolism and bioenergetics, synaptic plasticity and neuroprotection, and multi-target therapeutics [19]. These funding opportunities integrate with the the NIA AD Translational Program, which is discussed in Chapter 45.

48.6 Examples of Companies Funded by the NIA's Small Business Programs

The recent increase in funding for the small business programs, along with other enhancement efforts, expands the programs' potential impact. The programs are already resulting in innovations that have advanced to clinical trials or even to market. The following examples demonstrate how start-ups used NIA small business funding to reach key inflection points and advance toward commercialization.

AgeneBio. AgeneBio, Inc., is a private biopharmaceutical company developing innovative therapeutics aimed at preserving and restoring brain function. This work, led by the company's founder, Michela Gallagher, PhD, began after clinical research found that treatment of mild cognitive impairment (MCI) patients with the atypical anti-epileptic levetiracetam showed efficacy in normalizing heightened hippocampal activation and improving memory performance [20]. AgeneBio's therapeutic programs have since been designed to normalize the condition of aberrant neural activation and prevent or limit disease progression with small-molecule therapeutics. The company's lead asset, AGB101 (low-dose extended-release levetiracetam), is in a Phase 2/3 clinical trial for treatment of MCI due to AD.

The company also has a discovery-stage program that targets neural overactivity through a different mechanism: gamma-aminobutyric acid A receptor, alpha 5 (GABA-A α5). This program, led by AgeneBio Vice President of Research and Development, Sharon Rosenzweig-Lipson, PhD, receives funding through the NIH Blueprint Neurotherapeutics Network to support lead-compound drug development and through the NIA SBIR program for follow-on compound preclinical drug development.

"Our lead GABA-A α5 PAM [positive allosteric modulator] compound offers optimal precision for addressing cognitive impairment due to neural overactivity," said Dr. Gallagher. "This class of drugs shows great promise, not only for their potential to treat the early symptoms of AD but also for their ability to address other unmet patient needs in autism and schizophrenia. We are grateful for the continued support from the NIH and the Alzheimer's Drug Discovery Foundation (ADDF) for this research and are tremendously excited about the opportunity to advance development to clinical stage." AgeneBio demonstrates how a small company can harness NIH funding programs and venture philanthropy to bring a set of compounds through Phase 2 clinical trials.

Alector. Alector is a biotechnology company operating under the hypothesis that the immune system plays a critical role in the development of neurodegenerative diseases. Alector's research focuses on "immuno-neurology" as a strategy to treat neurodegeneration, with the idea that targeting immune genes tied to neurodegeneration can delay and ultimately halt disease progression (https://alector.com/our-science/).

Alector's lead candidate, AL001, acts by targeting sortilin (SORT1), a protein that promotes the degradation of progranulin (PGRN). PGRN haploinsufficiency causes frontotemporal dementia (FTD), while a subtler reduction in PGRN levels has been identified as a risk factor for other neurodegenerative diseases. Alector's therapeutic acts as a SORT1 inhibitor, ultimately elevating levels of PGRN (see www.globaldata.com).

With a $1.3 million Fast Track award from the NIA small business programs in 2015, Alector produced key data that enabled it to attract additional funding for preclinical testing, investigational new drug (IND) submission, and ultimately entry into clinics.

In 2019, the FDA granted AL001 Fast Track designation as an investigational therapeutic for the treatment of FTD. Alector initiated a Phase 3 trial for FTD in July 2020.

Avid Radiopharmaceuticals. Avid Radiopharmaceuticals, a spin-off out of the University of Pennsylvania, was founded as a molecular imaging diagnostics company. Strategically using the small business programs to fund feasibility and proof-of-concept studies helped Avid commercialize a diagnostic tool called Amyvid™. Amyvid is a radioactive tracer that detects beta-amyloid plaque density via positron emission tomography (PET) scans in patients with cognitive impairment [4]. It is widely used in clinical trials and became the first FDA-approved method of directly detecting the pathology of AD to reach the market.

Small business funding was critical in the development of Amyvid. As a small business awardee, Avid gained scientific credibility that attracted $100 million in venture capital funding to further test and develop its tool, as well as securing a partnership with PETNET Solutions, Inc. which allowed Avid to manufacture Amyvid. In 2010, Avid was acquired by Eli Lilly.

Founder, Daniel M. Skovronsky, MD, PhD, stated that initial SBIR support "was the most important part, because it's always hard to get a company started," adding that small business funding provided him the "confidence and time" to start his company [4].

Cognition Therapeutics. A drug discovery and development company, Cognition Therapeutics has had success with its lead candidate, CT1812, a novel first-in-class small molecule. Initial clinical studies have shown that CT1812 normalizes the protein-trafficking and lipid-metabolism pathways that are disrupted in AD. CT1812 has also been proven to enable the protection and restoration of synapses from amyloid-beta-oligomer-induced neurotoxicity.

Cognition Therapeutics focuses on developing a pipeline of disease-modifying small-molecule drugs that target AD and other neurocognitive disorders. With funding through the NIA R01 grant mechanism, the company ran early IND studies to confirm the safety of CT1812, setting the groundwork for future clinical trials to be funded by the SBIR program. In 2017, CT1812 received Fast Track designation from the FDA for treatment of AD patients.

To secure partnerships for the clinical development of CT1812, Cognition Therapeutics needed a deeper understanding of the mechanism of action. An NIA Fast Track award of $1 million allowed the company to demonstrate proof of concept, which supported its three ongoing Phase 2 clinical trials, making it attractive for outside partnerships. In June 2020, the company partnered with the Alzheimer's Clinical Trials Consortium to conduct a Phase 2 study via a $75.8 million NIA award [21]. Susan Catalano, PhD, co-founder and chief science officer, noted, "NIA support has been critical for CT1812's discovery and development. The commitment of the NIA to innovative and diverse approaches to treating AD is unequalled in the private sector and a critical linchpin in the fight against this devastating disease" [4].

Tetra Therapeutics. BPN-14770 is a novel, small-molecule drug developed by Tetra Therapeutics, a drug-development company whose research focuses on restoring clarity of thought in AD patients. BPN-14770 works by modulating, rather than inhibiting, the phosphodiesterase 4D enzyme. This mechanism of action prolongs cyclic adenosine monophosphate (cAMP) activity while maintaining safe levels of the enzyme, which, when mutated, alters cAMP signaling and causes impaired cognitive function.

With a $1.9 million Phase 1 grant from the NIA SBIR program, Tetra kick-started critical early-stage research, evaluating the safety and tolerability of BPN-14770 in a multiple ascending-dose study. This study's outcomes led to Phase 2 studies to test the applications in AD.

To develop and commercialize BPN-14770 for the treatment of AD, Tetra leveraged successful outcomes from its Phase 1 and Phase 2 studies to form a strategic alliance with Shionogi & Co., Ltd., which subsequently acquired Tetra for up to $500 million in upfront fees, regulatory, and commercialization milestones [22].

Mark Gurney, PhD, chairman and chief executive officer, recognizes the value SBIR funds had for early-stage research: "We have made significant progress over the last four years, advancing from initial discovery of BPN-14770 through the completion of a sequence of Phase 1 clinical studies in young and elderly volunteers. We sincerely thank our investors and the National Institutes of Health for their ongoing support of our efforts" [4].

48.7 Impact of the NIH's Small Business Programs and Lessons Learned

These company snapshots demonstrate how small business funding from the NIH can help translate academic discoveries into commercial solutions. Since private financing for start-up companies in the early stages of AD drug development is limited, the funding from the NIH's small business programs is critical. SBIR and STTR funding can help start-up companies reach critical value inflection points that could lead to additional capital to support further development. The high levels of funding since 2015 reflect a significant source of capital (estimated total of about $70 million in the NIA FY2020 small business funds provided for AD/

ADRD early-stage R&D) that could significantly increase the number of early-stage innovations that reach critical value inflection points.

Although funding for early-stage drug development is critical, the NIH recognizes that funding alone will not enable the full gamut of innovators to reach critical value inflection points. Therefore, the NIA launched the Office of Small Business Research (OSBR) in 2018, to proactively manage the small business programs, identifying and addressing gaps that could limit programmatic impact. The NIA OSBR ensures that the programs are structured to meet the needs of the innovator community. Recognizing that AD development can be costly even at the early stage, the NIA increased the budget limits on SBIR Phase I and Phase II awards to $500,000 and $2.5 million, respectively. These limits are significantly higher than the limits for typical NIH SBIR awards. Additionally, the NIA recognized that small businesses may not possess the specialized equipment or expertise to conduct all critical early-stage development activities and allows applicants to include fee-for-service activities, such as assays conducted at contract research organizations, as part of the small business's effort, if the small business is conducting specialized experimental design and data analysis activities.

The NIH's small business programs are designed to be part of the NIH's funding continuum. The NIH's translational funding programs, including the SBIR and STTR programs, can leverage the NIH funding programs geared toward academic innovators. In 2019, the NIH launched the Small Business Education and Entrepreneurial Development (SEED) office. SEED programs help develop collaborative relationships and build opportunities for NIH-funded innovators to further their product development efforts. SEED leads initiatives in three areas: academic innovation, management and enhancement of the NIH's small business programs, and support for academic and small business innovators.

The academic innovation team develops and facilitates programs that move innovations from academic laboratories to the marketplace. The team coordinates the NIH's proof-of-concept center consortium, which enables academic innovators to validate the potential health impacts of promising scientific discoveries and advance them into healthcare products and services. The team also helps coordinate the National Institute of General Medical Sciences–funded accelerator hubs in each of the four Institutional Development Award regions (Central, Northeastern, Southwestern, and Western). Like the small business programs, these accelerator hubs are an NIH effort to stimulate entrepreneurship, technology transfer, management, small business finance, and other skills needed to transition discoveries and technologies from the laboratory into commercial products that improve human health.

The SEED small business programs team works with NIH institutes and centers to optimize NIH small business funding programs and serve as a central source of information on NIH's small business programs and resources. The innovator support team delivers product development guidance from industry veterans to NIH-funded academic and small business innovators, and provides entrepreneurial training to the NIH awardees and program staff. This team also helps small business awardees present to potential investors and strategic partners, and at various industry showcases, as the NIH recognizes that private funding leveraging the NIH's earlier funding is usually necessary to achieve commercialization. SEED's work in each area enhances the NIA's efforts to facilitate the commercialization of products to advance prevention, treatment, diagnosis, management, and caregiving for AD/ADRD [4].

By design, the NIA SBIR and STTR portfolio includes a diverse group of companies. Unlike the portfolios of many private funders, it includes a significant percentage of companies led by first-time entrepreneurs. The NIH has learned that entrepreneurial training programs are critical for ensuring that funded companies are positioned for success when data demonstrate their proposed solution's merit. Since 2014, the NIH has launched a variety of entrepreneurial training programs.

The Innovation Corps (I-Corps™) at NIH program, launched in 2014, uses experiential learning to help investigators develop skills and strategies that will reduce risk during commercialization. Using a systematic, hands-on approach, teams of company personnel and advisors focus on customer discovery to optimize technology development and improve the company's odds of commercialization. Teams conduct more than 100 customer interviews during the 8-week program. Between 2017 and 2019, four NIA-funded small businesses completed the program. Longitudinal metrics for the I-Corps at NIH program have demonstrated a substantial impact thus far. A survey of

13 NIH awardees, 3 years after completion of the pilot program, revealed that these companies had secured a total of $78 million in follow-up funding, 8 strategic partnerships, 18 patents, and 2 spin-off companies [23].

The Concept to Clinic: Commercializing Innovation (C3i) Program is a 24-week entrepreneurial commercialization assistance training experience that NIH uses primarily to support medical-device innovators. The program uses a curriculum established by the Wallace H. Coulter Foundation to accelerate academic innovations to the marketplace. The C3i Program provides investigators with specialized business frameworks and tools that drive translation of medical devices from laboratory to market. The goal is to engage innovators who want to better understand the value of technologies under development and assess their commercial viability and potential business opportunities. Recognizing the importance of this resource for small business program awardees, the NIA joined this effort in 2019 and is now one of six institutes offering the C3i Program. Four NIA-supported companies have completed the program.

Training programs such as I-Corps at the NIH and C3i provide a foundational understanding of entrepreneurial, development, and commercialization challenges, but innovators supported by the NIH's small business programs also face business development challenges and needs as they advance toward and reach key value inflection points. In an effort to provide some support to innovators facing such needs, the NIH has retained Entrepreneurs-in-Residence (EIRs) to provide guidance to supported innovators. The NIH EIRs are highly experienced life-science ventures and business executives who work, one on one, with select SBIR companies to help them prepare for private follow-on financing or reach partnering objectives. In fall 2020, the NIA retained an EIR with a strong entrepreneurial, investor, and entrepreneurial training background to hold continual entrepreneurial training sessions, provide on-demand coaching, and facilitate connections between innovators and potential partners. In 2020, the NIA supported several innovators developing AD therapeutics to showcase their therapeutics at industry partnering conferences, and initial feedback indicated that the effort is leading to significant partnership discussions. In February 2021, the NIA hosted its inaugural virtual Longevity Innovations and Neurodegeneration Company Showcase, in which

funded innovators presented to potential investors and strategic partners.

To better understand grantees' and applicants' needs, the OSBR conducted a survey in January through March 2020. The survey was tailored to three audiences: current and past grantees, current applicants, and potential applicants. A total of 191 individuals completed the survey. In addition, the OSBR conducted in-depth interviews with 14 respondents. The market research survey and in-depth interviews revealed that respondents benefited from the NIA's SBIR and STTR program and resources, website, and existing communications efforts, such as webinars, conference presentations and exhibits, emails, and Twitter posts. Respondents wanted more in-depth information about the application process and aspects of navigating grants and entrepreneurship as well as additional training and resource materials. In response to these findings, the OSBR created a virtual workshop series that covers all aspects of grants from the peer-review process to grantsmanship and regulatory requirements, began assisting applicants through a dedicated Application Assistance Program (AAP), designed an array of targeted outreach efforts to engage women and minority-owned businesses and states with lower applicant success rates, created a LinkedIn page to reach additional research professionals eligible to apply, and helped applicants and awardees through events and one-on-one support. The OSBR is committed to continuing to listen to stakeholders' needs.

The resources that the NIA offers were designed to address gaps – beyond funding gaps – for early-stage innovators. Funding programs must complement and leverage the non-funding resources. Recognizing the need for funding to support commercialization-relevant activities beyond pure research, the NIH/NIA released a new iteration of the Commercialization Readiness Pilot (CRP) program in 2019. The CRP funding opportunities can support technical assistance and late-stage R&D activities that are essential to bringing innovations to the marketplace. Since 2016, the NIA has used the first NIH iteration of the CRP to award six companies a total of $11 million. This increased support is critical in research areas with high commercial risk, such as AD/ADRD [24].

The funding and resources provided by NIH small business programs can serve as a major vehicle for advancing early-stage AD therapeutics toward the clinic and even through early clinical development. However, the programs' impact will be limited by their ability to reach innovators. Thus, outreach to ensure that innovators know about NIH's small business programs and understand how to submit competitive applications is pivotal. In 2019, the NIA joined the AAP. The AAP is an NIH-wide 10-week coaching program that helps small businesses prepare Phase 1 applications for the NIH small business programs, at no cost to the applicant. Through one-on-one coaching from subject-matter experts, the program demystifies the federal grant application process and offers assistance in completing all components of the application. Although all small businesses may apply, the program encourages participation from under-represented small businesses, especially women-owned and socially and economically disadvantaged companies.

Since 2018, the NIA has dramatically increased its efforts to raise awareness of its small business programs and provide guidance to potential applicants. The number of attendees at NIA SBIR-focused outreach events increased more than eight-fold between FY2018 and FY2019, from approximately 230 attendees to approximately 2,000. This increase has helped to support a sustained increase in the number of AD- and ADRD-related applications. The NIA also is offering more in-person and virtual programs that provide application and programmatic guidance. In 2020, the NIA's webinars reached more than 1,500 potential applicants. Two webinars, one focused on Phase 2b and CRP funding programs and one focused on the NIH SBIR peer-review process, each reached more than 500 registrants. The increase in outreach and guidance available to applicants may have contributed to a significantly improved median score, provided to applicants by peer reviewers, in FY2020 compared with previous years [4].

In addition to direct outreach, stakeholder engagement has been critical in expanding the reach of the NIA's small business programs. Expanded presence at AD-relevant innovator conferences, such as the Alzheimer's Association International Conference and relevant pre-conferences, the Sachs Associates Neuroscience Innovation Forum, the Longevity Venture Summit, and the ADDF's International Conference on Alzheimer's Drug Discovery, has raised awareness of the programs in the community and helped raise the number of new applicants and awardees each year. The OSBR also teams up with non-profit trade associations, such as the Alzheimer's Association Business Consortium, the ADDF, and the Rainwater Charitable Foundation's Tau Consortium; state Biotechnology Innovation Organization associations; and regional innovation organizations to create a wider network and help our applicants access additional capital, potential partners, and other business services. In one example of the NIA and stakeholders' efforts to co-leverage each other's funding programs, the ADDF launched bridge funding opportunities to provide NIA SBIR/STTR Phase I awardees with interim funding. The ADDF funding will also enable investigators to continue to generate data as small business funding decisions are being finalized.

In addition to improving the quantity and quality of incoming applications, the increased focus on marketing the NIH's small business programs to the AD innovator community may have contributed to a diversified portfolio. In FY2019, 63% of NIA small business program recipients were receiving their first-ever NIA small business award (Figure 48.4). The diversity of approaches to treat AD has also significantly increased; the program has funded therapeutic approaches targeting approximately 12 molecular target categories since 2017. Target categories include synaptic plasticity, neurogenesis, inflammation, metabolism and bioenergetics, growth factors and hormones, and vasculature. Each of these efforts and the resulting expansion and diversification of the NIA small business programs' portfolio adds significant value in the fight against AD.

Developing effective treatments for AD/ADRD will require the most robust ecosystem imaginable. The NIA's small business programs play a pivotal role within that ecosystem, and the initial development of an expanded and more diverse set of resources and funding opportunities available to innovators may increase these programs' importance in the future. The NIA's efforts to proactively manage the programs, strategically provide funding, leverage the funding with resources that address challenges facing innovators, and ensure that diverse innovators across the country are poised to submit competitive solutions are all critical in maximizing the program's impact.

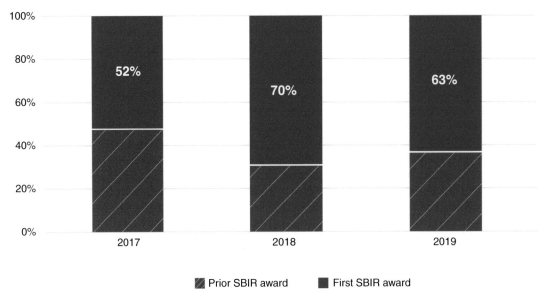

Figure 48.4 New companies awarded for AD/ADRD research: the graph represents the percentage of companies who received their first SBIR award during FY2017–FY2019.

Acknowledgments

Both first authors contributed equally. We acknowledge Amy Schneider of Palladian partners, Inc., for editorial support.

References

1. Deb A, Thornton JD, Sambamoorthi U, Innes K. Direct and indirect cost of managing Alzheimer's disease and related dementias in the United States. *Expert Rev Pharmacoecon Outcomes Res* 2017; **17**: 189–202.

2. Hurd MD, Martorell P, Delavande A, Mullen KJ, Langa KM. Monetary costs of dementia in the United States. *N Engl J Med* 2013; **368**: 1326–34.

3. US Department of Health and Human Services, Office of the Assistant Secretary for Planning and Evaluation. National plans to address Alzheimer's disease. 2012. Available at: https://aspe.hhs.gov/napa-national-plans (accessed December 7, 2021).

4. Ghazarian A, Haim T, Sauma S, Katiyar P. National Institute on Aging seed funding enables Alzheimer's disease startups to reach key value inflection points. *Alzheimers Dement* 2021;DOI: https://doi.org/10.1002/alz.12392.

5. Mauricio R, Benn C, Davis J, et al. Therapeutics for dementia: tackling gaps in developing life-changing treatments for dementia. *Alzheimers Dement (N Y)* 2019; **5**: 241–53.

6. Scott TJ, O'Connor AC, Link AN, Beaulieu TJ. Economic analysis of opportunities to accelerate Alzheimer's disease research and development. *Ann N Y Acad Sci* 2014; **1313**: 17–34.

7. Cummings J, Reiber C, Kumar P. The price of progress: funding and financing Alzheimer's disease drug development. *Alzheimers Dement (N Y)* 2018; **4**: 330–43.

8. US Small Business Administration. Birth and history of the SBIR program. Available at: www.sbir.gov/birth-and-history-of-the-sbir-program (accessed November 10, 2021).

9. Onken J, Miklos AC, Dorsey TF, et al. Using database linkages to measure innovation, commercialization, and survival of small businesses. *Eval Program Plann* 2019; **77**: 101710.

10. US Small Business Administration. About SBA. Available at: www.sba.gov/about-sba (accessed November 3, 2020).

11. US Small Business Administration. Performance benchmark requirements for Phase I. Available at: www.sbir.gov/performance-benchmarks (accessed November 10, 2020).

12. National Science Board. Science and Engineering Indicators. 2018: research and development – US trends and international comparisons. Available at: www.nsf.gov/statistics/2018/nsb20181/ (accessed November 10, 2020).

13. Jefferson RS. How the largest public funder of biomedical research in the world spends your money. Available at: www.forbes.com/sites/robinseatonjefferson/2018/12/21/how-the-largest-public-funder-of-biomedical-research-in-the-world-spends-your-money/?sh=69d3d48f27b9 (accessed November 23, 2020).

14. NIH Research Portfolio Online Reporting Tools (RePORT). Small business research (SBIR/STTR).

Available at: https://report.nih.gov/nihdatabook/category/8 (accessed November 23, 2020).

15. National Institutes of Health. Intellectual property and iEdison invention report requirements. Available at: https://sbir.nih.gov/policy/invention-reporting (accessed December 2, 2020).

16. Ben-Menachem G, Ferguson SM, Balakrishnan K. Doing business with the NIH. *Nat Biotechnol* 2006; **24**: 17–20.

17. National Institutes of Health. Advancing research on Alzheimer's disease (AD) and Alzheimer's-disease-related dementias (ADRD) (R41/R42). Available at: https://grants.nih.gov/grants/guide/pa-files/PAs-17-065.html (accessed November 10, 2020).

18. National Institutes of Health. Advancing research on Alzheimer's disease (AD) and Alzheimer's-disease-related dementias (ADRD) (R43/R44). Available at: https://grants.nih.gov/grants/guide/pa-files/PAs-17-064.html (accessed November 10, 2020).

19. Cole MA, Seabrook GR. On the horizon: the value and promise of the global pipeline of Alzheimer's disease therapeutics. *Alzheimers Dement (N Y)* 2020; **6**: e12009.

20. Bakker A, Krauss GL, Albert MA, et al. Reduction of hippocampal hyperactivity improves cognition in amnestic mild cognitive impairment. *Neuron* 2012; **74**: 467–74.

21. Cognition Therapeutics. Cognition Therapeutics receives $75.8 million NIA grant for 540-patient Phase 2 study of CT1812 in collaboration with the Alzheimer's Clinical Trials Consortium. Available at: https://cogrx.com/cognition-receives-nia-grant-for-actc-study/ (accessed December 2, 2020).

22. Businesswire. Tetra Therapeutics and Shionogi announce expanded alliance. Available at: www.businesswire.com/news/home/20200306005082/en/Tetra-Therapeutics-Shionogi-Announce-Expanded-Alliance (accessed December 2, 2021).

23. Canaria CA, Portilla L, Weingarten M. I-Corps at NIH: entrepreneurial training program creating successful small businesses. *Clin Transl Sci* 2019; **12**: 324–8.

24. Cummings J, Lee G, Ritter A, Sabbagh M, Zhong K. Alzheimer's disease drug development pipeline: 2019. *Alzheimers Dement (N Y)* 2019; **5**: 272–93.

Index

Printed in the United States
by Baker & Taylor Publisher Services